Neuro-Oncology for the Clinical Neurologist

Neuro-Oncology for the Clinical Neurologist

Roy E. Strowd, III
MD, MEd, MS
Associate Professor of Neurology and Oncology
Department of Neurology, Internal Medicine, and Translational Sciences Institute
Wake Forest Baptist Comprehensive Cancer Center
Wake Forest School of Medicine
Winston-Salem, North Carolina

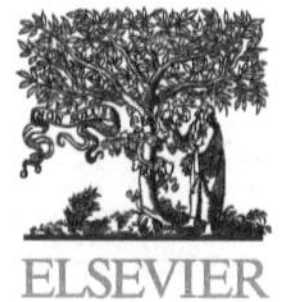
ELSEVIER

Elsevier
1600 John F. Kennedy Blvd.
Ste 1800
Philadelphia, PA 19103-2899

NEURO-ONCOLOGY FOR THE CLINICAL NEUROLOGIST ISBN: 978-0-323-69494-0

Library of Congress Control Number : 2020941988

Senior Content Strategist: Melanie Tucker
Content Development Specialist: Deborah Poulson
Publishing Services Manager: Deepthi Unni
Senior Project Manager: Manchu Mohan
Design Direction: Brian Salisbury

Printed in the United States of America

Last digit is the print number: 9 8 7 6 5 4 3 2 1

This book is dedicated to our patients and their caregivers—to those thriving after 20 years and those battling at 3 months; to those who have returned to fantastic trips around the world and to those who are struggling after having lost work, friends, and a former life; to caregivers who are excited by the opportunity of a clinical trial and to those who are estranged by a disease that can at times seem to take away the very soul. You asked that we tell your story and excite the world to find treatments, make advances, and improve care. It is a privilege and honor to humbly present these cases, tell parts of your story, and teach others.

Contributors List

Prakash Ambady, MD
Department of Neurology
Oregon Health and Science University
Portland, Oregon

Stephen J. Bagley, MD, MSCE
Assistant Professor
Department of Medicine, Division of Hematology/Oncology
University of Pennsylvania Perelman School of Medicine
Philadelphia, Pennsylvania

Jaishri Blakeley, MD
Department of Neurology
Johns Hopkins University School of Medicine
Baltimore, Maryland

Taylor Brooks, MD
Wake Forest Baptist Medical Center
Winston-Salem, North Carolina

Marc R. Bussière, MSc
Department of Radiation Oncology
Massachusetts General Hospital
Boston, Massachusetts

Jian L. Campian, MD, PhD
Department of Medicine
Division of Oncology
Washington University School of Medicine
St. Louis, Missouri

Michael D. Chan, MD
Department of Radiation Oncology
Co-Director, Gamma Knife Program
Wake Forest School of Medicine
Winston-Salem, North Carolina

Ugonma N. Chukwueke, MD
Center for Neuro-Oncology
Dana-Farber/Brigham and Women's Cancer Center
Boston, Massachusetts
and Harvard Medical School
Boston, Massachusetts

Christina K. Cramer, MD
Department of Radiation Oncology
Wake Forest School of Medicine
Winston-Salem, North Carolina

Daniel E. Couture, MD
Department of Neurosurgery
Wake Forest School of Medicine
Winston-Salem, North Carolina

Tiffany L. Cummings, PsyD
Department of Neurology
Wake Forest School of Medicine
Winston-Salem, North Carolina

Sonika Dahiya, MBBS, MD
Division of Neuropathology
Department of Pathology and Immunology
Washington University School of Medicine
St. Louis, Missouri

Peter de Blank, MD, MSCE
Associate Professor of Pediatrics
Department of Pediatrics
University of Cincinnati Medical Center
and
Cincinnati Children's Hospital Medical Center
Cincinnati, Ohio

Luisa A. Diaz-Arias, MD
Postdoctoral Research Fellow
Department of Neurology
Johns Hopkins University School of Medicine
Baltimore, Maryland

Federica Franchino, MD
Department of Neuro-Oncology
University and City of Health and Science Hospital
Turin, Italy

Jennifer L. Franke, BS
Department of Neurosurgery
Johns Hopkins University School of Medicine
Baltimore, Maryland

Carol Parks Geer, MD
Department of Radiology
Wake Forest School of Medicine
and
Department of Radiology
Wake Forest Baptist Medical Center
Winston-Salem, North Carolina

Elizabeth R. Gerstner, MD
Division of Neuro-Oncology
Department of Neurology
Massachusetts General Hospital
Boston, Massachusetts

Stuart Grossman, MD
Sidney Kimmel Comprehensive Cancer Center
Johns Hopkins University
Baltimore, Maryland

Jacob J. Henderson, MD
Section of Pediatric Hematology/Oncology
Mary Bridge Children's Hospital
Tacoma, Washington

Lauren L. Henke, MD, MSCI
Department of Radiation Oncology
Washington University School of Medicine
St. Louis, Missouri

Matthias Holdhoff, MD, PhD
The Sidney Kimmel Comprehensive Cancer Center at Johns Hopkins
The Johns Hopkins University School of Medicine
Baltimore, Maryland

Wesley Hsu, MD
Department of Neurosurgery
Wake Forest Baptist Health
Winston-Salem, North Carolina

Jiayi Huang, MD, MSCI
Department of Radiation Oncology
Washington University School of Medicine
St. Louis, Missouri

Christina Jackson, MD
Department of Neurosurgery
Johns Hopkins University School of Medicine
Baltimore, Maryland

Justin T. Jordan, MD, MPH
Stephen E. and Catherine Pappas Center for Neuro-Oncology
Massachusetts General Hospital
Boston, Massachusetts

David Olayinka Kamson, MD, PhD
Department of Neurology
Johns Hopkins Hospital
Baltimore, Maryland

Ahmad N. Kassem, MD
Resident Physician
Department of Internal Medicine
Metrohealth Medical Center
Cleveland, Ohio

Albert E. Kim, MD
Division of Neuro-Oncology
Department of Neurology
Massachusetts General Hospital
Boston, Massachusetts

Teddy E. Kim, MD
Department of Neurosurgery
Wake Forest Baptist Hospital
Winston-Salem, North Carolina

Molly Knox, MD
Department of Neurology
Mayo Clinic Arizona
Scottsdale, Arizona

David E. Kram, MD
Section of Pediatric Hematology-Oncology
Wake Forest School of Medicine
Winston-Salem, North Carolina

Priya Kumthekar, MD
Assistant Professor
Department of Neurology
Northwestern University Feinberg School of Medicine
Chicago, Illinois

Shannon Langmead, CRNP
Department of Neurology
Johns Hopkins University School of Medicine
Baltimore, Maryland

Adrian W. Laxton, MA, MD, FRCSC, FAANS
Department of Neurosurgery
Wake Forest School of Medicine
Winston-Salem, North Carolina

Emily S. Lebow, MD
Department of Radiation Oncology
Memorial Sloan Kettering Cancer Center
New York, New York

Michael Lim, MD
Department of Neurosurgery
Johns Hopkins University School of Medicine
Baltimore, Maryland

Mary Jane Lim-Fat, MD
Center for Neuro-Oncology
Dana-Farber/Brigham and Women's Cancer Center
Boston, Massachusetts and
Harvard Medical School
Boston, Massachusetts

K. Ina Ly, MD
Stephen E. and Catherine Pappas Center for Neuro-Oncology
Massachusetts General Hospital
Boston, Massachusetts

Sarah E. Mancone, MD
Department of Neurology
Yale School of Medicine
New Haven, Connecticut

Nimish Mohile, MD
Associate Professor of Neurology and Oncology
University of Rochester
Rochester, New York

Maciej M. Mrugala, MD, PhD, MPH
Department of Neurology and Medical Oncology
Mayo Clinic Cancer Center
Phoenix, Arizona

Carl M. Nechtman, MD
Department of Neurosurgery
Wake Forest Baptist Hospital
Winston-Salem, North Carolina

Sapna Pathak, MD
Department of Neurology
Wake Forest Baptist Medical Center
Winston-Salem, North Carolina

Joao Prola Netto, MD
Providence St Vincent's Medical Center
Portland, Oregon

David M. Peereboom, MD
Professor
Brain Tumor and Neuro-Oncology Center
Cleveland Clinic
Cleveland, Ohio

Alessia Pellerino, MD
Department of Neuro-Oncology
University and City of Health and Science Hospital
Turin, Italy

John C. Probasco, MD
Associate Professor of Neurology
Department of Neurology
Johns Hopkins University School of Medicine
Baltimore, Maryland

Amy Pruitt, MD
Department of Neurology
University of Pennsylvania
Philadelphia, Pennsylvania

Shakti Ramkissoon, MD, PhD
Department of Pathology
Wake Forest School of Medicine
Winston-Salem, North Carolina and
Foundation Medicine, Inc.
Morrisville, North Carolina

David Wayne Robinson, MD
Department of Radiology
Wake Forest Baptist Medical Center
Winston-Salem, North Carolina

Carlos G. Romo, MD
Department of Neurology
Brain Cancer Program
The Johns Hopkins University School of Medicine
Baltimore, Maryland

Roberta Rudà, MD
Department of Neuro-Oncology
City of Health and Science Hospital
Turin, Italy

Colette Shen, MD, PhD
Department of Radiation Oncology
UNC School of Medicine
Chapel Hill, North Carolina

Helen A. Shih, MD
Department of Radiation Oncology
Massachusetts General Hospital
Boston, Massachusetts

Mary Silvia, MD
Tuberous Sclerosis Clinic
Wake Forest Baptist Medical Center
Winston-Salem, North Carolina

Ananyaa Sivakumar
The Sidney Kimmel Comprehensive Cancer Center at Johns Hopkins
The Johns Hopkins University School of Medicine
Baltimore, Maryland

Riccardo Soffietti, MD
Department of Neuro-Oncology
University and City of Health and Science Hospital
Turin, Italy

Michael H. Soike, MD
Hazelrig-Salter Radiation Oncology Center
University of Alabama at Birmingham
Birmingham, Alabama

Roy E. Strowd, III, MD, MEd, MS
Associate Professor of Neurology and Oncology
Department of Neurology, Internal Medicine and Translational Sciences Institute
Wake Forest Baptist Comprehensive Cancer Center
Wake Forest School of Medicine
Winston-Salem, North Carolina

Shivani Sud, MD
Department of Radiation Oncology
UNC School of Medicine
Chapel Hill, North Carolina

Laszlo Szidonya, MD, PhD
Department of Diagnostic Radiology
Oregon Health and Science University
Portland, Oregon

Stephen B. Tatter, MD, PhD
Department of Neurosurgery
Wake Forest School of Medicine
Winston-Salem, North Carolina

Jigisha Thakkar, MD
Assistant Professor
Department of Neurology and Neurosurgery
Stritch School of Medicine
Loyola University Chicago
Maywood, Illinois

Kutluay Uluc, MD
Department of Neurology
Oregon Health and Science University
Portland, Oregon

Cristina Valencia-Sanchez, MD, PhD
Department of Neurology
Mayo Clinic Arizona
Scottsdale, Arizona

Courtney M. Vaughn, MPhil
Department of Radiation Oncology
UNC School of Medicine
Chapel Hill, North Carolina

Thuy M. Vu, MS, CGC
Department of Genetics
Wake Forest Baptist Medical Center
Winston-Salem, North Carolina

Andrea Wasilewski, MD
Assistant Professor of Neurology
University of Rochester,
Rochester, New York

Patrick Y. Wen, MD
Center for Neuro-Oncology
Dana-Farber/Brigham and Women's Cancer Center
Boston, Massachusetts and
Harvard Medical School
Boston, Massachusetts

Michelle Marie Williams, MD
Department of Neurosurgery
Wake Forest School of Medicine
Winston-Salem, North Carolina

Foreword

Neuro-oncology is an exciting field. Providers from across medicine work collaboratively to provide multidisciplinary care to patients who suffer from some of the most complex, life-changing, and at times devastating diseases. Tumors of the brain, spinal cord, and leptomeningeal space are among the most difficult to diagnose, refractory to treatment, and complex to manage. Patients and their caregivers who are afflicted by these tumors are amongst the most engaged in their care of any population that I have encountered. As new advances are made, novel techniques discovered, and models of care refined, it is critical that providers in all areas of medicine understand the practice of neuro-oncology and help provide unparalleled care to this population.

Who is this book for?

This book is intended for clinicians—providers who see patients in outpatient and inpatient medicine. While the title speaks to neurologists, the audience of the book is much broader and includes:

1. **Physicians**: internists, medical oncologists, radiologists, emergency medicine physicians
2. **Advanced practice providers**: physicians assistants and nurse practitioners
3. **Trainees**: medical students, residents in neurology, neurosurgery, radiation oncology, radiology, pathology, neuropsychology, pediatrics, and other fields

Importantly, while the text is focused on many aspects of tumor management in adults, selected chapters heavily represent the clinical scenarios that are relevant for pediatric patients. These sections (Chapters 7, 11, 16, 17, 18, 25, and 27) include both common tumors in pediatric patients, as well as late adult sequelae of pediatric brain tumor treatment that are critical for adult providers who manage these patients into adulthood.

How should this book be used?

This is a case-based review of neuro-oncology. Each chapter is organized into real world cases that reflect the diseases, clinical questions, and consultations that are encountered in clinical practice.

While the book is organized with the intention that you may read the text cover-to-cover, it is written more with the intention to provide a quick clinical reference that clinicians can use in the clinic just in time to manage new consultations, address patient care questions, and answer clinical conundrums. The text is formatted to allow providers to quickly reference case scenarios when they are referred a new patient with an abnormal MRI that might be tumor (Section 2); when they are seeing a brain tumor patient and need to integrate their recommendations into standard of care treatment algorithms (Section 3); when they are seeing a patient with a tumor syndrome that runs in the family (Section 4); or when they are sent a cancer patient who may have a suspected neurologic complication of cancer and its treatment (Section 5–8).

1. **Section 1 is a neuro-oncology primer.**
   This section reviews the foundational clinical principles for taking care of neuro-oncology patients. Read at your leisure or when you have the following questions:
   a. How do I interpret a neuropathology report? (Chapter 1)
   b. What are the surgical options for my patient with a new brain mass? (Chapter 2)
   c. What should I monitor when my patient is receiving radiation or chemotherapy? (Chapters 3–4)
2. **Section 2 is to be used when seeing a new imaging consult for a patient with an abnormal scan.**
   This section reviews common abnormal images. A new dural-based mass; is it a meningioma? A new spinal cord lesion; what is it? Each case provides a differential diagnosis and practical steps for managing the patient, including:
   a. Dural-based lesions (Chapter 5)
   b. Lesions in the brain parenchyma (Chapter 6)
   c. Lesions in the posterior fossa (Chapter 7)
   d. Lesions in the spinal cord (Chapter 8)
   e. Lesions of the peripheral nerves (Chapter 9)
3. **Section 3 is for managing patients with a known central nervous system tumor diagnosis.**
   This section summarizes the clinical scenarios that arise for patients with common tumors of the nervous system and discusses how these patients are evaluated and treated, including:
   a. Meningiomas (Chapter 10)
   b. Low-grade gliomas (Chapter 11)
   c. High-grade gliomas (Chapter 12)
   d. Central nervous system lymphomas (Chapter 13)
   e. Brain metastasis (Chapter 14)
   f. Leptomeningeal disease (Chapter 15)
4. **Section 4 focuses on familial tumor syndromes that affect the nervous system.**
   These patients often present first to a neurologist or primary care physician and require familiarity with the myriad manifestations that are often characteristic of these conditions. These chapters review common clinical scenarios for patients with:
   a. Neurofibromatosis type 1, type 2, and schwannomatosis (Chapter 16)
   b. Tuberous sclerosis (Chapter 17)
   c. Von Hippel Lindau disease (Chapter 18)
   d. Cowden syndrome (Chapter 18)
   e. Li-Fraumeni syndrome (Chapter 18)
   f. Lynch syndrome (Chapter 18)
5. **Sections 5–7 are for when providers are seeing consults of known cancer patients with neurologic complaints.**
   Neurologic symptoms are the second most common reason for a cancer patient to be admitted to the hospital (behind admission for scheduled chemotherapy!). Neurologic deficits can occur from the cancer itself (Section 5) or from treatment of the cancer (Sections 6 and 7).
   a. **Section 5** reviews neurologic complications of the cancer itself including direct effects of tumors that involve the nervous system and indirect effects of tumors that do not involve the nervous system. These latter disorders may contribute to neurologic deficits through paraneoplastic syndromes which are reviewed.
      i. Neurologic complications in brain tumor patients including seizures, cerebral edema, stroke, hydrocephalus **(Chapter 19)**
      ii. Non-neurologic complications to watch out for in brain tumor patients including endocrinopathy and hypercoagulability (Chapter 19)
      iii. Neurologic complications of hematologic malignancies including leukemia and lymphoma (Chapter 23)
      iv. Direct perineural cancer invasion causing cranial neuropathy in head and neck cancer patients (Chapter 21)
      v. Brachial plexopathy from cancer spread to the brachial plexus (Chapter 22)
      vi. Paraneoplastic neurologic syndromes (Chapter 20)

b. **Sections 6 and 7** review common neurologic complications of cancer treatment including radiation and systemic therapies. Both the central nervous system (CNS) and peripheral nervous system (PNS) can be affected. These chapters review common CNS symptoms (neurocognition), PNS symptoms (neuropathy), and other relevant complications including:
   i. Post-treatment radiation necrosis (Chapter 24)
   ii. Treatment-induced neurocognitive dysfunction (Chapter 25)
   iii. Chemotherapy induced peripheral neuropathy (Chapter 28)
   iv. Complications of systemic therapies (Chapter 27)
   v. Complications of immune-based therapies for cancer (Chapters 29–30)
   vi. And rare complications of radiation therapy (Chapter 26)

What is included in this book?

In addition to the chapters highlighted above, several additional resources are included to provide a quick review and reference of teaching points in neuro-oncology. These are intended to help the practicing clinician as a quick guide and include:

1. **Summary of clinical pearls**: this is a summary of all of the clinical teaching points from each chapter of the book. This is intended to be a quick reference guide on important, clinically relevant, actionable items for managing patients. This is a quick and easy read to jog your memory of key points in neuro-oncology.
2. **Reference list of clinical cases**: this is a list of the clinical cases that are covered in this book. Do you want to read a case about how to manage recurrent glioblastoma? Do you need a refresher case about how to diagnose a patient with tuberous sclerosis complex or neurofibromatosis? Do you need to review a case of the neurologic complications of immune checkpoint inhibitors? The list of cases is organized alphabetically by tumor type to serve as a quick reference to teaching cases that are covered in this book. Not all brain and spinal cord tumors are intended to be covered in this text and this reference list highlights the key and clinically relevant tumors that are included in these cases.

Acknowledgements

It is only through the generous efforts and tireless work of the authors and coauthors that this text is available and will improve care for patients. The future of our field lies in the next generation of practitioners. This text draws from the seasoned expertise of senior practitioners who have decades of experience, as well as from the excitement of early career clinicians and investigators—it is through these opportunities that the future of our field grows.

Contents

Section 5: Neurologic complications of cancer

Section 6: Neurologic complications of radiation therapy

Section 7: Neurologic complications of systemic therapy

Section 8: Neurologic complications of immune-based cancer therapies

Chapter 1

Fundamentals of neuropathology: introduction to neuropathology and molecular diagnostics

Sonika Dahiya and Shakti Ramkissoon

CHAPTER OUTLINE

Introduction

In typical cases, the clinical workflow for brain tumors begins with imaging studies; however, despite the increased sensitivity and capabilities of these methodologies, diagnosing brain tumors requires histopathologic evaluation of tissue. It is imperative for clinicians to understand how brain tumors are classified so that they can better counsel patients at the time of initial presentation, accurately describe prognosis, and prioritize management of medical or neurological comorbidities based on the anticipated behavior of the tumor.

Tumor classification has historically relied primarily upon morphologic features identified by light microscopy. In the past decade, integration of high-throughput genomic testing into routine clinical workflows has refined the approach to diagnosing brain tumors.[1] In this chapter, we explore tumor classification from traditional microscope-based approaches to currently available methodologies. We review genomic profiling and introduce the concept of an integrated diagnosis.

The chapter begins with a discussion of the histologic assessment of brain tumors, which is often the first data to be reported after a tumor surgery. This is followed by a discussion of molecular profiling, which is used to further classify these tumors, guide prognosis, and predict response to therapy. Molecular data typically returns in the weeks following surgery. Finally, we review a series of common case scenarios and integrate the histologic and molecular data into a final integrated diagnosis that clinicians can use to help manage and counsel these patients.

Histologic classification of central nervous system tumors

The primary method of diagnostic neuropathology and brain tumor classification remains microscopic evaluation of hematoxylin and eosin (H&E)–stained tissue sections by light microscopy. This approach has experienced relatively few changes over the past several decades with generations of pathologists still undergoing specialized training focused on learning to read or interpret stained sections on glass slides.

The process of converting a portion of resected brain tissue to an H&E stained section is the first step to achieve a tissue-based diagnosis. Brain tissues removed at the time of surgery can range from small biopsies, such as needle core biopsies, to large resections that often occur during a tumor debulking surgery. Once the fresh tissue reaches the laboratory, the sample is subjected to fixation in formalin-based solutions that serve to preserve tissues and cells.

Formalin-fixed tissues then undergo a series of steps, commonly referred to as tissue processing, which prepares the formalin-fixed tissues for embedding into a block of paraffin wax. Once the tissue fragment is embedded in paraffin and mounted into a cassette, this "block" serves as the final medium where the tissue can be safely stored for years (even decades). Importantly, this processing method preserves the integrity of the tissues for later use. Formalin-fixed paraffin-embedded (FFPE) samples are the mainstay of both traditional microscopic analysis and serve as the starting medium for most tissue-based molecular and genomic assays currently available.

Once a tissue sample is converted to an FFPE block, sections (5 microns thickness) can be cut from the block, placed onto glass slides, and subjected to staining with the dyes hematoxylin and eosin. Hematoxylin stains nucleic acids a deep blue-to-purple color, which readily highlights the nuclei of cells. Eosin stains other cellular components, like proteins, with a bright pink color that contrasts with the blue hematoxylin-stained nuclei—together these two dyes serve as the basis for all H&E-based tumor classification.

Brain tumor classification based on H&E features relies on the fact that the histologic appearance of these tumors is consistent from one patient to another. In fact, the features are so reproducible that they have been codified into the World Health Organization (WHO) Classification of Tumors of the Central Nervous System, which outlines the microscopic features present in all brain tumors and serves as the central resource to ensure all patients around the world are diagnosed and graded using the same criteria.

Tumor Grading. Unlike other tumors, which are staged based on size, lymph node involvement, and presence or extent of metastases (e.g., TNM classification), staging is not used for gliomas, which rarely spread beyond the central nervous system (CNS). Instead, gliomas are graded from grade I to IV and are broadly divided into low- and high-grade tumors. Grade I and II are considered "low grade" and grade III and IV as "high grade"; of these, grade I tumors are generally well circumscribed, whereas grades II–IV are diffusely infiltrating, albeit with some exceptions such as ependymoma and pleomorphic xanthoastrocytoma which tend to be well circumscribed despite conforming to grade II. The histologic features assessed to establish glioma grading include atypia, mitoses, endothelial or microvascular proliferation, and necrosis. Grade I tumors such as pilocytic astrocytomas are most commonly encountered in the pediatric setting. Although such tumors do occur in the adult population, the use of the term "lower-grade gliomas" in adults largely refers to infiltrating grade II tumors such as diffuse astrocytoma and oligodendroglioma. Grade III tumors include anaplastic astrocytoma (AA3) and anaplastic oligodendroglioma (AO3), whereas glioblastoma (GBM) is considered a grade IV astrocytoma. Progression of brain tumors from low to high grade does occur, most commonly in adults from grade II diffuse astrocytoma to higher-grade gliomas such as AA3 or GBM, which are termed "secondary" GBM. Not all GBMs present as progression from a lower-grade neoplasm. In fact, the vast majority of GBMs present as de novo tumors without any prior history of a lower-grade glioma and are referred to as "primary" GBMs. Ependymomas are also considered a subtype of glioma, albeit with combined glial and epithelial lineage, and are graded from I–III; these are generally well circumscribed, with the exception of WHO grade III tumors.

Tumor Lineage. Tumor lineage is another important concept that goes hand in hand with grading. Lineage refers to the presumed cell of origin to which a tumor morphologically resembles. This designation then leads to broad categories of tumors such as astrocytoma, oligodendroglioma, and ependymoma among others.

When reviewing H&Es for tumor classification, the first step is determining whether tumor cells are present. An initial feature to assess is the overall cellularity of the tissue compartment (white matter, cortex, thalamus, cerebellum) being analyzed. This cellularity should then be compared to what is normally expected for these tissues. When a tumor is moderate-to-densely cellular, this step can be trivial; however, in instances of low tumor content or scattered tumor cells infiltrating white matter (e.g., gliomatosis pattern), this step can be surprisingly difficult, as these tumors can be indistinguishable from reactive processes (gliosis) seen in the brain.

Once tumor cells are recognized, a grade must be assigned. Among diffuse gliomas, this is accomplished by cataloging the presence or absence of low- and high-grade histologic features, including nuclear atypia, presence/absence of mitotic figures, microvascular proliferation, and necrosis. Grade II diffuse gliomas are typically moderately cellular tumors that can occur as both solid lesions with diffuse infiltration of adjacent brain tissues or as largely diffusely infiltrating tumors. Grade II diffuse gliomas by definition lack mitoses, microvascular proliferation, and necrosis but show increased cellularity and nuclear atypia. The presence of mitoses (a marker of cell division) in a diffuse glioma warrants upgrading to an anaplastic glioma (grade III), and if necrosis and/or microvascular proliferation are present in astrocytic lineage tumors, a diagnosis of GBM (grade IV) would be warranted.

It should be noted that there are differences in grading based on tumor lineage. For example, oligodendrogliomas are restricted to grade II and III tumors, with no grade I or IV oligodendroglioma categories; in contrast, astrocytomas are graded on a scale of I to IV. Oligodendrogliomas with necrosis and microvascular proliferation are grade III, whereas astrocytomas with the same features are considered grade IV.

In addition to features important to grading, other histologic features readily apparent on H&E sections include tumor cell morphology and growth features, which are characteristic of certain lineages. Oligodendroglioma tumor cells are classically associated with round nuclei within cells that have clear cytoplasm, resulting in a "fried egg" appearance. These tumor cells are often distributed within a network of fine capillary-like vessels reminiscent of a "chicken wire" pattern. Astrocytomas often have irregularly shaped nuclei that may be eccentrically displaced (or pushed to the side of the cell); when associated with abundant amounts of pink cytoplasm, it is commonly referred to as gemistocytic morphology.

For many decades, the assessment of histologic features by H&E has been the foundation by which tumors were defined and served as the basis for much of our current understanding of natural history of diseases. Although this approach has proven invaluable, it is not without known limitations. Such challenges include tumors that demonstrate overlapping features between different lineages, thereby creating a challenge when attempting to assign a diagnosis and grade. Additionally, classification is entirely dependent on the tissue sampled, which introduces the concept of "under sampling." In some cases wherein neuroimaging studies highlight tumors that likely represent high-grade gliomas, on H&E sections the resected tissue may only demonstrate low-grade glioma characteristics. The discrepancy frequently results from undersampling of the more overtly malignant portions of the tumor.

In practice, H&E analysis is paired with immunohistochemistry (IHC) to support tumor classification particularly for lineage assignment and, more recently, to identify specific mutations that can be detected at the protein level. IHC is a method of applying antibodies against specific protein antigens that are evaluated using light microscopy. Common markers that are assessed by IHC include GFAP (glial fibrillary acidic protein), a cytoplasmic marker of astrocytes and glial cells, NeuN (neuronal nuclei), a marker of neuronal differentiation, and OLIG2 (oligodendrocyte transcription factor 2), a nuclear marker of glial lineage. In recent years, antibodies capable of detecting specific mutant proteins, such as H3F3A(K27M), BRAF(V600E), and IDH1(R132H), have become widely available for routine clinical use. Integrating IHC results with histologic features provides neuropathologists with critical information that is used to accurately assign a tumor lineage and grade. Additionally, as we will discuss below, determining mutational status can also provide therapeutic and prognostic information for the patient and clinical providers.

Molecular characterization of central nervous system tumors

Understanding the genomic drivers of each patient's tumor is important to achieving the goals of precision medicine. Traditional methodologies for understanding oncogenic drivers have been limited to single gene sequencing methods that interrogate hotspot mutations in specific genes such as *BRAF* or *IDH1/2*. Moreover, fluorescence in situ hybridization (FISH) analyses allow for gene level or arm-level evaluation to identify copy number alterations commonly associated with CNS tumors such as *EGFR* amplification in GBMs or chromosome 1p/19q co-deletion in oligodendrogliomas. Although these methodologies provide powerful insights into the molecular mechanisms driving gliomagenesis, they require significant tumor input if multiple probes need to be tested, and need specialized personnel for interpretation, all of which can limit the availability of testing.

The ability to extract nucleic acids (DNA and RNA) from FFPE samples has revolutionized integration of genomic data into diagnostic algorithms. Extracted FFPE DNA can now be used in massively paralleled or next-generation sequencing (NGS) assays that have largely replaced the need for single gene assays or FISH testing in brain tumors. Common approaches to NGS testing of DNA range from targeted panels that interrogate 30–500 cancer-related genes to whole-exome (WES) or whole-genome sequencing (WGS). RNA testing options range from gene expression profiling to whole transcriptome RNA sequencing. In many cases, the amount of tissue (and DNA) needed to perform a single gene assay is equivalent to that needed for a large panel that includes over 300 genes. The benefit of panel-based sequencing or WES lies in the ability to identify single nucleotide variants, small insertion-deletions (indels), rearrangements, and even, in some cases, copy number alterations in hundreds of genes in parallel compared to single gene assays.

Application of these advanced technologies has identified key genomic signatures of specific tumor lineages.

Seminal studies from The Cancer Genome Atlas demonstrated that adult gliomas are driven more by copy number alterations than mutations contrary to what is observed in other malignant tumors such as lung, colon, or breast carcinomas. Indeed, adult GBMs are typically characterized by polysomy of chromosome 7, *EGFR* amplification, *CDKN2A/B* deletion, and monosomy of chromosome 10 (leading to single copy loss of *PTEN*).[2] Conversely, oligodendroglial lineage tumors harbor *IDH1/2* mutations in association with chromosome 1p/19q co-deletion and frequent alterations involving *CIC* and *FUBP1*. Young adult diffuse astrocytomas are characterized by a combination of *IDH1/2*, *TP53*, and *ATRX* mutations. In the pediatric setting, grade I pilocytic astrocytomas are frequently characterized by *BRAF* alterations, including point mutations (*BRAF* V600E) or gene fusions *(KIAA1549-BRAF)*. Pediatric midline high-grade gliomas are now categorized based on their mutational profile. The presence of an *H3* mutation (e.g., *H3F3A* K27M) in a midline diffuse glioma now warrants a grade IV designation independent of other histologic features. Focused analysis of rare glioma subtypes has also identified novel oncogenic drivers, as is the case with angiocentric gliomas, which are essentially defined by the presence of *MYB* alterations such as *MYB-QKI* fusions.

By recognizing that many brain tumors can be readily distinguished from each other based on genomic signatures, tumor classification has been refined to incorporate these data. The field is moving toward a model of an "integrated diagnosis" that combines histologic findings with those of genomic/molecular data. In this approach, tumors are classified and graded first based on H&E and IHC features which yields a histopathologic diagnosis. In parallel, a portion of tissue is subjected to NGS testing that yields genomic characteristics such as mutations, fusions, and copy number alterations identified in the tumor. The histologic and genomic findings are then collected together into a unified final and integrated diagnosis—often several weeks after a histopathologic diagnosis has been rendered.[3]

Given the time required to perform genomic testing, treatment is typically initiated based on the histopathologic diagnosis; however, the value of additional genomic and molecular data is to enhance diagnostic accuracy, provide prognostic biomarkers (e.g., *IDH1/2* mutational status), and refine the treatment plan to better align with the patient's genomic profile. In this approach, the integrated diagnosis serves to overcome limitations associated with traditional histopathology diagnoses and ensures optimal clinical management.

Clinical cases

In the following case presentations, we will explore how histopathologic findings can be combined with genomic data to support diagnosis and prognosis, and guide clinical decision-making.

CASE 1.1 CHARACTERISTIC HISTOPATHOLOGICAL AND MOLECULAR FEATURES OF GLIOBLASTOMA

Case. A 69-year-old male presented to the emergency department with new onset seizures and rapidly progressive right sided weakness. Brain MRI with contrast revealed a centrally necrotic, multifocal ring-enhancing lesion in the left posterior frontal lobe (Fig. 1.1).

Histology. Microscopic examination of H&E sections (Fig. 1.2 A,B) demonstrates a densely cellular glial neoplasm composed of cells with irregular and hyperchromatic nuclei associated with moderate amounts of eosinophilic cytoplasm. Mitoses are readily identified. Multifocal microvascular proliferation is present, as well as areas of multifocal necrosis including palisading necrosis (Fig. 1.2B, black arrows). Immunohistochemistry reveals positive staining in tumor cells for GFAP (Fig. 1.2F), retained expression of ATRX (Fig. 1.2D), and negative staining for IDH1(R132H) (Fig. 1.2C).

Genomic and molecular analyses. Genomic profiling of tumor DNA by NGS reveals *EGFR*vIII amplification, *TERT* promoter mutation and homozygous deletion of *CDKN2A/B*. Alterations were not detected in the following genes: *IDH1*, *IDH2*, *BRAF*, *ATRX*, *TP53*, *PDGFRA*. Arm-level copy number analysis revealed polysomy of chromosome 7 and monosomy of chromosome 10. There was no evidence of 1p/19q co-deletion. Additionally, *MGMT* promoter methylation analysis demonstrated no evidence of methylation.

Integrated Diagnosis: GLIOBLASTOMA, WHO Grade IV, *IDH1/2* wild-type, *EGFRvIII* amplified; *MGMT* promoter unmethylated

Teaching Points. This case illustrates the classic clinical, histologic, and genomic presentation of adult glioblastoma. Patients present with neurologic symptoms, typically nonspecific but which can include new-onset seizures in the fifth to seventh decades of life. Imaging studies reveal important characteristics such as location, size, enhancement, and involvement of adjacent brain tissues. The histologic analysis of the tumor in this case demonstrated characteristic features of GBM including increased cellularity, cells with irregular nuclei, and high-grade features (mitoses, microvascular proliferation, and necrosis). Immunohistochemical stains for GFAP, OLIG2, and SOX2 support a glial lineage. The genomic profile of this tumor also demonstrates the classic alterations associated with adult GBM, notably gains of chromosome 7, single copy loss of chromosome 10, and homozygous deletion of *CDKN2A/B*. Amplification of *EGFR* is detected in approximately 40% of adult GBMs and the *EGFR*vIII variant is seen in half of these cases. The *EGFRvIII* variant results from deletion of exons 2–7, which generates a constitutively activated, ligand-

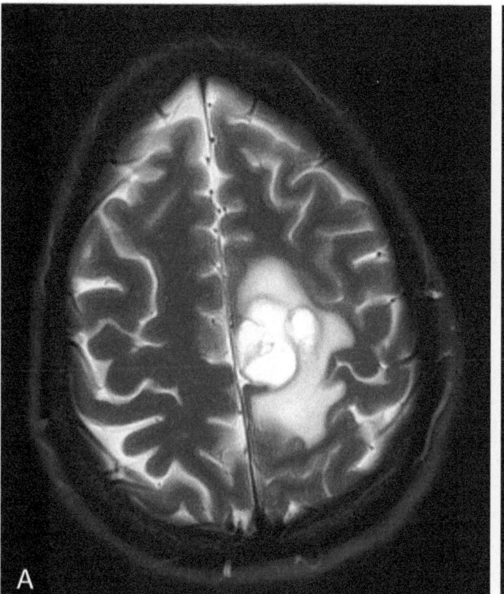

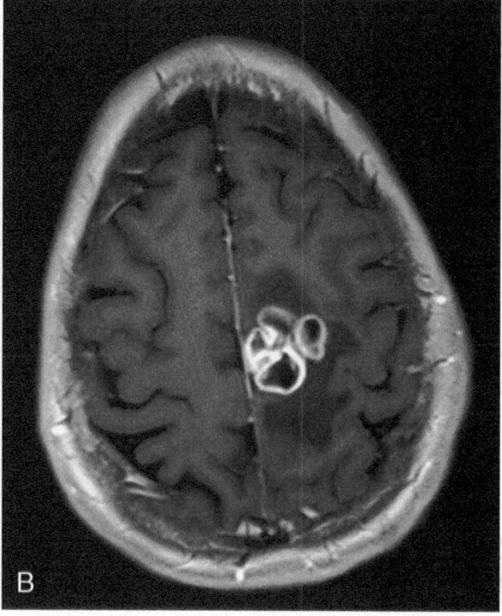

Fig. 1.1 MRI Brain including (A) axial T2-weighted sequence showing a 2.9 × 2.4 cm mass with surrounding edema in the left posterior frontal lobe, and (B) axial T1-weighted gadolinium enhanced sequence showing multiple foci of ring-enhancement with central necrosis concerning for a diagnosis of high-grade glioma.

independent kinase that promotes cell proliferation through the PI3 kinase, RAS, and MAPK signaling pathways. Although no specific therapies have demonstrated utility against *EGFRvIII*, it is an active area of investigation and serves as a key player of tumor growth. Loss of one copy of chromosome 10 is the most frequently detected genomic alteration in GBM, occurring in 60–80% of cases.[2] The tumor suppressor *PTEN* is located at 10q23.3 and considered a critical candidate gene in gliomagenesis as it is an important negative regulator of the PI3 kinase pathway. *TERT* promoter mutations are detected in 70–80% of GBMs and are associated with a worse prognosis in the absence of *IDH1/2* mutations.

As standard of care, patients diagnosed with GBM are treated with combination chemo- and radiation (adjuvant) therapy (see Chapters 4 and 12 for further discussion of treatment regimens for GBM). Analysis of the *MGMT* promoter is typically performed to evaluate the tumor's sensitivity to the alkylating agent temozolomide. O6-methylguanine methyltransferase (MGMT) is a DNA repair enzyme that is associated with resistance to alkylating agents when expressed. Methylation of the *MGMT* promoter leads to reduced protein expression in tumor cells allowing for accumulation of alkylating-induced DNA damage that promotes cell death. In this tumor, the absence of *MGMT* promoter methylation (unmethylated) indicates decreased responsiveness to temozolomide.

In summary, this case highlights the classic pathologic features of adult GBM and illustrates how the genomics can inform the signaling pathways driving gliomagenesis and provide potential therapeutic targets and important prognostic information that can inform clinical decision-making.

Clinical Pearls

1. Microvascular proliferation and palisading necrosis are pathologic hallmarks of glioblastoma and, when present, establish the diagnosis of GBM.
2. *IDH1/2* gene mutation is rare in glioblastoma; *EGFR* amplification and MGMT promoter methylation are observed in approximately 40% of GBMs.

CASE 1.2 USE OF MOLECULAR TESTING TO DEFINE THE DIAGNOSIS OF WHO GRADE 2, OLIDOENDROGLIOMA

Case. A 39-year-old female presenting with new onset headaches. Brain MRI reveals a nonenhancing temporal lobe lesion (Fig. 1.3).

Histology. Microscopic examination of H&E sections (Fig. 1.4A) reveals a moderately cellular glial neoplasm composed of cells with centrally located round nuclei associated with modest amounts of clear cytoplasm. Mitoses are not readily identified and occur in less than 1 per 10 high-power fields (HPFs). High-grade features including microvascular proliferation and necrosis are not detected. Immunohistochemistry reveals positive staining in tumor cells for IDH1 (R132H) (Fig. 1.4B) and OLIG-2 (Fig. 1.4D), and negative staining for TP53 (image not shown), with low Ki-67 proliferation index (Fig. 1.4E). An immunostain for ATRX shows positive staining in tumor nuclei (Fig. 1.4C).

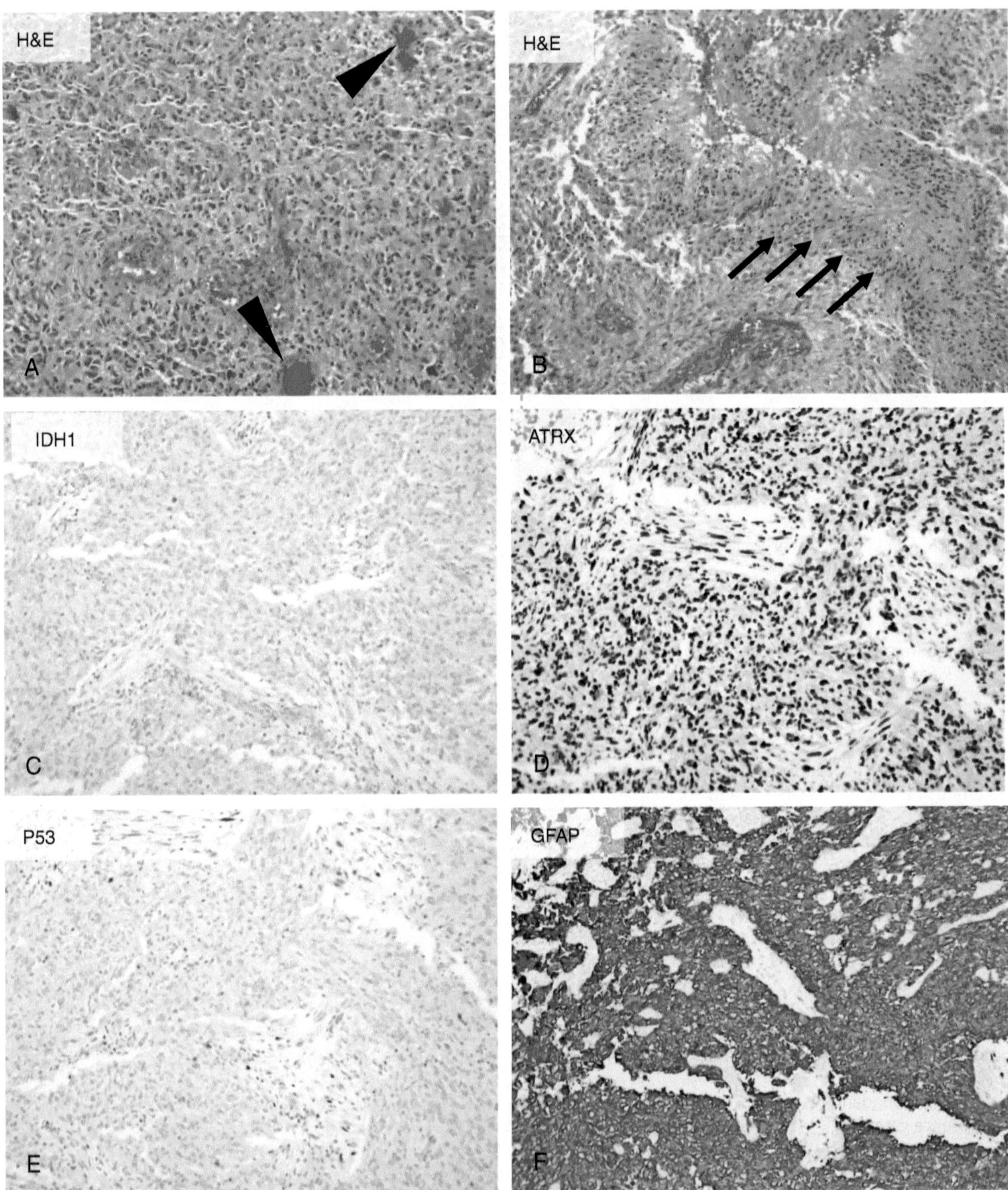

Fig. 1.2 Microscopic examination showing histologic features consistent with glioblastoma including H&E stained sections (A,B) showing microvascular proliferation (A, *black arrowheads*), and palisading necrosis (B, *black arrows*). Immunohistochemistry shows negative staining for IDH1(R132H) (C), retained expression of ATRX (D), negative staining for p53 (E), and positive staining in tumor cells for GFAP (F).

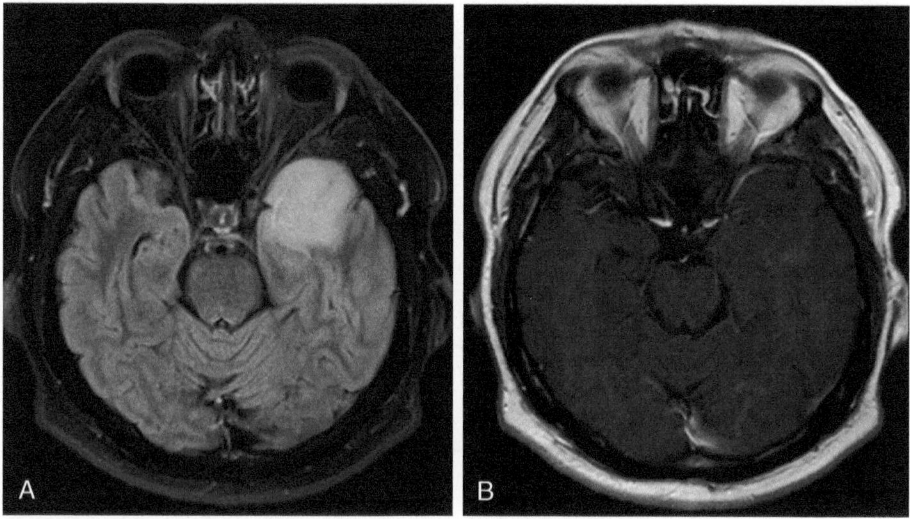

Fig. 1.3 MRI Brain including (A) axial fluid attenuation inversion recovery sequence showing a nonenhancing mass with minimal surrounding edema in the left anterior temporal pole, and (B) axial T1-weighted gadolinium enhanced sequence showing no evidence of contrast enhancement.

Genomics and molecular analysis. Genomic profiling of tumor cells reveals *IDH1* p.R132H and *CIC* p.R215W mutations. Alterations were not detected in the following genes: *IDH2, BRAF, ATRX, TP53*, or *EGFR*. Arm-level copy number analysis revealed co-deletion of chromosomes 1p/19q without evidence of deletions involving *CDKN2A/B*. *MGMT* promoter methylation was detected.

Integrated Diagnosis. OLIGODENDROGLIOMA, WHO Grade II, *IDH1*(R132H)-mutant, 1p/19q co-deleted; *MGMT* promoter methylated

Teaching Points. This case illustrates the classic histologic and genomic presentation of oligodendroglioma. In contrast to glioblastoma, these tumors typically present at younger ages, with a peak incidence in the fourth decade. Clinical symptoms can vary greatly but often include headaches, seizures, and other signs of increased cranial pressure. Combined CT and MRI studies frequently demonstrate well-circumscribed lesions often associated with calcifications. Histologic analysis revealed the classic cellular appearance of oligodendroglial lineage tumor cells, with round nuclei surrounded by abundant clear cytoplasm. A low mitotic index and absence of microvascular proliferation and necrosis support classification as a lower-grade glioma. The genomic profile is diagnostic of an oligodendroglial neoplasm as evidenced by 1p/19q co-deletion and presence of an *IDH1* (R132H) mutation. In addition to the diagnostic alterations, *CIC* mutations are typically observed in oligodendrogliomas and rarely present in astrocytic tumors. CIC functions as a transcriptional repressor to counteract activation of genes that are targets of receptor tyrosine kinase pathways. The absence of an *ATRX* mutation, and therefore retained ATRX protein expression, also supports an oligodendroglial lineage tumor. In general, oligodendrogliomas are slow-growing tumors and have relatively favorable prognostic indications compared to diffuse astrocytic tumors; however, recurrence and progression to a more malignant neoplasm can occur. The detection of *MGMT* promoter methylation indicates a more favorable response to alkylating chemotherapy agents.

In summary, this case illustrates how the presence of specific genomic alterations now defines a tumor diagnosis. Classification of oligodendrogliomas now requires presence of 1p/19q co-deletion and an *IDH1/2* mutation. Given the overlapping histologic features or limitations of sampling, incorporation of molecular data provides critical information for diagnosis and, importantly, prognosis.

Clinical Pearls

1. When molecular profiling of a brain tumor reveals the presence of 1p/19q co-deletion and *IDH1/2* mutation, a diagnosis of oligodendroglioma is made.
2. Histologically, oligodendrogliomas are characterized by the presence of round nuclei and perinuclear halo that has a "fried egg" appearance.
3. Grading of oligodendrogliomas is restricted to grade II and III tumors; there is no grade I or IV oligodendroglioma; oligodendrogliomas with necrosis and microvascular proliferation are grade III.

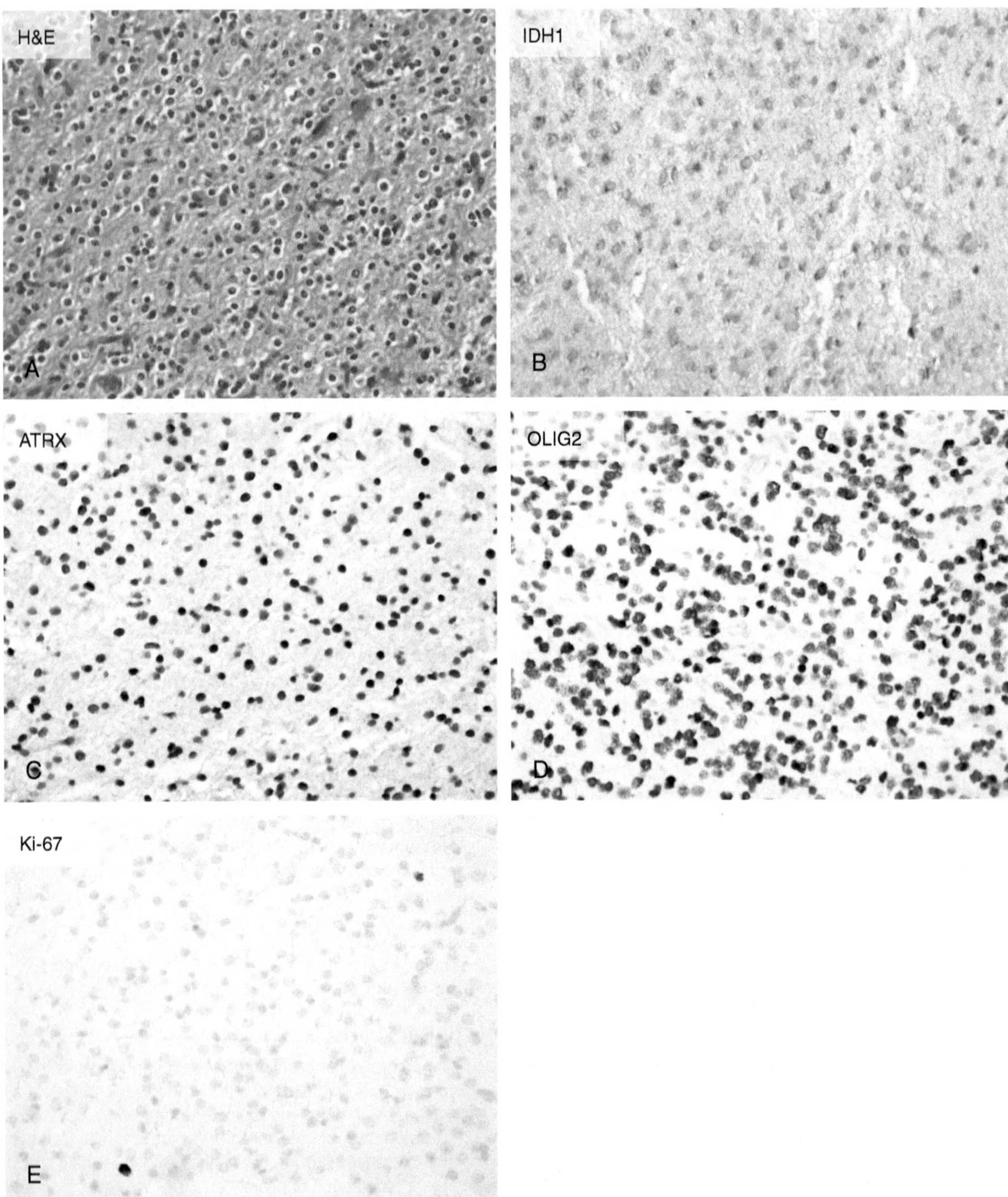

Fig. 1.4 Microscopic examination showing histologic features consistent with low-grade oligodendroglioma including H&E stained sections (A) demonstrating infiltrating tumors cells with circular nuclei and perinuclear halos (A). Immunohistochemistry shows positive staining for IDH1(R132H) (B), retained expression of ATRX (C), positive staining in tumor cells for OLIG2 (D), and low Ki-67 proliferation index (E).

CASE 1.3 USE OF GENOMIC PROFILING TO ESTABLISH A DIAGNOSIS OF WHO GRADE 2, ASTROCYTOMA

Case. 24-year-old male who presented with new-onset seizures. Imaging studies reveal a large right frontal lobe lesion with no enhancement (Fig. 1.5A–C).

Histology. Microscopic examination of H&E sections (Fig. 1.6A) reveal a moderately cellular glial neoplasm composed of cells with irregular-to-ovoid eccentric nuclei and associated with abundant amounts of eosinophilic cytoplasm. Mitoses, microvascular proliferation, and necrosis are not detected. Immunohistochemistry reveals positive staining in tumor cells for p53 (Fig. 1.6D) and IDH1 (R132H) (Fig. 1.6B), and negative staining for ATRX (loss of nuclear staining in tumor cells, Fig. 1.6C). The overall Ki-67 proliferation index is low (Fig. 1.6E).

Genomic and molecular analyses. Genomic profiling of tumor cells identifies *IDH1* (R132H), *TP53* (R273H), and *ATRX* (R1426*) mutations. Alterations were not detected in the following genes: *IDH2, BRAF, CIC, FUBP1*, or *EGFR*. Arm-level copy number analysis revealed no evidence of 1p/19q co-deletion, polysomy 7 or monosomy 10. *MGMT* promoter methylation was detected.

Integrated Diagnosis. DIFFUSE ASTROCYTOMA, WHO Grade II, *IDH1*(R132H)-mutated; *MGMT* promoter methylated; Negative for 1p/19q co-deletion

Teaching Points. This case highlights a typical presentation of an adult low-grade diffuse astrocytoma. Similar to oligodendrogliomas, these tumors present earlier in life, with a peak incidence in the third and fourth decades. On CT and MRI scans, tumors present as low-density masses with little or no contrast enhancement. Histologically low-grade diffuse astrocytomas demonstrate moderately increased cellularity and the presence of nuclear atypia. Mitotic indices are

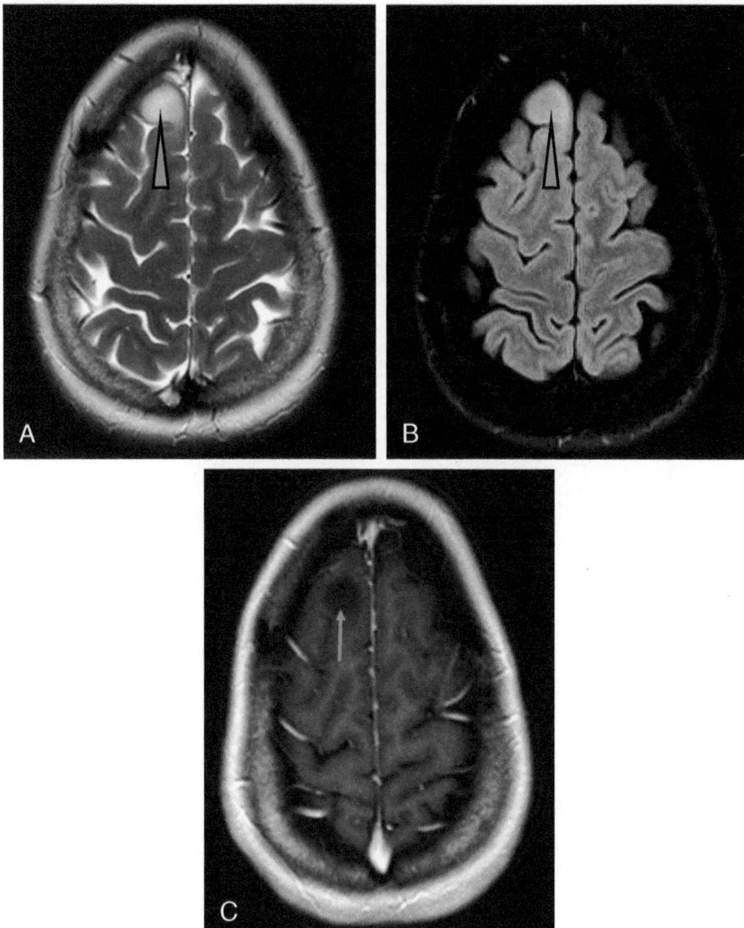

Fig. 1.5 MRI Brain including (A) axial T2-weighted sequence showing a small right anterior frontal mass with minimal surrounding edema *(arrowhead)*, and (B) axial fluid attenuation inversion recovery sequence showing this same mass *(arrowhead)*, and (C) axial T1-weighted gadolinium enhanced sequence showing no associated contrast enhancement *(arrow)*.

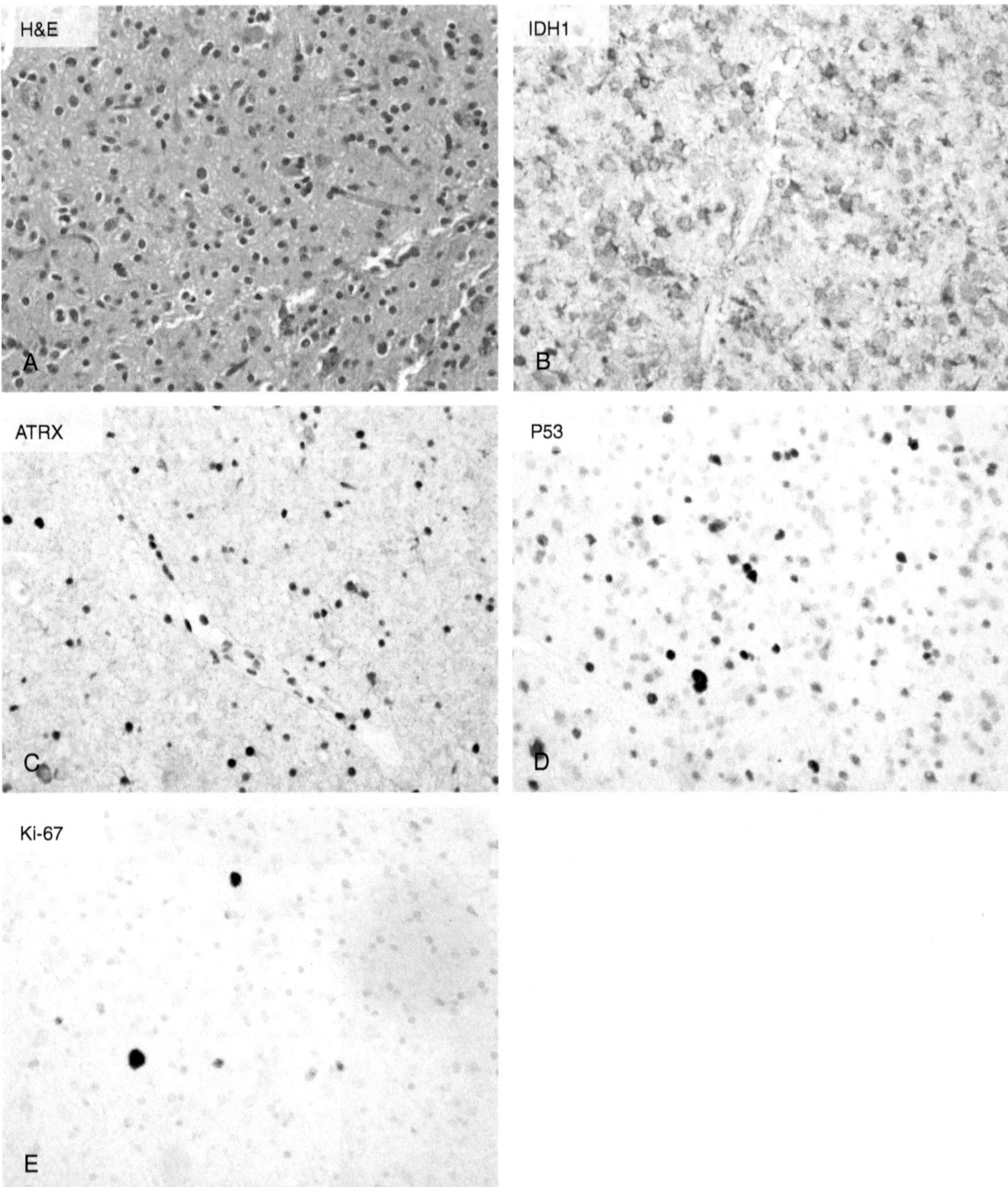

Fig. 1.6 Microscopic examination showing histologic features consistent with a low-grade astrocytoma including H&E stained sections (A) showing infiltrating irregularly shaped tumor cells with pleomorphic irregularly shaped nuclei. Immunohistochemistry shows positive staining for IDH1(R132H) (B), loss of nuclear staining in tumors cells of ATRX (C), positive staining for p53 (D), and low Ki-67 proliferation index (E).

typically low and high-grade features (microvascular proliferation and necrosis) are not observed. As these tumors tend to be diffusely infiltrating and atypical features can be subtle, incorporating genomics can significantly aid in diagnosis and classification. Although *IDH1/2* mutations are detected in >80% of low-grade astrocytic tumors, they are not lineage-defining as oligodendroglial tumors also harbor mutations in these genes; however, when *IDH1/2* mutations co-occur with *TP53* and *ATRX* mutations, this profile is associated with an astrocytic lineage tumor.[4] Of note, although immunohistochemical data support the genomic profile, it should not be used in isolation, as ATRX protein expression does not always correlate with mutational status; therefore both methodologies should be employed. *MGMT* promoter methylation is detected in almost 50% of diffuse astrocytomas and confers a better response to temozolomide; however, these tumors inevitably progress to higher-grade gliomas (see Chapter 11 for further discussion of the approach to low-grade gliomas).

In summary, this case highlights the importance genomic profiling and how the mutational profile aids in tumor classification. As low-grade tumors frequently exhibit subtle or nonspecific features, integrating the mutational profile provides significant diagnostic and prognostic information.

Clinical Pearls

1. Grade I gliomas are generally well circumscribed, whereas grades II–IV are diffusely infiltrating.
2. Low-grade diffusely infiltrating gliomas that lack co-deletion of chromosomes 1p and 19q are molecularly defined as astrocytomas.
3. Although *IDH1/2* gene mutation is common in low-grade diffuse astrocytomas, this is not a molecularly defining event and *IDH* wild-type low-grade diffuse astrocytomas also occur.
4. Low-grade gliomas can progress to higher-grade neoplasms and, when they recur as glioblastoma, are considered "secondary" GBMs.

CASE 1.4 HISTOPATHOLOGICAL AND MOLECULAR FINDINGS FOR WHO GRADE 3, ANAPLASTIC ASTROCYTOMA

Case. 40-year-old female who presented with headache, confusion, and blurred vision. Imaging studies demonstrate a large mass involving the frontal lobe associated with focal enhancement (Fig. 1.7A,B).

Histology. Microscopic examination of H&E sections (Fig. 1.8A) reveals a moderate-to-densely cellular glial neoplasm composed of cells with irregular and tapered nuclei and associated with moderate amounts of eosinophilic cytoplasm. Mitoses are present. Microvascular proliferation and necrosis are not detected. Immunohistochemistry reveals positive staining in tumor cells for GFAP (Fig. 1.8B), and ATRX (Fig. 1.8D), and negative staining for p53 (Fig. 1.8E) and IDH1 (R132H) (Fig. 1.8C) with an elevated Ki-67 proliferation index (Fig. 1.8F).

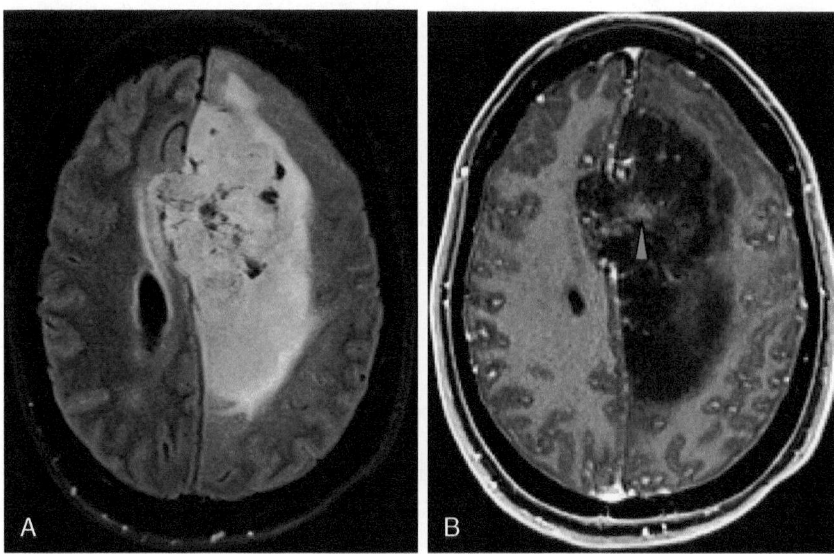

Fig. 1.7 MRI Brain including (A) axial fluid attenuation inversion recovery sequence showing a large mass arising from the left frontal lobe and crossing the corpus callosum with rightward midline shift and surrounding edema, and (B) axial T1-weighted gadolinium enhanced sequence showing a small area of patchy contrast enhancement *(orange arrowhead)*.

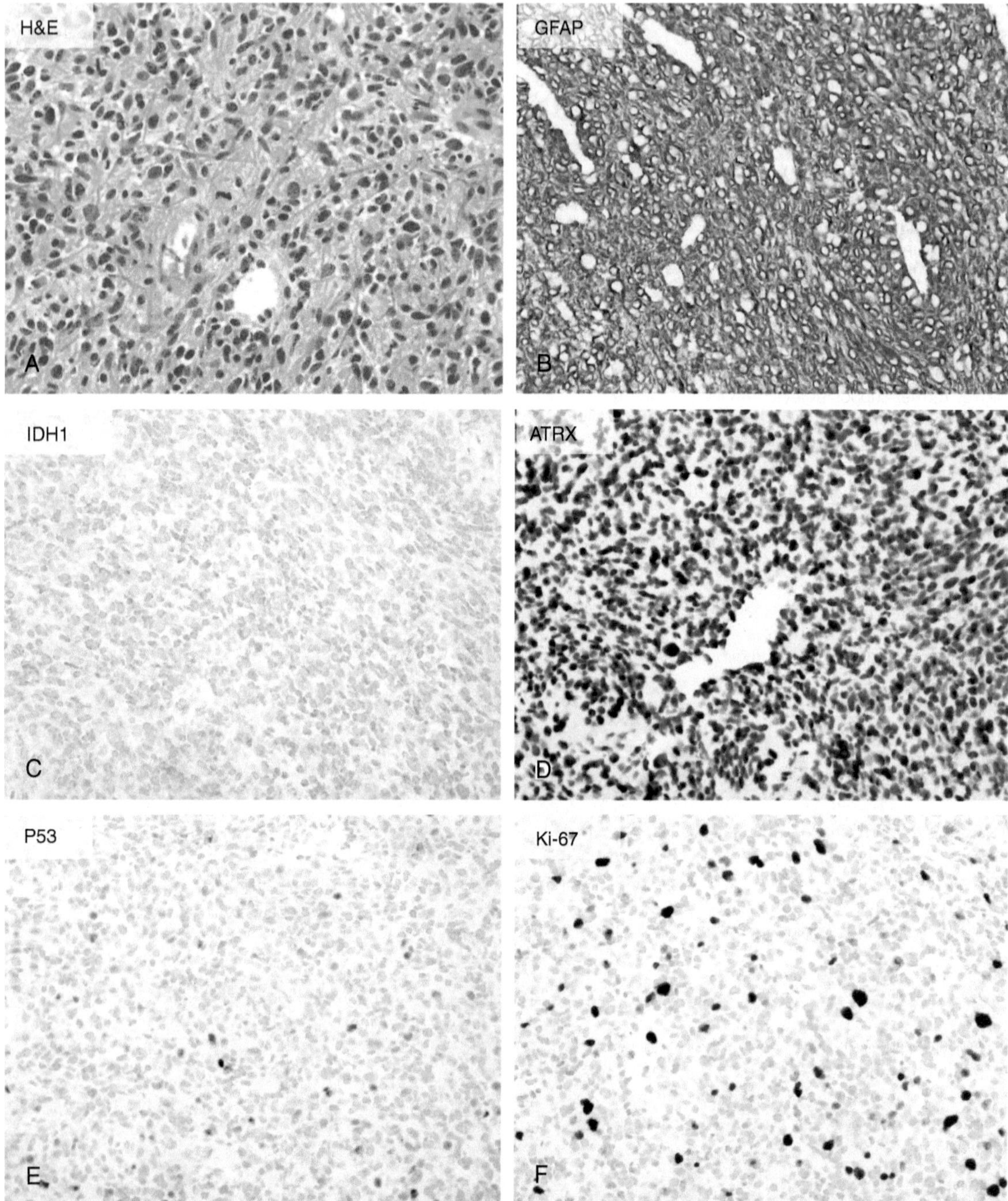

Fig. 1.8 Microscopic examination showing histologic features consistent with anaplastic astrocytoma including H&E stained sections (A) showing an infiltrating hypercellular tumor with irregular, pleomorphic nuclei and the presence of mitoses. Immunohistochemistry shows positive staining in tumor cells for GFAP (B) and ATRX (D) and negative staining for IDH1(R132H) (C) and p53 (E) with elevated Ki-67 proliferation index (F).

Genomic and molecular analyses. Genomic profiling of tumor cells reveals an *EGFR* (R108K) mutation but no mutations were detected in *IDH1, IDH2, TP53, ATRX, CIC,* or *FUBP1*. Copy number analysis revealed gains of chromosome 7, single copy deletion of *CDKN2A/B* (chr 9p21.3); 10q loss; and no evidence of 1p/19q co-deletion. *MGMT* promoter methylation was unmethylated.

Integrated Diagnosis. HIGH-GRADE GLIOMA at least ANAPLASTIC ASTROCYTOMA, WHO Grade III, *IDH1/2*-wild type; *MGMT* promoter unmethylated; Negative for 1p/19q co-deletion

Teaching Points. Whereas a majority of young adult diffuse gliomas harbor *IDH1/2* mutations, this case highlights an *IDH1/2*-wild type *de novo* or newly diagnosed diffuse astrocytic glioma with anaplastic features without prior history of a lower grade astrocytoma. IHC demonstrating positive staining for GFAP and OLIG2 align with an astrocytic lineage glioma, which is further supported by the presence of chromosome 7 gains and absence of 1p/19q co-deletion. The presence of *CDKN2A/B* loss is frequently seen in high grade gliomas. Furthermore, the presence of *PTEN*/10q loss combined with polysomy of chromosome 7 favors a molecular diagnosis of a higher-grade glioma (glioblastoma) despite the lack of histologic evidence of microvascular proliferation and/or necrosis.

Notably, patchy enhancement was detected on imaging studies; however, histologic examination revealed no definitive evidence of microvascular proliferation. Endothelial proliferation that occurs in high-grade gliomas is often irregular, disorganized vascular structures that result from abnormal vascular endothelial growth factor (VEGF)-induced angiogenesis. The leakiness of these abnormal vessels contributes to the contrast enhancement noted on MRI studies. If the tissue sampled in this case was limited (e.g., needle biopsy only), the discordance between enhancement by imaging and lack of microvascular proliferation by microscopic examination raises the possibility that the tumor may be under sampled; therefore, the final histologic grade assigned may not fully represent the underlying grade of the tumor. Although this tumor did not progress from a lower-grade glioma, the vast majority of anaplastic astrocytomas will progress and develop features of GBM. These lesions will not only acquire histologic hallmarks of GBM but also gain additional mutations and copy number changes typically associated with GBM.

Most patients diagnosed with *IDH1/2*-wild type anaplastic astrocytomas will go on to receive standard of care treatment for high-grade gliomas (chemoradiotherapy); however, it should be noted that the lack of a definitive tissue diagnosis of GBM can often be prohibitive for accessing some clinical trials.

Clinical Pearls

1. The presence of mitoses (a marker of cell division) in a diffuse glioma warrants upgrading to an anaplastic glioma (grade III).
2. The presence of chromosome 10q loss combined with polysomy of chromosome 7 favors a molecular diagnosis of a higher-grade glioma.

CASE 1.5 PATHOLOGIC ASSESSMENT OF DURAL-BASED MENINGIOMA

Case. 55-year-old female presenting with headaches and loss of smell. Imaging studies demonstrate a planum sphenoidale dural-based extra-axial mass (Fig. 1.9).

Histology. Microscopic examination of H&E sections (Fig. 1.10A) reveals a moderate-to-densely cellular neoplasm composed of cells with pale ovoid-to-tapered nuclei that are associated with moderate amounts of eosinophilic cytoplasm. Mitoses are rare and number less than 1 per 10 HPFs. There is no evidence of brain invasion, small cell change, prominent nucleoli, sheet-like growth or necrosis. Immunohistochemistry for Ki-67 (Fig. 1.10B), a marker of cell proliferation, shows a proliferation index of less than 1%.

Genomic and molecular analyses. Genomic profiling reveals a single *NF2* p.R160fs mutation. Copy number analysis reveals monosomy for chromosome 22 in a background of an otherwise neutral genome.

Integrated Diagnosis. MENINGIOMA, WHO Grade I, meningothelial subtype, *NF2* (R160fs) mutant.

Teaching Points. Meningiomas are the most common primary intracranial neoplasm in adults. Whereas most meningiomas are considered benign (WHO grade I), a subset of tumors can behave aggressively and are associated with invasion into adjacent tissues (including brain), recurrence, and progression (grade II and III). A majority (85–95%) of meningiomas are classified as WHO grade I, whereas grade II and III occur less frequently at 5–10% and 1–5%, respectively. Grading of meningiomas is critical to understanding long-term clinical behavior as anaplastic tumors are associated with poorer overall survival and progression-free rates after 10 years compared to grade I tumors.

There are many different morphologic subtypes of meningiomas based on histologic features. Grade I tumors include meningothelial, fibrous, microcystic, psammomatous, angiomatous, secretory, metaplastic, and lymphoplasmacyte-rich subtypes. Grade II include clear cell and chordoid subtypes, brain-invasive meningiomas, as well as tumors classified as atypical based on histologic criteria. Grade III tumors include rhabdoid and papillary subtypes, as well as those classified as anaplastic based on histologic criteria.

Meningiomas are graded based on the presence or absence of WHO defined histologic features. Grade I tumors by definition show less than 4 mitoses per 10 HPFs. Atypical meningiomas (WHO grade II) demonstrates 4–19 mitoses/10 HPFs and brain invasion or contain three of five atypical features including high nuclear/cytoplasmic ratio, prominent nucleoli, sheet-like growth, hypercellularity, or spontaneous necrosis. Anaplastic meningiomas (WHO grade III) show at least 20 mitoses/10 HPFs or display overtly malignant appearance like that seen in sarcoma. As noted above, some histologic subtypes are by definition associated with specific grades. For example, chordoid and clear cell meningiomas are by definition grade II, whereas rhabdoid and papillary subtypes are by definition grade III.

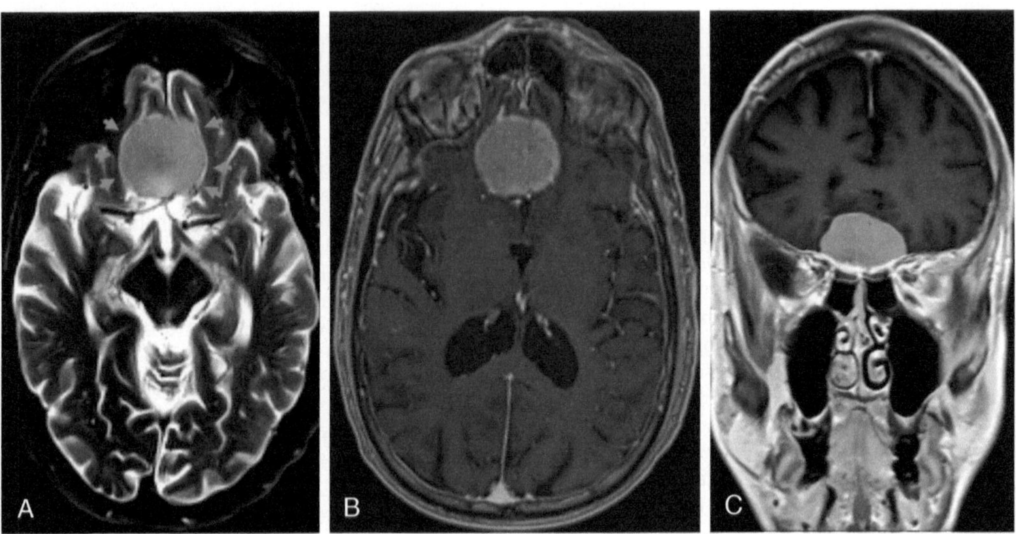

Fig. 1.9 MRI Brain including (A) axial T2-weighted sequence showing a 3.5 × 3.5 cm^2 mass lesion that is extra-axial in location as supported by the small rim of white cerebrospinal fluid surrounding the lesion *(orange arrows)*, and (B) axial T1-weighted gadolinium enhanced sequence highlighting this lesion, which (C) on coronal T1-weighted gadolinium enhanced images arises from the planum sphenoidale consistent with meningioma.

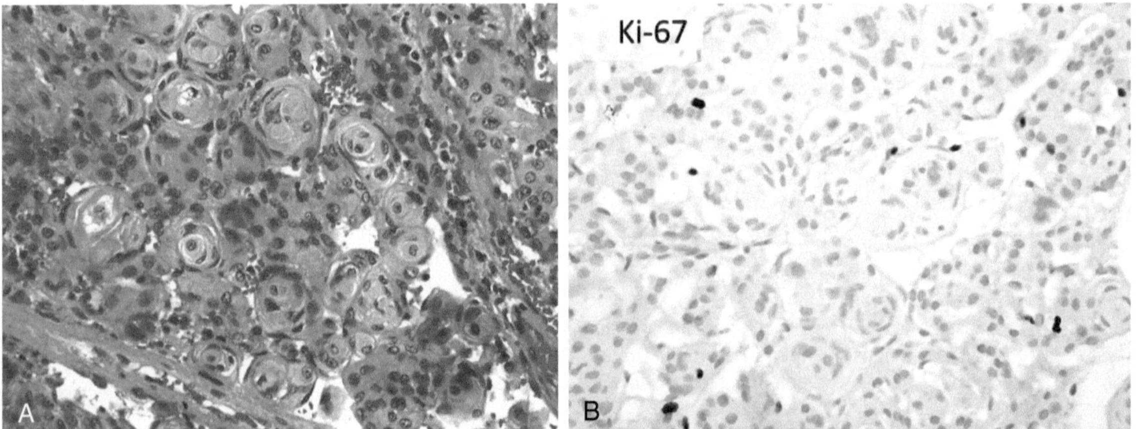

Fig. 1.10 Microscopic examination including H&E stained sections (A) showing a moderate-to-densely cellular neoplasm composed of whorls of tumor cells. Immunohistochemistry for Ki-67 shows a low proliferation index (B).

Meningioma represents one of the first tumors to be associated with a genomic driver when neurofibromin *(NF2)* was identified as the cause of neurofibromatosis 2 (NF2), wherein 50–75% of patients develop meningiomas (see Chapter 16 for further discussion of the approach to managing NF2). Sporadic meningiomas also harbor *NF2* mutations, with loss of NF2 protein observed in 40–60% of these cases. Collectively, mutations in *NF2*, *TRAF7*, *AKT1*, *KLF4*, *PIK3CA*, and *SMO* account for over 80% of recurrent alterations seen in grade I meningiomas. Currently, genomic profiling of meningiomas not only aids in the diagnosis and grading but also is used for clinical management regarding the risk of recurrence following surgical resection. For patients with grade II meningiomas, recent studies demonstrated that increased copy number changes are associated with a higher risk of recurrence and may benefit from increased monitoring. Additionally, the identification of *AKT*, *PIK3CA*, and *SMO* mutations provide opportunities for targeted therapies under investigation for

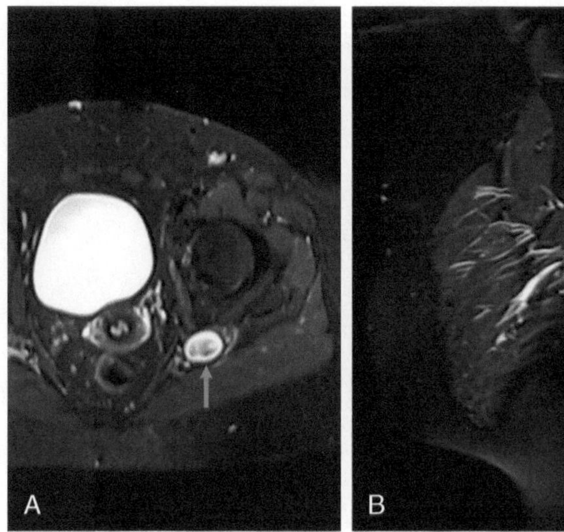

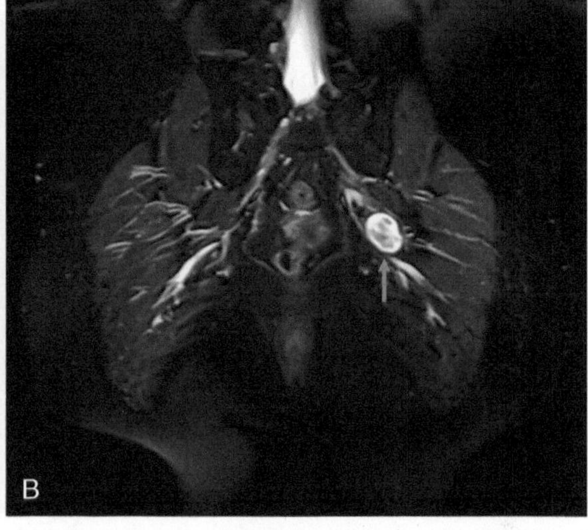

Fig. 1.11 MRI Lumbar Spine including (A) axial T2-weighted sequence showing a 2.5 × 2.1 cm² mass arising along the left sciatic nerve *(orange arrow)*, and (B) corresponding coronal T2-weighted sequence also showing the same T2 hyperintense lesion with targetoid appearance arising along the course of the left sciatic nerve consistent with peripheral nerve sheath tumor.

these tumors (see Chapter 10 for further discussion of the approach to managing meningioma).

Clinical Pearls

1. Meningiomas are the most common primary brain tumor and appear as dural-based lesions often with an area of adjacent thickened dura, termed a dural "tail."
2. Up to 95% of meningiomas are benign WHO grade I lesions, but rarely grade II and grade III tumors can present and require additional treatment.

CASE 6 HISTOPATHOLOGY OF A BENIGN PERIPHERAL NERVE SHEATH TUMOR: SCHWANNOMA VS NEUROFIBROMA

Case. 34-year-old female presenting with worsening low back and leg pain radiating down the posterior left lower leg with leg weakness. Contrast-enhanced MRI scans reveal a lesion arising along the left sciatic nerve (Fig. 1.11).

Histology. Microscopic examination of H&E sections (Fig. 1.12A) reveals a moderate-to-densely cellular spindle cell neoplasm composed of cells with ovoid-to-tapered nuclei. The tumor growth pattern is biphasic with some areas showing more dense or compact cellularity (Antoni A pattern, Fig. 1.12A "a" region), whereas other areas show a more hypocellular pattern (Antoni B, Fig. 1.12A "b" region) characterized by microcystic and/or myxoid features. Scattered Verocay bodies are noted in Antoni A areas characterized by prominent nuclear palisading. Tumor cells are dispersed within a background with abundant collagen fibers. Mitoses are not detected. Immunohistochemistry for Ki-67 (Fig. 1.12C), a marker of cell proliferation, shows a proliferation index of less than 1%. Tumor cells stain diffusely positive for S100 (Fig. 1.12B), a marker of calcium binding proteins. Silver stain (Bodian stain) and immunohistochemistry for neurofilament protein (NFP) typically show no evidence of interstitial or entrapped axons.

Genomics and molecular analysis. Genomic profiling of tumor cells reveals an *NF2* p.Y192* mutation and copy number analysis reveals a copy neutral genome.

Integrated Diagnosis. SCHWANNOMA, WHO Grade I, *NF2*-Y192* mutant

Teaching Points. Schwannomas are benign peripheral nerve sheath tumors that resemble Schwann cells. Although they most commonly involve peripheral nerves in the head and neck region, they can occur in the extremities, cranial nerves, and spinal nerve roots. Most schwannomas are asymptomatic; however, as they increase in size, they may present with pain and/or neurological deficits. Schwannomas are associated with NF2 where they classically present as bilateral tumors involving cranial nerve VIII (often referred to as acoustic neuromas; see Chapter 16 for further discussion of NF2-associated vestibular schwannomas). Large multinodular schwannomas or plexiform variants are also generally seen in association with NF2.

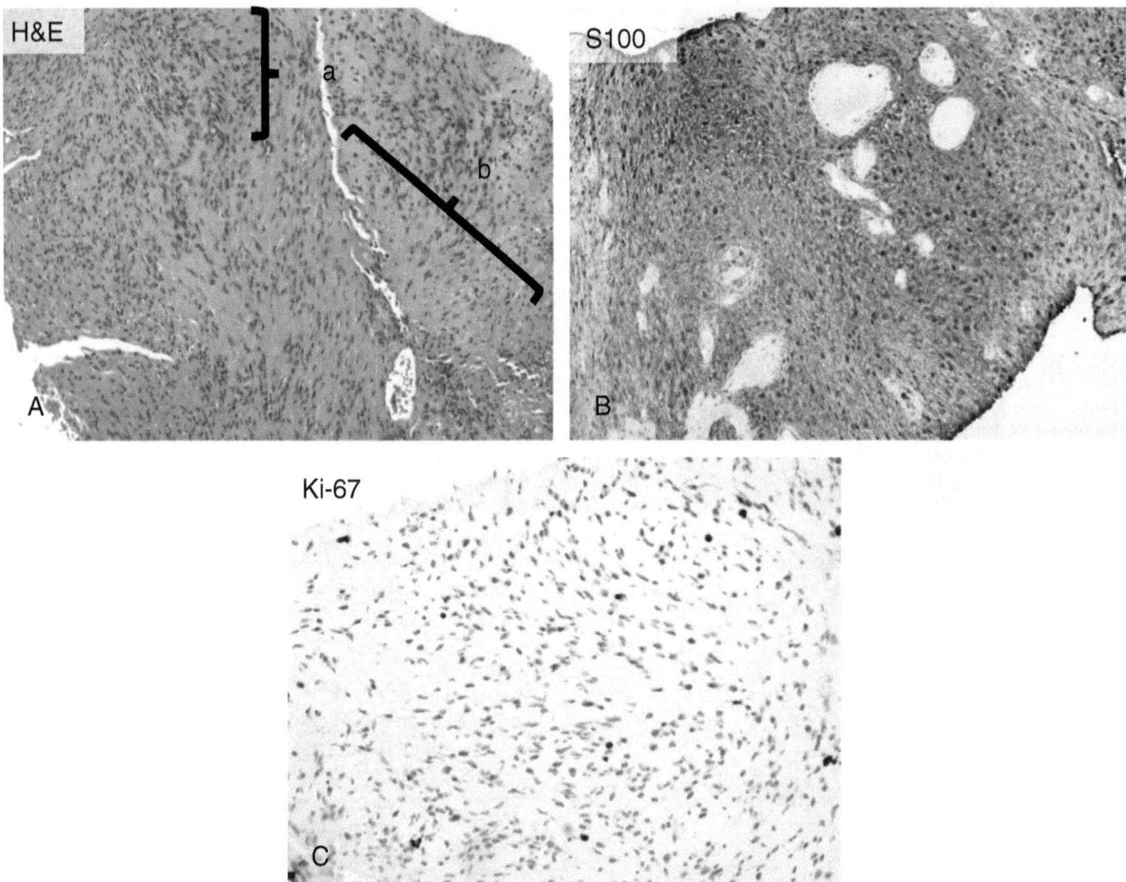

Fig. 1.12 Microscopic examination including H&E stained sections (A) showing a biphasic pattern of tumor with predominant areas of densely compact cellularity (Antoni A pattern) as well as minimal hypocellular areas (Antoni B pattern). Immunohistochemistry shows diffusely positive staining for S100, a marker of calcium binding proteins (B), and a low Ki-67 proliferation index (C).

Microscopically, the tumors vary significantly in cellular density, nuclear pleomorphism, and growth patterns; however, the prognosis for these schwannomas is excellent and often curable with surgical resection. Hallmark features include a biphasic growth pattern composed of dense (Antoni A) and loose (Antoni B) regions, as well as Verocay bodies where tumor nuclei appear stacked or lined up in rows (palisading). Malignant transformation of schwannomas is very rare.

Genomic analysis of schwannomas largely demonstrates mutations in *NF2* with a subset showing deletions of chromosome 22q. Patients presenting with schwannomatosis often harbor multiple peripheral and spinal schwannomas with mutations in *SMARCB1* and *LZTR1* rather than *NF2*.

A key differential diagnosis for schwannomas is neurofibroma. Whereas both arise in association with peripheral nerves, schwannomas tend to push aside or displace the normal nerve and can therefore be surgically excised while preserving nerve function. In contrast, neurofibromas, which can occur sporadically or in association with neurofibromatosis 1 (NF1), often have entrapped axons of the associated peripheral nerve coursing through the tumor (see Chapter 16 for further discussion of NF1-associated neurofibromas).

Conclusion

In summary, histopathological assessment is a crucial initial step in establishing a diagnosis, informing prognosis, and selecting optimal treatment for patients with brain tumors. For surgeons, this classification is the language for relaying postoperative tumor diagnoses. For neuro-oncologists and radiation oncologists, understanding the differences in glioma classification guides treatment decisions and patient management, while neurologists can incorporate the information in management decisions and discussions with patients about prognosis. Clinicians use their understanding of brain tumor diagnoses, likelihood of response to treatment, and prognosis to prioritize when to urgently manage seizures, cerebral edema, or other complications that will help keep a high-grade brain tumor patient on treatment; or when to pursue longer-term symptom directed management such as seizure surgery or neurocognitive evaluations for patients suffering late neurological complications of brain tumor survivorship.

References

1. Louis DN, Perry A, Reifenberger G, et al. The 2016 World Health Organization Classification Of Tumors Of The Central Nervous System: a summary. *Acta Neuropathol.* 2016;131(6):803–820. https://doi.org/10.1007/s00401-016-1545-1.
2. Brennan CW, Verhaak RGW, McKenna A, et al. The somatic genomic landscape of glioblastoma. *Cell.* 2013;155(2):462–477. https://doi.org/10.1016/j.cell.2013.09.034.
3. Wen PY, Huse JT. 2016 World Health Organization Classification of Central Nervous System Tumors. *Continuum (Minneap Minn).* 2017;23(6, Neuro-oncology):1531–1547. https://doi.org/10.1212/CON.0000000000000536.
4. Hartmann C, Meyer J, Balss J, et al. Type and frequency of IDH1 and IDH2 mutations are related to astrocytic and oligodendroglial differentiation and age: a study of 1,010 diffuse gliomas. *Acta Neuropathol.* 2009;118(4):469–474. https://doi.org/10.1007/s00401-009-0561-9.

Chapter | 2 |

Surgical considerations for brain and spine tumors

Michelle Marie Williams, Stephen B. Tatter, and Adrian W. Laxton

CHAPTER OUTLINE

Introduction to brain and spine tumor surgery

For tumors affecting the brain and spinal cord, surgical resection is the fastest and most definitive treatment. In some cases, it is also the safest, such as when mass effect from the tumor compresses vital structures or when cerebral edema causes a life-threatening rise in intracranial pressure (ICP). Before making the decision to operate, the surgeon must weigh the risks and benefits to the patient. Possible complications of surgery include infection, hemorrhage, cerebrospinal fluid flow disruption, and sequelae of damage to the nervous system, including weakness, loss of sensation, aphasia, coma, or death. Not all patients are good surgical candidates, because of high systemic disease burden, short expected survival time, or medical problems precluding anesthesia. For patients who undergo radiation, the ability to heal at an in-field surgical incision is another consideration. In this chapter, we will review key clinical principles in the surgical management of several different types of brain and spine tumors including: posterior fossa masses, unresectable and resectable high-grade gliomas, spinal cord tumors, and central nervous system metastases.

Clinical cases

CASE 2.1 ELEVATED INTRACRANIAL PRESSURE FROM A POSTERIOR FOSSA MASS

Case. An 11-year-old, previously healthy male presented with 5 weeks of headaches and dizziness. These headaches were worst in the morning and were also associated with nausea. Neurological examination showed mild dysmetria of the right upper extremity, truncal ataxia, and subtle bilateral cranial nerve VI palsies concerning for elevated ICP. MRI Brain demonstrated a 6 × 7 cm^2 cystic mass in the right cerebellum with an enhancing mural nodule (Fig. 2.1, large white arrows) and enlarged ventricles with transependymal flow consistent with hydrocephalus (Fig. 2.1, small white arrows). Due to the clinical and imaging signs of hydrocephalus, he was taken to the operating room emergently. A right suboccipital craniotomy was performed for gross total resection of the mass. Pathology was consistent with World Health Organization (WHO)

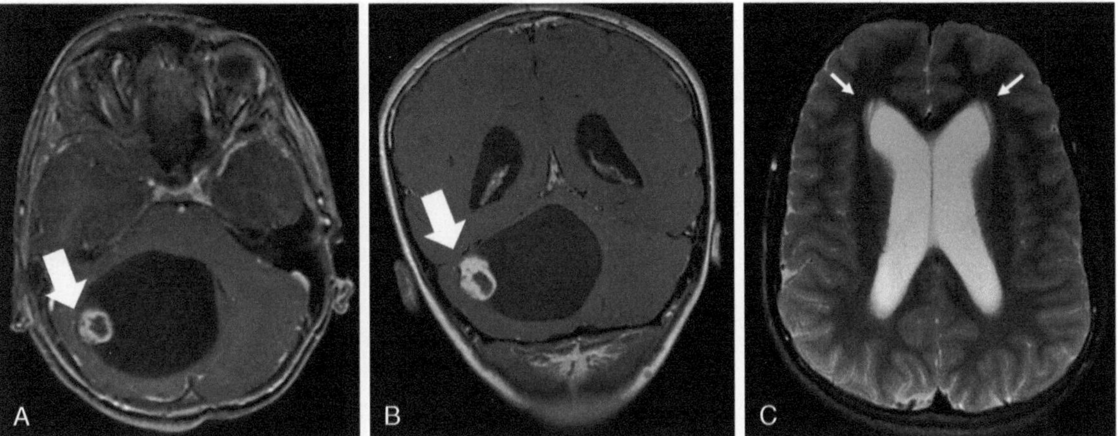

Fig. 2.1 Contrast-enhanced MRI scan of a right cerebellar juvenile pilocytic astrocytoma. (A) Contrast-enhanced Tl-weighted axial view. Arrow indicates enhancing mural nodule. (B) Contrast-enhanced Tl-weighted coronal view. Arrow indicates enhancing mural nodule. (C) T2-weighted axial view. Arrows indicate transependymal flow.

grade 1 pilocytic astrocytoma. Postoperatively, he recovered well and was followed in clinic with serial MRIs and has had no recurrence of his tumor.

Teaching Points: Posterior Fossa Tumors. This case highlights two important principles including: (1) the management of increased ICP and (2) outcomes for pediatric patients with pilocytic astrocytoma. Patients with posterior fossa masses frequently present with obstructive hydrocephalus because of mass effect on the fourth ventricle. Clinical symptoms of elevated ICP include headache that awakens the patient in the early morning, unexplained nausea, and vision changes. Bilateral cranial nerve VI palsies or papilledema may be present on examination. The presence of hydrocephalus is an important surgical consideration, as it indicates that the mass should be resected in a more urgent or even emergent fashion. In most cases, the ICP increases slowly over time, which allows the patient to accommodate it. However, if the fourth ventricle becomes acutely obstructed, there may be sudden and dangerous increases in ICP. If a patient is acutely herniating, an external ventricular drain should be placed first as a temporizing measure before proceeding to the operating room for resection of the mass. In most cases, the hydrocephalus resolves postoperatively and patients do not require permanent ventricular shunt placement.

Another important surgical consideration is the extent of resection that is achieved for juvenile pilocytic astrocytomas. Gross total resection has been shown to improve progression-free survival and, in some cases, provide a surgical cure.[1] When feasible, the surgeon should aim for total resection of the mass rather than just decompression of the posterior fossa. Pilocytic astrocytomas that are not completely resected have a higher rate of recurrence and are either observed or, in some cases, radiation therapy is considered.

Clinical Pearls

1. Clinicians must be aware of symptoms of increased ICP including early morning headache, unexplained nausea, vision changes, bilateral cranial nerve VI palsies, and papilledema.
2. Obstructive hydrocephalus from a posterior fossa mass requires urgent or emergent surgical evaluation for resection or ventricular decompression.
3. Children with posterior fossa pilocytic astrocytomas generally have excellent outcomes, particularly when gross total resection is achieved.

CASE 2.2 NEW SYMPTOMATIC SUPRATENTORIAL HIGH-GRADE LESION

Case. A 64-year-old male presented with 4 days of confusion and left hemibody weakness. On examination, his left hemibody motor strength was 4+/5 with left pronator drift. MRI Brain showed a 3 × 6 cm^2 lobulated, multifocal ring-enhancing mass in the right temporal lobe, with surrounding cerebral edema (Fig. 2.2). Past medical history was significant for both bladder and prostate cancer—the bladder cancer was recently diagnosed and thought to be superficial; the prostate cancer had been previously treated with cryoablation.

One surgical option in this case is to obtain a tissue diagnosis via biopsy. However, based on the large size of the mass and the degree of surrounding cerebral edema, it was decided that the patient would benefit from surgical resection. The left-sided weakness noted in this patient was thought to be

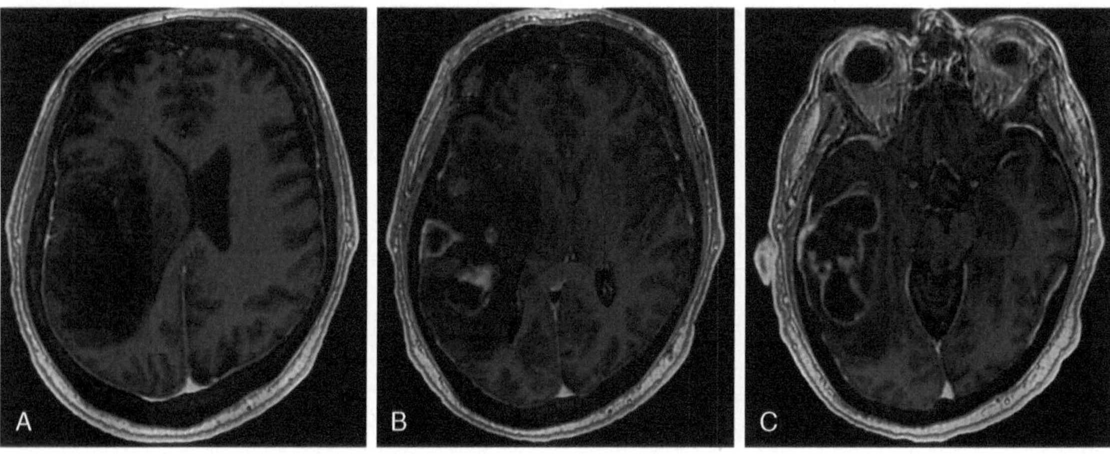

Fig. 2.2 Contrast enhanced Tl-weighted axial MRI view of a right temporal high-grade glioma. (A) Superior cut in which no tumor is visualized, but rather hypointense cerebral edema extending up to the frontal lobe. (B) Superior aspect of the enhancing mass is visualized in the temporal lobe. (C) Body of the mass is visualized in the inferior temporal lobe.

due to cerebral edema that extended up into the right motor cortex rather than direct tumor involvement. The patient was started on dexamethasone 10 mg intravenous once followed by 4 mg oral every 6 hours for management of edema and levetiracetam for seizure prevention given the location of the mass in the temporal lobe. A right temporal craniotomy was performed with gross total resection of the mass on the day after admission, and pathology was consistent with a WHO grade 4 glioblastoma (GBM).

Teaching Points: Surgical Management of Resectable Supratentorial Masses. This case highlights the role of surgery for (1) tissue diagnosis, (2) cytoreduction of a tumor, and (3) symptom relief from cerebral edema. Though it would be rare to have prostate cancer or superficial bladder cancer metastasis to the brain with this appearance, it is impossible to make a definitive diagnosis based on imaging characteristics alone. In general, any patient who presents with a new brain mass and no established primary cancer needs tissue for diagnosis.[2] In rare cases, a single brain mass with imaging findings concerning for high-grade glioma will be found histologically to be the first presentation of a brain metastasis even if no other masses are visualized on systemic imaging. In addition, histologic determination of WHO grade and molecular profiling of tumor tissue help guide treatment and prognosis discussions and cannot be determined without tissue (see Chapter 1 for further discussion of molecular classification of brain tumors).

In general, surgical options for a supratentorial mass include biopsy or resection. Biopsy is often performed stereotactically, though in selected cases, open biopsy may be pursued. The extent of resection is determined to be either gross total (e.g., no residual tumor) or subtotal resection based on postoperative imaging typically performed between 24–72 hours after surgery. The decision to pursue resection is guided by multiple factors, including the size of the mass, superficial location, proximity to eloquent cortex or white matter tracts, and overall patient prognosis. Greater extent of surgical resection is associated with improved functional outcomes for patients with high-grade gliomas, although not necessarily with greater survival.[2] Factors that favor tumor resection are size >3 cm, location in non-eloquent brain tissue, superficial or easily surgically accessible location, or a patient who is expected to survive long enough to recover and benefit from surgery.

Clinical Pearls

1. Gross or near gross total resection with >90% of tumor resected is consistently associated with improved outcomes in uncontrolled studies of glioma.
2. In general, surgery plays three roles in the management of glioma patients including: (1) tissue diagnosis, (2) cytoreduction of tumor, and (3) symptom relief from cerebral edema.

CASE 2.3 RECURRENT UNRESECTABLE HIGH-GRADE GLIOMA

Case. A 57-year-old male was diagnosed 14 years ago with a left frontal astrocytoma (WHO grade 2) and underwent gross total resection followed by radiation therapy. He now re-presents with a breakthrough generalized tonic-clonic seizure. On examination, he is bradyphrenic with slowed verbal and motor responses, but no focal neurological deficits. MRI Brain shows a 7 × 6 cm^2 heterogeneously enhancing mass crossing the corpus callosum (Fig. 2.3). The patient was not a candidate for repeat gross total resection due to the deep location of the tumor compressing the corpus callosum and extending across

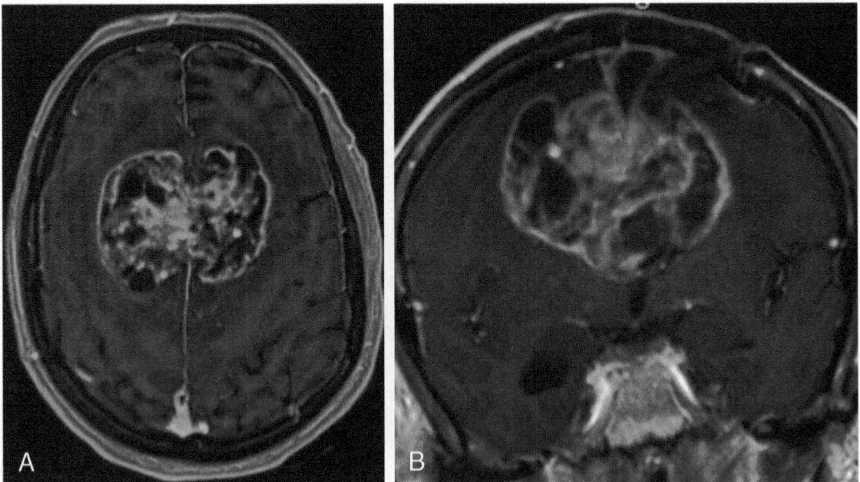

Fig. 2.3 Contrast-enhanced MRI scan of a high-grade glioma centered in the corpus callosum. (A) Contrast-enhanced Tl-weighted axial view. (B) Contrast-enhanced Tl-weighted coronal view.

the midline. The mass was in the vicinity of the deep cerebral veins and the body of the mass was adjacent to the anterior cerebral arteries, increasing perioperative risk of hemorrhage. He was started on dexamethasone 10 mg intravenous once followed by 4 mg oral every 6 hours for cerebral edema. He underwent open biopsy, which confirmed a diagnosis of WHO grade 4 GBM. Radiation oncology and medical oncology were consulted for further management (see Chapter 3 and Chapter 4 for further background on the principles of radiation and medical neuro-oncology).

Teaching Points: Unresectable Brain Mass. As discussed in the preceding case, a greater extent of surgical resection correlates with improved functional status for patients with high-grade glioma.[2] However, surgeons must consider subtotal resection or biopsy for lesions that are in close proximity to or involve critical structures, such as the brainstem or major blood vessels. In cases where the mass involves or abuts eloquent but resectable brain tissue, such as the occipital lobe or speech areas, the surgeon will consider preoperative deficits before considering surgical resection. For example, if a patient already has a fixed hemiparesis, the benefits of achieving gross total resection for a lesion adjacent to the motor cortex outweighs the postoperative risk of weakness. This may not be the case if the patient retains functional brain tissue.

Laser Interstitial Thermal Therapy. An additional surgical option for deep tumors that are not amenable to open surgical resection is laser interstitial thermal therapy (LITT). This surgical procedure is performed through a small burr hole and can be performed at the time of a stereotactic biopsy. A probe is inserted via MRI guidance into the tumor and thermal heating is used to ablate the tissue using laser technology. Current uses include gliomas, brain metastases, radiation necrosis, and seizure surgery. Postoperative recovery is often minimal, and patients are typically discharged the day after the procedure. Multifocal tumors, large lesions (e.g., diameter greater than about 3 cm), or inaccessible locations may preclude the use of LITT. For the patient described in this case, the large tumor size and crossing of the midline prohibited the use of LITT.

Clinical Pearls

1. Tumors in deep locations, adjacent to eloquent structures, or crossing the midline may not be amenable to open resection.
2. In selected cases, LITT is a surgical option for tissue ablation and can be performed at the time of tissue biopsy.

CASE 2.4 RECURRENT SYMPTOMATIC INTRAMEDULLARY SPINAL CORD TUMOR

Case. A 12-year-old male with a WHO grade 3 right frontal anaplastic ependymoma previously underwent surgical resection. Staging at that time revealed metastasis to the right cerebellum and spinal cord at T3–4, both of which were previously resected, and pathology was WHO grade 2 for both tumors. The patient received craniospinal radiation therapy. During surveillance imaging, MRI spine demonstrated a new extramedullary lesion at the level of T11–T12 (Fig. 2.4). Neurological examination showed full strength with normal sensation and deep tendon reflexes. He was taken for T10–L1 laminectomy and gross total resection of the mass. Pathology confirmed recurrent WHO grade 2 ependymoma. Postoperatively, he remained with full strength, intact urination without neurogenic bladder, and was discharged home with plans for targeted radiation therapy and consideration of adjuvant chemotherapy.

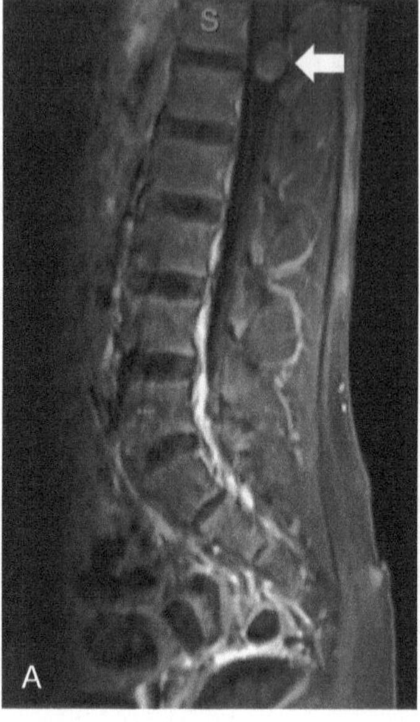

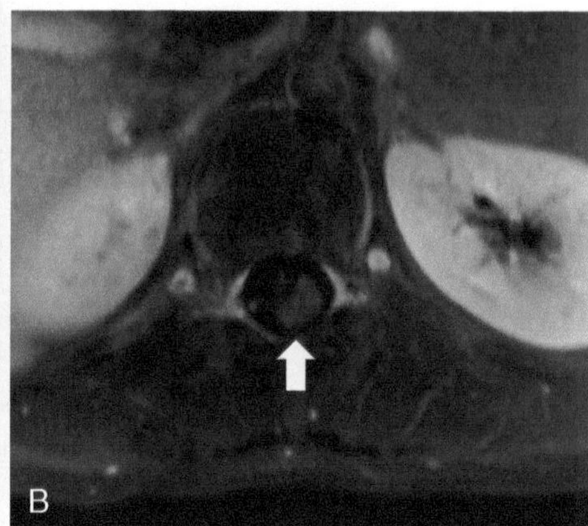

Fig. 2.4 Contrast-enhanced lumbar MRI scan of an ependymoma. (A) Sagittal view. *Arrow* indicates the ependymoma. (B) Axial view. *Arrow* indicates the ependymoma, which is eccentric to the left.

Teaching Points: Spinal Cord Ependymoma and Surgery. This case highlights several key principles including (1) the importance of gross total resection of ependymoma and (2) the importance of weighing tumor resection with perioperative risk for spinal cord tumors. Though this patient had no appreciable neurological deficits from his tumor, surgical resection of ependymomas is associated with improved outcomes and progression-free survival.[1] Outcomes are consistently more favorable in patients who receive gross total compared with lesser extents of resection.[3]

As with brain tumors, cytoreduction and relief of peritumoral edema associated with spine tumors can lead to improved functional outcomes. This must be weighed against the risks of causing neurological deficit, including paralysis of the upper and/or lower limbs, loss of sensation below the level of surgery, and loss of bowel and bladder function. Damage to the cervical spine in particular, either from the tumor itself or from surgery, has the potential to cause more severe side effects, including diaphragmatic paralysis requiring mechanical ventilation. Care must be taken to select a surgical approach that minimizes the risk of damage to normal tissue while allowing for maximal safe resection of the tumor. In the cervical spine, ventral lesions may be amenable to an anterior approach, whereas this is usually not possible in the thoracic spine.

Ease of resection also varies by tumor location. In general, extradural masses such as metastases, meningiomas, or schwannomas have the lowest risks of perioperative damage to the spinal cord or nerves. Intramedullary lesions such as astrocytoma, ependymomas, hemangioblastomas, or other intrinsic spinal cord tumors may necessitate manipulation of the spinal cord during the approach and resection. In the case of ependymomas, WHO grade 1 lesions are well circumscribed and often are more readily peeled away from the spinal cord, whereas WHO grade 2 and 3 tumors can be more adherent with poorly defined surgical planes, often making them difficult to separate from the normal adjacent spinal cord tissue.[1]

For spinal cord tumors, the surgical approach has potential to destabilize the spine. Posterior approaches often require removal of the bony posterior lamina and disruption of the posterior longitudinal ligament or interspinous ligaments. Depending on the extent of tumor involvement, partial or complete resection of the vertebral body may be required. Laminectomies must be done at enough levels to provide an adequate surgical corridor to access the most proximal and distal portions of the tumor, with appropriate visualization so as not to jeopardize surrounding neural and vascular tissue. In cases where substantial components of the spine's structural support have been compromised, it is necessary to perform a spinal fusion by placing screws and rods above and below the surgical levels. If the patient is likely to receive subsequent radiation therapy, the surgeon must consider whether this could further destabilize the spine. For instance, a mass with bony vertebral involvement that regresses after radiation could result in a compression fracture. In these cases, it may be prudent to perform a fusion during initial surgical resection even if the spine has adequate structural support at that time in anticipation of future compromise.

Clinical Pearls

1. Gross total resection is consistently associated with improved outcomes for patients with ependymoma and should be pursued aggressively.
2. Extramedullary tumors such as metastases, meningiomas, and schwannomas carry a different surgical risk from intramedullary lesions such as astrocytomas or ependymomas.

CASE 2.5 NEW SYMPTOMATIC MULTIFOCAL BRAIN LESION IN A KNOWN CANCER PATIENT

Case. A 52-year-old female has a history of melanoma metastatic to the liver, lungs, peritoneum, and brain. She previously received Gamma Knife stereotactic radiotherapy to multiple brain lesions, including right temporal and left cerebellar masses. She now presents with 2 days of progressive somnolence and unexplained emesis. On examination, she is somnolent and nonverbal but follows commands. MRI Brain shows multiple new intracranial lesions including a new lesion in the right posterior lateral frontal lobe (Fig. 2.5, large white arrow). This lesion measures 3 × 2 cm^2 and is contiguous with a 1.5 × 1 cm^2 more superior component. There is a large amount of surrounding vasogenic edema extending into the right temporal lobe and insular cortex. Dexamethasone 10 mg intravenous once and 4 mg intravenous every 6 hours, as well as mannitol, were initiated for management of cerebral edema. Continuous video electroencephalography was negative for subclinical seizure activity. She underwent a right frontal craniotomy for resection of the right frontal mass. Intraoperative preliminary pathology was read as malignant tumor and final pathology confirmed metastatic melanoma.

Teaching Points: Surgical Treatment of Brain Metastasis. For this case, the known prior cancer diagnosis and imaging evidence of multiple homogeneously enhancing lesions is consistent with an imaging diagnosis of brain metastasis. As in this case, brain metastases commonly appear at the cortical gray-white matter junction or in the cerebellum (see Chapter 14 for the approach to brain metastasis). In this case, definitive tissue diagnosis is not required and a presumptive diagnosis can inform clinical management.

The surgical management of brain metastases differs from that of primary brain tumors. Many patients with metastatic disease present with multiple brain lesions. As in this case, when multiple brain lesions are present, surgical resection of all lesions is neither possible nor feasible, and the surgeon must consider whether symptomatic relief of peritumoral edema around a specific lesion warrants surgical intervention. It is crucial to determine which lesion is likely to be causing the most severe symptoms. Oftentimes the largest lesion is the culprit, but not always. Lesion location is another important factor. A small tumor located directly in the motor cortex is likely the cause of contralateral hemiparesis even if there are other larger masses in other locations. In this case, the patient's symptoms were not explained by seizure, metabolic abnormality, ventriculomegaly, or hydrocephalus and were thought to be due to the large amount of vasogenic edema around the right frontotemporal mass.

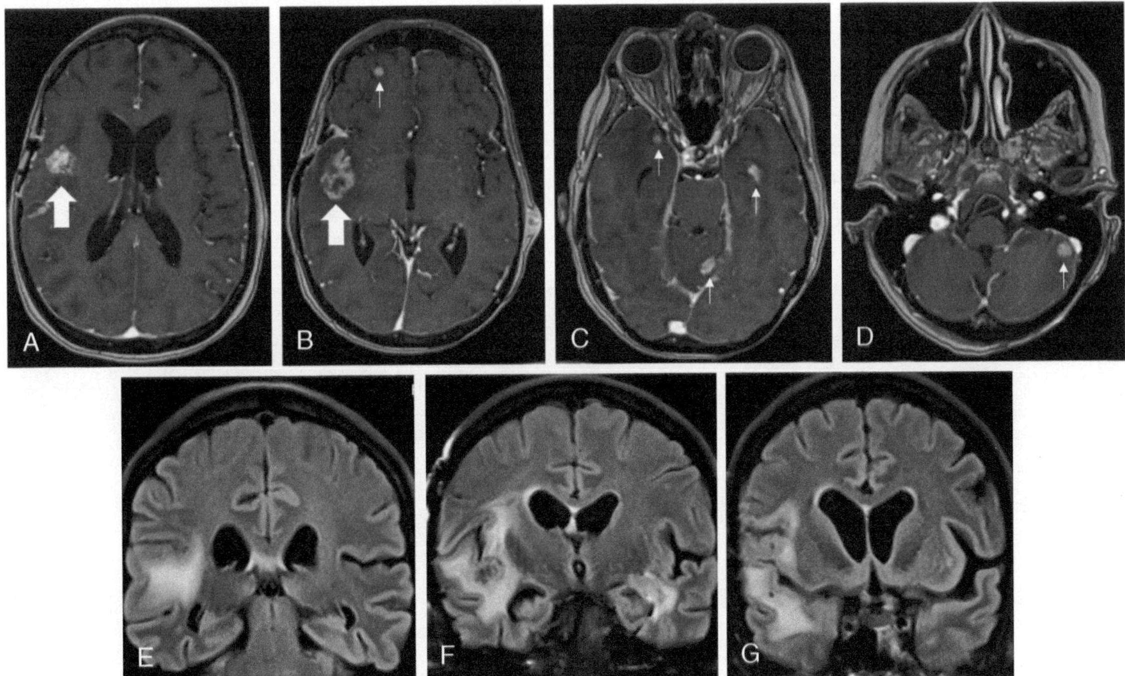

Fig. 2.5 Contrast-enhanced MRI scan of metastatic melanoma. (A–D) Contrasted Tl-weighted axial view. *Large arrows* indicate the symptomatic lesion. *Small arrows* indicate other metastatic lesions. (E–G) FLAIR (fluid attenuation inversion recovery) sequence, coronal view. Right temporal lobe edema is visualized.

Clinicians must consider the degree of vasogenic edema around a lesion. If there is a large amount of edema surrounding one particular lesion and the patient is having symptoms in the area of edema, or symptoms of elevated ICP, surgical resection may readily address this lesion and reduce the need for corticosteroids—particularly in patients receiving immune-directed systemic therapy. Additionally, if mass effect from one lesion is obstructing cerebrospinal flow causing hydrocephalus, surgery should be considered, and if the lesion is not resectable, then ventricular shunt should be placed. In emergent cases, external ventricular drain may be required as a life saving measure.

In general, metastatic lesions measuring >3 cm should be considered for operative resection. Small lesions may be amenable to LITT or Gamma Knife stereotactic radiosurgery (see Chapter 14 for further discussion of the approach to brain metastasis treatment). If there is no established cancer diagnosis and no clear primary lesion to biopsy, brain biopsy may be used for definitive diagnosis. Patients who have a high number of small metastatic lesions may benefit from whole brain radiation; however, increasingly stereotactic radiosurgery is the favored treatment for brain metastases.

Clinical Pearls

1. When evaluating a patient with a known cancer diagnosis and multiple brain lesions, surgery may be beneficial when there is a single, large (>3 cm) lesion with symptomatic cerebral edema.

CASE 2.6 LARGE DURAL-BASED LESION WITH SYMPTOMS

Case. A 75-year-old male with a history of cecal adenocarcinoma requiring prior hemicolectomy presented after multiple falls due to left leg weakness, progressive confusion, and inability to complete his activities of daily living. During evaluation for rib fractures, CT head showed a 6 × 5 cm^2 right parietal hyperdense mass with 1.5 cm of midline shift (Fig. 2.6). The patient left prematurely against medical advice. Upon re-presentation for pain control for his fractures, he was noted to be disoriented and with weakness in his left hand grip as well as decreased sensation throughout his left leg. Dexamethasone 10 mg intravenous once followed by 4 mg intravenously every 6 hours was initiated for cerebral edema. MRI Brain showed an avidly, homogeneously enhancing mass that was extra-axial and dural-based. The imaging findings favored meningioma, hemangiopericytoma, or dural-based metastasis. Given the history of cecal adenocarcinoma, a CT scan of the chest, abdomen, and pelvis was obtained and was negative for systemic mass lesions. He was deemed a candidate for surgical resection due to the large size of the tumor, resulting mass effect, and midline shift. Because of his confusion, this was also discussed with his family, who were in agreement. A right parietal craniotomy was performed and gross total resection was achieved. Pathology was consistent with a WHO grade 1 meningioma.

Teaching Points: Surgical Management of Meningioma. Surgery is a backbone of the management of meningioma. Although asymptomatic meningiomas can be observed with imaging, symptomatic lesions like the one in this case or those that present with mass effect, compression of adjacent structures, or brain infiltration on imaging should be surgically removed when possible.

Greater extent of resection directly correlates with lower recurrence rates.[4] Recurrence rates for WHO grade 1 meningioma depend on the grade of resection, which is determined using the Simpson grading scale (Table 2.1). This scale is determined intraoperatively by the surgeon and ranges from grade 1 (e.g., removal of all affected dura and underlying bone) to grade 5 (e.g., debulking only). Recurrence rates are as low as 5–10% for completely resected Simpson grade 1 meningiomas. If involved dura cannot safely be resected, coagulation of the remaining dura improves resection to a Simpson

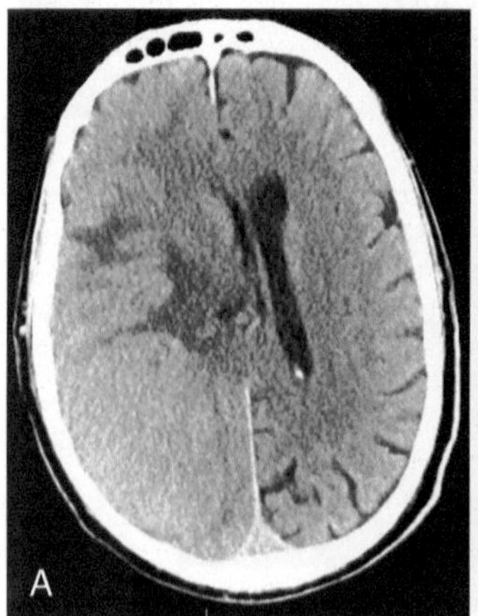

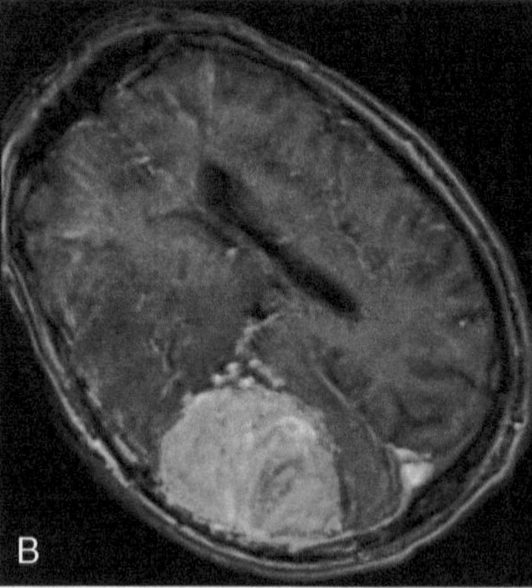

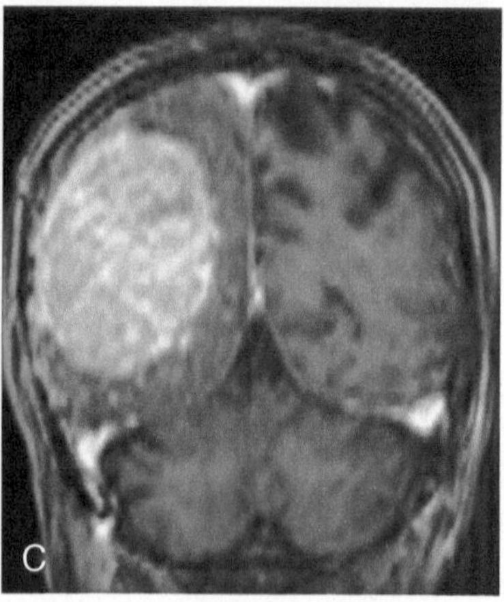

Fig. 2.6 Right parietal convexity meningioma. (A) Non-contrast CT scan, axial view. Right-sided edema causes sulcal effacement and right-to-left midline shift. (B) Contrast-enhanced Tl-weighted MRI, axial view. (C) Contrast-enhanced Tl-weighted MRI, coronal view.

Table 2.1 Simpson grade of meningioma resection

Simpson Grade	Description	10-Year Progression-Free Survival
Grade 1	Complete removal of all tumor tissue including underlying bone and associated dura	>90%
Grade 2	Complete removal of all tumor tissue and coagulation of dural attachment	~80%
Grade 3	Complete removal of the intracranial component of the tumor leaving the dural attachment and/or extradural tumor behind	~70%
Grade 4	Partial (e.g., subtotal) resection	~60%
Grade 5	Tumor decompression with or without biopsy	~0%

From Gousias K, Schramm J, Simon M. The Simpson grading revisited: aggressive surgery and its place in modern meningioma management. *J Neurosurg*. 2016;125:551–560; Nanda A, Bir SC, Maiti TK, Konar SK, Missios S, Guthikonda B. Relevance of Simpson grading system and recurrence-free survival after surgery for World Health Organization Grade 1 meningioma. *J Neurosurg*. 2017;126:201–211.

grade 2 with recurrence rates of 15–20%. Partial tumor resection alone is associated with recurrence rates as high as 30–40% by 10 years.[4]

As with the previously discussed cases, extent of resection is limited by proximity to other vital brain structures including the dural sinuses or adjacent structures in the skull-base. Convexity meningiomas are often more easily accessed than skull-based meningiomas. Meningiomas are highly vascularized tumors and, for large lesions, the surgeon may consider preoperative embolization of the feeding vessels to minimize blood loss. Tumors that are higher grade (e.g., grade 2–3) or recur after surgery are often treated with radiation therapy (see Chapter 10 for discussion of the approach to meningioma management).

Many patients with brain tumors are altered at the time of presentation and unable to consent for themselves. It is important to appreciate the social factors that affect these patients, and ensure that the appropriate decision makers are involved before proceeding with surgery.

Clinical Pearls

1. For meningiomas that cannot be observed, surgical resection should be considered, particularly when there is brain infiltration, mass effect, or clinical symptoms.
2. Extent of surgical resection for WHO grade 1 meningiomas is guided by the Simpson grade scale where greater extent of resection predicts lower rates of tumor recurrence.

CASE 2.7 BONY METASTATIC LESION WITH SPINAL CORD COMPRESSION

Case. A 52-year-old male with a history of right thigh pleomorphic undifferentiated sarcoma was previously treated with surgical resection, neoadjuvant chemotherapy, and radiation. He had known widespread metastases to the lung, abdomen, and spine. He previously underwent an L3 corpectomy with L1–5 posterior fusion for resection of a large metastatic lumbar spine lesion. He presented with worsening back pain and new right L3 radiculopathy. Neurological examination demonstrated stable chronic right lower extremity leg weakness and sensory changes that were unchanged since his primary tumor resection. He had no new neurological deficits. A contrasted MRI of the lumbar spine showed progression of the L3 lesion which invaded the right neural foramen and extended into the spinal canal, causing severe compression of the thecal sac (Fig. 2.7).

Given the extent of disease, a multidisciplinary conversation was held with the patient and his family regarding treatment options and hospice. He elected to proceed with aggressive surgical treatment and was taken to the operating room for repeat decompression of the recurrent mass via an L2 laminectomy. As he already had hardware in place from the previous resection, he did not require any further spinal instrumentation and arthrodesis with cadaveric bone graft was performed.

Teaching Points: Surgical Management of Spine Metastasis. Management of osseous metastasis to the spinal cord must include three considerations including (1) neurological status of the patient, (2) degree of spinal cord compression on imaging, and (3) treatment responsiveness of the tumor. One of the most important clinical considerations is the time course of new neurological deficits. A prospective trial in 2005 evaluated the role of surgery comparing corticosteroids and radiotherapy treatment to decompressive surgery with corticosteroids and postoperative radiotherapy for patients with lesions compressing the spinal cord and new neurological deficits.[5] In this study, new neurological deficits were defined as having been present for no more than 48 hours. Patients in this study treated with surgery had prolonged survival and were more likely to experience return of ambulation if plegic at the time of presentation. These patients were more likely to

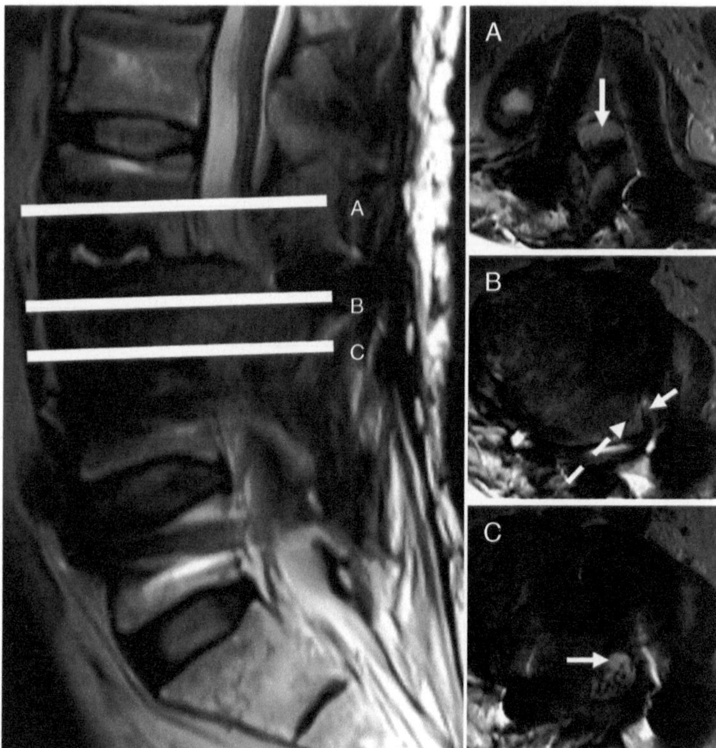

Fig. 2.7 Contrast-enhanced lumbar MRI scan showing metastatic sarcoma at the level of L3. (A) Axial view at the level of L2. *Arrows* indicate normal cerebrospinal fluid around uncompressed nerve roots. (B) Axial view at the level of L3. *Dashed arrow* shows sarcoma lesion causing compression and deviation of the nerve roots. *Solid arrow* shows thin rim of cerebrospinal fluid. (C) Axial view at the level of L3–4. *Arrow* indicates cerebrospinal fluid surrounding uncompressed nerve roots.

remain ambulatory compared with the nonsurgical treatment group. There was also a significant decrease in pain medication requirement for the surgical group. These data support the role of surgery for spinal decompression in patients with new or rapidly worsening neurological deficits from compressive spinal metastasis. Of note, bowel and bladder function is also an important symptom to consider in these patients. Acute cauda equina syndrome is an indication for emergent decompressive surgery.

Imaging criteria are also important in managing patients with osseous metastases to the spine and are guided by the degree of spinal cord compression (Table 2.2) (see Chapter 8 for the imaging evaluation of spinal lesions). Although most spinal metastases are confined to the bone, approximately 20% of patients develop malignant epidural cord compression where disease enters the spinal canal. Pure bony metastases that do not extend into the spinal canal may be more suitable for treatment with radiation alone. Mild cases where epidural disease is visible but not causing any symptoms or evidence of neural compression may also be amenable to radiotherapy. In these cases, the radiation oncologist may still request neurosurgical intervention to create a greater margin between normal neural tissue and the target lesion if the radiation dose is felt to threaten the spinal cord and nerves based on proximity. In severe cases, where there is compression of the spinal cord, surgical evaluation is a necessity. As discussed

Table 2.2 Spinal oncology study group criteria for grading epidural spinal cord compression

Grade[a]	Description
Grade 0	Tumor is confined to bone only
Grade 1	Tumor extension into the epidural space without deformation of the spinal cord
– 1a	– Epidural impingement but no deformation of the thecal sac
– 1b	– Deformation of the thecal sac but does not contact the spinal cord
– 1c	– Deformation of the thecal sac with contact of the cord but no cord compression
Grade 2	Spinal cord compression with visible cerebrospinal fluid signal around the cord
Grade 3	Spinal cord compression without visible cerebrospinal fluid signal

[a]Using axial T2-weighted images at the site of the most severe compression, this grading scale is used to guide treatment decisions for patients with osseous metastases to the spine.
From Laufer I, Rubin DG, Lis E, Cox BW, Stubblefield MD, Yamada Y, Bilsky MH. The NOMS framework: approach to the treatment of spinal metastatic tumors. *Oncologist*. 2013;18(6):744–751.

with the previous spinal cord tumor case, spinal stability following surgery is another major consideration. If significant structural elements are resected during surgery, the patient may require fusion, especially if further radiation is planned to the area.

Finally, clinicians must also take into account the treatment responsiveness of the tumor. Radiosensitive tumors such as lymphoma, multiple myeloma, germinoma, small cell lung cancer, or others may be rapidly responsive to radiation therapy and not require surgical intervention compared with less radiation sensitive histologies (see Chapter 3 for principles of radiation oncology). As such, multidisciplinary coordination of care across neurosurgical oncology, radiation oncology, medical oncology, and neurology is beneficial.

Clinical Pearls

1. Management of patients with osseous metastasis to the spinal cord should include assessment of new neurological symptoms, degree of spinal cord compression on axial T2-weighted MRI images at the point of greatest compression, and treatment responsiveness of the tumor type.
2. Spinal cord decompression improves neurological outcomes for patients with new deficits including paralysis, bowel or bladder dysfunction, or sensory loss that have been present for no more than 48 hours from onset.

Conclusions

Neurosurgical resection of brain and spine tumors is an important tool to establish a definitive tumor diagnosis, recover function in symptomatic patients, and, at times, improve outcomes when applied in optimal scenarios. In general, surgical intervention is considered in three situations including (1) when a definitive tissue diagnosis is needed, (2) to remove tumor tissue for surgical cure or cytoreduction prior to additional therapy, or (3) when symptomatic management of peritumoral edema, mass effect, or midline shift is beneficial. Every patient who is a potential surgical candidate should be evaluated on a case-by-case basis and, when appropriate, multidisciplinary assessment can be beneficial.

References

1. Batchelor TT, Nishikawa R, Tarbell NJ, Weller M, eds. *Oxford Textbook of Neuro-Oncology*. Oxford: Oxford University Press; 2017.
2. Altwairgi AK, Raja S, Manzoor M, et al. Management and treatment recommendations for World Health Organization Grade III and IV gliomas. *Int J Health Sci (Qassim)*. 2017;11(3):54–62.
3. Rodríguez D, Cheung MC, Housri N, Quinones-Hinojosa A, Camphausen K, Koniaris LG. Outcomes of malignant CNS ependymomas: an examination of 2408 cases through the Surveillance, Epidemiology, and End Results (SEER) database (1973–2005). *J Surg Res*. 2009;156(2):340–351. https://doi.org/10.1016/j.jss.2009.04.024.
4. Nanda A, Bir SC, Maiti TK, Konar SK, Missios S, Guthikonda B. Relevance of Simpson grading system and recurrence-free survival after surgery for World Health Organization Grade I meningioma. *J Neurosurg*. 2017;126(1):201–211. https://doi.org/10.3171/2016.1.JNS151842.
5. Patchell RA, Tibbs PA, Regine WF, et al. Direct decompressive surgical resection in the treatment of spinal cord compression caused by metastatic cancer: a randomised trial. *Lancet*. 2005;366(9486):643–648. https://doi.org/10.1016/S0140-6736(05)66954-1.

Chapter 3

Introduction to radiation therapy

Emily S. Lebow, Marc R. Bussière, and Helen A. Shih

CHAPTER OUTLINE

Background: radiation biology and physics overview

Radiation therapy treats cancer by causing DNA damage, most importantly double-strand breaks (DSBs). Although normal cells can efficiently detect and repair DSBs through homologous recombination or non-homologous end joining, malignant cells lack these mechanisms and DSBs are often lethal. As a result, malignant cells are more susceptible to radiation-induced DNA damage than normal cells. Importantly, normal cells can safely tolerate only a finite dose of radiation without risk of permanent damage. Radiation therapy is designed to maximize dose to the tumor while minimizing dose to normal surrounding structures.

Radiation dose represents the energy absorbed per unit mass, Gray (Gy). Alternatively, radiobiological equivalent dose, Gy(RBE), may be used to quantify biological damage increases resulting from different types of radiation. The total dose of radiation is typically divided into smaller daily doses, a technique termed fractionation. There are several biologic rationales to support fractionation of radiation therapy. Most importantly, fractionation provides opportunity for normal tissues to repair radiation-induced DNA damage, thereby reducing toxicity. Fractionation also allows time for malignant cells in relatively radioresistant phases of the cell cycle (S phase) to cycle to more radiosensitive phases of the cell cycle (G2 and mitosis). During the course of fractionated radiation therapy, hypoxic niches of the tumor are reoxygenated, thereby making those cells more sensitive to radiation.

Despite advances in radiation techniques that minimize dose to normal tissues, a number of early and late toxicities are common. Early radiation toxicity (during or within weeks of radiation treatment) occur in rapidly dividing tissues. Radiation accelerates cell loss while impairing cell proliferation, disrupting a precise equilibrium. Early radiation toxicity is generally reversible after completion of radiation treatment and return of equilibrium between cell replication and loss. Common examples include hair loss and mucositis but are dependent on the site irradiated. Late radiation toxicity occurs due to permanent loss of organ parenchymal cells and radiation-induced signaling (such as TGFβ) that promotes fibrosis. Examples include infertility, coronary artery disease, and bowel malabsorption. Late toxicities are generally irreversible. Rarely, radiation therapy may also cause a second primary tumor that can be benign or malignant, depending upon the irradiated tissue. Radiation exposure induces a mutator phenotype in which cells more readily acquire additional mutations that may be oncogenic.[1] The risk of secondary malignancy is higher in patients treated at younger ages (i.e., younger age confers increased risk due to longer follow-up duration), higher cumulative dose, site of irradiation, receipt of chemotherapy, and in those with tumor predisposition syndromes (e.g., neurofibromatosis; see Chapter 16 for further discussion of neurofibromatosis).

Types of radiation therapy

Radiation therapy is most commonly delivered from a source outside the patient, an approach termed *external beam radiation therapy* (EBRT). Radiation oncologists use several techniques to plan and deliver EBRT. Three-dimensional conformal radiation therapy (3D-CRT) refers to radiation planning that relies on high-definition CT images for planning, often with additional assistance by MRI. There are several types of advanced 3D-CRT techniques that enable more precise delivery of radiation. The implied form of 3D-CRT is the original that employs software that enables the planner to place any number of beams of radiation from different directions, custom-shaped from the sides, and with some ability to attenuate the beam with materials placed in the path of the beam. More common forms of radiation delivery that also require the same 3D-based planning CT scan, but which use different principles and more advanced software to plan, are intensity modulated radiation therapy (IMRT) and volumetric modulated arc therapy (VMAT). IMRT and VMAT are complex delivery techniques that use software optimization techniques to determine the ideal treatment parameters using multiple beam segments with nonuniform dose intensities that add together to create treatment plans that meet predefined constraints and objectives. The most desirable treatment plans deliver the prescribed radiation doses to the target (the tumor, tumor bed, or areas at risk of disease recurrence as defined by the radiation oncologist) while minimizing dose to surrounding normal tissues (prioritized for dose-sparing as defined by the physician). Multiple static beams (often 5–9 beams and sometimes more) are used with IMRT, whereas one or more arcs are used with VMAT, which delivers the radiation therapy using equipment that rotates around the patient.

Stereotactic radiosurgery (SRS) is a type of EBRT that delivers the entire dose of radiation in one single or several small fractions of RT. SRS may be delivered with any high conformity technique but most commonly utilizes multiple radiation arcs or beams to converge on a precisely defined target. This optimizes treatment to deliver high doses to a confined area with little radiation exposure to adjacent tissue (i.e., no margin). Radiation dose to critical intracranial structures must be carefully considered during the planning process. Radiation dose efficacy on tumor and tolerance of normal tissues is extremely dependent upon the number of fractions (e.g., how interspaced) used to deliver the RT dose. Cranial irradiation is complex because of the multiple radiation sensitive structures including the optic chiasm, optic nerves, cochlea, hippocampus, brainstem, pituitary, retina, lacrimal gland, and lens.[2] All EBRT techniques require careful patient positioning and target localization for treatment.

Radiation therapy most commonly utilizes photons but increasingly may utilize protons in certain clinical scenarios. Photons, or high energy x-rays, are generated by linear accelerators. Photons can also be harnessed in the form of gamma-rays emitted by multiple low-energy Cobalt-60 radioactive sources for SRS. In contrast, protons are generated from proton accelerators that are larger and more complex than linear accelerators. The therapeutic advantage of protons is not in the type of RT delivered, which is essentially the same for protons and photons, but in reducing damage to normal tissue around the tumor. The physical properties of protons allow for reduced dose of radiation to normal tissues adjacent to the tumor while maintaining therapeutic dose delivered to the tumor. The clinical benefit of protons relative to photons is thus far widely accepted for a number of diseases including uveal melanoma, skull base malignancies, sinonasal malignancies, and childhood malignancies such as medulloblastoma, craniopharyngioma, and rhabdomyosarcoma.[3] The benefit of proton therapy for many other disease sites (such as breast cancer and prostate cancer) remains an area of ongoing investigation. The main disadvantage of proton therapy is the expense of establishing and operating proton facilities, which has historically limited its availability.

Clinical cases

CASE 3.1 RADIATION THERAPY FOR HIGH-GRADE GLIOMA

Case. A 65-year-old male presented with left facial droop, difficulty ambulating, and emotional lability. An MRI showed a heterogeneously enhancing, well-circumscribed right temporal mass measuring 6.5 × 5.1 × 4.3 cm^3 with mass effect causing 1.1 cm leftward midline shift and uncal herniation (Fig. 3.1A). The patient underwent a craniotomy with near gross total resection of the tumor. Pathology showed WHO grade IV glioblastoma. Molecular analysis showed *MGMT* promoter hypermethylation, *IDH1* wildtype, *ATRX* retained, and *TP53* mutation. Postoperative imaging showed a residual nodular focus of enhancement and persistent fluid attenuated inversion recovery (FLAIR) hyperintensity surrounding the resection cavity. Following resection, the patient's neurologic deficits completely resolved, and he had an excellent performance status. The patient was treated with adjuvant photon EBRT to the resection cavity with a total dose of 60 Gy in 30 fractions (2 Gy per fraction) over 6 weeks (Fig. 3.1B). The patient was also treated with concurrent and adjuvant temozolomide

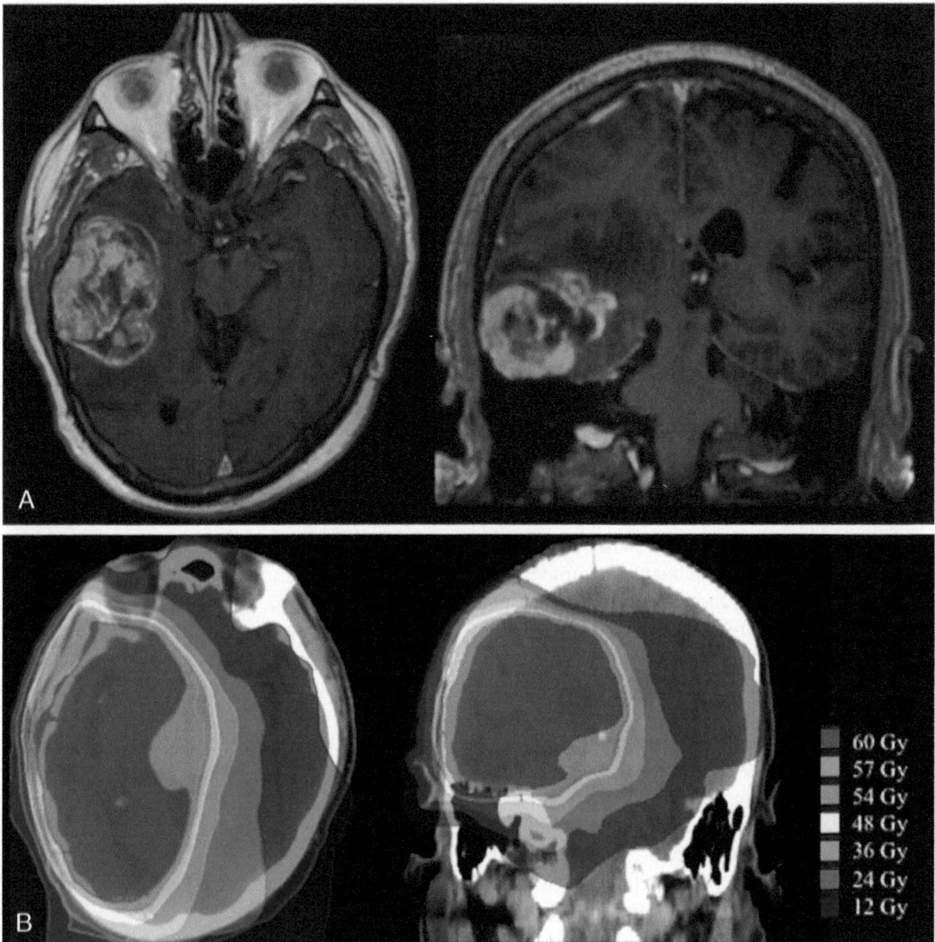

Fig. 3.1 The patient is a 68-year-old man with glioblastoma. (A) Preoperative T1 post-contrast MRI of the patient's right temporal glioblastoma measuring 6.5 cm × 5.1 cm × 4.3 cm. The tumor exerted profound mass effect including subfalcine herniation and a 1.1 cm leftward shift. (B) The patient was treated with external beam radiation therapy to a dose of 60 Gy in 30 fractions over 6 weeks with concurrent temozolomide. The treatment was planned with volumetric modulated arc therapy, a form of radiation therapy in which the radiation source rotates in arcs around the patient while the radiation beam is on. A custom margin was added to the resection cavity + T2/FLAIR-defined tumor to treat the microscopic disease of high-grade glioma known to infiltrate beyond the radiographically detectable abnormality. *FLAIR*, Fluid attenuation inversion recovery.

chemotherapy. The patient tolerated treatment well with only fatigue, mild appetite loss, and expected patchy partial alopecia.

Teaching Points. The standard of care for high-grade glioma is maximal safe resection followed by combined modality therapy consisting of adjuvant radiation therapy and temozolomide. Because of the infiltrative nature of high-grade glioma, microscopic disease extends beyond the radiographically defined tumor into the adjacent radiographically normal appearing brain parenchyma. As a result, radiation is delivered to the resection cavity plus a margin of adjacent brain parenchyma (most commonly between 1.0 and 2.5 cm depending on the physician) to provide coverage of infiltrative tumor cells. The typical radiation course for high-grade glioma is 60 Gy delivered in 30 fractions (2 Gy per fraction) over 6 weeks (Monday–Friday, no weekend or holiday treatments). Radiation can be planned and delivered with several EBRT techniques, including 3D-CRT, IMRT, and VMAT. Among patients with high-grade glioma, adjuvant radiation therapy improves disease control and survival but is not curative.[4]

A variety of treatment approaches should be considered for patients who are elderly or debilitated.[5] Among the elderly (generally defined as over the age of 60 or 65) and those with poor performance status, a shorter course of radiation therapy with concurrent and adjuvant temozolomide is well tolerated. These hypofractionated regimens include 40 Gy delivered in 15 fractions over 3 weeks or even 25 Gy delivered in 5 fractions over 1 week. Among patients who cannot tolerate combined modality therapy (i.e., radiation and chemotherapy), treatment with either radiation or temozolomide monotherapy should be considered depending on *MGMT* methylation status. Patients with *MGMT* unmethylated disease benefit greater from hypofractionated radiation therapy monotherapy over temozolomide monotherapy. In patients with *MGMT* methylated disease, temozolomide monotherapy can be appropriate in selected cases.[6–9]

Follow-up MRI should be performed 1 month after completion of radiation therapy and then every 2 to 4 months thereafter. Initial imaging 1 month after radiation therapy establishes a new baseline prior to continuation of additional adjuvant chemotherapy. It is important to consider the possibility of pseudoprogression (treatment-related imaging changes that resemble disease progression) in patients with apparent disease progression within the first several months after radiation therapy. In patients with pseudoprogression, imaging changes and new clinical symptoms will typically resolve without additional cancer-directed therapy. Patients with *MGMT* methylated glioblastoma treated with radiation therapy and concurrent temozolomide are at increased risk of pseudoprogression.[10] In these cases, serial imaging is recommended as advanced MRI-based imaging techniques, positron-emission tomography (PET) imaging, or other noninvasive tools cannot reliably differentiate pseudoprogression from true tumor progression. In selected cases, surgery may be needed (see Chapter 2 for approaches to surgery in brain tumor patients).

There are multiple acute and late toxicities of radiation therapy for high-grade glioma. The most common acute toxicities are alopecia, radiation dermatitis, fatigue, and loss of appetite. These toxicities are typically mild, managed with supportive care, and resolve after completion of radiation therapy. Late toxicities occur months to years after radiation therapy, may be irreversible, and most commonly include neurocognitive impairment, leukoencephalopathy, and endocrinopathies (e.g., thyroid disease).

Clinical Pearls

1. The standard of care for high-grade glioma is maximal safe resection followed by combined modality therapy consisting of adjuvant radiation therapy and temozolomide. The typical radiation regimen is 60 Gy in 30 fractions (2 Gy per fraction) delivered over 6 weeks.
2. Among the elderly or those with poor performance status, hypofractionated radiation therapy (for example, 40.05 Gy in 15 fractions delivered over 3 weeks) with temozolomide, radiation therapy alone, or temozolomide alone may be appropriate in certain patients. This decision is often guided by *MGMT* methylation status.
3. EBRT for high-grade glioma may be planned and delivered with 3D-CRT, IMRT, or VMAT.
4. Imaging follow-up should occur 1 month after completion of radiation therapy to establish a new baseline prior to continuation of additional adjuvant chemotherapy. The possibility of pseudoprogression instead of early disease progression should be considered, particularly in patients treated with concurrent temozolomide.

CASE 3.2 STEREOTACTIC RADIOSURGERY FOR A PATIENT WITH A SOLITARY BRAIN METASTASIS

Case. A 39-year-old female never-smoker presented with hemoptysis and a right hilar mass on imaging. Bronchoscopy showed lung adenocarcinoma that was positive for the *ROS1* translocation. Several days later, the patient developed left arm clumsiness and headache. MRI imaging revealed five small brain metastases, diffuse osseous metastases in the spine and ilium, and multiple hepatic metastases. The patient was treated with crizotinib and pemetrexed with good response including in the brain. Approximately 1 year later, routine staging brain MRI showed a punctate focus of enhancement in the right cerebellum which subsequently enlarged to 5 mm in size on follow-up imaging. This was the only site of disease progression. At the time of evaluation for radiation therapy, the patient was asymptomatic from the brain metastasis and neurologically intact on examination. She had excellent performance status limited only by fatigue related to systemic therapy. The lesion was treated with single fraction SRS of 18 Gy (Fig. 3.2). Follow-up MRI 2 months after SRS showed complete radiographic resolution of the right cerebellar metastasis, but a new punctate enhancing lesion appeared in the right temporal lobe. The right temporal lesion enlarged to 4 mm on imaging 4 months later. The right temporal lesion was then treated with SRS to 18 Gy (Fig. 3.2). The patient experienced no side effects from either SRS treatment. Neither brain metastases recurred on follow-up imaging available 2 years post-treatment.

Teaching Points. Among patients with a single or limited number of brain metastases and good prognosis, SRS is preferred relative to whole brain radiation therapy (WBRT). SRS achieves excellent rates of local disease control with minimal side effects.[11–15] Whereas WBRT delivers radiation dose to the entire brain parenchyma, SRS delivers a high dose of radiation with high precision to a small target. As a result of sparing radiation dose to most of the brain, patients treated with SRS have improved cognitive function and quality of life following treatment compared with patients treated with WBRT.[12,16] Because SRS is very localized, its primary disadvantage is the risk of developing new brain metastases in the untreated region of the brain,[17–19] as occurred with the patient in this case. As a result, short-interval follow-up images is recommended around every 2–3 months following SRS. Longer intervals between imaging can be considered subsequently as the patient achieves longer time in stability of intracranial disease. A limited number of new brain metastases may be amenable to salvage

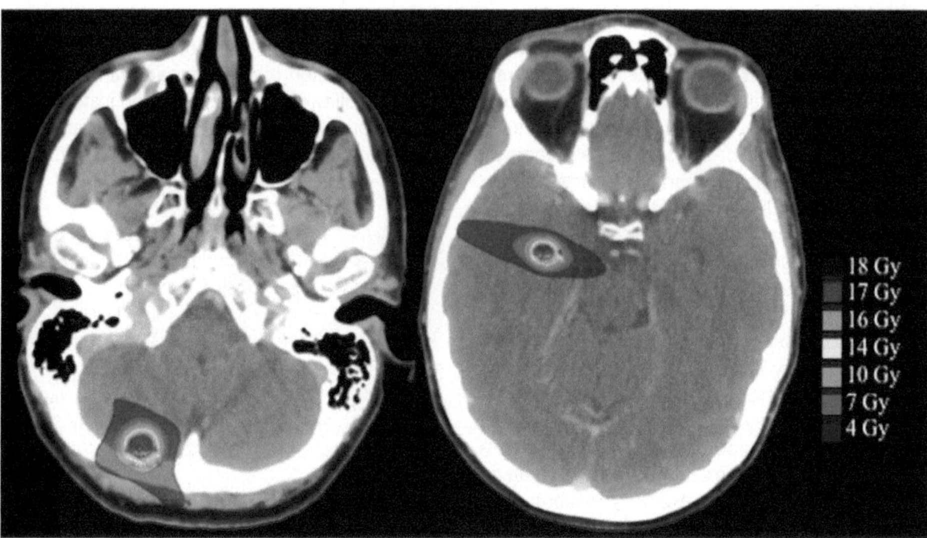

Fig. 3.2 The patient is a 39-year-old woman with non–small-cell lung cancer brain metastases. Both the cerebellar and temporal brain metastases were treated with stereotactic radiosurgery to a dose of 18 Gy in one fraction. Both lesions demonstrated durable disease control and did not recur on available follow-up imaging 2 years after SRS. *SRS*, Stereotactic radiosurgery.

SRS, whereas diffuse progression of intracranial disease may require WBRT.

SRS is generally well tolerated and with few acute toxicities. The most important late complication of SRS is radiation necrosis, an inflammatory reaction that may cause headache, seizures, focal neurologic deficit, or neurocognitive symptoms. Radiation necrosis may develop months to years after treatment with SRS. The risk of radiation necrosis is associated with higher SRS dose, lesion size, location, and receipt of prior radiation therapy. Larger lesions are associated with increased risk of radiation necrosis. SRS delivered to the brainstem, deep gray matter (such as the thalamus or basal ganglia), motor strip, or proximal to cranial nerves is more likely to cause symptomatic radiation necrosis compared with other areas of brain parenchyma.[20,21] Prior treatment with WBRT or SRS to the same lesion also increases risk of radiation necrosis.[17] Corticosteroids, bevacizumab, surgical resection, or laser interstitial thermal therapy (i.e., laser interstitial thermal therapy [LITT]; see Chapter 2 for further discussion of LITT) are used to treat symptomatic radiation necrosis.[18]

There are several approaches to mitigate the likelihood of radiation necrosis in high-risk brain metastases. Fractionated EBRT (delivered in 2–3 Gy fractions over a few weeks) is preferred for very high-risk lesions that are poor candidates for stereotactic techniques due to size or location. SRS may also be delivered in multiple fractions (generally between two and five) rather than as a large dose in a single fraction. Finally, the total radiation dose for SRS may be adjusted. The dose generally ranges from 15 Gy to 24 Gy.[17] Larger lesions or those located next to eloquent structures are treated with lower doses to reduce the risk of toxicity.

Clinical Pearls

1. Among patients with a limited number of brain metastases and good prognosis, SRS is preferred over WBRT. SRS achieves high rates of local control and is associated with improved cognitive function and quality of life compared with WBRT.
2. Because of the risk of developing new brain metastases after SRS, patients should have routine surveillance imaging every 2–3 months following treatment and with longer intervals with longer time of central nervous system (CNS) disease stability.
3. Radiation necrosis is a late toxicity of SRS that develops months to years after treatment and is most commonly asymptomatic but can have associated symptoms ranging from focal neurologic deficits to generalized cognitive symptoms depending upon the location. Steroids, bevacizumab, or surgical resection are used to treat symptomatic radiation necrosis.
4. The risk of radiation necrosis is associated with brain metastasis size and radiation dose. Fractionated radiation therapy should be considered for high-risk lesions. Alternatively, SRS can be delivered with a reduced dose or in few fractions (between two and five) to reduce risk of toxicity.

CASE 3.3 WHOLE BRAIN RADIATION THERAPY FOR DIFFUSE BRAIN METASTASES

Case. A 47-year-old male presented with a suspicious mole that was biopsied and found to be a 3.65-mm thick, non-ulcerated melanoma. The patient underwent a wide local excision with sentinel lymph node biopsy that showed one left axillary sentinel node (1/1) and one of two right axillary nodes (1/2) positive for disease. MRI and PET/CT showed no evidence of metastatic disease. Bilateral complete node dissection showed involvement of 0/18 nodes in the left axilla and 1/16 nodes in the right axilla. The patient was treated with adjuvant interferon therapy. PET/CT 1 year later showed interval disease progression with adrenal gland and splenic metastases. The patient was treated with seven cycles of pembrolizumab and had subsequent systemic and intracranial disease progression with four new brain metastases. The patient was started on ipilimumab and nivolumab combination therapy. Subsequent MRI showed eleven brain metastases that were new or increased in size from the prior study 2 months previously (Fig. 3.3A). The largest metastasis was a 1 cm left anterior cingulate lesion with surrounding vasogenic edema. The patient had an excellent performance status with no symptoms and with a completely intact neurologic examination. Given the volume and rate of disease progression, the patient was recommended for WBRT rather than multifocal SRS, which would leave the rest of the untreated brain at high risk for further new metastases. To reduce the risk of post-treatment cognitive dysfunction, the patient was treated with hippocampal avoidance whole brain radiation therapy (HA-WBRT) to a total of 30 Gy in 10 fractions (Fig. 3.3B). The dose to the patient's bilateral hippocampi was reduced. During treatment, the patient developed mild but persistent nausea for which he received dexamethasone with good symptomatic relief.

Teaching Points. WBRT is the recommended approach for patients with diffuse brain metastases. The most common treatment regimen is 30–37.5 Gy delivered in 10–15 fractions.[19] WBRT decreases the risk of new brain metastases compared with treatment with SRS, thereby reducing the need for salvage treatment and reducing risk of symptoms from intracranial disease progression.[20,21] Survival following WBRT is historically limited, ranging from 2 to 6 months.[22,23] However, groups of contemporary patients with positive prognostic factors may survive years after treatment.[24,25] WBRT is most likely to improve survival in younger patients (under 60 years of age) or in limited clinical scenarios, such as when combined with SRS or surgery in the setting of a solitary brain metastasis.[26] However, WBRT does not improve survival or quality of life for patients who are elderly, debilitated, or with progressive systemic disease. For these patients, best supportive care alone should be considered.[27]

WBRT is associated with significant early and late toxicity which can be debilitating. Early toxicities include fatigue, nausea, and headaches. Late toxicities may occur months to years after completion of radiation treatment, are often progressive, and include progressive neurocognitive decline associated with leukoencephalopathy, progressive chronic fatigue and reduced stamina, possible permanent hair loss, hearing loss, and long-term hypopituitarism in long-term survivors. Several strategies are being explored to reduce WBRT-associated toxicity. Memantine, an oral NMDA inhibitor, is well-tolerated and improves time to development of cognitive decline.[28] WBRT with reduced dose to the hippocampus, termed hippocampal avoidance whole brain radiation therapy (HA-WBRT), also reduces the likelihood of post-treatment neurocognitive impairment.[29,30] HA-WBRT is delivered using IMRT or VMAT planning, allowing for selective dose reduction to the hippocampus while maintaining adequate dose coverage of the remaining brain parenchyma.

Clinical Pearls

1. WBRT is generally recommended for patients with diffuse brain metastases and reduces the risk of new brain metastases compared with management by SRS.
2. WBRT improves survival for only limited sets of patients. Patients who are elderly, debilitated, or with a very poor prognosis may not benefit from WBRT in terms of survival or quality of life. Best supportive care is a reasonable alternative for these groups of patients.
3. WBRT is most commonly delivered as 30 Gy in 10 fractions over 2 weeks.
4. WBRT harbors significant risk of toxicity, the most severe of which is irreversible cognitive decline that may occur months to years after treatment.
5. Delivery of WBRT with IMRT and/or VMAT allows dose adjustment to specific intracranial structures, including dose reduction to the hippocampus. This approach is termed hippocampal avoidance whole brain radiation therapy (HA-WBRT) and may reduce cognitive decline following treatment.

CASE 3.4 RADIATION THERAPY FOR A PRIMARY INTRAMEDULLARY SPINAL CORD TUMOR

Case. A 68-year-old woman with a history of obesity presented with weakness, numbness, back pain, and episodes of urinary incontinence. Spine MRI showed an ovoid mildly T2 hyperintense and T1 heterogeneously enhancing intramedullary mass at the level of the T9 vertebral body (Fig. 3.4A). The patient underwent a T8–T10 laminectomy for intradural microsurgical exploration and radical subtotal resection of tumor. Pathology showed a low-grade infiltrating glioma with features of ependymoma. Postoperatively, the patient's performance status was limited by chronic hip pain attributed to obesity, arthritis, and deconditioning. Her neurologic examination was notable for decreased sensation in her left lower extremity. The patient was treated with proton therapy to reduce radiation exposure to surrounding structures, including the esophagus, bone marrow, and lungs. The patient was treated with 50.4 Gy to the T8–T10 spinal cord in 28 fractions (1.8 Gy per fraction) over 5.5 weeks (Fig. 3.4B). The patient experienced transient mild fatigue and erythema in the treatment field.

Teaching Points. Primary spinal cord tumors are rare, accounting for only between 2% and 4% of primary central nervous system tumors. Primary spinal cord tumors may be intramedullary, intradural-extramedullary, or extradural. Here, we focus our discussion on primary intramedullary spinal cord

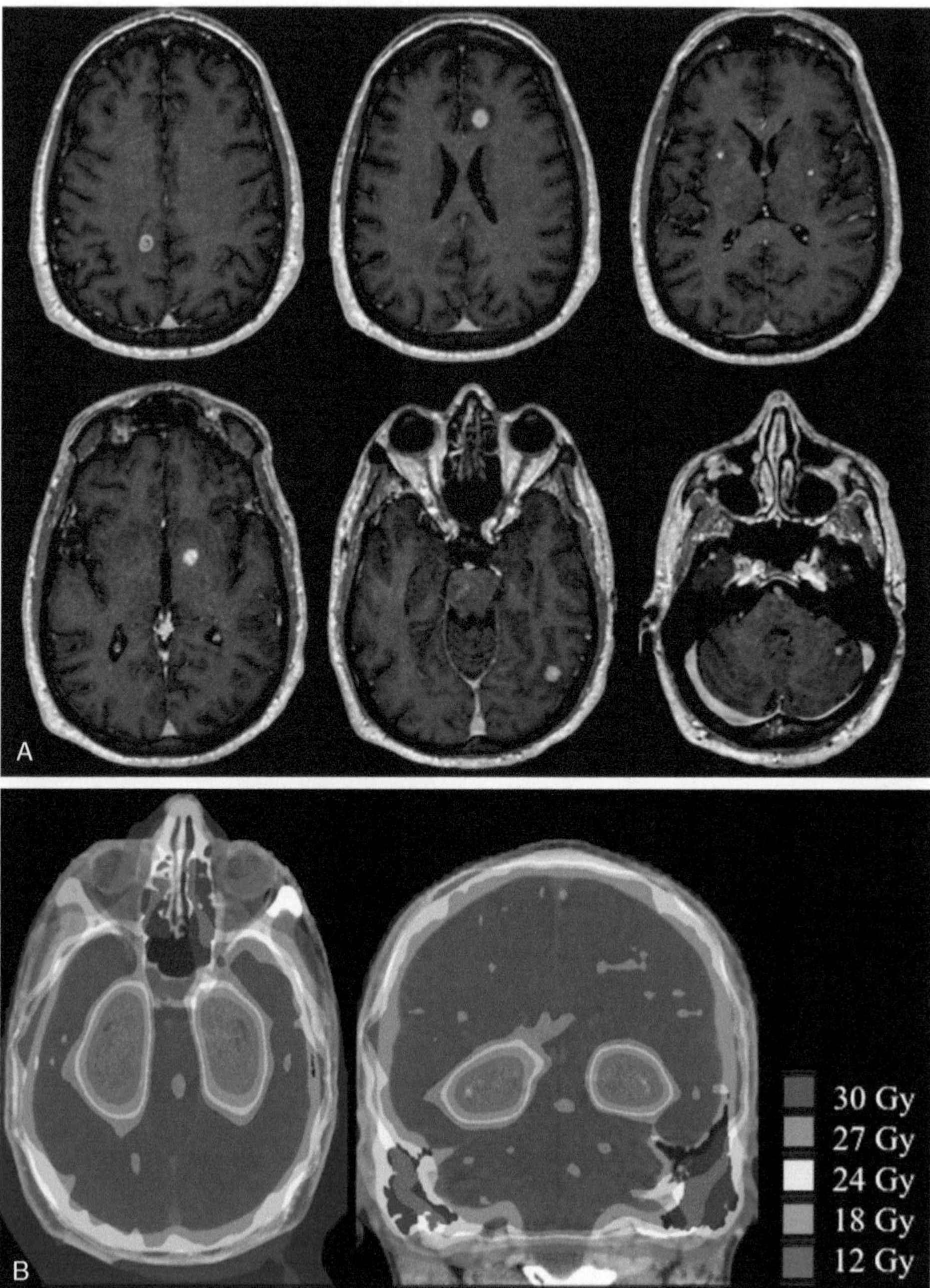

Fig. 3.3 The patient is a 47-year-old man with melanoma brain metastases. (A) MRI demonstrates numerous brain metastases throughout the bilateral cerebral hemispheres and cerebellum. (B) The patient was treated with hippocampal avoidance whole brain radiation therapy to a dose of 30 Gy in 10 fractions over 3 weeks. The radiation was planned with volumetric modulated arc therapy, which allowed for selective dose reduction to the bilateral hippocampi while maintaining adequate coverage of the surrounding brain parenchyma.

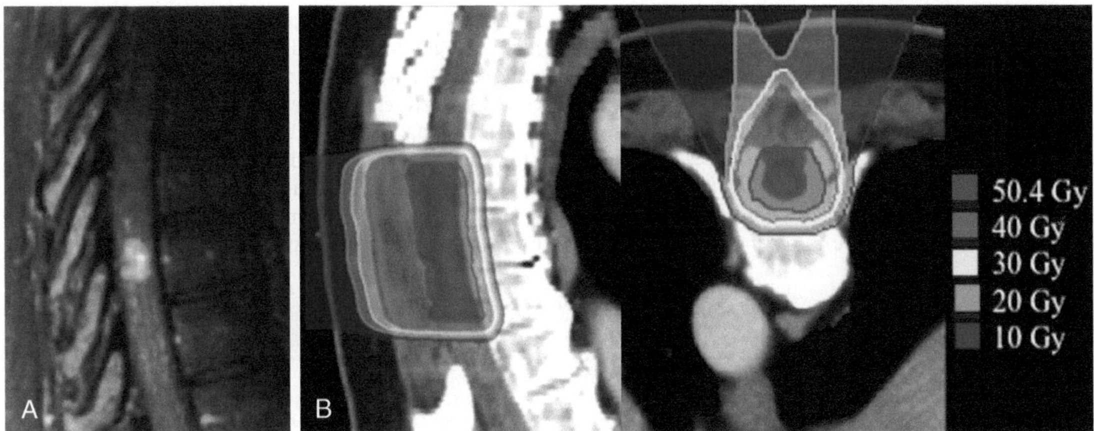

Fig. 3.4 The patient is a 68-year-old woman with a thoracic intramedullary low-grade glioma. (A) Preoperative spine MRI shows a T1 hyperintense heterogenous intramedullary mass at the approximate level of the T9 vertebral body. (B) The patient was treated with external beam radiation therapy to a dose of 50.4 Gy(RBE) to the T8–T10 cord in 28 fractions (1.8 Gy(RBE) per fraction) over nearly 6 weeks. Proton therapy was utilized to reduce radiation exposure to adjacent normal tissues, including the esophagus, bone marrow, and lungs.

tumors, which comprise approximately 10% of primary spinal cord tumors.[31] Gliomas are the most common type of intramedullary tumors, which includes ependymomas, astrocytomas, and oligodendrogliomas. Upfront treatment of intramedullary spinal cord tumors consists of maximal safe resection, which is often limited to a biopsy or conservative subtotal resection given the high risk of surgical morbidity. Gross total resection is difficult to achieve among intramedullary gliomas given their infiltrative nature and location within the spinal cord (see Chapter 2 for discussion of surgical approaches to CNS tumors).[31]

Radiation therapy is generally recommended for patients, either upfront (including after biopsy or subtotal resection), especially in cases of aggressive disease histology, or at time of radiographic or symptomatic disease progression. Patients are treated with doses ranging from 45 to 54 Gy in 1.8 Gy daily fractions over the course of 5–6 weeks. EBRT for intramedullary tumors is planned with 3D-CRT or techniques of IMRT or VMAT can be used to reduce dose to anterior normal tissues. Given the rarity of these tumors, evidence supporting postoperative radiation therapy is less clear and based upon retrospective series rather than randomized trials.[31–34]

Radiation therapy of intramedullary spinal cord tumors is challenging in that the spinal cord is both the target of radiation and the structure most at risk for toxicity. The dose tolerance of the spinal cord depends on a number of factors, including dose per daily fraction and the length of spinal cord irradiated. Spinal cord toxicity includes a transient radiation-induced myelopathy in which patients experience an electric-shock sensation during neck flexion, termed Lhermitte's sign.[35] The most feared complication of spinal cord irradiation is a chronic progressive myelopathy, which results in permanent and progressive neurologic deficits. These range from minor sensory or motor impairments to complete paraplegia. The average onset is 18 months after radiation exposure.[36]

Local normal tissue toxicity following spinal irradiation depends on the level of spinal cord irradiation. For example, irradiation of cervical cord tumors puts the laryngeal airway and pharyngeal mucosa at risk of symptoms. In contrast, irradiation of thoracic cord tumors places organs such as the esophagus, lungs, heart, and liver at risk. Irradiation of lumbar tumors places the kidney, bowel, ovary, and uterus at risk. Some patients may benefit from proton radiation therapy for intramedullary spinal cord tumors to reduce dose to adjacent normal tissues. Proton therapy for ependymomas has been studied particularly in the pediatric population, given the high likelihood of cure and increased risk for long-term toxicities among childhood cancer survivors.[37]

Clinical Pearls

1. Radiation therapy for intramedullary spinal cord tumors is standard after surgery or at the time of progressive disease.
2. Patients are most commonly treated with a dose between 45 to 54 Gy in 1.8 Gy daily fractions over the course of 5–6 weeks.
3. Chronic progressive myelopathy is the most serious complication of spinal cord irradiation. It results in permanent and often progressive neurologic deficits, ranging from minor sensory and motor deficits to complete paraplegia in severe cases. There are no proven effective treatments.
4. Proton therapy for intramedullary spinal cord tumors may be considered in some clinical scenarios, particularly for children who are at highest risk of long-term treatment-associated toxicity.

Conclusions

Radiation therapy is an integral component in the management of most brain and spinal cord tumors. 3D-conformal radiation therapy provides the benefit of treating infiltrative lesions such as gliomas and including a margin of perilesional tissue that may give rise to recurrence. Stereotactic radiosurgery provides surgical precision to optimally deliver higher single doses of radiation with limited surrounding margin that is commonly used for treating discrete, well-circumscribed lesions like brain metastases, meningioma, osseous spinal metastases, and other lesions. Toxicity is often related to the location of the tumor and treatment field, with numerous techniques available for the selected cases described for maximizing the dose delivered to the tumor and minimizing damage to surrounding tissues.

References

1. Allan JM, Travis LB. Mechanisms of therapy-related carcinogenesis. *Nat Rev Cancer*. 2005;5(12):943–955.
2. Scoccianti S, Detti B, Gadda D, et al. Organs at risk in the brain and their dose-constraints in adults and in children: a radiation oncologist's guide for delineation in everyday practice. *Radiother Oncol*. 2015;114(2):230–238.
3. Allen AM, Pawlicki T, Dong L, et al. An evidence based review of proton beam therapy: the report of ASTRO's emerging technology committee. *Radiother Oncol*. 2012;103(1):8–11.
4. Kirkpatrick JP, Laack NN, Shih HA, Gondi V. Management of GBM: a problem of local recurrence. *J Neuro Oncol*. 2017;134(3):487–493.
5. Cabrera AR, Kirkpatrick JP, Fiveash JB, et al. Radiation therapy for glioblastoma: executive summary of an American Society for Radiation Oncology evidence-based clinical practice guideline. *Pract Radiat Oncol*. 2016;6(4):217–225.
6. Perry JR, Laperriere N, O'Callaghan CJ, et al. Short-course radiation plus temozolomide in elderly patients with glioblastoma. *N Engl J Med*. 2017;376(11):1027–1037.
7. Wick W, Platten M, Meisner C, et al. Temozolomide chemotherapy alone versus radiotherapy alone for malignant astrocytoma in the elderly: the NOA-08 randomised, phase 3 trial. *Lancet Oncol*. 2012;13(7):707–715.
8. Malmström A, Grønberg BH, Marosi C, et al. Temozolomide versus standard 6-week radiotherapy versus hypofractionated radiotherapy in patients older than 60 years with glioblastoma: the Nordic randomised, phase 3 trial. *Lancet Oncol*. 2012;13(9):916–926.
9. Roa W, Kepka L, Kumar N, et al. International Atomic Energy Agency randomized phase III study of radiation therapy in elderly and/or frail patients with newly diagnosed glioblastoma multiforme. *J Clin Oncol*. 2015;33(35):4145–4150.
10. Brandsma D, Stalpers L, Taal W, Sminia P, van den Bent MJ. Clinical features, mechanisms, and management of pseudoprogression in malignant gliomas. *Lancet Oncol*. 2008;9(5):453–461.
11. Kocher M, Soffietti R, Abacioglu U, et al. Adjuvant whole-brain radiotherapy versus observation after radiosurgery or surgical resection of one to three cerebral metastases: results of the EORTC 22952-26001 study. *J Clin Oncol*. 2011;29(2):134–141.
12. Brown PD, Jaeckle K, Ballman KV, et al. Effect of radiosurgery alone vs radiosurgery with whole brain radiation therapy on cognitive function in patients with 1 to 3 brain metastases: a randomized clinical trial. *J Am Med Assoc*. 2016;316(4):401–409.
13. Aoyama H, Shirato H, Tago M, et al. Stereotactic radiosurgery plus whole-brain radiation therapy vs stereotactic radiosurgery alone for treatment of brain metastases: a randomized controlled trial. *J Am Med Assoc*. 2006;295(21):2483–2491.
14. Jensen CA, Chan MD, McCoy TP, et al. Cavity-directed radiosurgery as adjuvant therapy after resection of a brain metastasis. *J Neurosurg*. 2011;114(6):1585–1591.
15. Brennan C, Yang TJ, Hilden P, et al. A phase 2 trial of stereotactic radiosurgery boost after surgical resection for brain metastases. *Int J Radiat Oncol Biol Phys*. 2014;88(1):130–136.
16. Chang EL, Wefel JS, Hess KR, et al. Neurocognition in patients with brain metastases treated with radiosurgery or radiosurgery plus whole-brain irradiation: a randomised controlled trial. *Lancet Oncol*. 2009;10(11):1037–1044.
17. Shaw E, Scott C, Souhami L, et al. Single dose radiosurgical treatment of recurrent previously irradiated primary brain tumors and brain metastases: final report of RTOG protocol 90-05. *Int J Radiat Oncol Biol Phys*. 2000;47(2):291–298.
18. Chao ST, Ahluwalia MS, Barnett GH, et al. Challenges with the diagnosis and treatment of cerebral radiation necrosis. *Int J Radiat Oncol Biol Phys*. 2013;87(3):449–457.
19. Tsao MN, Xu W, Wong RK, et al. Whole brain radiotherapy for the treatment of newly diagnosed multiple brain metastases. *Cochrane Database Syst Rev*. 2018;1: CD003869.
20. Flickinger JC, Kondziolka D, Lunsford LD, et al. Development of a model to predict permanent symptomatic postradiosurgery injury for arteriovenous malformation patients. Arteriovenous Malformation Radiosurgery Study Group. *Int J Radiat Oncol Biol Phys*. 2000;46(5):1143–1148.
21. Stafford SL, Pollock BE, Leavitt JA, et al. A study on the radiation tolerance of the optic nerves and chiasm after stereotactic radiosurgery. *Int J Radiat Oncol Biol Phys*. 2003;55(5):1177–1181.
22. Suh JH, Stea B, Nabid A, et al. Phase III study of efaproxiral as an adjunct to whole-brain radiation therapy for brain metastases. *J Clin Oncol*. 2006;24(1):106–114.
23. Mehta MP, Rodrigus P, Terhaard CH, et al. Survival and neurologic outcomes in a randomized trial of motexafin gadolinium and whole-brain radiation therapy in brain metastases. *J Clin Oncol*. 2003;21(13):2529–2536.
24. Tsakonas G, Hellman F, Gubanski M, et al. Prognostic factors affecting survival after whole brain radiotherapy in patients with brain metastasized lung cancer. *Acta Oncol*. 2018;57(2):231–238.
25. Jeene PM, de Vries KC, van Nes JGH, et al. Survival after whole brain radiotherapy for brain metastases from lung cancer and

breast cancer is poor in 6325 Dutch patients treated between 2000 and 2014. *Acta Oncol*. 2018;57(5):637–643.

26. Andrews DW, Scott CB, Sperduto PW, et al. Whole brain radiation therapy with or without stereotactic radiosurgery boost for patients with one to three brain metastases: phase III results of the RTOG 9508 randomised trial. *Lancet*. 2004;363(9422):1665–1672.
27. Mulvenna P, Nankivell M, Barton R, et al. Dexamethasone and supportive care with or without whole brain radiotherapy in treating patients with non-small cell lung cancer with brain metastases unsuitable for resection or stereotactic radiotherapy (QUARTZ): results from a phase 3, non-inferiority, randomised trial. *Lancet*. 2016;388(10055):2004–2014.
28. Brown PD, Pugh S, Laack NN, et al. Memantine for the prevention of cognitive dysfunction in patients receiving whole-brain radiotherapy: a randomized, double-blind, placebo-controlled trial. *Neuro Oncol*. 2013;15(10):1429–1437.
29. Gondi V, Pugh SL, Tome WA, et al. Preservation of memory with conformal avoidance of the hippocampal neural stem-cell compartment during whole-brain radiotherapy for brain metastases (RTOG 0933): a phase II multi-institutional trial. *J Clin Oncol*. 2014;32(34):3810–3816.
30. Gondi V, Deshmukh S, Brown PD, et al. Preservation of neurocognitive function with conformal avoidance of the hippocampus during whole-brain radiotherapy for brain metastases: preliminary results of phase III trial NRG Oncology CC001. 2018;102:1607.
31. Chamberlain MC, Eaton KD, Fink JR, Tredway T. Intradural intramedullary spinal cord metastasis due to mesothelioma. *J Neuro Oncol*. 2010;97(1):133–136.
32. Lee SH, Chung CK, Kim CH, et al. Long-term outcomes of surgical resection with or without adjuvant radiation therapy for treatment of spinal ependymoma: a retrospective multicenter study by the Korea Spinal Oncology Research Group. *Neuro Oncol*. 2013;15(7):921–929.
33. Abdel-Wahab M, Etuk B, Palermo J, et al. Spinal cord gliomas: a multi-institutional retrospective analysis. *Int J Radiat Oncol Biol Phys*. 2006;64(4):1060–1071.
34. Minehan KJ, Brown PD, Scheithauer BW, Krauss WE, Wright MP. Prognosis and treatment of spinal cord astrocytoma. *Int J Radiat Oncol Biol Phys*. 2009;73(3):727–733.
35. Leung WM, Tsang NM, Chang FT, Lo CJ. Lhermitte's sign among nasopharyngeal cancer patients after radiotherapy. *Head Neck*. 2005;27(3):187–194.
36. Wong CS, Fehlings MG, Sahgal A. Pathobiology of radiation myelopathy and strategies to mitigate injury. *Spinal Cord*. 2015;53(8):574–580.
37. Amsbaugh MJ, Grosshans DR, McAleer MF, et al. Proton therapy for spinal ependymomas: planning, acute toxicities, and preliminary outcomes. *Int J Radiat Oncol Biol Phys*. 2012;83(5):1419–1424.

Chapter | 4 |

Evidence-based approaches to chemotherapy for gliomas

Alessia Pellerino, Federica Franchino, Roberta Rudà, and Riccardo Soffietti

CHAPTER OUTLINE

Introduction

Chemotherapy has a crucial role in the management of gliomas. Traditionally, the management is characterized by an extensive surgery followed by a combination of radiotherapy (RT) and chemotherapy. In general, chemotherapy has been used as a neoadjuvant, adjuvant, or concurrent treatment, and our understanding of optimal use has continued to evolve over time. *Neoadjuvant* chemotherapy is administered prior to the main or definitive treatment, which is usually surgery (i.e., before surgery). *Adjuvant* chemotherapy is administered after the main or definitive treatment. For brain or spinal cord tumors, this is typically after radiation therapy (i.e., adjuvant to radiation). In some cases, *concurrent* chemotherapy may be administered simultaneously with radiation therapy. Different chemotherapeutic regimens have been investigated in both low-grade gliomas (LGGs) and high-grade gliomas (HGGs). Overall, the impact of chemotherapy for disease control still remains modest as compared with surgery or RT. New compounds are needed, and searching for novel druggable pathways is the current mission of basic and translational research in neuro-oncology.

Chemotherapy regimens

Here, we describe the traditional chemotherapeutic schedules used in daily clinical practice according to the results from the most important clinical trials in both LGGs and HGGs. First, we review common chemotherapy regimens used in clinical practice. Then, we present a series of cases and summarize the landmark clinical trials that inform the use of chemotherapy in patient management.

Temozolomide

Temozolomide (TMZ) is an oral agent converted by the liver to the active metabolite 5-(3-methyltriazen-1-yl)-imidazole-4-carboxamide (MTIC). The antineoplastic effect results from alkylating the middle guanine residue of DNA, leading to defective mismatch repair and cell death. TMZ is used commonly in many central nervous system (CNS) regimens due to its many favorable characteristics including good oral bioavailability, limited protein binding, and good CNS penetration with measurable levels being achieved in the cerebrospinal fluid (CSF) and in brain parenchyma following oral administration.[1] Considering these properties, TMZ may be used with different schedules and timing for treating many gliomas, CNS lymphoma, or selected brain or leptomeningeal metastases.

Treatment Schedules. TMZ is often administered concurrently and/or adjuvant to radiation therapy.

Concurrent Temozolomide. The most frequent regimen consists of TMZ administered at 75 mg/m^2 per day for 6 consecutive weeks along with conformal RT according to the Stupp regimen.[2,3] The aim of this treatment is to increase in a synergistic way the effect of combined radiation and chemotherapy with acceptable tolerability, possibly as a result of a radiosensitizing effect of TMZ during radiation. Several trials have demonstrated a significant benefit of TMZ in newly diagnosed glioblastoma (GBM). Thus, chemoradiation represents the standard of care (SOC) for GBM in clinical practice[2–4] and the main control arm in clinical trials with experimental drugs.

Adjuvant Temozolomide. TMZ may also be administered adjuvantly or in the recurrent setting. Several different schedules may be employed. The most frequent schedule following chemoradiation consists of 150–200 mg/m^2 per day for day 1–5 every 28 days for six cycles. Cycle 1 is administered at 150 mg/m^2 per day and, if there is no unacceptable toxicity, this is escalated to 200 mg/m^2 per day for the remaining cycles. The O-6-methylguanine-DNA methyltransferase *(MGMT)* gene plays an important role in the clinical response to TMZ. The MGMT enzyme is involved in repairing DNA following alkylating-induced damage such as those caused by TMZ. As a result, silencing of this gene (e.g., through methylation of the *MGMT* promoter) limits the cancer cells ability to survive TMZ-induced DNA damage and is associated with improved responses. Methylation of the *MGMT* promoter is associated with a better overall survival (OS) in newly diagnosed GBM.[5] Clinical trials have also studied the use of "intensified" protocols to increase the total dose of TMZ delivered, deplete the amount of MGMT in the cell, and overcome treatment resistance.[6,7] These dose-dense regimens include schedules such as 75–100 mg/m^2 per day for 3 weeks-on and 1 week-off, or 120–150 mg/m^2 per day for 1 week-on and 1 week-off, or "continuous" administration at 50 mg/m^2 per day for 28-out-of-28 days (e.g., metronomic). These schedules did not show improvement in OS as compared with standard schedules with a major risk of toxicity (see Case 4.4: Newly diagnosed glioblastoma, later).

Other Temozolomide Regimens. Other regimens have also been studied. TMZ has been investigated in the neoadjuvant setting (before conformal RT) in both grade III astrocytomas and GBM. There was no advantage in OS in GBM. Neoadjuvant TMZ in grade III astrocytoma resulted in a longer survival at 5 years.[8] Preoperative TMZ in LGGs has also been suggested in order to decrease the tumor volume, amount of tumor infiltration, and facilitate a safer, more radical resection.[9–12]

Toxicity. In general, TMZ is well tolerated by most patients. The most frequent side effects are nausea/vomiting and fatigue. However, approximately 20% of patients discontinue TMZ due to myelosuppression, in particular for thrombocytopenia (<100,000/mm^3). Severe thrombocytopenia as defined by the common terminology criteria for adverse events (CTCAE) as grades 3 or 4 and prolonged thrombocytopenia occurs in about 5% of patients.[13] Moreover, a rare idiosyncratic reaction may appear during chemoradiation with a severe decrease of red blood cells (<2 × 10^6/mm^3), hemoglobin (<8.0 g/dL), thrombocytes (<75,000/mm^3), and febrile neutropenia (<1,000/mm^3).[14]

PCV chemotherapy: procarbazine, CCNU, and vincristine

Procarbazine (PC), lomustine (CCNU), and vincristine is a combined therapy administered in a 6-week cycle with CCNU on day 1, vincristine on days 8 and 29, and PC on days 8–21.

PC is an oral alkylating drug with modest efficacy in HGGs when used as monotherapy. Fatigue, anorexia, and myelosuppression are the most frequent adverse events. Patients must follow a tyramine-free diet to avoid an excess tyramine catecholamine reaction.

CCNU is an oral nitrosourea that is also the standard second-line chemotherapy in progressive HGGs in Europe. Toxicity includes cumulative myelosuppression, nausea/vomiting, fatigue, and, in rare cases, pulmonary fibrosis.

Vincristine is a vinca alkaloid that interferes with microtubule formation and disrupts the tumor cytoskeleton. Typical side effects are a dose-dependent sensorimotor peripheral neuropathy, myelosuppression and constipation. Vincristine is commonly used in pediatric brain cancers because of the high sensitivity of glioma cells,[15] whereas in adults it has a minor impact due to a poor penetration through the blood-brain barrier (BBB).[16]

Typically, PC + CCNU + vincristine (PCV) chemotherapy is administered as an adjuvant treatment following RT in high-risk grade II and anaplastic gliomas (see Case 4.1: Anaplastic gliomas with 1p19q co-deletion and Case 4.3: Low-grade gliomas, later) or as a second-line chemotherapy in cases of recurrent of HGGs (see Case 4.6: Treatment for recurrent high-grade gliomas, later) .

Nitrosourea chemotherapy

In addition to lomustine, fotemustine (diethyl 1-{1-[3-(2-chloroethyl)-3-nitro-soureido]ethyl} phosphonate (FTM) and carmustine (1,2-bis(2-chloroethyl)-1-nitrosourea; BCNU) are intravenous nitrosoureas used for treating CNS gliomas. These agents have favorable CNS characteristics, including high lipophilicity and low molecular weight, which makes, it easier to cross the BBB. The antitumor effect is based on alkylation of DNA and generation of cytotoxic damage. Similar to TMZ, the presence of methylation of MGMT confers a major sensitivity to FTM and BCNU. After intravenous infusion, the steady state is achieved within 45 minutes with a median half-life of 3 hours and a CSF concentration about 23% of plasma levels. The most important side effects are thrombocytopenia, leucopenia, and anemia.[17] In contrast to cytopenias with temozolomide, which often remain reversible with blood counts returning to their pre-cycle baseline with each round of treatment, cytopenias with the nitrosourea compounds can be cumulative where blood counts fail to recover to their pre-cycle baseline prior to the next treatment.

Currently, CCNU, BCNU, and FTM are employed as a second-line chemotherapy in recurrent HGGs with CCNU/BCNU used in the United States and FTM used in some European countries (including Italy). They are also used as a single agent or in combination with targeted therapy (e.g., bevacizumab) in an off-label setting (see Case 4.6: Treatment for recurrent high-grade gliomas, later).

Clinical cases

CASE 4.1 ANAPLASTIC (WHO GRADE 3) GLIOMA WITH 1P/19Q CO-DELETION

Case. A 42-year-old woman with a history of depression and chronic pain on sertraline and tramadol presented with a new contrast-enhancing lesion in the deep left frontal lobe with downward displacement of the corpus callosum and lateral ventricles. Stereotactic biopsy was performed and revealed a grade III oligodendroglioma (*IDH1* mutated, 1p/19q co-deleted, *MGMT* methylated). The patient was treated with radiation therapy (RT 59.4 Gy/33 fr) followed by adjuvant PCV chemotherapy. Prior to adjuvant chemotherapy, her antidepressant and tramadol were withheld due to concern about precipitating a tyramine-reaction from drug-drug interactions with procarbazine. She was instructed in a tyramine-free diet and chemotherapy was initiated. She suffered moderate treatment-induced nausea without emesis that responded to ondansetron premedication and she completed four cycles of adjuvant therapy with partial radiographic response to treatment. Despite normal blood counts prior to treatment, she experienced gradual onset of myelosuppression such that after cycle 4, her white blood cell count was 2.0 cells/mm^3, platelet count was 75,000 cells/mm^3, and further chemotherapy was withheld.

Teaching Points. This case highlights several important principles in the chemotherapeutic management of anaplastic gliomas including (1) the chemosensitivity of oligodendrogliomas, and (2) important treatment related toxicities of PCV chemotherapy. *IDH* mutant, 1p19q co-deleted oligodendrogliomas are among the most chemosensitive gliomas with several clinical trials having demonstrated prolonged median survival of more than 10 years with adding PCV chemotherapy to RT (see the next section). PCV chemotherapy is associated with important treatment-related toxicities and drug-drug as well as drug-diet interactions. Clinicians should be aware of the risk of a tyramine reaction in patients taking procarbazine. This catecholamine-like reaction can occur in patients who ingest or consume tyramine-containing foods or pharmacologic agents while taking PC. Patients become hypertensive often with diaphoresis, mydriasis, palpitations, headache, and chest pain. The reaction typically resolves within several hours but can be severe and require hospitalization. Patients should be counseled to avoid tyramine-containing foods including preserved meat, fish, cheese, alcohol, and other protein-rich foods.

Review of trials for co-deleted anaplastic oligodendroglioma

Interest in chemotherapy for oligodendrogliomas increased in the 1990s when responses to PCV were initially reported in small series of patients with recurrent oligodendrogliomas and oligoastrocytomas.[18,19] This was subsequently confirmed in prospective trials later.[20,21] Based on these findings, several clinical trials were designed to determine the role of PCV chemotherapy for managing anaplastic oligodendrogliomas.

RTOG 9402 Trial. The RTOG 9402 trial[22] randomized patients with anaplastic gliomas to RT alone or neoadjuvant PCV followed by RT. It demonstrated that patients with anaplastic 1p/19q co-deleted oligodendrogliomas (i.e., co-deleted) live longer than those with absence of 1p/19q co-deletion (i.e., non–co-deleted) after the addition of PCV to RT. For patients who received PCV/RT, those with co-deleted oligodendrogliomas had a median survival of 14.7 years compared with only 2.6 years with non–co-deleted tumors (hazard ratio [HR] 0.36; 95% confidence interval [CI] 0.23–0.5; $p < .001$). Similarly, in patients randomized to RT alone, those with co-deleted oligodendrogliomas had a longer median survival of 7.3 years compared with only 2.7 years in non–co-deleted tumors (HR 0.40; 95% CI 0.27–0.60; $p < .001$). The addition of PCV significantly improved overall survival in co-deleted anaplastic oligodendrogliomas. Median OS for patients treated with PCV/RT (14.7 years) was twice that of patients receiving RT alone (7.3 years; HR 0.59; 95% CI 0.37–0.95; $p = 0.03$).

EORTC 26951 Trial. The European Organization for Research and Treatment of Cancer (EORTC) 26951 trial[23] similarly randomized patients with anaplastic glioma to RT alone or RT followed by adjuvant PCV. This study showed a prolonged

OS in the RT/PCV arm (42.3 months) compared with RT alone (30.6 months; HR 0.75; 95% CI 0.60–0.95). In co-deleted tumors, OS was not reached in the RT/PCV group as compared with 112 months in the RT group (HR 0.56; 95% CI 0.31–1.03).These studies established the role of PCV chemotherapy for anaplastic oligodendrogliomas with 1p19q co-deletion.

Interestingly, in the EORTC 26951 trial, only 30% of patients completed the planned six cycles of PCV due to hematologic toxicity. Considering the safety profile of PCV schedule, two surveys have shown that clinicians prefer to use TMZ rather than PCV.[24,25] Although the German NOA-4 trial on grade II gliomas did not display any difference between PCV chemotherapy and TMZ,[26,27] it is still not known whether TMZ may replace PCV. This is currently under investigation by the CODEL trial (ClinicalTrials.gov Identifier: NCT00887146), which compares RT plus PCV versus RT plus concomitant and adjuvant TMZ for co-deleted oligodendrogliomas (both grade II and grade III).

A critical issue with regard to chemoradiation is the risk of cognitive dysfunctions in long-term survivors due to radiation neurotoxicity.[28] Oligodendroglial tumors are considered chemosensitive. Median survival with maximum therapy is >10 years. Thus, toxicity from treatment is a major patient and provider concern. Neoadjuvant chemotherapy with alkylating agents could be used as the initial up-front treatment in 1p/19q co-deleted oligodendrogliomas in order to delay salvage RT to progression.[29–31] This is currently being investigated in the POLCA trial, which compares initial treatment with RT and PCV versus PCV alone (RT being postponed at the time of progression) in 1p/19q co-deleted anaplastic oligodendrogliomas (ClinicalTrials.gov Identifier: NCT02444000).

Clinical Pearls and Treatment Recommendations in Daily Practice

Taken together, the long-term results of the RTOG 9402 and the EORTC 26951 trials suggest that 1p/19q co-deletion identifies slow-growing tumors that respond to chemotherapy and may be controlled for many years with RT plus PCV. Hence, combined treatment with RT and PCV should be the SOC in co-deleted anaplastic oligodendrogliomas as defined by the recent WHO 2016 classification (see Chapter 1 for more discussion of histopathologic classification). Some have also suggested that diffuse gliomas with astrocytic phenotype (that by definition are *IDH 1-2* mutated) should be treated similar to 1p/19q co-deleted anaplastic oligodendrogliomas.

CASE 4.2 ANAPLASTIC (WHO GRADE 3) GLIOMAS WITHOUT 1P/19Q CO-DELETION

Case. A 35-year-old woman presented with a tonic-clonic seizure on the left side. Brain MRI showed a bilateral frontal T2/fluid attenuated inversion recovery (FLAIR) lesion without contrast enhancement. The patient underwent a subtotal resection (Fig. 4.1A) and was started an antiepileptic therapy with levetiracetam 2000 mg/day. The histological examination revealed a grade III astrocytoma (*IDH1* mutated, 1p/19q non–co-deleted, *MGMT* unmethylated). The patient was enrolled in the CATNON trial and was randomized for the arm 3 (RT 59.4 Gy/33 fr plus adjuvant TMZ 150–200 mg/m^2 for 5 consecutive days/28 days for 12 cycles). The brain MRI after the completion of 12 cycles of chemotherapy displayed a partial response on T2/FLAIR sequences without contrast enhancement on T1-weighted sequence and lower relative cerebral blood volume (rCBV) value on perfusion MRI (Fig. 4.1B).

Teaching Points. This case highlights the fact that, unlike co-deleted anaplastic oligodendrogliomas which tend to be extremely chemosensitive, similar results have not been observed for non–co-deleted anaplastic astrocytomas. The majority of these tumors will be *IDH* mutated with variable *MGMT* promoter methylation. As in this case, following maximal safe resection, radiation therapy remains the backbone of adjuvant treatment. The role of chemotherapy has been and continues to be investigated in clinical trials with initial results suggesting a benefit, particularly in *IDH* mutant gliomas.

Review of trials for non–co-deleted anaplastic astrocytoma

RTOG 9402 and EORTC 26951. The use of PCV chemotherapy for non–co-deleted anaplastic gliomas was assessed in both the RTOG 9402 and EORTC 26951 trials. Both studies did not show a statistically significant OS benefit of adjuvant RT plus PCV as compared with RT alone in patients without 1p/19q co-deletion. Median OS was similar for both treatment groups in the RTOG 9402 trial (2.6 years vs 2.7 years, respectively; HR 0.85; 95% CI 0.58–1.23; $p = 0.39$) and in the EORTC 26951 trial (25 months vs 21 months; HR 0.83; 95% CI 0.62–1.10). These data highlight the conventional opinion that non–co-deleted tumors are characterized by a lower sensitivity to chemotherapy and worse prognosis than 1p/19q co-deleted gliomas.

CATNON. Following these studies, the role of chemotherapy in newly diagnosed non–co-deleted anaplastic gliomas was further investigated by the phase III EORTC 26053-22054 CATNON trial (Concurrent and Adjuvant Temozolomide Chemotherapy in Non-1p/19q Deleted Anaplastic Glioma, ClinicalTrials.gov Identifier: NCT00626990). This trial was designed to address the role of adjuvant TMZ for the treatment of non–co-deleted anaplastic gliomas. In this study, patients were randomized 1:1:1:1 into four different treatment arms: (1) RT alone (59.4 Gy in 33 fractions); (2) RT plus adjuvant TMZ (12 4-week cycles of 150–200 mg/m^2 per day); (3) RT plus concomitant TMZ (75 mg/m^2 per day during radiotherapy); (4) RT plus concomitant and adjuvant TMZ (Stupp regimen). The first interim analysis of the CATNON trial showed a significant advantage in progression-free survival (PFS) for patients receiving adjuvant TMZ (42.8 months; 95% CI 28.6–60.6; 5-year PFS 43.1%) over those not receiving adjuvant TMZ (19.0 months; 95% CI 14.4–24.6; 5-year PFS 24.3%). The same was true for OS (not reached; 5-year OS 55.9% vs 41.1 months; 95% CI 36.6–60.7; 5-year OS 44.1%). The multivariable analysis showed that age >50 years (HR 4.04; 95% CI 2.78–5.87;

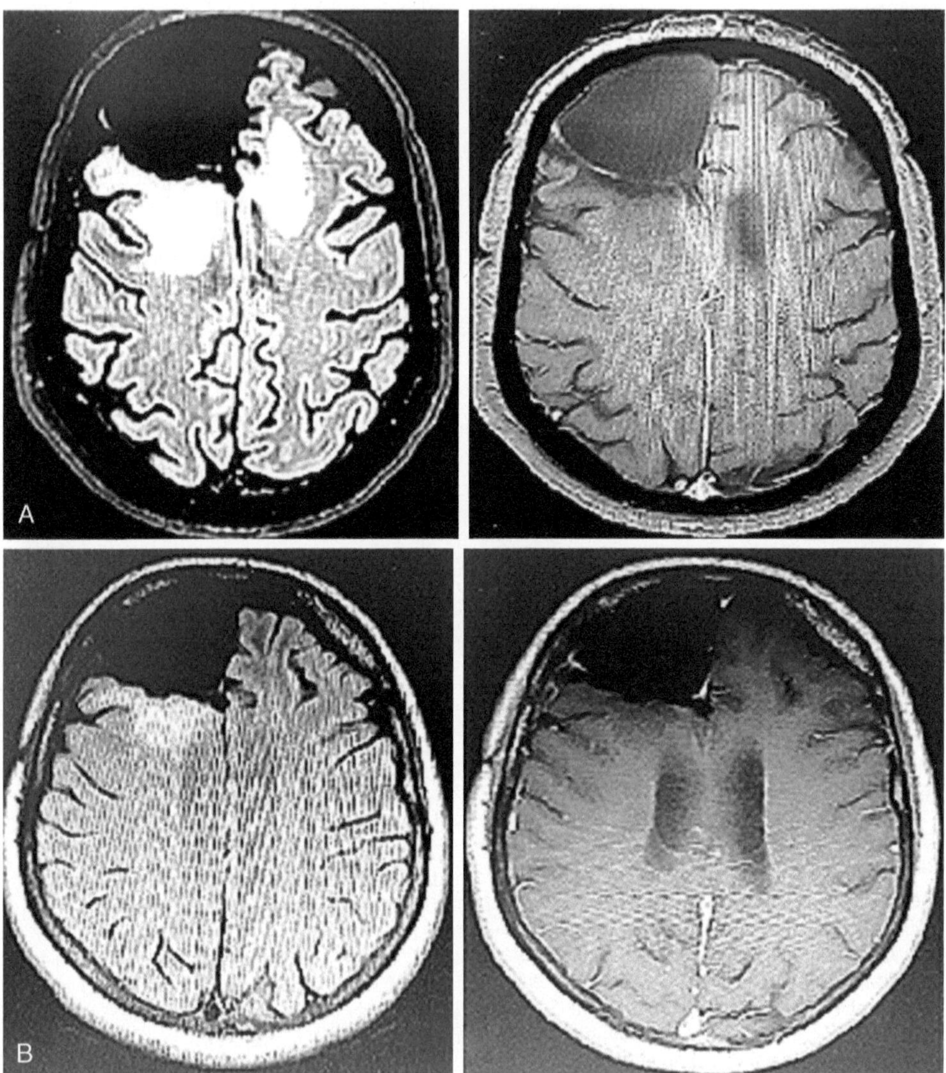

Fig. 4.1 (A) Brain MRI before (A) and after radiotherapy combined with adjuvant temozolomide for 12 cycles. (B) Partial response on T2/FLAIR sequences without contrast enhancement on T1-weighted sequence.

$p = 0.0001$) was a risk factor for poorer survival, whereas administration of adjuvant TMZ (HR 0.65; 95% CI 0.45–0.93; p 0.0014) and *MGMT* promoter methylation (HR 0.49; 95% CI 0.26–0.93; p = 0.0031) were associated with longer survival.[32]

Clinical Pearls and Treatment Recommendations in Daily Practice

The SOC for 1p/19q non–co-deleted anaplastic gliomas includes maximal safe resection, RT, and TMZ-based chemotherapy. Some questions still remain, including the specific timing and sequence of TMZ and the role of molecular profiling, to inform personalization of treatment.

In current practice, these patients may receive RT followed by 12 cycles of adjuvant TMZ or RT with concurrent TMZ followed by 6 cycles of adjuvant TMZ. A meta-analysis on GBM has suggested that the efficacy of 6 rather than 12 cycles of adjuvant TMZ are equivalent.[33] However, it is unknown whether six cycles of TMZ may lead to the same outcome in PFS and OS for anaplastic grade III gliomas. Moreover, prior trials were started before the identification of the isocitrate dehydrogenase (*IDH*) 1/2 mutations as a marker of glioma of prognostic significance.[34] Further retrospective molecular analysis, including *IDH1/2* and *MGMT* methylation status, may help to identify those patients who will benefit most from TMZ. Lastly, further follow-up is needed to evaluate the impact of concomitant TMZ in improving OS. In particular, the second-interim analysis of the CATNON trial revealed that concurrent chemoradiation does not provide a significant increase in OS. However, a trend toward a benefit of concomitant chemoradiation is observed in *IDH* mutated tumors, but not in *IDH* wild-type tumors.[35]

CASE 4.3 LOW-GRADE (WHO GRADE 2) GLIOMAS

Case. In June 2005, a 50-year-old man had partial seizures with secondary generalization. Brain MRI showed a mild patchy enhancing lesion on the right temporo-insular lobe without significant mass effect (Fig. 4.2A). The patient was started on antiepileptic therapy (oxcarbazepine 900 mg/day and levetiracetam 2000 mg/day) and underwent a subtotal resection. The histological examination revealed a grade II oligodendroglioma (*IDH1* mutated, 1p/19q co-deleted, *MGMT* methylated). Considering the favorable molecular profile and the presence of residual tumor, the patient received up-front chemotherapy with 1 week-on/1 week-off TMZ (150 mg/m^2 per day). The patient achieved a significant reduction of seizure frequency, as well as a complete response on contrast enhanced T1-weighted sequence and minor response on T2/FLAIR sequence in brain MRI (RANO criteria) (Fig. 4.2B) after 12 cycles of chemotherapy. The clinical and radiological response lasted until December 2015.

Teaching Points. Low-grade gliomas are a heterogeneous group of tumors that include pure oligodendrogliomas, *IDH* mutant astrocytomas, and *IDH* wild-type astrocytomas. Mixed oligoastrocytomas have essentially been removed by integrating molecular assessment into glioma classification (see Chapter 1, Cases 1.2 and 1.3 for further discussion of molecular classification of low-grade gliomas). This case highlights the role of chemotherapy for low-grade gliomas. Historically, LGGs were thought to not be chemosensitive to alkylating therapy due to their slow-growing biology. However, recent clinical trials have demonstrated favorable outcomes in patients with 1p19q co-deleted oligodendrogliomas and frequently for *IDH* mutant astrocytomas, compared with *IDH* wild-type low-grade gliomas which have largely not been responsive to chemotherapy.

Review of trials for low-grade glioma

Three pivotal phase III trials inform the chemotherapy management of LGGs including EORTC 22845, RTOG 9802, and EORTC 22033-26033. Historically, RT was the initial treatment for all low-grade gliomas.

EORTC 22845 Trial. This phase III trial addressed the question of timing of radiation for LGGs. Patients with LGG were randomized to early versus delayed RT. Early RT improved median PFS compared with delayed RT at tumor progression (early RT: 5.3 years; delayed RT: 3.4 years; HR 0.59; 95% CI 0.45–0.77; $p < .0001$) and improved seizure control at 1 year. However, median OS was not different (early: 7.4 years; delayed RT: 7.2 years; HR 0.97; 95% CI 0.71–1.34; $p = 0.872$.[36]

RTOG 9802 Trial. In 1998, the phase III RTOG 9802 trial was launched by the Radiation Therapy Oncology Group comparing RT with or without adjuvant PCV. The publication of a preliminary analysis of this trial in 2012 did not report an OS advantage with the addition of chemotherapy despite an improvement of PFS.[37] Notably, OS and PFS curves matched for all patients between years 0 and 2, but separated significantly after 2 years, favoring RT + PCV. A similar trend was noted for OS. With a longer follow-up, a statistically significant benefit in OS for the RT plus PCV arm was observed (13.3 years, 95% CI 10.6–not reached; 5-year OS 72%, 95% CI 64–80) as compared with RT alone (7.8 years, 95% CI 6.1–9.8; 5-year OS 63%, 95% CI 55–72; HR 0.59, $p = 0.003$). In parallel, patients who received RT plus PCV displayed a longer PFS (median PFS 10.4 years, 95% CI 6.1–not reached) than those treated with RT alone (median PFS 4.0 years, 95% CI 3.1–5.5; HR 0.50; $p < 0.001$). Patients with *IDH1* mutation had a longer OS (13.1 years, 95% CI 10.1–not reached) than those without *IDH1* mutation (5.1 years, 95% CI 1.9–11.5). The longest survival was observed in *IDH1* mutant gliomas who received RT and PCV. Multivariable analysis revealed that age <40 years, oligodendroglial tumor, and chemoradiation are favorable prognostic factors for both PFS and OS. *IDH1* mutation was correlated with a better PFS, but not statistically significant for OS.[38]

EORTC 22033-26033. The risk of a neurocognitive impairment in long-term survivors after 8–12 years following RT[39] led a number of clinicians to postpone the use of RT in favor of up-front chemotherapy. In this regard, the aim of the phase III EORTC 22033-26033 study investigated whether the dose-dense TMZ was superior to standard radiation therapy in high-risk LGGs. No difference in median PFS was observed between the two arms (TMZ arm: 39 months; 95% CI 35–44; RT arm: 46 months; 95% CI 40–56; HR 1.16; 95% CI 0.9–1.5, $p = 0.22$). For patients with *IDH1/2* mutation and 1p/19q co-deletion, outcomes were similar (TMZ arm: 55.0 months; RT arm: 61.6 months). However, for patients with *IDH1/2* mutation and absence of 1p/19q co-deletion, median PFS was longer for those receiving RT (55 months, 95% CI 48–66) compared with TMZ (36 months, 95% CI 28.4–47; HR 0.53; 95% CI 0.35–0.82; $p = 0.0043$).[40] These results suggest that RT may be superior to chemotherapy in astrocytomas. However, data on OS are needed to confirm this preliminary analysis.

A retrospective analysis conducted by the US National Cancer Database showed that chemotherapy alone may be more effective compared with RT alone in oligodendroglial tumors, but not in astrocytomas.[41] Furthermore, a retrospective study of the US National Cancer Database has reported that chemotherapy alone confers a similar OS compared with chemoradiation,[42] but the median follow-up was short (4.6 years) with inability to reveal the late effect of chemoradiation.

TMZ alone after surgery may represent an option, especially in oligodendroglial tumors that are more chemosensitive, in order to delay RT and the risk of cognitive impairment. Wahl

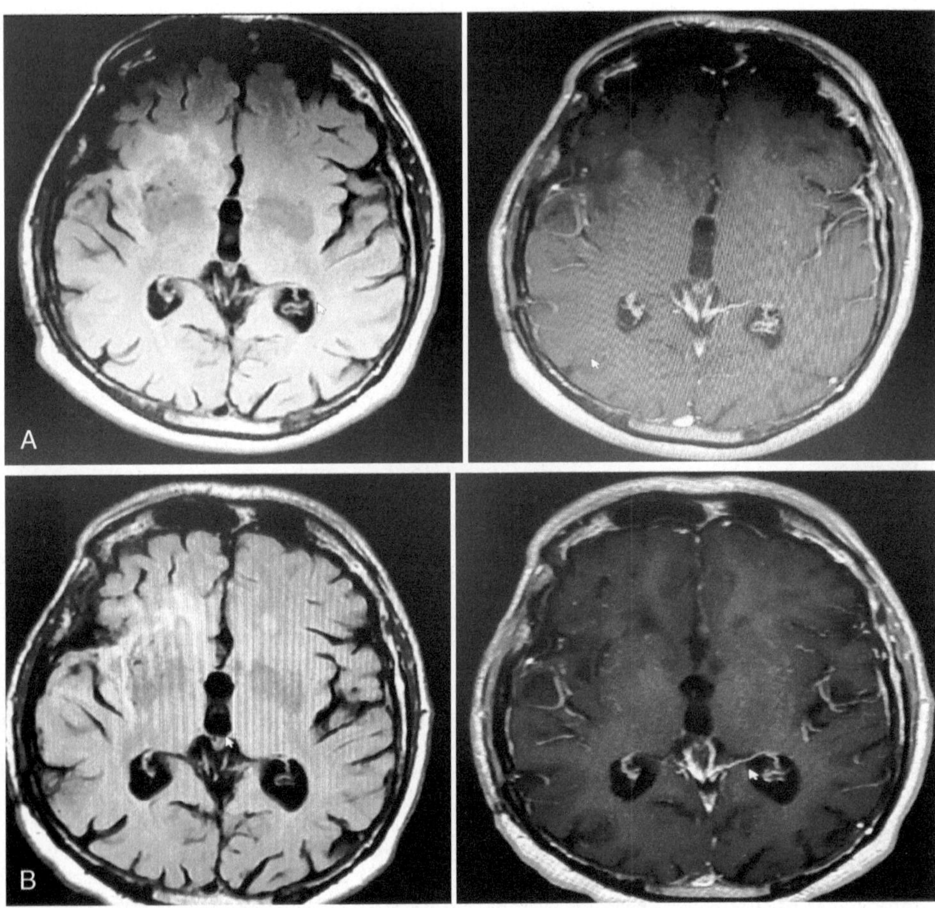

Fig. 4.2 Brain MRI before (A) and after 1 week-on/1 week-off chemotherapy with temozolomide (B): a complete response on contrast T1-weighted sequence and minor response on T2/FLAIR sequence in brain MRI.

and colleagues reported a median PFS and OS of 4.2 and 9.7 years, respectively, in a cohort of high-risk LGGs treated with TMZ alone following initial surgery.[43] Similarly, the phase II AINO study showed a PFS of 4.2 years and an OS of 9.8 years in oligodendrogliomas *IDH*-mutant and 1p/19q co-deleted, which are comparable to the EORTC (4.6 years) and Wahl (4.9 years) studies.[44] Interestingly, both studies demonstrated a median time to delay of RT of 5.8 and 8.2 years, respectively.

Clinical Pearls and Treatment Recommendations in Daily Practice

Like anaplastic gliomas, certain histomolecular LGG subtypes are chemotherapy responsive. The recent phase II and III trials provide helpful guidance. First, RT alone may be comparable to TMZ alone as initial therapy for certain LGGs, particularly those with *IDH* mutation, given that PFS of patients receiving TMZ alone in the EORTC 22033-26033 is similar to that of patients treated with RT alone in EORTC 22845 and RTOG 9802 trials. Second, PCV with RT should be considered SOC for LGGs, particularly oligodendrogliomas. However, the impact of combined treatment on neurocognitive functions and quality of life is still unknown. Whether a sequential approach, consisting of TMZ as initial treatment with reoperation and/or RT plus PCV at tumor relapse, has the same impact of early RT plus PCV in balancing survival and cognitive preservation for patients with high-risk co-deleted oligodendrogliomas is unsolved, and can justify the use of chemotherapy alone as initial therapy. Lastly, both TMZ and PCV may favorably impact seizures and are considered as a biomarker of treatment efficacy.[31,45,46]

CASE 4.4 NEWLY DIAGNOSED GLIOBLASTOMA

Case. In March 2015, a 57-year-old man reported mental confusion, memory impairment, and blurred vision on the left eye. Karnofsky Performance Status (KPS) was 80/100 (i.e., normal activity, some signs and symptoms of disease). Brain MRI showed an enhancing lesion in the left temporal lobe with surrounding edema (Fig. 4.3A). The patient underwent a subtotal resection. Pathology was read as glioblastoma, WHO grade IV, *IDH* wild type, *MGMT* promoter methylated. An MRI performed after 1 month from surgery showed a conspicuous residual tumor (Fig. 4.3B). The patient started conformal RT (60 Gy/30 fr) associated with concomitant TMZ (75 mg/m^2) and adjuvant TMZ for six cycles according to the Stupp regimen. Brain MRI after the concomitant and adjuvant treatment displayed a complete response on the gadolinium T1-weighted sequence and a partial response on T2/FLAIR sequences (RANO Criteria; Fig. 4.3C), respectively.

Teaching Points. This case presents the typical chemotherapeutic treatment regimen for patients with GBM, which includes concurrent chemotherapy followed by six cycles of adjuvant chemotherapy. Methylation of the *MGMT* promoter is both prognostic of improved survival as well as predictive

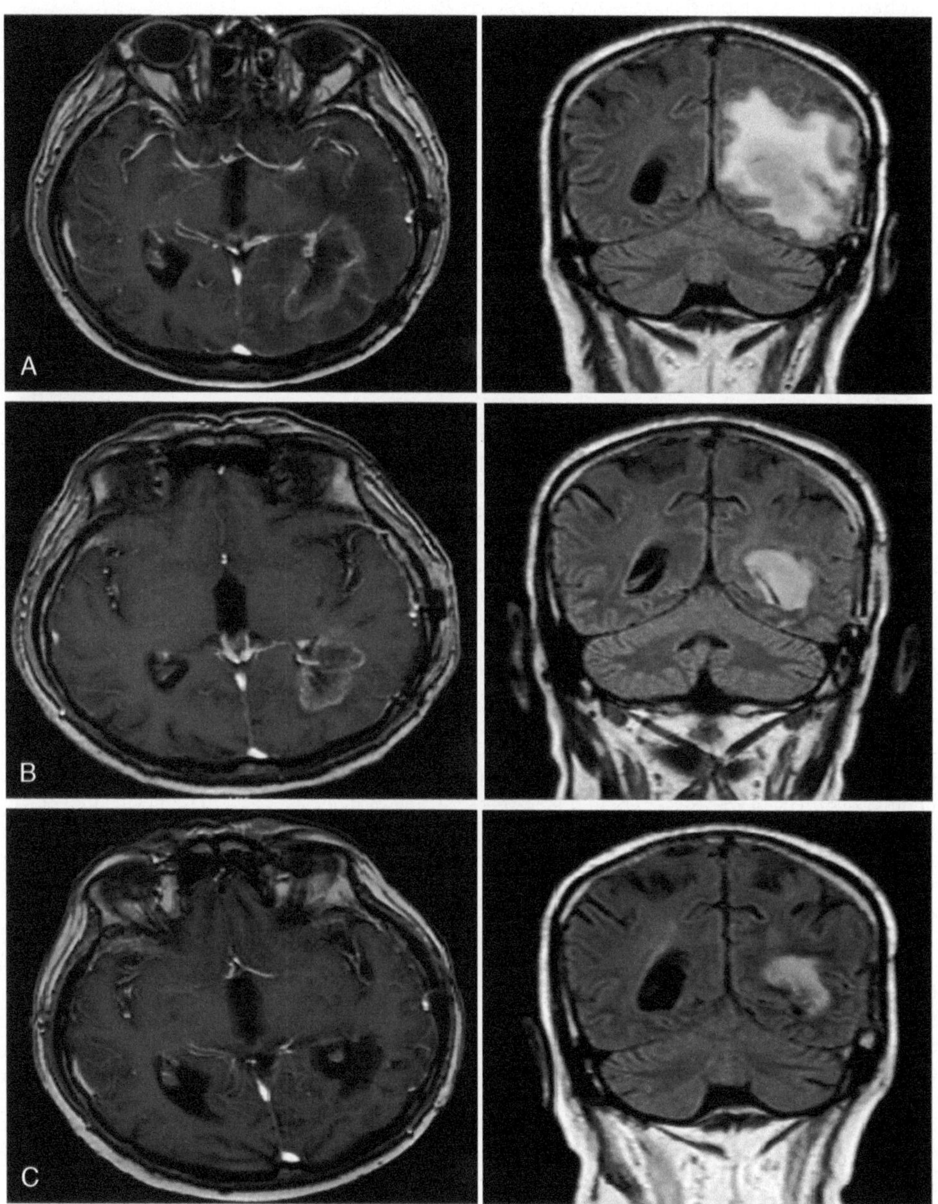

Fig. 4.3 Brain MRI before surgery (A), after 1 month from subtotal resection (B) and following chemoradiation according to Stupp protocol (C): a complete response on the gadolinium T1-weighted sequence and a partial response on T2/FLAIR sequences.

of a more favorable response to chemotherapy. In this case, imaging showed complete resolution of the enhancing disease and partial response of the infiltrative T2-hyperintense disease.

Review of Trials for Glioblastoma

Although a pooled analysis of six randomized trials of RT versus no RT after surgery showed a significant survival advantage for RT,[47,48] the survival benefit of RT in GBM still remains limited with a low rate of long-term survivors. The addition of nitrosoureas after RT confers a modest improvement of OS (1-year OS 35%) according to a meta-analysis of 12 randomized trials.[49] Based on the antitumor activity of TMZ in the treatment of recurrent HGG[50–52] and the encouraging data from a pilot phase II study on the association of RT and TMZ,[2] in 2004 the European Organization for Research and Treatment of Cancer (EORTC) 26981-22981/National Cancer Institute of Canada Clinical Trial Group (NCIC) conducted a randomized phase III study.

EORTC 26981-22981. This study was designed to evaluate the addition to RT (60 Gy/30 fractions for 5 days per week for 6 consecutive weeks) of concomitant (75 mg/m^2 from the first to the last day of radiotherapy) and adjuvant TMZ (150–200 mg/m^2 for 5 days every 28 days for six cycles).[3] The median survival benefit was 2.5 months with a median OS of 14.6 months (95% CI 13.2–16.8) and a 2-year OS of 26.5% (95% CI 21.2–31.7) in the chemoradiation arm as compared with 12.1 months (95% CI 11.2–13.0) and 10.4% (95% CI 6.8–14.1) for RT alone. A similar advantage was achieved in median PFS (6.9 months; 95% CI 5.8–8.2) following chemoradiation versus RT alone (5.0 months; 95% CI 4.2–5.5). Furthermore, patients whose tumors had *MGMT* promoter methylation displayed a longer OS following chemoradiation (median OS 21.7 months; 2-year OS 46.0%) than those patients with unmethylated *MGMT* promoter (median OS 12.7 months; 2-year OS 13.8%).[5] The 5-year analysis of the EORTC/NCIC trial confirmed the benefit of chemoradiation in terms of OS in *MGMT* methylated patients (median OS 23.4 months; 2-year OS 48.9%; 3-year OS 27.7%; 4-year OS 22.1%) as compared with the *MGMT* unmethylated patients (median OS 12.6 months; 2-year OS 14.8%; 3-year OS 11.1%; 4-year OS 11.1%). Thus, the methylation of *MGMT* promoter has been considered as a strong predictive factor for response to alkylating agents.[4]

In many countries, the Stupp regimen is extended over six adjuvant cycles of TMZ with the expectation to delay tumor recurrence. However, continuing TMZ beyond six cycles has slightly improved PFS (12.2 months for > 6 cycles vs 10.4 months for ≤ 6 cycles), especially among patients with MGMT methylation, but has no impact on OS (27.0 months vs 24.9 months, respectively).[53] Considering the cumulative risk of TMZ side effects and the onset of resistance to alkylating agents,[54] an extension of adjuvant TMZ beyond six cycles is not currently recommended for GBM. Similarly, the use of intensified TMZ, such as dose-dense TMZ (7 days on–7 days off) or "metronomic" schedule (50 mg/m^2 per day continuously), has not improved OS compared with TMZ standard schedule, regardless of the *MGMT* methylation status.[55,56]

AVAGLIO & RTOG-0825. The activity of bevacizumab (BEV), a human monoclonal antibody targeting vascular endothelial growth factor (VEGF)-A, has been investigated in combination with Stupp regimen in newly diagnosed GBM in two different phase III trials (AVAGLIO and RTOG-0825).[57,58] In both trials, PFS was prolonged in the BEV arm (median PFS 10.6 vs 7.2 months in AVAGLIO; 10.7 months vs 7.3 months in RTOG-0825), whereas no advantage in OS was reported in newly diagnosed GBM.[59,60]

Clinical Pearls and Treatment Recommendations in Daily Practice

The SOC for GBM consists of maximal safe resection followed by RT plus concomitant and adjuvant TMZ for six cycles (Stupp regimen), regardless of *MGMT* methylation status. Although *MGMT* methylated patients achieve a longer PFS and OS after chemoradiation, outside of clinical trials, there is lack of alternative treatments for *MGMT* unmethylated patients.

CASE 4.5 GLIOBLASTOMA IN ELDERLY PATIENTS

Case. In January 2018, a 78-year-old woman presented with headache, aphasia, and severe right hemiparesis. KPS was 60/100 (i.e., requires occasional assistance, able to care for most of personal needs). Brain MRI showed a contrast-enhancing lesion on the left fronto-temporal lobe with surrounding edema (Fig. 4.4A). The patient refused surgery. An MRI spectroscopy was performed with evidence of a choline peak and a reduction of N-acetyl aspartate (NAA) associated with higher perfusion values (rCBV >4.0 in comparison with normal tissue). These findings suggested a diagnosis of GBM. The patient began hypofractionated conformal RT (40 Gy/15 fr) associated with concomitant TMZ (75 mg/m^2) and adjuvant TMZ for six cycles according to Perry schedule. Brain MRI following treatment displayed a partial response (RANO Criteria; Fig. 4.4B) with a reduction of tumor on both T2/FLAIR and gadolinium T1-weighted sequences. The patient had a neurological improvement with disappearance of aphasia and right strength deficit, achieving a KPS of 90.

Teaching Points. Whereas in general glioma is a disease of younger adults in the fourth to seventh decades, elderly patients whose age at diagnosis is >65 years are also affected. These patients are frequently not included in many clinical trials and may not tolerate aggressive therapy similarly to younger patients. This case highlights the treatment options and controversies in managing elderly patients with GBM including (1) whether to pursue shorter course hypofractionated radiation therapy (e.g., 40 Gy) compared with full dose radiation (e.g., 60 Gy, see Chapter 2 for principles of radiation therapy), and (2) how to incorporate TMZ chemotherapy in elderly patients with GBM, which has been studied in several clinical trials.

Review of trials for elderly GBM

Management of GBM in elderly patients (>65 years) is more difficult due to a poor prognosis, frequent coexistence of

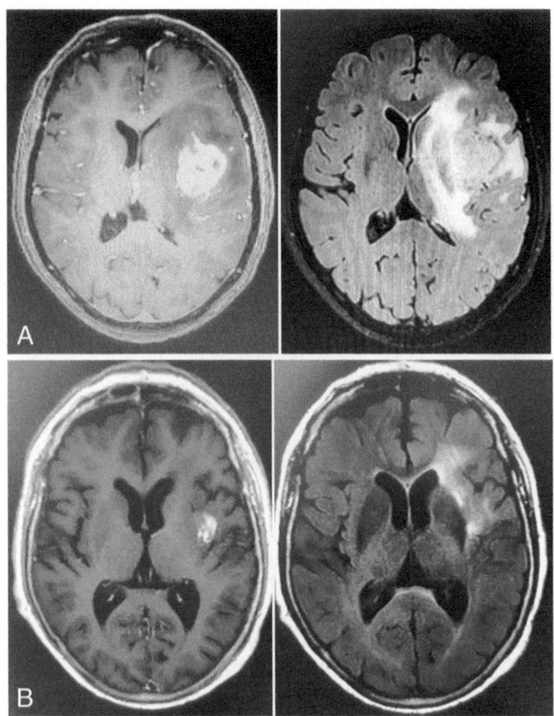

Fig. 4.4 Brain MRI before (A) and after short-course radiation associated with concomitant and adjuvant temozolomide for six cycles (B): a partial response with a reduction of alteration in both T2/FLAIR and gadolinium T1-weighted sequences.

comorbidities and concomitant medications, and an increased risk of side effects from antineoplastic therapy.[61] One trial reported that OS is significantly longer among elderly patients who received RT alone than those treated with palliative care,[62] whereas another two studies (NOA-08 and Nordic trials) showed that RT alone or TMZ alone confer a similar outcome in terms of OS,[63,64] suggesting that these patients could be treated with hypofractionated RT alone, leaving TMZ monotherapy for those with *MGMT* promoter methylation.

Hypofractionated RT and Temozolomide in the Elderly. A new SOC in elderly GBM has been recently validated by Perry and colleagues with the NCT00482677 trial, which studied short-course hypofractionated radiation (40 Gy/15 fractions) combined with concomitant and adjuvant TMZ. This trial showed an improvement of OS in patients treated with RT plus TMZ as compared with RT alone (median OS 9.3 months vs 7.6 month, respectively). Interestingly, *MGMT* unmethylated tumors also had some benefit in OS from combined treatment (median OS 10.0 months).[65] This trial enrolled a so-called fit elderly population, characterized by good cognitive performance (median Mini-Mental State Examination [MMSE] 27) and Eastern Cooperative Oncology Group (ECOG) score (0–1 76.8%) and who had undergone extensive surgery (gross-total resection 68.3%) prior to treatment. It is unknown whether the Perry schedule has similar impact in frail elderly patients with worse prognostic factors.

Clinical Pearls and Treatment Recommendations in Daily Practice

Short-course hypofractionated radiation therapy along with concomitant and adjuvant TMZ is recommended in elderly patients who undergo gross-total or subtotal resection with a good performance. For frail elderly patients with poor performance status, treatment based on MGMT promoter methylated status may be considered, i.e., TMZ monotherapy for patients with methylated MGMT, and RT alone or best supportive care for MGMT unmethylated frail elderly patients.

CASE 4.6 TREATMENT FOR RECURRENT HIGH-GRADE GLIOMAS

Case. A 66-year-old woman with a diagnosis of GBM (*IDH1/2* wild type, *MGMT* methylated) received standard chemoradiation according to Stupp protocol from April 2016 to January 2017. Brain MRI following six cycles of standard schedule of TMZ showed progressive disease (Fig. 4.5A). Clinical trials were considered but not available, and the patient started fotemustine (FTM, Addeo schedule for five administrations, induction phase).[66] Brain MRI following the induction phase displayed a significant reduction of the enhancing lesion (partial response according to RANO criteria), as well as a decrease of T2/FLAIR hyperintensity in the frontal lobes (Fig. 4.5B). The patient underwent maintenance phase of FTM for a total of 7 monthly infusions.

Teaching Points. This case demonstrates the therapeutic options for patients with recurrent HGG and highlights the importance of timing of recurrence in selecting optimal treatments.

The main therapeutic options for recurrent HGGs include (1) rechallenge with TMZ either at standard dose or dose intensified TMZ, (2) nitrosourea-based regimens, and (3) BEV (off-label).[67] Responses to alkylating regimens are generally more favorable in patients with MGMT methylated tumors. Several phase II trials (RESCUE, NCT00657267, and BR12) have not demonstrated a survival advantage with using dose-intensified TMZ in recurrent GBM, regardless of the type of schedule.[68]

Temozolomide for Recurrent HGG. Patients who progress months to years after completing adjuvant TMZ can be re-challenged with TMZ particularly for *IDH* mutated or *MGMT* promoter methylated HGGs. In contrast, patients who progress during or within 3 months of completing TMZ often show poor response to continued TMZ-based therapy or TMZ rechallenge. In these patients, second-line or salvage regimens are considered.

Nitrosourea for Recurrent HGG. Although CCNU is considered the SOC after the failure of TMZ and the control arm in clinical trials focused on recurrent HGGs, the response rate ranges from 4.3% to 8.9% with a median PFS of 7–10 months and 6 month-PFS of 19.9–24.5%.[69,70] In Europe, FTM is the second-line chemotherapy in recurrent grade III

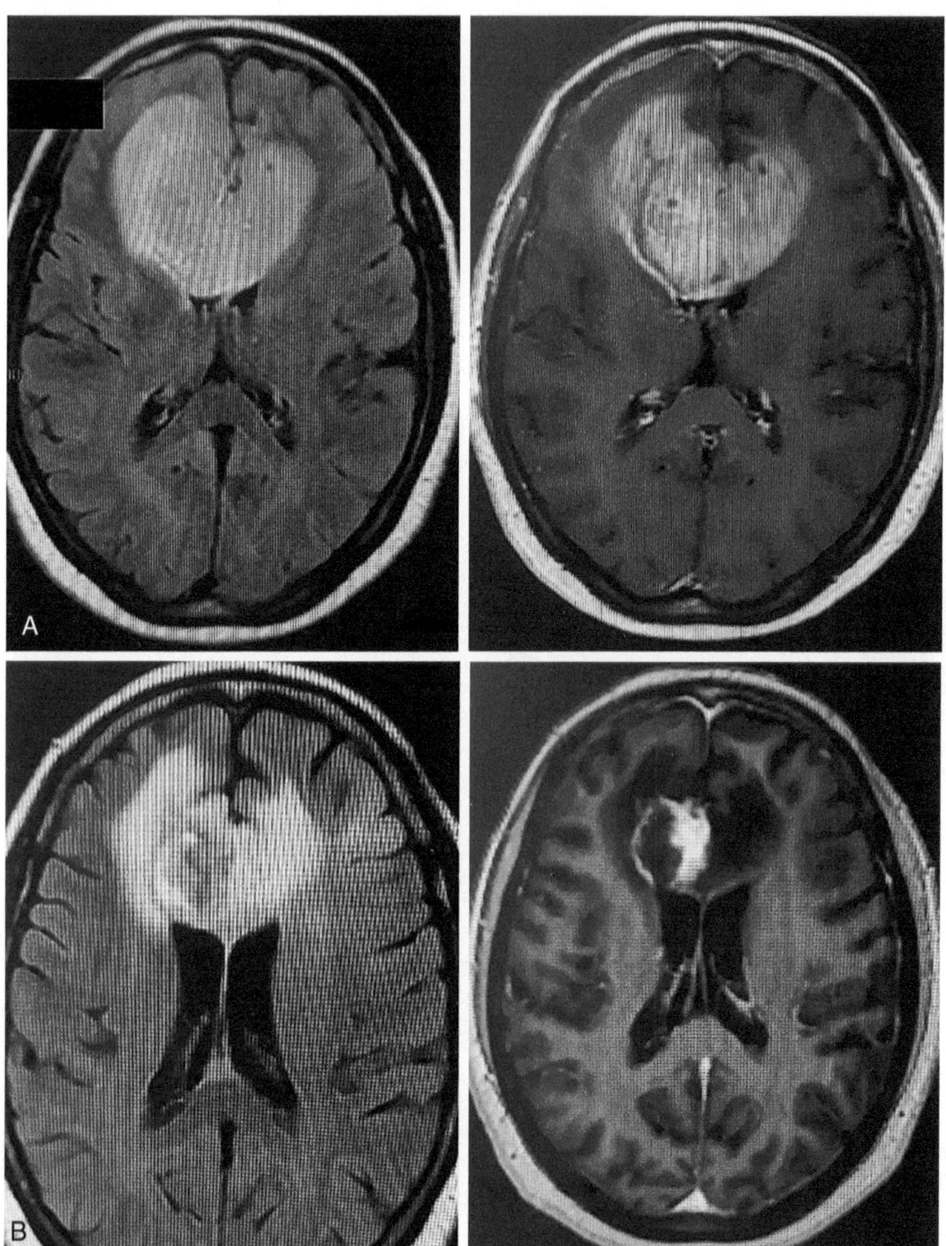

Fig. 4.5 Brain MRI before (A) and following fotemustine 80 mg/m^2 biweekly according to Addeo schedule (induction phase) (B): a significant reduction of the enhancing lesion, as well a decrease of T2/FLAIR hyperintensity in the frontal lobes.

astrocytomas and GBM. The dosage may range from 60 to 100 mg/m^2 every 2 weeks (induction phase) or 4 weeks (maintenance phase) achieving a 6-month PFS of 20.9–61%, a median PFS of 6.0–6.7 months, and a median OS of 9.5–11.1 months. Table 4.1 summarizes the most important studies on FTM used alone or in association with other compounds.

Bevacizumab for Recurrent HGG. In the US, BEV may be used in recurrent GBM based on results of the BRAIN trial, which displayed a benefit in terms of OS as a single agent (median OS 9.2 months) or in combination with irinotecan (median OS 8.7 months) with a good tolerability.[84]

Table 4.1 Studies on fotemustine used alone or in combination with other drugs in recurrent high-grade gliomas

Authors	Number of patients	Types of gliomas	FTM schedule	PFS	OS
Scoccianti et al., 2008[70]	27	GBM	Standard[a]	5.7 months	9.1 months
Silvani et al., 2008[71]	54	GBM	PC 450 mg day 1–2, 300 mg day 3; FTM 110 mg/m^2 day 3 every 5 weeks	4.8 months	7.2 months
Brandes et al., 2009[72]	43	GBM	Standard[a]	1.7 months	6 months
Fabrini et al., 2009[73]	50	GBM	Standard[a]	6.1 months	8.1 months
Fabi et al., 2010[74]	40	GBM Grade III gliomas	FTM 60 mg/m^2 weekly for 3 cycles followed by a 5-week rest period; then FTM 75 mg/m^2 every 3 weeks	3.0 months	6 months
Addeo et al., 2011[65]	40	GBM	FTM 80 mg/m^2 every 2 weeks for 5 cycles followed by a 5-week rest period; then FTM 80 mg/m^2 every 4 weeks	6.7 months	11 months
Soffietti et al., 2012[75]	32	Grade III gliomas	FTM 75 mg/m^2 day 1–8 + BEV 10 mg/kg day 1–15 followed by a 3-week rest period; then FTM 75 mg/m^2 + BEV 10 mg/day 1 every 3 weeks	5 months	8.6 months
Santoni et al., 2013[76]	65	GBM	Standard[a]	4.2 months	7.1 months
Soffietti et al., 2014[77]	54	GBM	FTM 75 mg/m^2 day 1–8 + BEV 10 mg/kg day 1–15 followed by a 3-week rest period; then FTM 75 mg/m^2 + BEV 10 mg/day 1 every 3 weeks	5.2 months	9.1 months
Liu et al., 2015[78]	176	GBM	FTM 75 mg/m^2 day 1–8 + BEV 10 mg/kg day 1–15 followed by a 3-week rest period; then FTM 75 mg/m^2 + BEV 10 mg/day 1 every 3 weeks	5.0 months	8.0 months
Perez-Segura et al., 2016[79]	114	GBM Grade III gliomas	80 mg/m^2 bi-weekly for 5 consecutive administrations (induction phase); 80 mg/m^2 monthly (maintenance phase)	3.0 months	5.2 months
Brandes et al., 2016[80]	91	GBM	FTM 75 mg/m^2 on day 1-8-15 (induction phase); 100 mg/m^2 every 3 weeks or BEV 10mg/m^2 biweekly	3.45 months (FTM) 3.38 months (BEV)	8.7 months (FTM) 7.3 months (BEV)
Lombardi et al., 2016[81]	38	GBM	80 mg/m^2 bi-weekly for five consecutive administrations (induction phase); 80 mg/m^2 monthly (maintenance phase)	4.1 months	7.0 months
Marinelli et al., 2018[82]	37	GBM	FTM 120–140 mg/m^2 biweekly	12.1 weeks	19.7 months

[a]Standard: FTM 100 mg/m^2 every week for 3 consecutive weeks followed by a 5-week rest period; then, an infusion every 3 weeks
BEV, Bevacizumab; *FTM*, fotemustine; *GBM*, glioblastoma; *OS*, overall survival; *PC*, procarbazine; *PFS*, progression-free survival.

Conclusion

Traditional chemotherapy is the mainstay of treatment in both LGGs and HGGs. Most of the available drugs for gliomas used in clinical practice belong to alkylating agents, whose action seems to be strongly correlated with the molecular profile of the tumor. Although the role of TMZ and nitrosoureas has been clarified in GBM, the optimal schedule and timing of chemotherapy need to be further investigated in LGGs. Both LGGs and HGGs tend to recur, and no other effective chemotherapy is validated thus far. New compounds are needed, and searching for novel druggable pathways is the current mission of basic and translational research in neuro-oncology.

References

1. Ostermann S, Csajka C, Buclin T, et al. Plasma and cerebrospinal fluid population pharmacokinetics of temozolomide in malignant glioma patients. *Clin Cancer Res*. 2004;10:3728–3736.
2. Stupp R, Dietrich PY, Ostermann Kraljevic S, et al. Promising survival for patients with newly diagnosed glioblastoma multiforme treated with concomitant radiation plus temozolomide followed by adjuvant temozolomide. *J Clin Oncol*. 2002;20:1375–1382.
3. Stupp R, Mason WP, van den Bent MJ, et al. Radiotherapy plus concomitant and adjuvant temozolomide for glioblastoma. *N Engl J Med*. 2005;352:987–996.
4. Stupp R, Hegi ME, Mason WP, et al. Effects of radiotherapy with concomitant and adjuvant temozolomide versus radiotherapy alone on survival in glioblastoma in a randomized phase III study: 5-year analysis of the EORTC-NCIC trial. *Lancet Oncol*. 2009;10(5):459–466.
5. Hegi ME, Diserens AC, Gorlia T, et al. MGMT gene silencing and benefit from temozolomide in glioblastoma. *N Engl J Med*. 2005;352:997–1003.
6. Spiro TP, Liu L, Majka S, Haaga J, Willson JK, Gerson SL. Temozolomide: the effect of once- and twice-a-day dosing on tumor tissue levels of the DNA repair protein O6-alkylguanine-DNA-alkyltransferase. *Clin Cancer Res*. 2001;7:2309–2317.
7. Tolcher AW, Gerson SL, Denis L, et al. Marked inactivation of O6-alkylguanine-DNA-alkyltransferase activity with protracted temozolomide schedules. *Br J Cancer*. 2003;88:1004–1011.
8. Malmström A, Poulsen HS, Grønberg BH, et al. Postoperative neoadjuvant temozolomide before radiotherapy versus standard radiotherapy in patients 60 years or younger with anaplastic astrocytoma or glioblastoma: a randomized trial. *Acta Oncol*. 2017;56(12):1776–1785.
9. Voloschin AD, Louis DN, Cosgrove GR, Batchelor TT. Neoadjuvant temozolomide followed by complete resection of a 1p- and 19q-deleted anaplastic oligoastrocytoma: case study. *Neuro Oncol*. 2005;7:97–100.
10. Duffau H, Taillandier L, Capelle L. Radical surgery after chemotherapy: a new therapeutic strategy to envision in grade II glioma. *J Neurooncol*. 2006;80:171–176.
11. Blonski M, Pallud J, Gozé C, et al. Neoadjuvant chemotherapy may optimize the extent of resection of World Health Organization grade II gliomas: a case series of 17 patients. *J Neurooncol*. 2013;113:267–275.
12. Jo J, Williams B, Smolkin M, et al. Effect of neoadjuvant temozolomide upon volume reduction and resection of diffuse low-grade glioma. *J Neurooncol*. 2014;120(1):155–161.
13. Gerber DE, Grossman SA, Zeltzman M, et al. The impact of thrombocytopenia from temozolomide and radiation in newly diagnosed adults with high-grade gliomas. *Neuro Oncol*. 2007;9:47–52.
14. Grossman SA, Desideri S, Ye X, et al. Iatrogenic immunosuppression in patients with newly diagnosed high-grade gliomas. ASCO Annual Meeting Proceedings Part I. *J Clin Oncol*. 2007;25:2012.
15. Thorarinsdottir HK, Rood B, Kamani N, et al. Outcome for children < 4 years of age with malignant central nervous system tumors treated with high-dose chemotherapy and autologous stem cell rescue. *Pediatr Blood Cancer*. 2007;48:278–284.
16. Boyle FM, Eller SL, Grossman SA. Penetration of intra-arterially administered vincristine in experimental brain tumor. *Neuro Oncol*. 2004;6:300–305.
17. Lombardi G, Farina P, Della Puppa A, et al. An overview of fotemustine in high-grade gliomas: from single agent to association with bevacizumab. *Biomed Res Int*. 2014;2014:698542.
18. Cairncross JG, Macdonald DR. Successful chemotherapy for recurrent malignant oligodendroglioma. *Ann Neurol*. 1988;23:360–364.
19. Kim L, Hochberg FH, Thornton AF, et al. Procarbazine, lomustine, and vincristine (PCV) chemotherapy for grade III and grade IV oligoastrocytomas. *J Neurosurg*. 1996;85:602–607.
20. Cairncross G, Macdonald D, Ludwin S, et al. Chemotherapy for anaplastic oligodendroglioma: National Cancer Institute of Canada Clinical Trials Group. *J Clin Oncol*. 1994;12:2013–2021.
21. van den Bent MJ, Kros JM, Heimans JJ, et al. Response rate and prognostic factors of recurrent oligodendroglioma treated with procarbazine, CCNU and vincristine chemotherapy: Dutch Neuro-Oncology Group. *Neurology*. 1998;51:1140–1145.
22. Cairncross G, Wang M, Shaw E, et al. Phase III trial of chemoradiotherapy for anaplastic oligodendroglioma: long-term results of RTOG 9402. *J Clin Oncol*. 2013;31(3):337–343.
23. van den Bent MJ, Brandes AA, Taphoorn MJ, et al. Adjuvant procarbazine, lomustine, and vincristine chemotherapy in newly diagnosed anaplastic oligodendroglioma: long-term follow-up of EORTC brain tumor group study 26951. *J Clin Oncol*. 2013;31:344–350.
24. Abrey LE, Louis DN, Paleologos NA, et al. A survey of practice patterns for anaplastic oligodendroglioma. *Neuro Oncol*. 2007;9:314–318.
25. Panageas KS, Iwamoto FM, Cloughesy TF, et al. Initial treatment patterns over time for anaplastic oligodendroglial tumors. *Neuro Oncol*. 2012;14:761–767.
26. Wick W, Hartmann C, Engel C, et al. NOA-04 randomized phase III trial of sequential radiochemotherapy of anaplastic glioma with procarbazine, lomustine, and vincristine or temozolomide. *J Clin Oncol*. 2009;27:5874–5880.

27. Brada M, Stenning S, Gabe R, et al. Temozolomide versus procarbazine, lomustine, and vincristine in recurrent high-grade glioma. *J Clin Oncol*. 2010;28:4601–4608.
28. Douw L, Klein M, Fagel SS, et al. Cognitive and radiological effects of radiotherapy in patients with low-grade glioma: long-term follow-up. *Lancet Neurol*. 2009;8:810–818.
29. Donovan LE, Lassman AB. Chemotherapy treatment and trials in low-grade gliomas. *Neurosurg Clin N Am*. 2019;30(1):103–109.
30. Rudà R. New developments and new dilemmas in lower-grade gliomas. *Neuro Oncol*. 2019;21(7):828–829.
31. Rudà R, Bruno F, Soffietti R. What have we learned from recent clinical studies in low-grade gliomas? *Curr Treat Options Neurol*. 2018;20(8):33.
32. van den Bent MJ, Baumert B, Erridge SC, et al. Interim results from the CATNON trial (EORTC study 26053-22054) of treatment with concurrent and adjuvant temozolomide for 1p/19q non-co-deleted anaplastic glioma: a phase 3, randomised, open-label intergroup study. *Lancet*. 2017;390(10103):1645–1653.
33. Blumenthal DT, Gorlia T, Gilbert MR, et al. Is more better? The impact of extended adjuvant temozolomide in newly diagnosed glioblastoma: a secondary analysis of EORTC and NRG Oncology/RTOG. *Neuro Oncol*. 2017;19(8):1119–1126.
34. Yan H, Parsons DW, Jin G, et al. IDH1 and IDH2 mutations in gliomas. *N Engl J Med*. 2009;360(8):765–773.
35. van den Bent MJ, Erridge S, Vogelbaun MA, et al. Second interim and first molecular analysis of the EORTC randomized phase III intergroup CATNON trial on concurrent and adjuvant temozolomide in anaplastic glioma without 1p/19q codeletion. *J Clin Oncol*. 2019;37(suppl 15):2000.
36. van den Bent MJ, Afra D, de Witte O, et al. Long-term efficacy of early versus delayed radiotherapy for low-grade astrocytoma and oligodendroglioma in adults: the EORTC 22845 randomised trial. *Lancet*. 2005;366(9490):985–990.
37. Shaw EG, Wang M, Coons SW, et al. Randomized trial of radiation therapy plus procarbazine, lomustine, and vincristine chemotherapy for supratentorial adult low-grade glioma: initial results of RTOG 9802. *J Clin Oncol*. 2012;30(25):3065–3070.
38. Buckner JC, Shaw EG, Pugh SL, et al. Radiation plus procarbazine, CCNU, and vincristine in low-grade glioma. *N Engl J Med*. 2016;374(14):1344–1355.
39. Klein M, Heimans JJ, Aaronson NK, et al. Effect of radiotherapy and other treatment-related factors on mid-term to long-term cognitive sequelae in low-grade gliomas: a comparative study. *Lancet*. 2002;360(9343):1361–1368.
40. Baumert BG, Hegi ME, van den Bent MJ, et al. Temozolomide chemotherapy versus radiotherapy in high-risk low-grade glioma (EORTC 22033-26033): a randomised, open-label, phase 3 intergroup study. *Lancet Oncol*. 2016;11:1521–1532.
41. Wu J, Neale N, Huang Y, et al. Comparison of adjuvant radiation therapy alone and chemotherapy alone in surgically resected low-grade gliomas: survival analyses of 2253 cases from the National Cancer Data Base. *World Neurosurg*. 2018;112:e812–e822.
42. Jhaveri J, Liu Y, Chowdhary M, et al. Is less more? Comparing chemotherapy alone with chemotherapy and radiation for high-risk grade 2 glioma: an analysis of the National Cancer Data Base. *Cancer*. 2018;124(6):1169–1178.
43. Wahl M, Phillips JJ, Molinaro AM, et al. Chemotherapy for adult low-grade gliomas: clinical outcomes by molecular subtype in a phase II study of adjuvant temozolomide. *Neuro Oncol*. 2017;19(2):242–251.
44. Rudà R, Pellerino A, Pace A, et al. Efficacy of initial temozolomide for high-risk low-grade gliomas in a phase II AINO (Italian Association for Neuro-Oncology) study: a post-hoc analysis within molecular subgroups of WHO 201. *J Neurooncol*. 2019;145(3):593.
45. Koekkoek JA, Dirven L, Heimans JJ, et al. Seizure reduction is a prognostic marker in low-grade glioma patients treated with temozolomide. *J Neurooncol*. 2016;126(2):347–354.
46. Avila EK, Chamberlain M, Schiff D, et al. Seizure control as a new metric in assessing efficacy of tumor treatment in low-grade glioma trials. *Neuro Oncol*. 2017;19(1):12–21.
47. Walker MD, Green SB, Byar DP, et al. Randomized comparisons of radiotherapy and nitrosoureas for the treatment of malignant glioma after surgery. *N Engl J Med*. 1980;303:1323–1329.
48. Lapierre N, Zuraw L, Cairncross G. Radiotherapy for newly diagnosed malignant glioma in adults: a systematic review. *Radiother Oncol*. 2002;64:259–273.
49. Stewart LA. Chemotherapy in adult high-grade glioma: a systematic review and meta-analysis of individual patient data from 12 randomized trials. *Lancet*. 2002;359:1011–1018.
50. Newlands ES, Stevens MFG, Wedge SR, Wheelhouse RT, Brock C. Temozolomide: a review of its discovery, chemical properties, pre-clinical development and clinical trials. *Cancer Treat Rev*. 1997;23:35–61.
51. Stupp R, Gander M, Leyvraz S, Newlands E. Current and future developments in the use of temozolomide for the treatment of brain tumors. *Lancet Oncol*. 2001;2:552–560.
52. Yung WK, Albright RE, Olson J, et al. A phase II study of temozolomide vs procarbazine in patients with glioblastoma multiforme at first relapse. *Br J Cancer*. 2000;83:588–593.
53. Happold C, Roth P, Wick W, et al. Distinct molecular mechanisms of acquired resistance to temozolomide in glioblastoma cells. *J Neurochem*. 2012;122:444–455.
54. Gilbert MR, Wang M, Aldape KD, et al. Dose-dense temozolomide for newly diagnosed glioblastoma: a randomized phase III clinical trial. *J Clin Oncol*. 2013;31(32):4085–4091.
55. Clarke JL, Iwamoto FM, Sul J, et al. Randomized phase II trial of chemoradiotherapy followed by either dose-dense or metronomic temozolomide for newly diagnosed glioblastoma. *J Clin Oncol*. 2009;27:3861–3867.
56. Chinot OL, Wick W, Mason W, et al. Bevacizumab plus radiotherapy-temozolomide for newly diagnosed glioblastoma. *N Engl J Med*. 2014;370:709–722.
57. Gilbert MR, Dignam JJ, Armstrong TS, et al. A randomized trial of bevacizumab for newly diagnosed glioblastoma. *N Engl J Med*. 2014;370:699–708.
58. Taal W, Oosterkamp HM, Walenkamp AM, et al. Single-agent bevacizumab or lomustine versus a combination of bevacizumab plus lomustine in patients with recurrent glioblastoma (BELOB trial): a randomized controlled phase II trial. *Lancet Oncol*. 2014;15:943–953.
59. Wick W, Gorlia T, Bendszuz M, et al. Lomustine and bevacizumab in progressive glioblastoma. *N Engl J Med*. 2017;377:1954–1963.
60. Brandes AA, Franceschi E, Tosoni A, et al. Temozolomide concomitant and adjuvant to radiotherapy in elderly patients with glioblastoma: correlation with MGMT promoter methylation status. *Cancer*. 2009;115:3512–3518.
61. Keime-Guibert F, Chinot O, Taillandier L, et al. Radiotherapy for glioblastoma in the elderly. *N Engl J Med*. 2007;356:1527–1535.

62. Wick W, Platten M, Meisner C, et al. Temozolomide chemotherapy versus radiotherapy alone for malignant astrocytoma in the elderly: the NOA-08 randomised, phase 3 trial. *Lancet Oncol.* 2012;13:707–715.
63. Malmström A, Grønberg BH, Marosi C, et al. Temozolomide versus standard 6-week radiotherapy versus hypofractionated radiotherapy in patients older than 60 years with glioblastoma: the Nordic randomized, phase 3 trial. *Lancet Oncol.* 2012;13:916–926.
64. Perry JR, Laperriere N, O'Callaghan CJ, et al. Short-course radiation plus temozolomide in elderly patients with glioblastoma. *N Engl J Med.* 2017;376(11):1027–1037.
65. Addeo R, Caraglia M, De Santi MS, et al. A new schedule of fotemustine in temozolomide-pretreated patients with relapsing glioblastoma. *J Neurooncol.* 2011;102(3):417–424.
66. Weller M, van den Bent M, Hopkins K, et al. European Association for Neuro-Oncology (EANO) task force on malignant glioma. EANO guideline for the diagnosis and treatment of anaplastic gliomas and glioblastoma. *Lancet Oncol.* 2014;15:e395–e403.
67. Pellerino A, Franchino F, Soffietti R, Rudà R. Overview on current treatment standards in high-grade gliomas. *Q J Nucl Med Mol Imaging.* 2018;62(3):225–238.
68. Wick W, Puduvalli VK, Chamberlain MC, et al. Phase III study of enzastaurin compared with lomustine in the treatment of recurrent intracranial glioblastoma. *J Clin Oncol.* 2010;28:1168–1174.
69. Batchelor TT, Mulholland P, Neyns B, et al. Phase III randomized trial comparing the efficacy of cediranib as monotherapy, and in combination with lomustine, versus lomustine alone in patients with recurrent glioblastoma. *J Clin Oncol.* 2013;31:3212–3218.
70. Scoccianti S, Detti B, Sardaro A, et al. Second-line chemotherapy with fotemustine in temozolomide-pretreated patients with relapsing glioblastoma: a single institution experience. *Anticancer Drugs.* 2008;19(6):613–620.
71. Silvani A, Lamperti E, Gaviani P, et al. Salvage chemotherapy with procarbazine and fotemustine combination in the treatment of temozolomide treated recurrent glioblastoma patients. *J Neurooncol.* 2008;87(2):143–151.
72. Brandes AA, Tosoni A, Franceschi E, et al. Fotemustine as second-line treatment for recurrent or progressive glioblastoma after concomitant and/or adjuvant temozolomide: a phase II trial of Gruppo Italiano Cooperativo di Neuro-Oncologia (GICNO). *Cancer Chemother Pharmacol.* 2009;64(4):769–775.
73. Fabrini MG, Silvano G, Lolli I, et al. A multi-institutional phase II study on second-line fotemustine chemotherapy in recurrent glioblastoma. *J Neurooncol.* 2009;92(1):79–86.
74. Fabi A, Metro G, Vidiri A, et al. Low-dose fotemustine for recurrent malignant glioma: a multicenter phase II study. *J Neurooncol.* 2010;100(2):209–215.
75. Soffietti R, Trevisan E, Bosa C, Bertero L, Rudà R. Phase II trial of bevacizumab and fotemustine in recurrent grade III gliomas. *J Clin Oncol.* 2012;30:2075.
76. Santoni M, Scoccianti S, Lolli I, et al. Efficacy and safety of second-line fotemustine in elderly patients with recurrent glioblastoma. *J Neurooncol.* 2013;113(3):397–401.
77. Soffietti R, Trevisan E, Bertero L, et al. Bevacizumab and fotemustine for recurrent glioblastoma: a phase II study of AINO (Italian Association of Neuro-Oncology). *J Neurooncol.* 2014;116(3):533–541.
78. Liu Z, Zhang G, Zhu L, et al. Retrospective analysis of bevacizumab in combination with fotemustine in Chinese patients with recurrent glioblastoma multiforme. *Biomed Res Int.* 2015;2015:723612.
79. Pérez-Segura P, Manneh R, Ceballos I, et al. GEINOFOTE: efficacy and safety of fotemustine in patients with high-grade recurrent gliomas and poor performance status. *Clin Transl Oncol.* 2016;18(8):805–812.
80. Brandes AA, Finocchiaro G, Zagonel V, et al. AVAREG: a phase II, randomized, noncomparative study of fotemustine or bevacizumab for patients with recurrent glioblastoma. *Neuro Oncol.* 2016;18(9):1304–1312.
81. Lombardi G, Bellu L, Pambuku A, et al. Clinical outcome of an alternative fotemustine schedule in elderly patients with recurrent glioblastoma: a mono-institutional retrospective study. *J Neurooncol.* 2016;128(3):481–486.
82. Marinelli A, Lamberti G, Cerbone L, et al. High-dose fotemustine in temozolomide-pretreated glioblastoma multiforme patients: a phase I/II trial. *Medicine (Baltimore).* 2018;97(27):e11254.
83. Friedman HS, Prados MD, Wen PY, et al. Bevacizumab alone and in combination with irinotecan in recurrent glioblastoma. *J Clin Oncol.* 2009;27:4733–4740.
84. Picca A, Di Stefano AL, Sanson M. Current and future tools for determination and monitoring of isocitrate dehydrogenase status in gliomas. *Curr Opin Neurol.* 2018;31(6):727–732.

Chapter | 5 |

Evaluation of a dural-based lesion

David Wayne Robinson and Carol Parks Geer

CHAPTER OUTLINE

Introduction

There is significant overlap in the imaging appearance and presentation of dural-based mass lesions. The differential diagnosis includes both benign lesions (such as meningioma—WHO grade I) and more aggressive, malignant lesions (such as dural-based metastasis, atypical or malignant meningioma—WHO grade II and III, and lymphoma). Also included are inflammatory pathologies, such as IgG4-related disease (RD) and granulomatous disease (e.g., sarcoid). This chapter reviews several patient case studies of common and important dural-based mass lesions utilizing a structured framework that allows the reader to generate findings and a differential diagnosis. The case outcomes are then presented, and key teaching points are reviewed. An emphasis is placed on imaging and the interpretation of central findings. Treatment considerations are mentioned for continuity of thought, but most diagnoses have dedicated chapters later in this text that cover treatment in greater detail.

Imaging of the meninges

Imaging of the meninges relies primarily on MRI, although CT can provide important information. The meninges are not well visualized normally, so conspicuity on any imaging modality should prompt close evaluation.

When evaluating dural-based lesions, it is helpful to examine not only the appearance of the lesion but also the effect the lesion is having on surrounding structures. For example, a characteristic feature of meningiomas is hyperostosis or infiltration of the adjacent calvarium. Not all meningiomas have this feature (estimated incidence ranges from 4.5–44%),[1] but its presence should weight the differential toward a meningioma and away from other diagnoses. The characteristics of the lesion are, of course, also instructive. The presence of intralesional calcifications can be a feature of meningiomas (occurs in 20–30%).[2] Both of these imaging findings are best appreciated on CT and illustrate why CT can be helpful in the workup for any dural-based lesion.

MRI is most helpful in evaluating for characteristic imaging features of a dural-based lesion, for the full extent of the lesion, and for the effect on the adjacent brain parenchyma. Each MRI imaging sequence provides information about the lesion, which helps rank the differential diagnosis. Although WHO grade I[3] meningiomas are the most common extra-axial dural-based lesion,[4] other pathologic entities such as dural-based metastasis, lymphoma, malignant meningiomas, and granulomatous diseases need to be excluded, as these can be more aggressive and need urgent treatment. Developing a differential diagnosis for a new dural-based lesion is essential, as errors in management can occur if one decides too early that a lesion is a benign meningioma (e.g., WHO grade I).

Clinical pearls for evaluating dural-based lesions

Some rules of thumb to consider when evaluating a new dural-based lesion include:

1. Most are T1 iso-hypointense on MRI. If they are T1 hyperintense, consider etiologies that contain methemoglobin (subacute hemorrhage), high protein, fat, melanin, or calcium.
2. Some dural-based lesions are T2 hyperintense due to high water content. Others are T2 hypointense due to their high cellularity (particularly if the tumor cells have a high nuclear to cytoplasmic ratio, such as lymphoma).[5] Some meningiomas can be fibrous and these have lower T2 signal.
3. Diffusion restriction in dural-based lesions is variable. Diffusion restriction is an evaluation of how freely water molecules can move in a given medium. If restricted diffusion is present, then consider highly cellular tumors, such as lymphoma, cellular meningiomas, or metastases.
4. Enhancement is a product of disruption of the blood–brain barrier. Extra-axial lesions do not have a blood–brain barrier and most avidly enhance. Meningiomas, the most common dural-based neoplasm, typically diffusely and homogeneously enhance. They often have adjacent dural enhancement/thickening, which is referred to as a "dural tail."[6] Most other dural-based neoplasms also avidly enhance, so the presence of enhancement does not exclude more aggressive neoplasms. If the enhancement pattern is heterogenous, a low-grade meningioma is less likely.
5. Evaluate the relationship of the dural-based lesion with the brain. To establish the lesion is truly extra-axial, look for cerebrospinal fluid (CSF) between the margins of the tumor and the adjacent brain parenchyma (also called a CSF cleft).[7] If there is an indistinct interface between the dural-based mass and the brain or if there is a large amount of edema in the brain, there is a higher likelihood that the mass will be a higher meningioma grade or a more aggressive neoplasm.

Clinical cases

CASE 5.1 SMALL INCIDENTALLY DISCOVERED DURAL-BASED MENINGIOMA

Case. A 61-year-old female presented to the ED with vague constitutional complaints. A CT head was ordered as part of a vertigo workup. She was seen by Neurology 2 weeks later for persistent vertigo and an MRI Brain was ordered.

Imaging findings. CT without contrast demonstrates a partially calcified (Fig. 5.1), extra-axial lesion overlying the left frontal convexity (Fig. 5.2) with extension into the adjacent calvarium and associated hyperostosis (Fig. 5.1). The lesion is isointense to grey matter on T1 (Fig. 5.3). The lesion is heterogeneous on T2 with very dark components consistent with calcification (Fig. 5.4). The lesion is avidly enhancing (Fig. 5.5).

Primary differential diagnosis.

1. Meningioma
2. Dural-based metastasis

Other studies/testing needed or recommended. Follow-up brain MRI with and without contrast in approximately 3 months to document stability.

Referrals to consider. Neurosurgery.

Diagnosis. Incidental meningioma

Treatment considerations. Given the relatively small size of the lesion, absence of edema in the adjacent brain

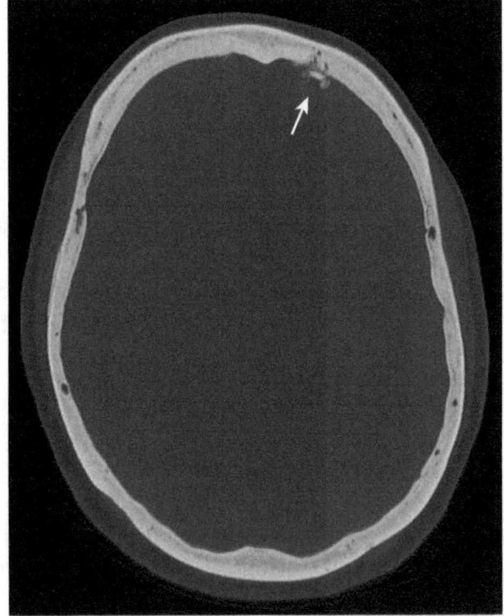

Fig. 5.1 CT without contrast, bone window (3000/700).

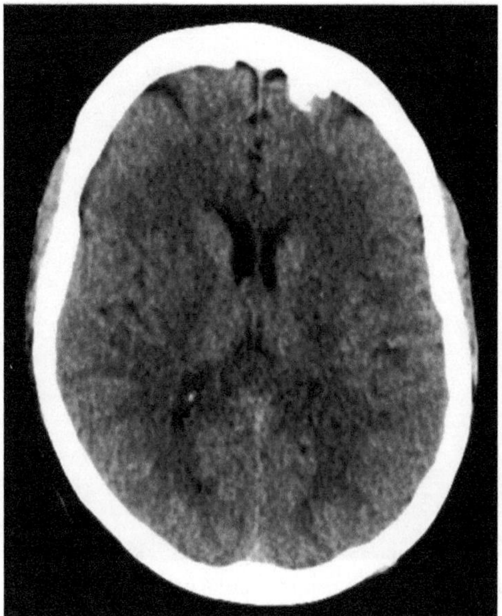

Fig. 5.2 CT without contrast, subarachnoid hemorrhage (SAH) window (95/60).

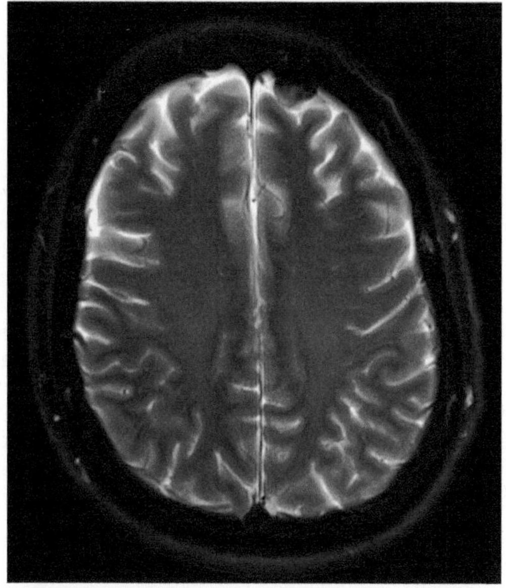

Fig. 5.4 T2 weighted.

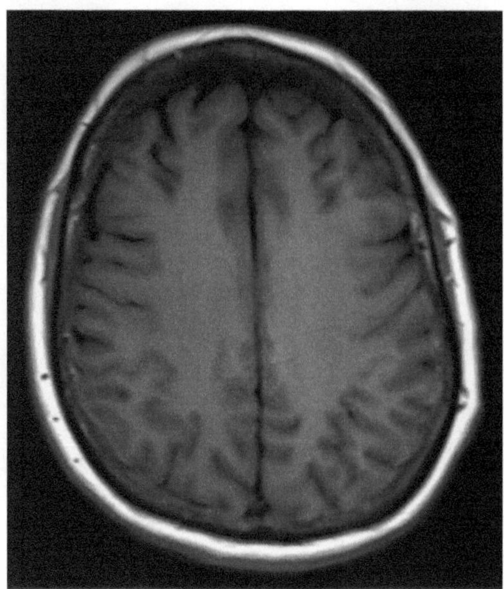

Fig. 5.3 T1 weighted.

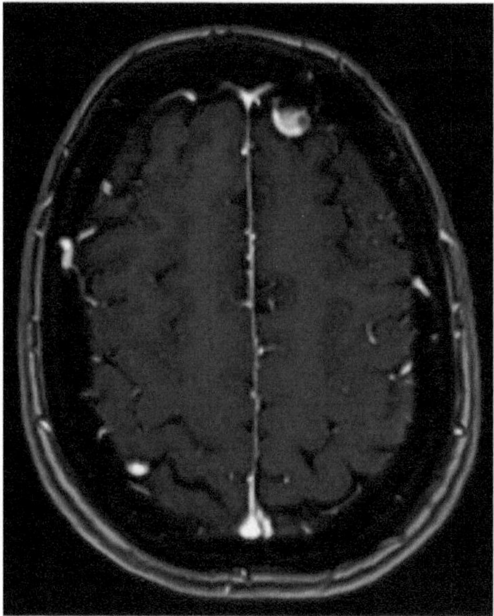

Fig. 5.5 Volumetric interpolated brain examination (T1 weighted) with contrast.

parenchyma, and absence of symptoms that could be attributed to the lesion, treatment should primarily involve observant monitoring with periodic imaging to evaluate for growth. Consider performing initial follow-up imaging with MRI in 3 months given that dural-based metastasis is on the differential. If the lesion is unchanged, follow-up imaging could be performed at 6–12 months and then every year to assess for growth.[8] If there is evidence of interval growth, the patient should be referred for neurosurgical consultation.

What happened in the case presented. Patient received treatment related to probable benign positional vertigo with no specific treatment for the incidental meningioma. Serial follow-up imaging over the last 2 years has demonstrated continued stability of the lesion, making it most compatible with an incidental meningioma.

Teaching Points: Diagnosing an Incidental Lesion as Meningioma Based on Imaging Features. With incidental dural-based masses such as this one, there can be features that strongly suggest that the mass is a meningioma, such as hyperostosis and internal calcifications. However, only follow-up imaging can determine if the mass is almost certainly a benign meningioma (e.g., WHO grade I) rather than a higher-grade meningioma, dural-based metastasis, or other less common dural-based lesions, such as lymphoma or granulomatous disease. If the incidental, asymptomatic lesion is stable on follow-up imaging, it is reasonable to continue to follow the lesion with serial imaging. Alternatively, neurosurgical consultation would also be reasonable (see Chapter 10 for discussion of meningioma management).

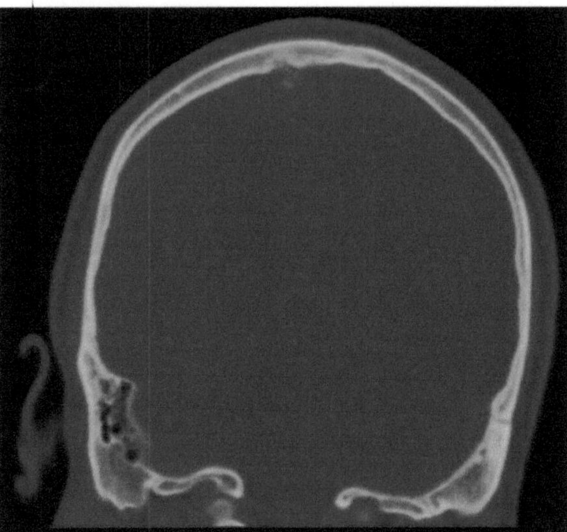

Fig. 5.6 CT with contrast, bone window (3000/700).

CASE 5.2 LARGE ATYPICAL DURAL-BASED MENINGIOMA

Case. A 39-year-old male who presented to an urgent care facility with a chief complaint of a 1-week history of left leg tremors lasting 3–4 minutes, which progressed to numbness the night before. A CT and subsequent MRI were obtained.

Imaging findings. CT with contrast demonstrates a partially calcified (Fig. 5.6), avidly enhancing, extra-axial lesion overlying the right parietal lobe (Fig. 5.7) with extension into the adjacent calvarium and associated hyperostosis (Fig. 5.6). The lesion is iso-hypointense to grey matter on T1 (Fig. 5.8), heterogenous on T2 (Fig. 5.9), and diffusely enhancing with an adjacent enhancing dural tail (arrow) (Figs 5.10 and 5.11).

Differential diagnosis.

1. Meningioma
2. Hemangiopericytoma
3. Dural metastasis

Other studies/testing needed or recommended. None.

Referrals to consider.

1. Neurosurgery
2. Potentially radiation Oncology after neurosurgical resection (depending on WHO grade of tumor)

Diagnosis. Meningioma (atypical, grade II)

Treatment considerations. Treatment of large meningiomas, particularly those that are symptomatic and demonstrating more aggressive features, is primarily surgical excision with follow-up imaging to monitor for recurrence. If surgical pathology indicates a high-grade tumor, adjuvant external beam radiation should be considered.

What happened in the case presented. Patient underwent right parietal craniotomy and gross-total resection of the meningioma, which he tolerated without complication. Pathology confirmed an anaplastic meningioma (WHO grade II), and the patient was referred to radiation oncology for external beam radiation. At 3-year follow-up, patient has memory and concentration problems, but no evidence of disease recurrence.

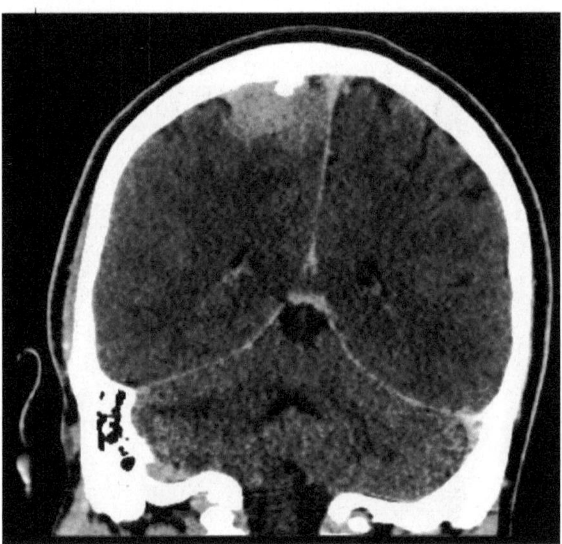

Fig. 5.7 CT with contrast, SAH window (95/60).

Teaching Points: Imaging Features Suggestive of a Higher-Grade Meningioma. As discussed in the previous case, differentiating meningiomas from other dural-based pathology on the initial imaging study can be challenging. The presence of hyperostosis of the adjacent calvarium or

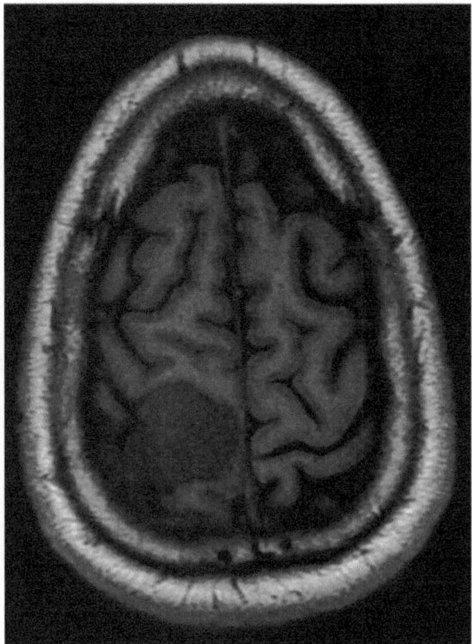

Fig. 5.8 T1 weighted.

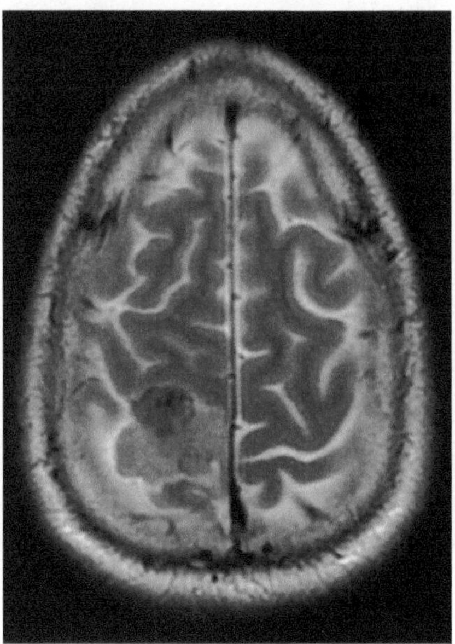

Fig. 5.9 T2 weighted.

intralesional calcifications favor meningiomas. Although this case ultimately turned out to be an anaplastic meningioma, it is not possible to reliably differentiate WHO grade I–III by imaging alone. Invasion of the mass into the adjacent brain is concerning for a higher-grade meningioma (grade II or III),[9] dural-based metastasis, or hemangiopericytoma.

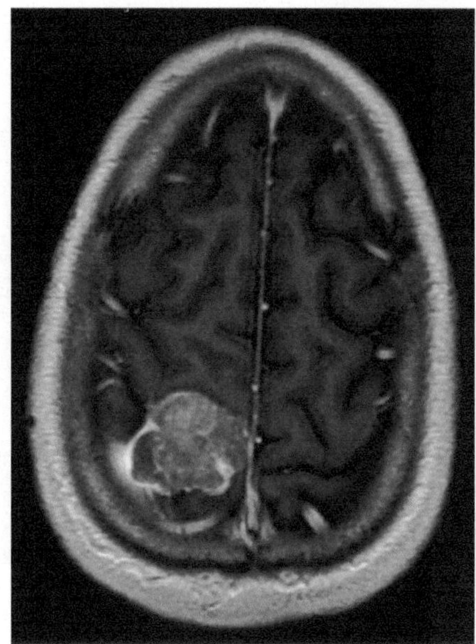

Fig. 5.10 T1 weighted with contrast.

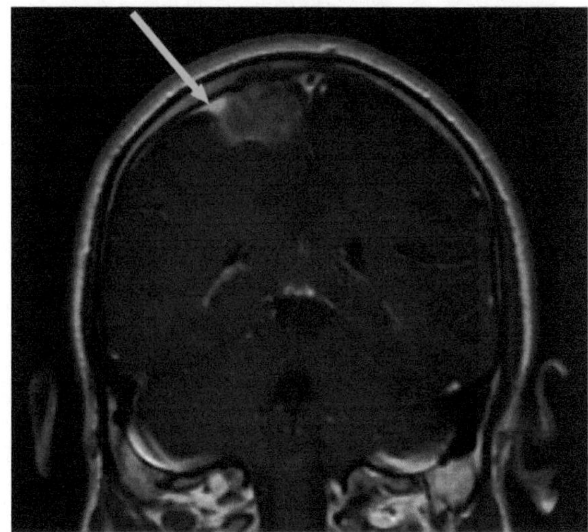

Fig. 5.11 T1 weighted with contrast (coronal).

CASE 5.3 SKULL-BASED LESION CONCERNING FOR MENINGIOMA VERSUS INFLAMMATORY LESION

Case. A 45-year-old female presents with 1-year history of progressive painless right-sided vision loss. She also describes some transient symptoms involving the right side of her face and neck.

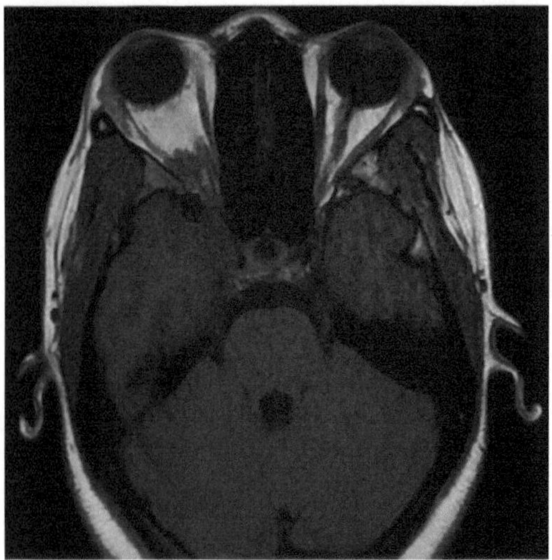

Fig. 5.12 T1 weighted.

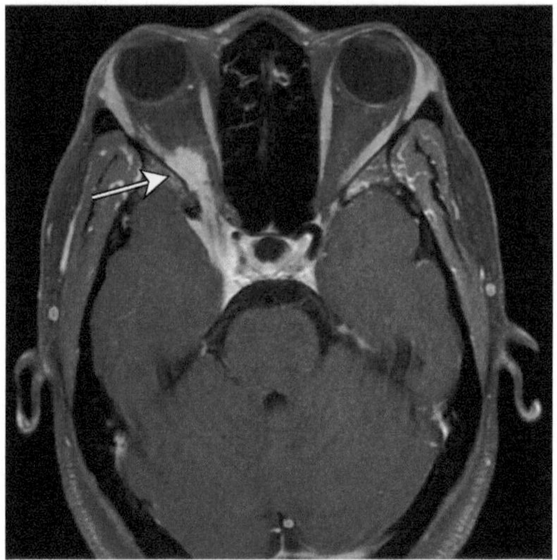

Fig. 5.14 T1 weighted with contrast.

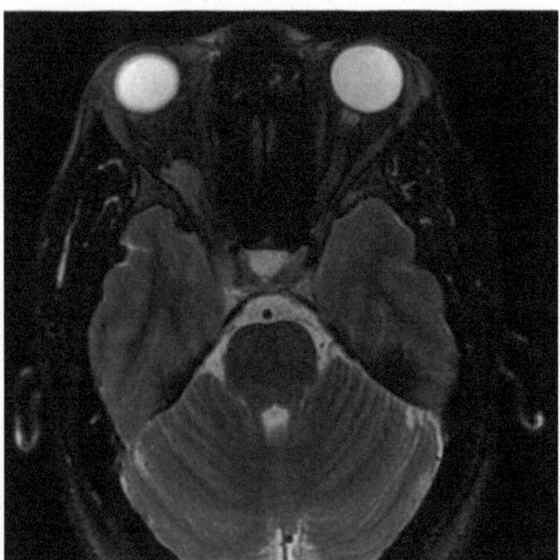

Fig. 5.13 T2 weighted.

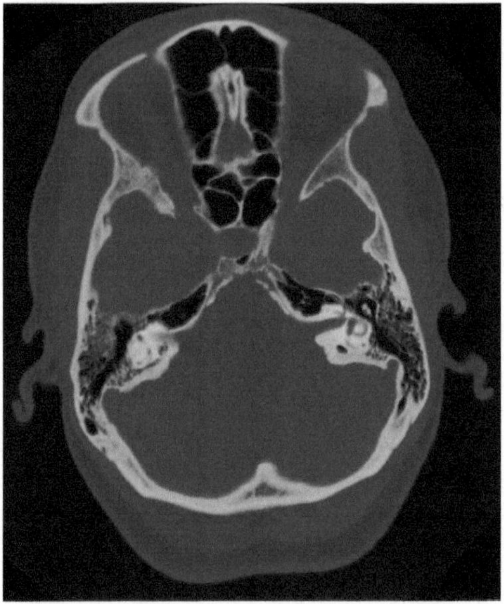

Fig. 5.15 CT without contrast, bone window (3890/800).

Imaging findings. Soft tissue mass centered in the right posterolateral orbit extending through the superior orbital fissure into the right cavernous sinus and along the dural margin of the right middle cranial fossa. The lesion is T1 isointense (Fig. 5.12), relatively isointense to grey matter on T2 (Fig. 5.13), and avidly enhances (Fig. 5.14). On CT, there is asymmetric sclerosis and expanded appearance of the right sphenoid bone (Fig. 5.15).

Differential diagnosis.

1. Meningioma
2. IgG4-RD
3. Idiopathic orbital inflammation (Tolosa Hunt)
4. Orbital sarcoidosis
5. Orbital lymphoma
6. Orbital metastasis
7. Perineural spread of head and neck squamous cell carcinoma

Referrals to consider.

1. Ophthalmology
2. Neurosurgery
3. Potentially Radiation Oncology if the lesion is likely a meningioma or metastasis

Diagnosis. Meningioma

Treatment considerations. An inflammatory etiology (IgG4-RD or idiopathic orbital inflammation—"pseudotumor") is usually treated with steroid therapy.[10] However, idiopathic orbital pseudotumor typically presents with orbital pain,[11] and IgG4- RD typically presents with headache. Serum IgG4 can be elevated in patients with IgG4-RD[12] but is nonspecific.[13] In this case of painless orbital symptoms, biopsy/excision should be considered as orbital lymphoma can initially improve on steroid therapy and be difficult to detect on delayed biopsy after steroid treatment.[14] Pathology can be determined with a targeted biopsy or at the time of surgical resection/debulking. The intracranial portion will likely be treated with adjuvant therapy due to difficulty with surgical resection of a lesion involving the cavernous sinus. Sarcoid can also involve the orbit. This possible diagnosis should be considered in the appropriate patient population. The presence of sclerosis and expansion of the adjacent sphenoid wing (hyperostosis) strongly favors a meningioma over the other entities in the differential for this case.

What happened in the case presented. Laboratory workup was negative for inflammatory markers. Given the progressive nature of her symptoms, surgical debulking of the intraorbital portion of the mass, followed by gamma knife therapy of the intracranial portion was recommended. The lesion was confirmed to be a meningioma (WHO grade I) at resection.

Teaching Points: Differentiating Skull-Based Meningioma From Orbital Inflammatory Lesion. The presence of adjacent sclerosis of the sphenoid bone (hyperostosis) is more suggestive of a meningioma rather than other orbital neoplasms such as lymphoma. Lack of orbital pain is also more consistent with a neoplasm rather than inflammation.

CASE 5.4A CEREBELLOPONTINE ANGLE (CPA) VESTIBULAR SCHWANNOMA

Case. A 46-year-old male presented to the ED after a fall in the shower resulting in a fractured rib and complaint of progressive blurry vision. On fundoscopic examination, he was found to have papilledema. Further investigation revealed right-sided hearing loss.

Imaging findings. Large T1 isointense (Fig. 5.16), heterogeneous signal on T2 (Fig. 5.17), and avidly enhancing mass (Fig. 5.18) in the right cerebellopontine angle (CPA) with extension into/from the right internal auditory canal. There is no restricted diffusion (Fig. 5.19). This mass exerts significant mass effect on the adjacent pons, cerebellar peduncle, and right cerebellar hemisphere with effacement of the fourth ventricle. This has resulted in moderate obstructive hydrocephalus (Fig. 5.20). The mass has a characteristic "ice-cream on a cone" appearance.

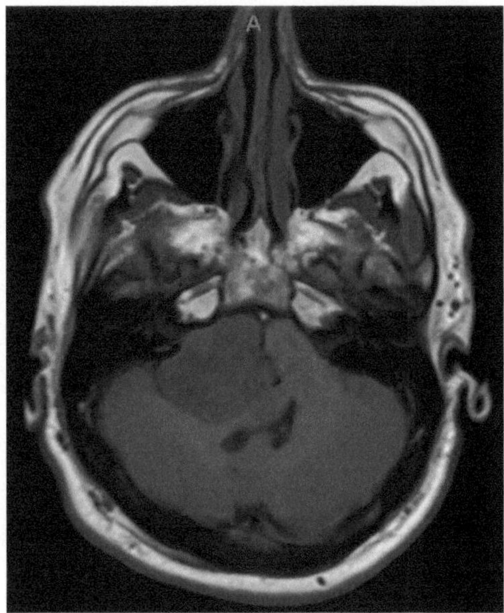

Fig. 5.16 T1 weighted.

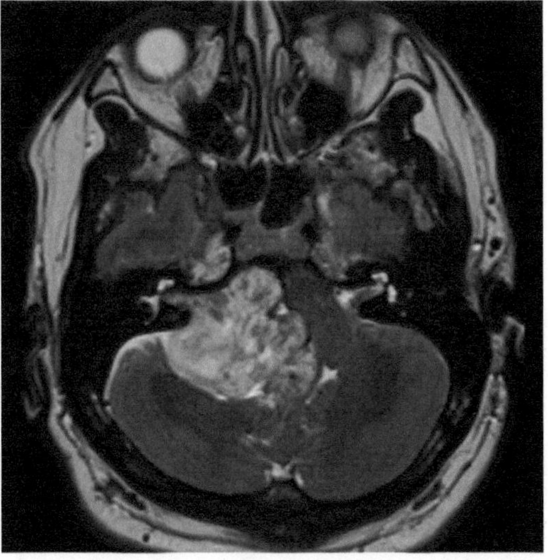

Fig. 5.17 T2 weighted.

Differential diagnosis.

1. Schwannoma
2. Meningioma
3. Epidermoid Cyst

Other studies/testing needed or recommended. None

Referrals to consider.

1. Neurosurgery
2. ENT

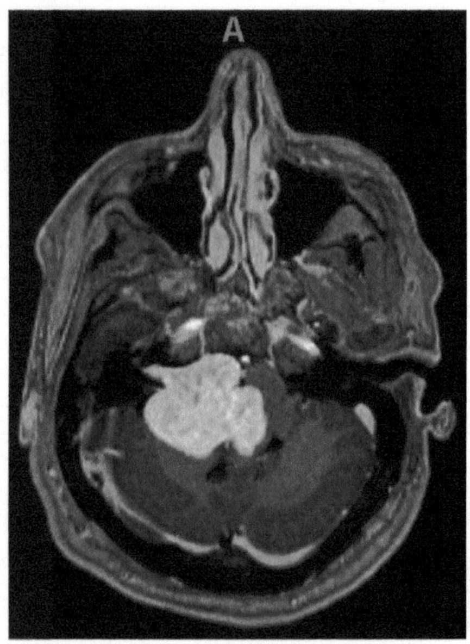

Fig. 5.18 T1 weighted with contrast.

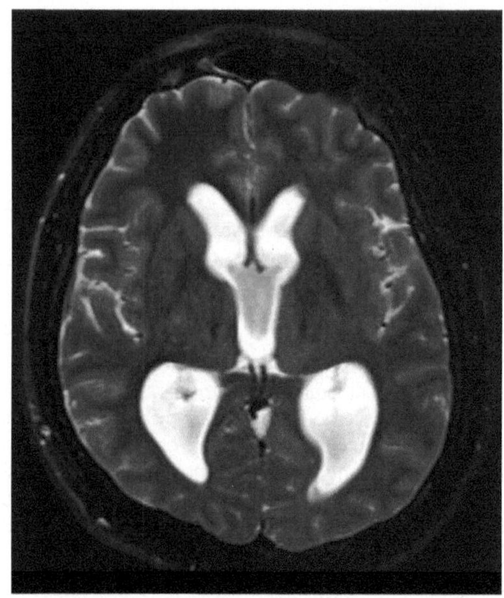

Fig. 5.20 T2 weighted.

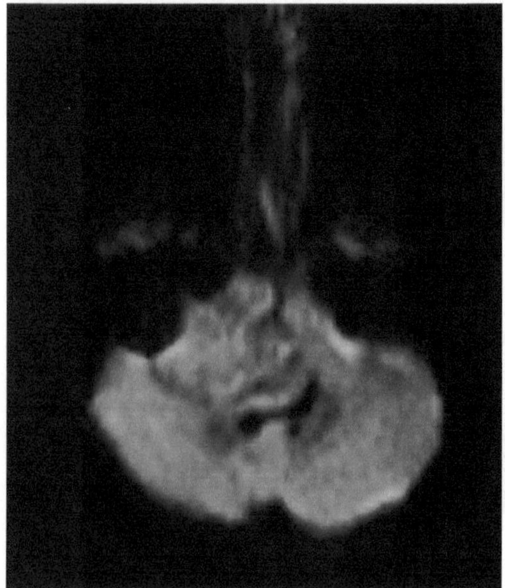

Fig. 5.19 Diffusion-weighted imaging.

Diagnosis. Vestibular Schwannoma

Treatment considerations. The obstructive hydrocephalus and associated vision changes are the most immediate concern and warrant prompt surgical intervention. Smaller vestibular schwannomas can be treated surgically, followed observantly for growth, or treated with gamma knife/stereotactic radiosurgery depending on associated symptoms, age of patient, and patient co-morbidities.

What happened in the case presented. Patient initially underwent emergent placement of a ventriculoperitoneal shunt to salvage his vision followed by staged retromastoid craniotomy and tumor resection by neurosurgery and ENT. Pathology confirmed a vestibular schwannoma.

Teaching Points: Evaluation and Management of Vestibular Schwannoma. A vestibular schwannoma is a benign tumor that typically arises near the transition point of the glial and Schwann cells within the internal auditory canal (IAC). More than 90% of these tumors arise from the inferior division of the vestibular nerve.[15] As this tumor grows, it eventually extends into the CPA cistern. This pattern of growth gives the mass its characteristic "ice-cream on a cone" appearance.[16] When vestibular schwannomas become large, they can cause mass effect on the adjacent brainstem and cerebellum.CT is usually the first modality employed in the workup of intracranial pathology and, after identification of a mass within the CPA, pay particular attention to the presence or absence of calcifications. A vestibular schwannoma typically will not have calcifications. Their presence should make you consider other pathology on your differential, namely a meningioma.

MRI with and without gadolinium contrast is the preferred modality to work up intracranial masses. A vestibular schwannoma should be isointense to slightly hypointense to surrounding brain on T1-weighted imaging but enhance avidly with gadolinium. On T2-weighted imaging, the tissue itself will be somewhat hyperintense to brain, but any cystic areas will be isointense to CSF. Vestibular schwannomas will typically expand the IAC when they become large. Finally, these tumors do not typically restrict diffusion, which helps to differentiate them from another CPA mass, an epidermoid cyst.[17]

CASE 5.4B CEREBELLOPONTINE ANGLE (CPA) MENINGIOMA

Case. A 49-year-old male with a 6-month history of progressive right-sided ear and throat pain, and intermittent tingling in the right V2 and V3 distributions.

Imaging findings. Dural-based mass in the right cerebellopontine cistern with faint intralesional calcifications (Fig. 5.21). The lesion is T1 isointense (Fig. 5.22), T2 iso-hypointense to grey matter (Fig. 5.23), and avidly enhancing (Fig. 5.24). Note the presence of a dural tail anteriorly along the clivus (arrow). The lesion causes mass effect on the medulla, pons, and middle cerebellar peduncle, which are displaced posteriorly and to the left. There is no edema in the adjacent brainstem or cerebellum.

Differential diagnosis.

1. Meningioma
2. Schwannoma
4. Dural-based metastasis

Other studies/testing needed or recommended. None

Referrals to consider.

1. Neurosurgery
2. Radiation oncology

Diagnosis. Meningioma

Treatment considerations. Treatment options include observation with serial imaging, open surgical excision, and radiation therapy.

What happened in the case presented. The patient was initially evaluated by ENT and referred to Neurosurgery. He was offered observation with serial imaging, open surgical resection, and gamma knife radiosurgery. Given the progressive nature of his symptoms, he opted to proceed with gamma knife radiosurgery. This procedure was well-tolerated, and at 3-year follow-up he is symptom free. Subsequent imaging demonstrated a decrease in the tumor size consistent with radiation treatment response.

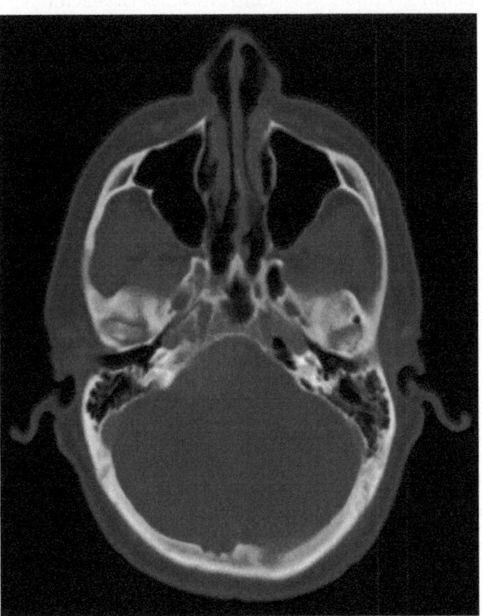

Fig. 5.21 CT without contrast, bone window (3000/700).

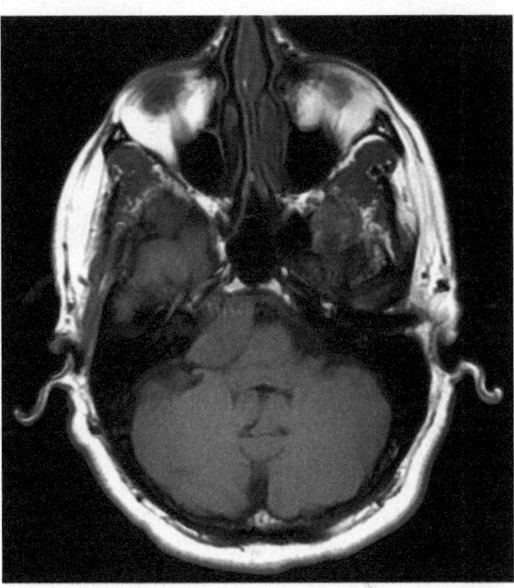

Fig. 5.22 T1 weighted.

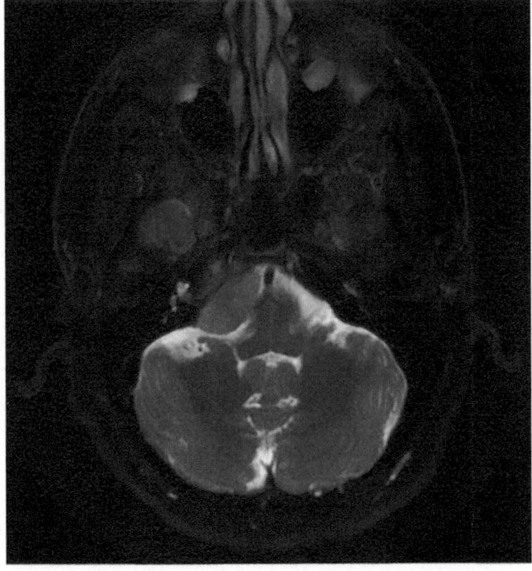

Fig. 5.23 T2 weighted.

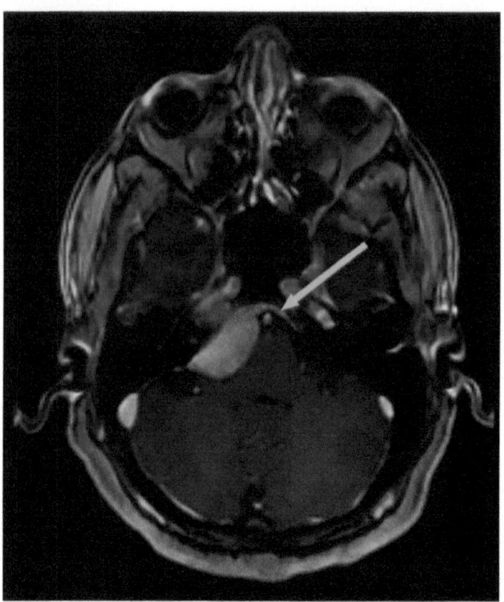

Fig. 5.24 T1 weighted with contrast.

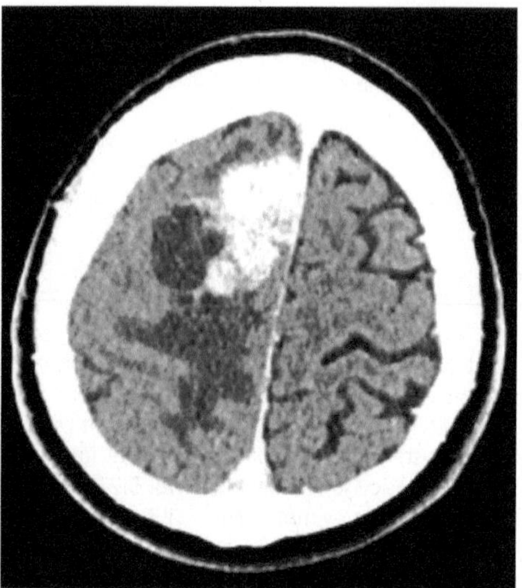

Fig. 5.25 CT contrast-enhanced.

Teaching Points: Imaging Features That Favor Diagnosis of Meningioma for CPA Mass. The differential diagnosis for a CPA mass includes both dural-based and non–dural-based pathology. Note the different appearance of the meningioma in this case with the vestibular schwannoma in the previous case. The meningioma is clearly dural-based and has a "dural tail." Intralesional calcifications would be more common with a meningioma. This case did not have hyperostosis, but this would be a helpful imaging feature suggesting meningioma if it were present. There is no expansion of the adjacent internal auditory canal in this case, which would be a typical feature of a vestibular schwannoma.

CASE 5.5 DURAL-BASED LESION DIAGNOSED AS HEMANGIOPERICYTOMA

Case. A 62-year-old male with a 2-month history of progressive left-arm weakness, tremor, and memory problems. An initial workup by his primary care provider (PCP) was unrevealing, but a central nervous system etiology was suspected, and a CT and subsequent brain MRI was ordered.

Imaging findings. High right paramedian frontal dural-based extra-axial mass with cystic and solid components that demonstrates avid enhancement on both CT and MRI (Figs 5.25–5.29). The solid component of the mass is heterogenous on T1- (Fig. 5.26) and T2-weighted imaging (Fig. 5.27) with surrounding vasogenic edema seen best on T2 and fluid attenuated inversion recovery (FLAIR; Fig. 5.28). The cystic component is seen more clearly on T2-weighted imaging as hyperintense (Fig. 5.27). There is no restricted diffusion (Fig. 5.30).

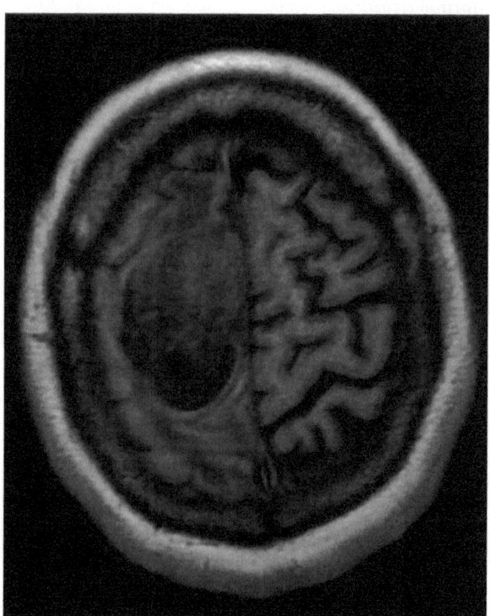

Fig. 5.26 T1 weighted.

Differential diagnosis.

1. Meningioma
2. Dural-based metastasis
3. Hemangiopericytoma
4. Dural-based lymphoma

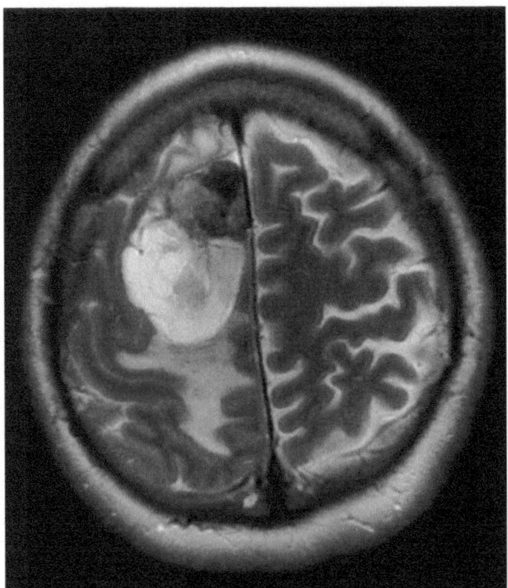

Fig. 5.27 T2 weighted.

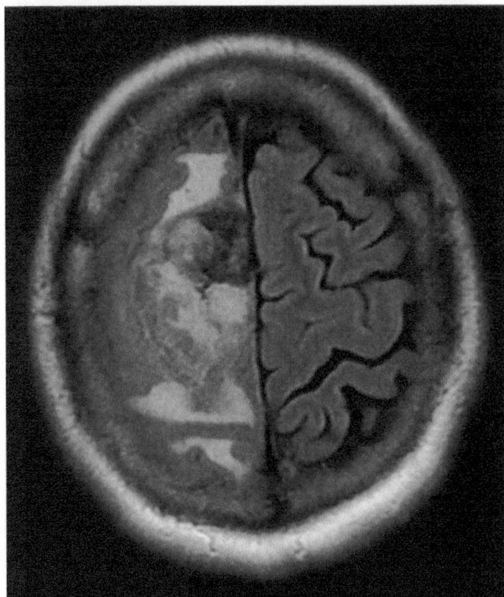

Fig. 5.28 T2 fluid attenuation inversion recovery (FLAIR).

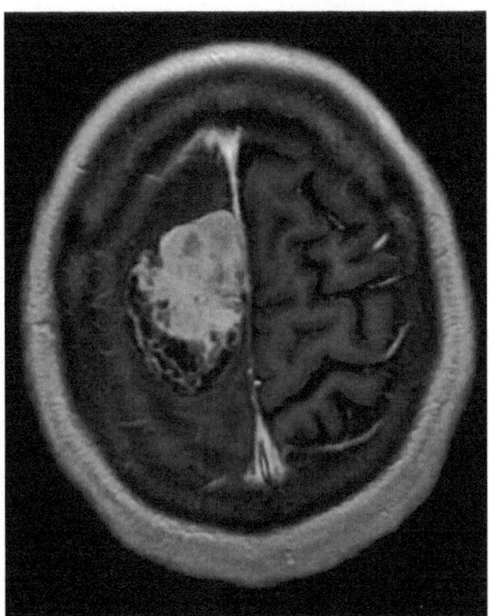

Fig. 5.29 T1 weighted with contrast.

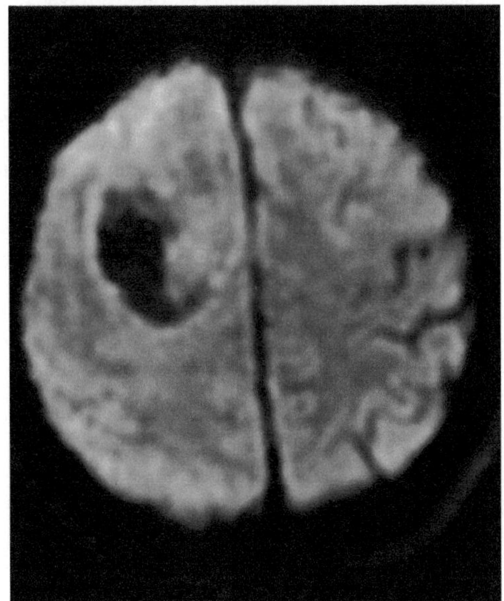

Fig. 5.30 Diffusion-weighted imaging.

Other studies/testing needed or recommended. Angiography

Referrals to consider.

1. Neurosurgery
2. Radiation oncology

Diagnosis. Hemangiopericytoma

Treatment considerations. Hemangiopericytomas are highly vascular tumors, and surgical planning with catheter angiography and possible preoperative embolization can be helpful.[18] Ultimately the treatment of choice is complete surgical excision, which can be augmented with adjuvant radiation therapy.

What happened in the case presented. Patient underwent right frontal craniotomy and maximal safe resection of the tumor (presumed meningioma). A small portion had invaded the superior sagittal sinus, which was not resected. Surgical pathology revealed the tumor to be a hemangiopericytoma (WHO grade II), and the patient received external beam radiotherapy and a CT chest/abdomen/pelvis to evaluate for metastatic disease (negative). Follow-up brain MRIs have shown no residual or recurrent disease. Clinically, he reports significant improvement in preoperative symptoms, including no residual left upper extremity weakness or memory problems.

Teaching Points: Imaging Features of Hemangiopericytoma. The imaging features of a hemangiopericytoma are often indistinguishable from an atypical or malignant meningioma. This diagnosis should be suspected in cases of atypical or more aggressive appearing suspected meningiomas, such as those with adjacent bone erosion (although this feature was not seen in this case), brain parenchymal invasion, a large amount of edema in the adjacent brain, or the presence of large flow voids, which indicates a highly vascular tumor.[19]

CASE 5.6 DURAL-BASED METASTASIS

Case. A 76-year-old female with a 1-month history of progressive worsening intermittent confusion. She has a history of atrial fibrillation not on anticoagulation.

Imaging findings. MRI demonstrates a T1 hypointense (Fig. 5.31), T2 heterogeneous/slightly hyperintense (Fig. 5.32), avidly enhancing (Fig. 5.33) dural-based mass in the anterior left middle cranial fossa (Fig. 5.34), with associated vasogenic edema in the left temporal lobe (Fig. 5.33). The mass mildly restricts diffusion (Figs 5.34 and 5.35).

Differential diagnosis.

1. Meningioma
2. Metastatic disease
3. Hemangiopericytoma
4. Dural-based lymphoma
5. Granulomatous disease (sarcoid)

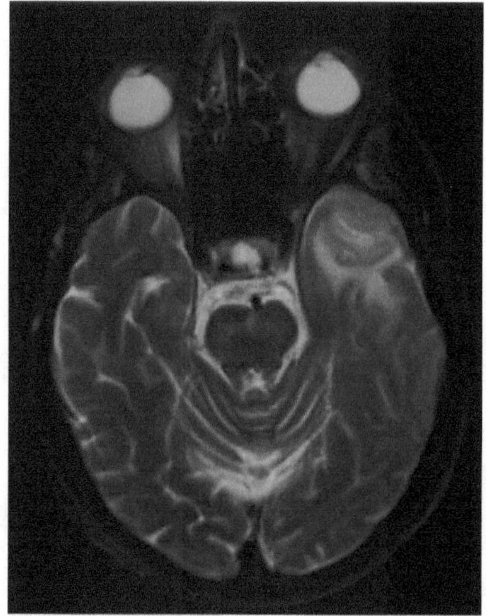

Fig. 5.32 T2 weighted.

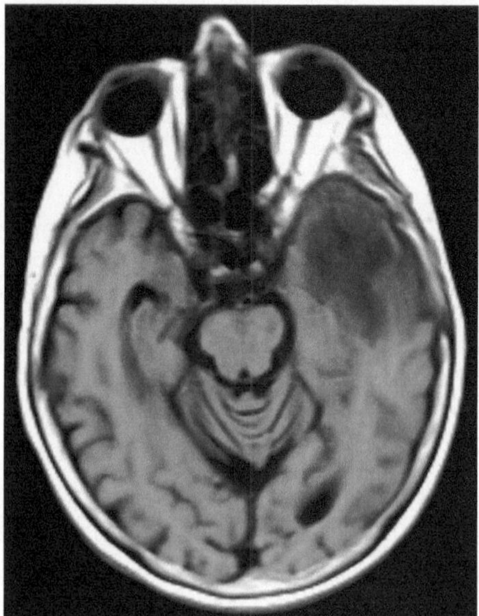

Fig. 5.31 T1 weighted.

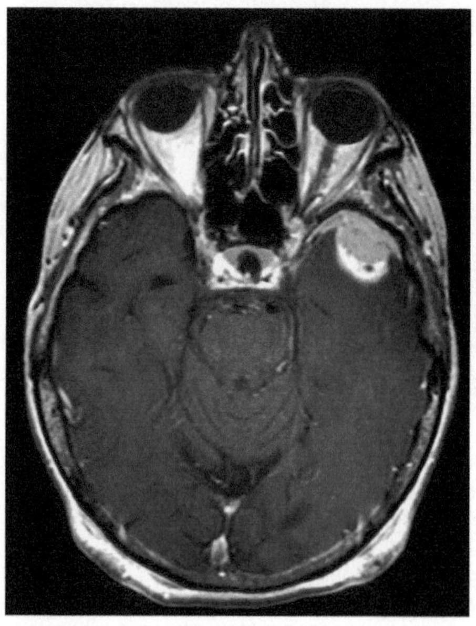

Fig. 5.33 T1 weighted with contrast.

Other studies/testing needed or recommended.
1. CT Chest, Abdomen, Pelvis with contrast
2. PET CT

Referrals to consider.
1. Neurosurgery
2. Hematology/Oncology
3. Radiation Oncology

Diagnosis. Dural-based metastatic adenocarcinoma of lung primary

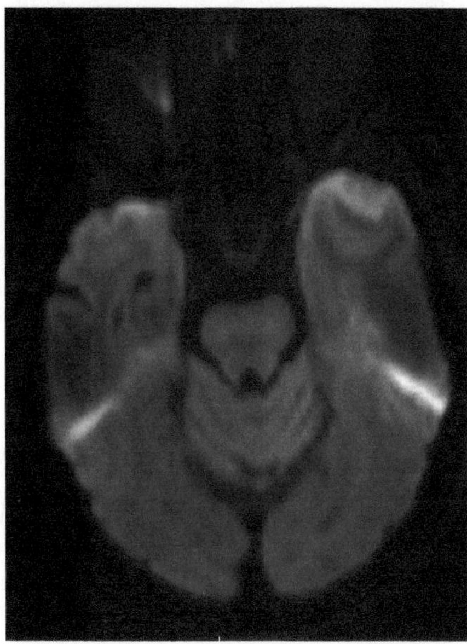

Fig. 5.34 Diffusion-weighted imaging.

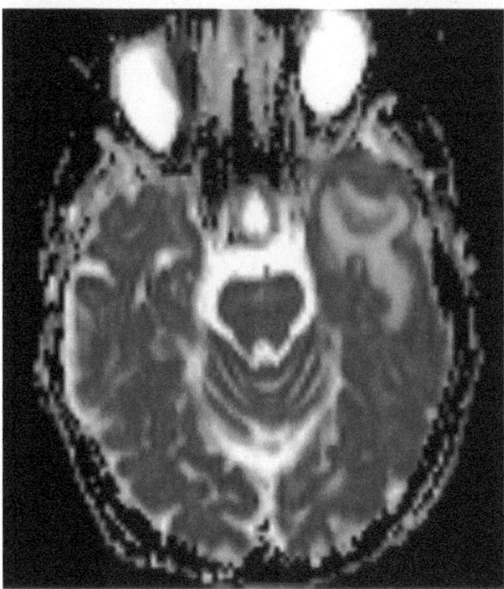

Fig. 5.35 Apparent diffusion coefficient.

Treatment considerations. Although this lesion could be a meningioma, the presence of edema in the adjacent brain parenchyma and symptoms that likely are related to the edema warrants more urgent workup for the diagnosis, as opposed to observant monitoring with a repeat brain MRI in 3 months. Neurosurgical consultation should be obtained. Neurosurgery may elect to resect this lesion or may want a chest-abdomen-pelvic CT and mammogram to evaluate for a primary malignancy given that dural-based metastasis is in the differential. Sarcoid would be less likely as a new diagnosis in this age group.[20] Lymphoma would also be less likely given that the patient did not have a history of lymphoma. Once a tissue diagnosis is made, additional treatment options may be considered, including chemotherapy and/or radiation therapy.

What happened in the case presented. Patient underwent left temporal craniotomy for total resection of brain mass, and the pathology was consistent with poorly differentiated adenocarcinoma of lung origin. Further intervention with gamma knife stereotactic radiosurgery to the tumor resection region was performed and well tolerated. Chest-abdomen-pelvic CT demonstrated a right lower lobe lung cancer. The patient was treated with adjuvant chemotherapy. However, 2 months post gamma knife treatment, she developed expressive aphasia. MRI was obtained and showed multiple new dural-based lesions. Two additional rounds of gamma knife therapy were performed before the patient and family decided to transition to comfort care.

Teaching Points: Imaging Features that Suggest Dural-Based Metastasis. Dural-based metastases can look exactly like a meningioma on imaging. Although dural-based metastasis should be high on the differential diagnosis in the setting of multiple lesions, they must also be considered with a solitary lesion (as in this case). This is an example of why solitary dural-based, enhancing lesions that look like meningiomas need to be followed closely initially to establish stability so that more aggressive pathology is not missed. If this left middle cranial fossa mass did not have associated edema in the temporal lobe, it would be appropriate to obtain a follow-up brain MRI in 3 months to document stability, assuming that this is a possible meningioma.

CASE 5.7 DURAL-BASED LYMPHOMA

Case. A 60-year-old female with a history significant for work-limiting fatigue and drenching night sweats for the last 10 months, a chronic daily headache for the last 4 months, and blurred vision in her left eye for the last 2 months. A palpable lump was present on her left thigh. This was excised, and pathology was significant for natural killer (NK)/T-cell lymphoma. She also has a past medical history significant for autoimmune hepatitis.

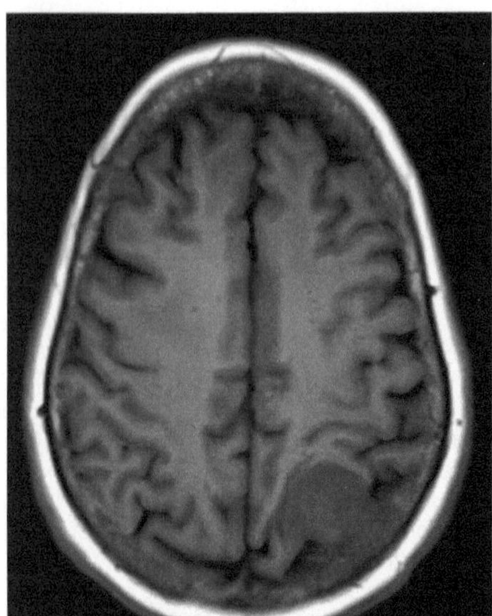

Fig. 5.36 T1 weighted.

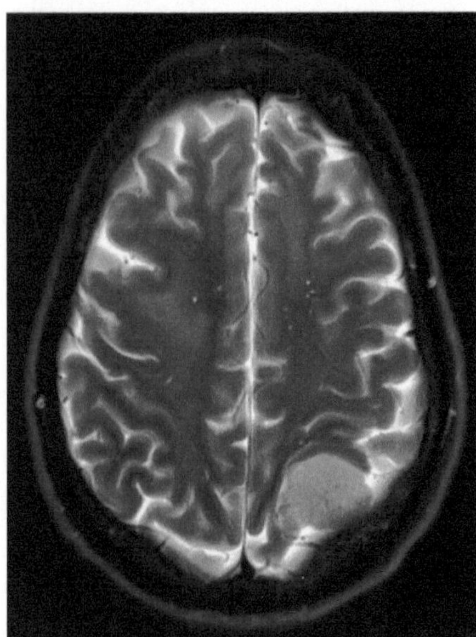

Fig. 5.37 T2 weighted.

Imaging findings. MRI demonstrates a T1 isointense (Fig. 5.36), T2 mildly hyperintense (Fig. 5.37), avidly enhancing (Fig. 5.38) dural-based mass along the left parietal convexity. The lesion mildly restricts diffusion (Figs 5.39 and 5.40).

Differential diagnosis.

1. T-cell lymphoma
2. Meningioma
3. Metastatic disease

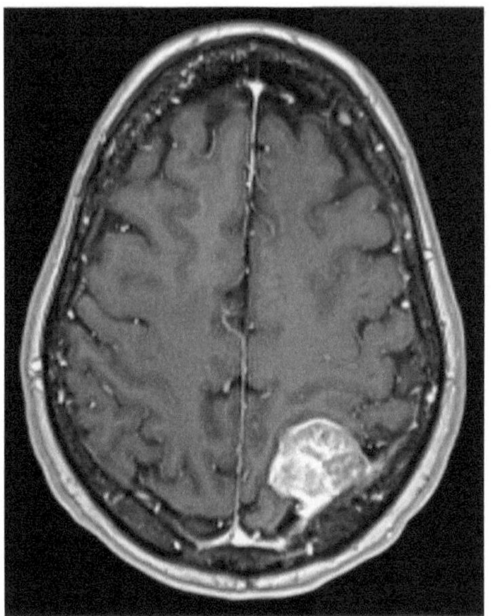

Fig. 5.38 T1 weighted with contrast.

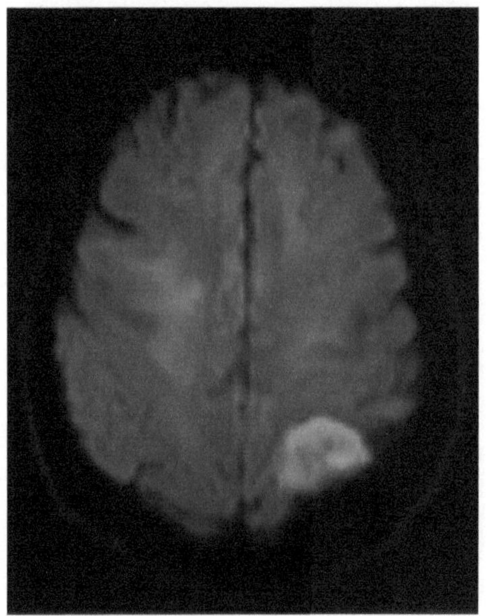

Fig. 5.39 Diffusion-weighted imaging.

Other studies/testing needed or recommended.

1. CT Chest, Abdomen, Pelvis with contrast
2. PET CT

Referrals to consider.

1. Neurosurgery
2. Hematology-Oncology

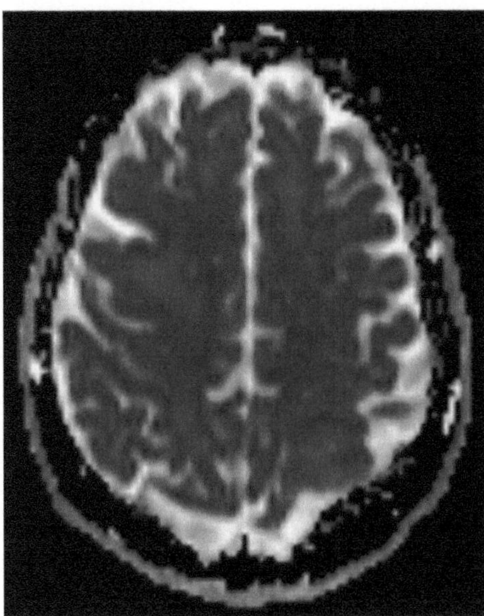

Fig. 5.40 Apparent diffusion coefficient.

Diagnosis. Dural-based Lymphoma (putative)

Treatment considerations. Although the patient has a tissue diagnosis of peripheral T-cell lymphoma and the imaging findings are consistent with dural-based lymphoma, the imaging is nonspecific, and a coexisting, incidental meningioma is possible. A tissue diagnosis is warranted. Treatment with chemotherapy should be pursued for the peripheral T-cell lymphoma, but if the dural-based lesion is confirmed to be lymphoma, consideration should be given for adding intrathecal methotrexate and radiation therapy.

What happened in the case presented. A left parietal craniotomy for both diagnosis and cytoreduction was recommended once the patient was stable from a medical perspective. Unfortunately, the patient's clinical status worsened, and she elected to be transitioned to comfort care.

Teaching Points: Imaging Features of a Dural-Based Lymphoma. A dural-based lesion, even a solitary one, in a patient with a history of lymphoma should raise concern for CNS lymphoma. The appearance may mimic a meningioma, so tissue diagnosis may be necessary. The characteristic imaging features in an immunocompetent patient are hyperdense and enhancing on CT, isointense on T1, iso-hypointense on T2, diffusely enhancing, and restricted diffusion due to high cellularity.[5] In immunocompromised patients, lymphoma is usually peripherally enhancing on both MRI and CT.[21]

Conclusion

There is significant overlap in the imaging appearance and presentation of dural-based mass lesions. The differential includes both benign lesions such as meningioma (WHO grade I) and more aggressive, malignant lesions such as dural-based metastasis, atypical or malignant meningioma (WHO grade II and III), and lymphoma. The differential also includes inflammatory pathology, such as IgG4-RD and granulomatous disease (sarcoid). Because it is usually not possible to determine if a dural-based lesion is benign or more aggressive, these lesions need short-term follow-up imaging at a minimum, so that a dural-based metastasis is not ignored thinking that it is a benign meningioma.

References

1. Arana E, Martí-Bonmatí L. CT and MR imaging of focal calvarial lesions. *AJR. Am J Roentgenology.* 1999;172(6):1683–1688.
2. Greenberg H, Chandler WF, Sandler HM. *Brain Tumors.* New York: Oxford University Press; 1999.
3. Louis DN, Perry A, Reifenberger G, et al. The 2016 World Health Organization classification of tumors of the central nervous system: a summary. *Acta Neuropathol.* 2016;131(6):803–820.
4. Louis DN, et al. Meningiomas. Pathology and genetics of tumors of the nervous system. In: Kleihues P, Cavenee WK, eds. *World Health Organization Classification of Tumors.* Lyon: IARC Press; 2000:176–184.
5. Mansour A, Qandeel M, Abdel-Razeq H, Abu Ali HA. MR imaging features of intracranial primary CNS lymphoma in immune competent patients. *Canc Imag.* 2014;14(1):22.
6. Takeguchi T, Miki H, Shimizu T, et al. The dural tail of intracranial meningiomas on fluid-attenuated inversion-recovery images. *Neuroradiology.* 2004;46(2):130–135.
7. Takeguchi T, Miki H, Shimizu T, et al. Evaluation of the tumor-brain interface of intracranial meningiomas on MR imaging including FLAIR images. *Magn Reson Med Sci.* 2003;2(4):165–169.
8. Zeng L, Liang P, Jiao J, Chen J, Lei T. Will an asymptomatic meningioma grow or not grow? A meta-analysis. *J Neurol Surg Cent Eur Neurosurg.* 2015;76:341–347.
9. Lin BJ, Chou KN, Kao HW, et al. Correlation between magnetic resonance imaging grading and pathological grading in meningioma. *J Neurosurg.* 2014;121(5):1201–1208.
10. Swamy BN, McCluskey P, Nemet A, et al. Idiopathic orbital inflammatory syndrome: clinical features and treatment outcomes. *Br J Ophthalmol.* 2007;91(12):1667–1670.
11. Weber AL, Romo LV, Sabates NR. Pseudotumor of the orbit. Clinical, pathologic, and radiologic evaluation. *Radiol Clin North Am.* 1999;37(1):151–168,xi.
12. Fujita A, Sakai O, Chapman MN, Sugimoto H. IgG4-related disease of the head and neck: CT and MR imaging manifestations. *Radiographics.* 2012;32(7):1945–1958.

13. McNab AA, McKelvie P. IgG4-related ophthalmic disease. Part II: clinical aspects. *Ophthalmic Plast Reconstr Surg.* 2015;31(3):167–178.
14. Char DH, Miller T. Orbital pseudotumor: fine-needle aspiration biopsy and response to therapy. *Ophthalmology.* 1993;100(11):1702–1710.
15. Silk PS, Lane JI, Driscoll CL. Surgical approaches to vestibular schwannomas: what the radiologist needs to know. *Radiographics.* 2009;29(7):1955–1970.
16. Koontz NA, Seltman TA, Kralik SF, Mosier KM, Harnsberger HR. Classic signs in head and neck imaging. *Clin Radiol.* 2016;71(12):1211–1222.
17. Tsuruda JS, Chew WM, Moseley ME, Norman D. Diffusion-weighted MR imaging of the brain: value of differentiating between extraaxial cysts and epidermoid tumors. *AJR Am J Roentgenol.* 1990;155(5):1059–1065.
18. Duffis EJ, Ganchi CD, Prestigiacomo CJ, et al. On behalf of the American Society of Interventional and Therapeutic Neuroradiology. Head, neck, and brain tumor embolization. *AJNR Am J Neuroradiol.* 2001;22(suppl 8):S14–S15.
19. Chiechi MV, Smirniotopoulos JG, Mena H. Intracranial hemangiopericytomas: MR and CT features. *AJNR Am J Neuroradiol.* 1996;17(7):1365–1371.
20. Kornienko VN, Pronin IN. *Diagnostic Neuroradiology.* Berlin: Springer Verlag; 2008.
21. Kleinschmidt-DeMasters BK, Damek DM, Lillehei KO, Dogan A, Giannini C. Epstein Barr virus-associated primary CNS lymphomas in elderly patients on immunosuppressive medications. *J Neuropathol Exp Neurol.* 2008;67(11):1103–1111.

Chapter 6

Evaluation of a supratentorial parenchymal lesion

Albert E. Kim and Elizabeth R. Gerstner

CHAPTER OUTLINE

Introduction

Central nervous system (CNS) tumors encompass histologically diverse entities with widely varying prognostic and therapeutic implications. Within the brain, tumors can be divided into two main categories: primary and secondary brain tumors. Primary brain tumors arise from the brain parenchyma, meninges, nerves, or glands within the cranial cavity. In order to uniformly classify these tumors, the World Health Organization (WHO) has established an internationally accepted nomenclature and criteria based on histopathologic analysis of tumor tissue. The most recent update (WHO 2016 classification) has integrated molecular markers, which reflect genetic changes that are felt to underlie tumorigenesis, with well-established histologic criteria to classify gliomas (see Chapter 1 for molecular classification of brain tumors).[1] Secondary brain tumors metastasize to the brain from another part of the body and are more common than primary brain tumors. The most common types of cancer that metastasize to the brain include lung, kidney, melanoma, and breast cancer.

Although ultimately an exact diagnosis frequently requires tissue confirmation, neuro-imaging is the initial step in the evaluation of patients with suspected CNS tumors. On initial presentation, patients often have clinical symptoms, such as seizures or hemiparesis, attributable to the location of the lesion or mass effect. Correlation of the patient's neurologic symptoms with imaging is a critical step to initial management (i.e., steroid and anti-epileptic administration; surgical resection versus biopsy), as the ease of obtaining MRI these days has increased the risk of incidental findings. Furthermore, imaging can aid in creating an initial differential diagnosis of the suspected tumor and surgical planning.

This chapter provides an approach for the general neurologist or related practitioner to use when conducting an initial encounter of patients with different types of brain tumors. We focus on tumors that are commonly encountered in clinical practice. First, we present an overview of currently used standard and advanced imaging modalities in the evaluation of suspected brain tumors. Next, we present four clinical vignettes, each with a different type of tumor, in which we review imaging, prognosis, and initial management. Internists and neurologists are on the "front lines" of evaluating these patients and are often the first to identify patients with a suspected brain tumor. Our hope is that this chapter will improve familiarity with recognizing the characteristic radiographic appearance of common brain tumors, facilitating diagnostic testing in an expeditious fashion, as well as informing prognosis and different therapeutic strategies.

Imaging techniques

A CT or MRI of the head or brain is generally the first step in the evaluation of a patient who presents with neurologic symptoms. Although MRI is more sensitive for identifying

CNS tumors, CT is usually much faster, cheaper, and more widely available—and therefore usually the first screening test for a brain tumor. In this section, we review pitfalls and pearls of both CT and MRI in the evaluation of brain tumors at time of diagnosis.

Computed tomography. A CT scan combines a series of x-ray images taken from different angles, and then processes these images through digital geometry processing to generate a three-dimensional cross-sectional view of the intended object.[2] In addition to tumors, CT scans of the head are also used to detect hemorrhage, infarction, or bone trauma. Hyperdense structures (i.e., blood, calcifications) attenuate x-rays to a greater degree and will appear brighter on CT, whereas hypo-dense substances (i.e., air, infarction, edema) are radiolucent and will appear darker on CT.[2] One important distinction is that of cytotoxic versus vasogenic cerebral edema. Cytotoxic edema, commonly seen in cerebral ischemia, is the result of an inability to maintain the ATP-dependent sodium/potassium membrane pumps on cell surface, which are responsible for the high extracellular and low intracellular Na+ gradient.[3] When these pumps fail, Na+ accumulates within the cell and therefore draws in chloride (Cl−) and water, along an osmotic gradient—which in turn results in cellular swelling.[3] There is no compromise of the blood-brain barrier (BBB). Imaging reveals effacement of cerebral sulci and edema affecting both grey and white matter. Vasogenic edema, seen in malignant brain tumors and cerebral abscesses, is the result of BBB disruption and resultant extracellular edema via leakage of fluid from capillaries.[3] This generally affects white matter only and spares the outer cortical gray matter. On imaging, grey-white matter differentiation is maintained. In cases of persistent neurologic symptoms, hyperosmolar therapy (i.e., mannitol, hypertonic saline) is beneficial for cytotoxic edema, whereas corticosteroids are helpful for vasogenic edema.

The use of iodinated contrast with CT can improve detection of tumors, as abnormal enhancement can reflect disruption of the BBB and increased vascularity, which can be seen in malignant tumors.[2] Despite these advantages, MRI is generally preferred over CT due to limitations with CT such as posterior fossa beam hardening artifact, poor soft tissue characterization, and inferior resolution (compared with MRI). CT, however, remains a reasonable alternative in patients with contraindications to MRI (i.e., MRI-incompatible implants [Autoimatic Implantable Cardioverter Defibrillator (AICD), pacemaker]; inability to lie still for a prolonged period).

Magnetic resonance imaging. MRI is based off of the magnetization properties of protons in the water molecules of tissue being examined. During an MRI scan, a powerful magnetic field is first used to align protons, which are normally randomly oriented, into one plane.[4] This alignment is then perturbed by an externally applied radiofrequency (RF) pulse. After some time, the protons eventually return to their resting alignment through various relaxation processes and, in doing so, emit RF energy. These emitted signals are collected and processed through Fourier transformation to create a specific MRI pulse sequence.[4] By varying the sequence of RF pulses applied and collected, different sequences are created.[4] Different pulse sequences measure different aspects of molecular behavior, which in turn characterize various nervous system structures, such as grey and white matter, cerebrospinal fluid (CSF), and meninges.

The most common MRI sequences are T1-weighted and T2-weighted images. On T1-weighted images, grey matter is darker than white matter, and CSF is dark. On T2-weighted images, grey matter is brighter (i.e., more hyperintense) than white matter, and CSF is bright. The T2-fluid attenuated inversion recovery (FLAIR) sequence is a T2-weighted image with an additional RF pulse that suppresses the bright signal of CSF.[4] Inflammation (i.e., edema, demyelination) is dark on T1-weighted images and bright on T2-weighted and FLAIR images. In clinical practice, the T2-weighted or FLAIR images are useful to track treatment response in low-grade gliomas, or to qualitatively assess for vasogenic edema in high-grade gliomas and lymphomas.

T1-weighted images can also be performed while injecting gadolinium, a paramagnetic contrast enhancement agent.[4] In general, fat, protein, hemorrhage, melanin, and gadolinium contrast will be bright on T1-weighted images. The use of gadolinium with MRI is helpful in evaluating BBB breakdown, which is implicated in high-grade gliomas and lymphomas. Longitudinal comparison of T1-weighted post-contrast MRIs is the current standard of care in evaluating treatment efficacy in high-grade gliomas and lymphomas. This method, however, is not always reliable in brain tumor evaluation, as increasing contrast enhancement can be seen in both true tumor progression (i.e., active tumor) and post-treatment inflammatory changes associated with radiation, targeted therapy, or immunotherapy (i.e., dying tumor). The latter is known as pseudoprogression, and is commonly seen in MGMT-methylated gliomas that have recently undergone treatment with radiation and temozolomide. Imaging changes may also lead to tumor pseudoresponse—which reflects a rapid decrease in contrast enhancement and edema after administration of anti-angiogenic therapy (i.e., bevacizumab). In such cases, there is generally no real change in actual tumor size as seen on T2-weighted imaging but contrast enhanced sequences are dramatically improved. Due to these issues, several radiographic response criteria including the Response Assessment in Neuro-Oncology criteria (RANO)[5] and Immunotherapy Response Assessment in Neuro-Oncology criteria (iRANO)[6] have been developed to standardize assessment of tumor response and progressive disease. Additional advanced imaging modalities that reflect an underlying tumor's physiologic response or genomic and molecular changes are under development and may be a solution for this response assessment conundrum in the future.

Diffuse-weighted and susceptibility weighted MRI. Two advanced MRI sequences frequently encountered in clinical practice are diffusion-weighted imaging (DWI) and susceptibility-weighted imaging (SWI). DWI is a measure of the random Brownian motion of water molecules within different tissues.[4] This free movement of water is restricted in several pathologic conditions, such as acute ischemic stroke, abscess, and hypercellular tumors such as lymphoma and, occasionally, high-grade gliomas. On imaging, "restricted diffusion" manifests as high signal on isotropic images (DWI) and corresponding low apparent diffusion coefficient (ADC) values for the voxel in question. SWI is an MRI sequence that is particularly sensitive to compounds with paramagnetic and diamagnetic properties that distort the local magnetic field. The most common clinical use of SWI is for detection of small amounts of blood products or calcifications that may not be picked up on other MRI sequences or CT. The presence of a microhemorrhage within a brain tumor can be associated with high-grade gliomas, or with parenchymal tumors recently treated with radiation.[2] Calcifications within tumors can be seen in lower-grade meningiomas or oligodendrogliomas,[2] as these entities are more indolent and chronic in nature. Notably, different MRI vendors have different names for these sequences and there may be slight differences in how the images are acquired. For example, a gradient echo (GRE) sequence provides similar information as an SWI sequences.

Positron emission tomography (PET). Due to increasing awareness that standard post-contrast anatomic MRI can be misleading for brain tumor assessment, other imaging modalities are currently being explored. Positron emission tomography (PET) is a nuclear medicine functional imaging technique that can illustrate aspects of tumor metabolism. At present, there are two main classes of radiotracers: glucose metabolism tracers and amino acid transport tracers. ^{18}F-2-fluoro-2-deoxy-D-glucose (^{18}F-FDG) is a widespread and relatively cheap glucose metabolism tracer that was previously felt to be useful in delineating high-grade gliomas, given a positive correlation between glycolysis rate and malignancy.[7] Unfortunately, due to high physiologic glucose metabolism within the brain, ^{18}F-FDG has poor spatial and diagnostic accuracy for gliomas. Due to relatively low tracer uptake in normal grey matter, amino acid PET tracers (i.e. ^{11}C-methyl-methionine [^{11}C-MET] and 3,4-dihydroxy-6-^{18}F-fluoro-L-phenylalanine [^{18}F-DOPA]) can detect gliomas with greater sensitivity and may be helpful in differentiating progression from pseudoprogression.[7,8] These tracers, which are still under development, currently have major limitations (i.e., short half-life requiring close proximity to cyclotron,[7] nonspecific uptake in other areas)[8] that limit clinical use.

MR spectroscopy (MRS) and perfusion MRI (pMRI). Other sequences that are currently incorporated in clinical practice are MR spectroscopy (MRS) and perfusion MRI (pMRI). MRS is used to study the metabolic changes within the tissue in question. This sequence determines relative concentrations of a variety of cellular metabolites, such as choline (associated with membrane turnover and synthesis), creatine (associated with energy metabolism), *N*-acetyl-aspartate (NAA, associated with neuronal health), and lactate (associated with anaerobic glycolysis).[9] High-grade gliomas are associated with a low NAA and creatine peak, and elevated choline peak—which correlate with increased membrane turnover and neuronal loss.[9] In clinical practice, although MRS does correlate with tumor type and grade, it is not sufficiently sensitive or specific enough to replace histologic diagnosis, nor is it able to reliably differentiate between pseudoprogression and true tumor progression. pMRI assesses cerebral microvasculature by modeling the concentration of blood in different voxels. Kinetic analysis of this data enables quantitation of several physiologic biomarkers, such as cerebral blood flow, cerebral blood volume, and mean transit time.[10] These measures are sometimes helpful in directing brain biopsy to the most aggressive portion of a lesion, distinguishing radiation necrosis from progressive tumor, and assessing response to anti-angiogenic agents (i.e., bevacizumab). In clinical practice, even with perfusion imaging, tissue analysis is still frequently required, and guidelines for pMRI data acquisition and processing have not been standardized across centers.

Clinical cases

CASE 6.1 RIM-ENHANCING PARENCHYMAL LESION

Case. A 71-year-old female has a history of localized non–small-cell lung cancer under remission. She presents to medical attention after a first-time generalized tonic-clonic seizure. She denies fevers or recent infections. From a lung cancer perspective, this was diagnosed 5 years ago, and she underwent a video-assisted thoracoscopic surgery with right middle lobe resection. Staging systemic imaging revealed no sites of metastases. Since then, she has been monitored with surveillance imaging, which has demonstrated continued remission.

After the patient presented to the emergency department (ED) for new seizure, a brain MRI with and without gadolinium contrast was obtained. This revealed an intra-axial right frontal lobe lesion that measured approximately 3.9 × 3.6 × 4.2 cm, and was associated with vasogenic edema (Fig. 6.1). The radiologic differential was felt to include a high-grade glioma versus less likely a metastasis or abscess. After imaging, a neurosurgical consultation was requested. The patient was started on levetiracetam 750 mg bid and dexamethasone 4 mg bid, and admitted to the hospital. Three days later, she was taken to the operating room for a gross total resection of contrast-enhancing disease. Histopathologic analysis revealed a glioblastoma (GBM). She was discharged from the hospital 2 days afterwards, and was referred to Radiation Oncology and Neuro-oncology for consideration of fractionated radiation and chemotherapy.

Teaching Points: Imaging Features of Supratentorial GBM. This case illustrates several classic features of GBM. GBM is a WHO grade IV malignant astrocytic tumor characterized by necrosis and neovascularity. It is the most common primary malignant intracranial neoplasm, and has an estimated incidence of 15,000 new cases yearly in the United States.[11] Headaches (50–60%), seizures (20–50%), and focal neurologic deficits (10–40%) are the most common presenting signs of a GBM.[12] Fig. 6.1 is a characteristic appearance of a GBM. T2/FLAIR imaging often demonstrates a heterogenous and hyperintense mass with adjacent tumor infiltration and vasogenic edema, although it can be difficult to distinguish infiltrative tumor from perilesional edema. T1 post-contrast imaging generally illustrates thick, irregular ring-enhancement surrounding an area of central necrosis. Although not seen in this case, there is often involvement of the corpus callosum, which signifies involvement of the white matter tracts and spread to the contralateral hemisphere (e.g., "butterfly" lesion). Corpus callosal involvement is more commonly associated with GBM and lymphoma, and rarely for metastases or strokes. There is usually no diffusion restriction. SWI often has artifact that correlates to the area of central necrosis seen on T1 post-contrast imaging.

Imaging differential for HGG. Other considerations on the imaging differential for GBM include a solitary brain metastasis, abscess (given ring-enhancing lesion, though should have prominent diffusion restriction), HIV-related primary CNS lymphoma, "tumefactive" demyelination, or subacute ischemia. This patient's history of lung cancer does increase clinical suspicion for metastasis; however, she had a locally treated cancer that was likely cured. There are, however, some cancers such as melanoma or renal cell carcinoma that can appear years after a primary tumor has been treated and the patient is in remission. Although it can be difficult radiographically to discern a solitary metastasis from GBM, metastases are generally smaller, located in the grey-white junction, and do not have as much vasogenic edema. GBM tends to have irregularly shaped contrast enhancement and FLAIR hyperintensities due to its predilection for spread along white matter tracts.[13]

For this patient, we note the lack of diffusion restriction and rather thick contrast enhancement is not consistent with an abscess. A demyelinating lesion would be atypical in a patient of this age range. Additionally, there was not a history of an abrupt-onset neurologic deficit several days ago, and to have such extensive vasogenic edema would be uncommon for a stroke. This being said, unusual presentations of all the above can occur. To date, there is no advanced imaging modality (i.e., MRS, pMRI, diffusion tensor imaging) that can accurately diagnose a GBM and thus supplant the need for tumor tissue in diagnosis.[14]

Patient management. Standard of care for adjuvant treatment of GBM and other high-grade gliomas is covered in a separate section. On initial presentation, we emphasize the importance of an urgent neurosurgical consultation. The goal of surgery is to confirm a pathologic diagnosis and to achieve maximal safe resection consistent with preservation of neurologic function (see Chapter 2, Case 2.2 for further discussion of surgical management of high-grade brain tumors). Doing so provides the benefit of cytoreduction, prior to adjuvant radiation and chemotherapy, which has demonstrated improved outcomes—compared with a biopsy only.[13] Furthermore, maximal safe resection will provide adequate tissue through which molecular analyses can be run, and sampling bias can be avoided. Subtotal resection or stereotactic biopsy may be required, however, depending on the location and extent of the tumor and the patient's functional status. If the suspicion for a high-grade glioma is high, a CT chest/abdomen/pelvis (to assess for a systemic malignancy) can be deferred given the need for tissue diagnosis.[15] Once the diagnosis of GBM is confirmed, patients should start fractionated radiation and systemic therapy within 4–6 weeks of surgery, as per National Comprehensive Cancer Network guidelines.[16]

Clinical Pearls

1. The imaging differential for a single ring-enhancing supratentorial lesion includes high-grade glioma, solitary brain metastasis, cerebral abscess, tumefactive demyelination, and subacute stroke.
2. For such a lesion, surgical consultation and evaluation are required to establish a tissue diagnosis and guide treatment decisions.

CASE 6.2 NON-ENHANCING PARENCHYMAL LESION

Case. A 29-year-old female presented to medical attention after a first-time generalized tonic-clonic seizure. Brain MRI demonstrated an expansile left parietal T2/FLAIR lesion without enhancement, measuring approximately 3.3 × 3.9 × 3 cm and encompassing the post-central gyrus (Fig. 6.2). She was started on levetiracetam 500 mg bid and dexamethasone 4 mg bid. Six days after presentation, she was taken for a left parietal craniotomy and resection. Postoperative imaging demonstrated a subtotal resection, due to this lesion's proximity to the post-central gyrus. Tissue analysis revealed a WHO grade II, isocitrate dehydrogenase (IDH)-mutant, 1p/19q-co-deleted oligodendroglioma. Immediately after surgery, the patient had proprioceptive difficulties and numbness in her right upper extremity. She was discharged from the hospital 3 days afterwards with outpatient physical therapy, and referred to radiation Oncology and Neuro-oncology for consideration of adjuvant radiation and chemotherapy.

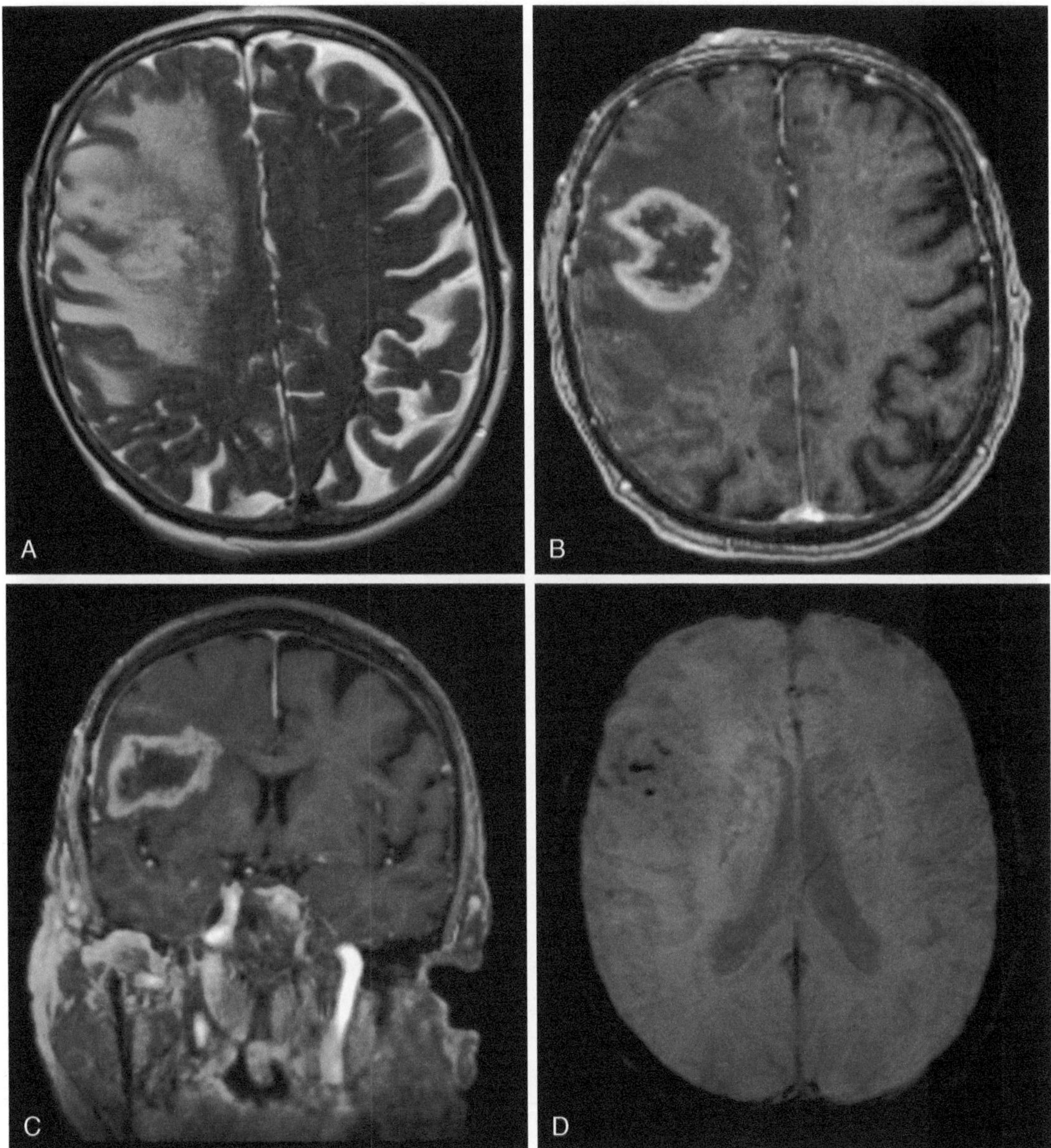

Fig. 6.1 Brain MRI for a patient with a newly diagnosed GBM, with T2-weighted sequence (A), T1 post-contrast sequence (B: axial slice, C: coronal slice), and SWI sequence (D). Imaging demonstrates thick, irregular enhancement surrounding an area of central necrosis in the right frontal lobe (B, C) with adjacent vasogenic edema (A). There was no diffusion restriction (not shown), and an area of susceptibility artifact (D) correlating to area of central necrosis. *GBM*, Glioblastoma, *SWI*, susceptibility-weighted imaging.

Teaching Points: Imaging Features of Supratentorial Low-Grade Glioma. This case illustrates many characteristic features of a low-grade glioma (LGG). Based on current epidemiological data, the incidence of LGGs is estimated at 2500 new cases yearly in the United States.[12] Within the classification of LGG, an oligodendroglioma is a WHO grade II glioma that is generally well differentiated, but diffusely infiltrative. The typical patient ranges in age from the late 20s to the mid-40s.[17] Whereas seizures are the most common presenting symptom, an increasing number of patients are diagnosed following presentation for unrelated issues (i.e., migraine, head trauma) due to widespread availability of CT and MRI. Due to an increased

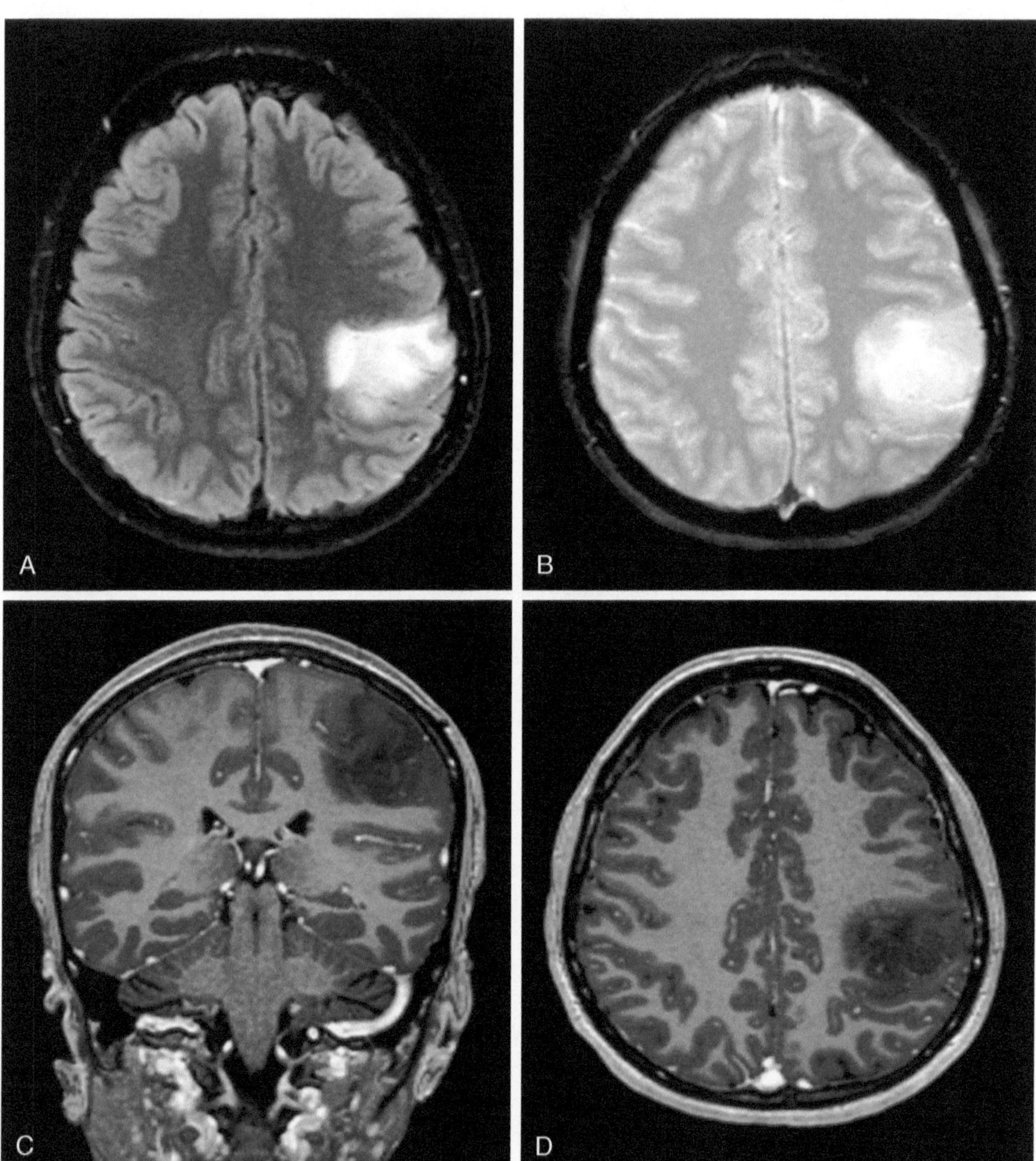

Fig. 6.2 Brain MRI for a patient with a newly diagnosed oligodendroglioma, with (A) T2/FLAIR sequence, (B) GRE sequence, and (C) and (D) T1 post-contrast sequence (C: coronal slice, D: axial slice). Imaging demonstrates an expansile left parietal T2/FLAIR-hyperintense mass (A) with no susceptibility artifact on the GRE sequence (B) and no contrast enhancement (C, D). There were no areas of diffusion restriction (not shown). *FLAIR*, Fluid attenuated inversion recovery; *GRE*, gradient echo.

understanding of a tumor's molecular changes and implications regarding prognosis and treatment sensitivity, the new WHO 2016 classification defines LGG by both histologic and molecular features (Chapter 1). Grade II gliomas with the IDH mutation and 1p/19q co-deletion are termed oligodendrogliomas regardless of morphology.[17] Those lacking 1p/19 co-deletion but with the IDH mutation are defined as diffuse astrocytomas.[17]

Neuroimaging can often be suggestive of a diagnosis of LGG. More than 95% of LGG are supratentorial, roughly equally split between frontal and temporal locations with few occipital lobe tumors.[17] On MRI, LGG typically manifests as a T1 hypointense and T2/FLAIR hyperintense lesion lacing contrast enhancement. Approximately 20% of LGG demonstrates calcification, which can manifest as areas of "blooming" on GRE or SWI imaging.

Oligodendrogliomas are generally well-circumscribed masses with minimal associated edema, whereas diffuse astrocytomas can be more infiltrative and have more associated edema. LGG will not have restricted diffusion. MRS will generally have an elevated 2-hydroxyglutarate and choline peak, and a low NAA peak, although these characteristics are not necessarily specific to LGG.

Imaging differential for low-grade glioma. Other considerations for a radiologic differential diagnosis include subacute ischemia, cerebritis, an arteriovenous malformation (AVM), or herpes encephalitis. Subacute ischemia will follow a specific vascular territory (i.e., middle cerebral artery, anterior cerebral artery, posterior cerebral artery) and are often times wedge-shaped. History of an abrupt-onset neurologic deficit would lend support to this possibility. The rather expansile nature of this lesion would be atypical for ischemia. Cerebritis is generally associated with patchy enhancement and restricted diffusion. This, too, can be associated with an abrupt neurologic change. A calcified or thrombosed AVM is generally associated with multiple enlarged flow voids. Vascular imaging (i.e., CT angiogram, catheter angiography) could be considered, depending on radiographic suspicion. Finally, herpes encephalitis is generally confined to the temporal lobes, and associated with SWI or GRE signal (signifying blood products) with contrast enhancement. History of seizures, fever, and altered mental status would be helpful.

Patient management. As with other tumors, a definitive diagnosis is only obtained via tissue confirmation. Once a suspicious lesion is discovered, an expeditious referral to neurosurgery is recommended. If clinical suspicion for an LGG is high, maximal safe resection is recommended.[16] Recent literature has suggested that extent of resection correlates significantly with overall survival (OS). A large series of 216 patients with LGG who underwent resection found a 5-year OS of 97% with an extent of resection greater than 90%, but only 76% with an extent of resection less than 90%.[18] Furthermore, surgical debulking improves diagnostic accuracy, as needle biopsies are at risk for misdiagnosis given the possibility of sampling bias due to the heterogenous nature of these tumors. The timing and choice of radiation and chemotherapy for LGG will be discussed in another section, but appropriate referrals to neuro-oncology and radiation oncology should be arranged prior to the patient's discharge.

Clinical Pearls

1. The differential diagnosis of a non-enhancing supratentorial lesion on MRI includes low-grade glioma and subacute ischemia, cerebritis, an arteriovenous malformation (AVM), or herpes encephalitis

CASE 6.3 HOMOGENEOUSLY ENHANCING PARENCHYMAL LESION

Case. A 70-year-old female who presented to medical attention after a 2-month history of progressive fatigue and somnolence. At baseline, the patient was independent with all activities of daily living. In the weeks preceding her admission, she was noted to have increased somnolence and progressive difficulty with dexterity in her left upper extremity while typing. A brain MRI demonstrated a 2.0 × 2.3 × 2.6 cm homogenously enhancing right lentiform nucleus lesion and a smaller right parietal lesion with surrounding edema (Fig. 6.3). The basal ganglia lesion had diffusion restriction. Due to radiographic concern for central nervous system lymphoma (CNSL), a neurosurgical consult was immediately requested and steroids were withheld to maximize the yield of biopsy. The next day, the patient underwent a stereotactic biopsy of the right basal ganglia contrast-enhancing lesion. Frozen pathology was concerning for lymphoma. She was started on dexamethasone after her biopsy to symptomatic cognitive and motor benefit, and near return to her prior baseline.

While awaiting permanent stains on tumor tissue, an extent-of-disease (EOD) staging evaluation was performed during that hospitalization. Testing included a serum HIV, whole body PET/CT scan (to exclude synchronous systemic disease), MRI spine, CSF analysis for cytology and flow cytometry, and slit-lamp ophthalmologic examination (to exclude vitreoretinal lymphoma)—all of which were negative. During the EOD evaluation, the biopsy was finalized as diffuse large B-cell lymphoma (DLBCL), non-germinal center subtype, with a Ki-67 proliferation index of 60%. She was started on high-dose methotrexate and rituximab, following completion of EOD evaluation. In all, chemotherapy was administered 3 days after her biopsy and on the same hospital admission as her initial presentation.

Teaching Points: Imaging Features of CNS Lymphoma and Its Mimics. Primary central nervous system lymphoma (PCNSL) is a highly aggressive, infiltrative extranodal non-Hodgkin's lymphoma (NHL) that is confined to the brain, eyes, spinal cord, or leptomeninges without systemic involvement at time of diagnosis. PCNSL accounts for approximately 2% of all brain tumors, with an annual incidence of 1,900 cases annually in the United States.[19] Approximately 95% of PCNSL is CD20+ DLBCL.[19] Synchronous CNS and systemic lymphoma, or secondary CNS lymphoma (SCNSL), is more common than PCNSL and usually associated with highly aggressive NHL, such as Burkitt's lymphoma or lymphoblastic lymphoma. Radiographic appearance and CNS-directed therapy is similar for both entities. The median age for PCNSL is 66 in immunocompetent individuals, and 37 in immunocompromised patients (i.e., HIV-positive, post-transplant).[19] Common presenting symptoms include cognitive changes, encephalopathy, focal neurologic deficits, and headaches. Seizures are relatively uncommon, given the predilection of CNSL for deep structures of the brain.

CNSL has characteristic features on MRI. Approximately 87% of CNSL is located within the supratentorium, with the deep grey nuclei generally affected.[20] There is frequently involvement of the corpus callosum. Leptomeningeal or dural involvement is rare, but more common in synchronous CNS and systemic lymphoma.[19] In immunocompetent individuals, PCNSL is associated with homogenous contrast enhancement with well-defined borders. Immunocompromised patients can

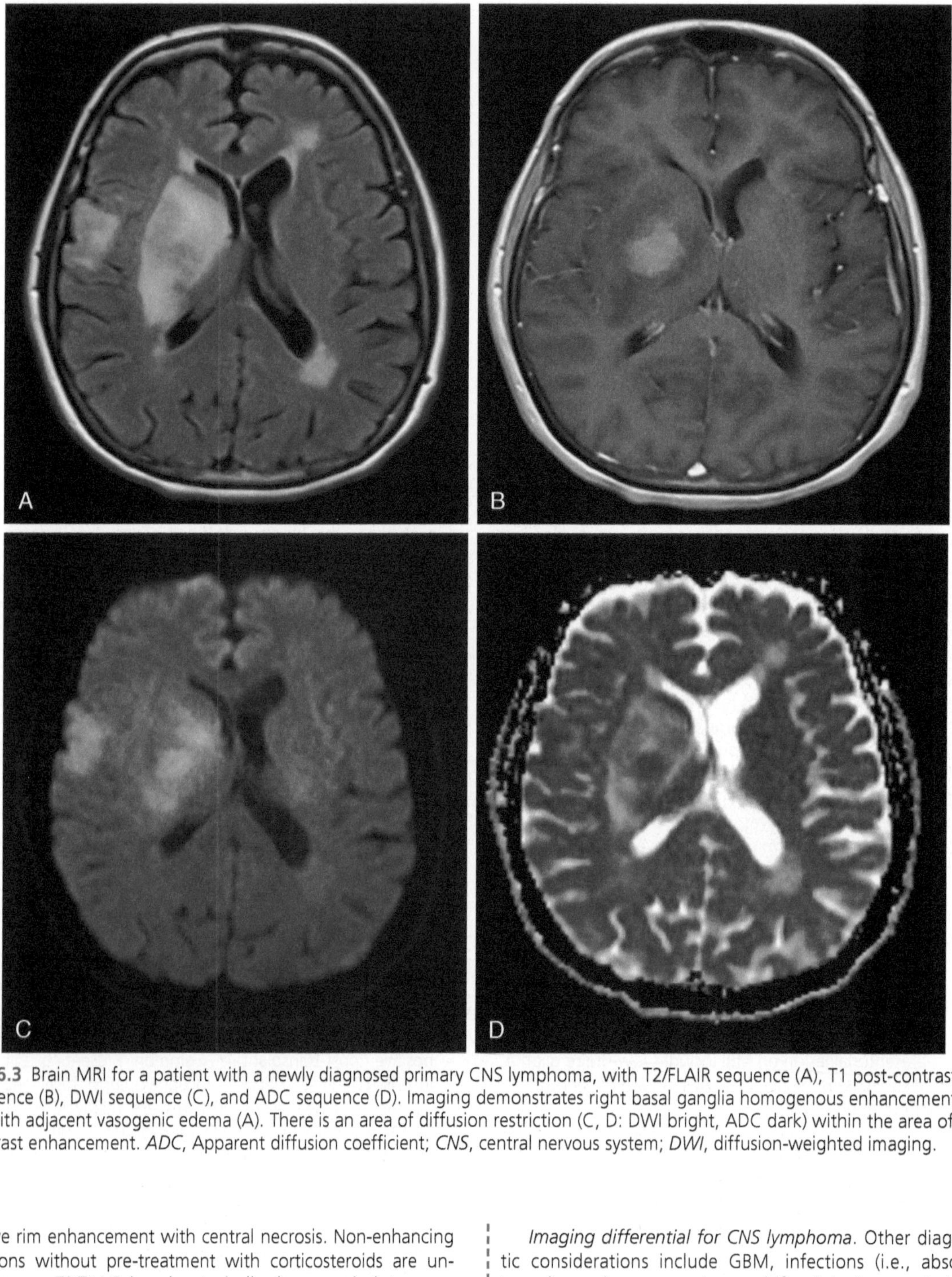

Fig. 6.3 Brain MRI for a patient with a newly diagnosed primary CNS lymphoma, with T2/FLAIR sequence (A), T1 post-contrast sequence (B), DWI sequence (C), and ADC sequence (D). Imaging demonstrates right basal ganglia homogenous enhancement (B) with adjacent vasogenic edema (A). There is an area of diffusion restriction (C, D: DWI bright, ADC dark) within the area of contrast enhancement. *ADC*, Apparent diffusion coefficient; *CNS*, central nervous system; *DWI*, diffusion-weighted imaging.

have rim enhancement with central necrosis. Non-enhancing lesions without pre-treatment with corticosteroids are uncommon. T2/FLAIR imaging typically shows an isointense or hypointense lesion with mild surrounding vasogenic edema. There is frequently restricted diffusion, which correlates with high cellularity and tightly compacted cells.

Imaging differential for CNS lymphoma. Other diagnostic considerations include GBM, infections (i.e., abscess, toxoplasmosis, progressive multifocal leukoencephalopathy [PML]), demyelinating disorders, or metastases. GBM generally has irregularly shaped contrast enhancement surrounding an area of central necrosis, which can be seen in immune-compromised PCNSL. An abscess usually has a T2 hypointense rim, a thin rim of enhancement with central necrosis, and prominent central diffusion restriction. Toxoplasmosis is associated with the "eccentric target sign" and usually involves the basal ganglia or corticomedullary junction. PML lesions are found in immunocompromised patients, usually non-enhance, and involve the subcortical U-fibers. Demyelinating lesions are usually found in younger patients, and can have "horseshoe-shaped" enhancement that are open toward the cortex. Metastases can have a similar radiographic appearance to PCNSL, but are generally located in the juxtacortical areas and associate with more vasogenic edema.

Patient management. In cases of suspected CNSL, we discourage empiric use of corticosteroids prior to obtaining tissue, due to its lymphocytotoxic response and risk of non-diagnostic brain biopsy.[21,22] For those with symptomatic mass effect, hyperosmolar therapy (i.e., mannitol or hypertonic saline) can be used in the short term as a bridge to surgery, after which steroids can be started while pathology is pending. If radiographic concern for CNSL is high, we recommend tissue analysis of a contrast-enhancing lesion as a first step rather than ancillary testing (i.e., CSF analysis or ophthalmologic examination), as concomitant vitreoretinal (present in 15–25% of cases)[23,24] or leptomeningeal involvement (present in 7–42% of cases)[21,23,24] are often not seen. Consequently, ancillary testing may delay diagnosis of CNSL.

In CNSL, there is controversy on optimal extent of surgery (biopsy versus aggressive surgery) and choice of systemic agents used for induction and consolidation regimens. For the purposes of initial management, our recommendation is for expeditious tissue analysis (given worse outcomes with delayed diagnosis of PCNSL or initiation of chemotherapy),[25] efficient EOD testing, and start of tumor-directed therapy. If tissue frozen section is concerning for lymphoma, we recommend an urgent medical oncology or neuro-oncology consultation for guidance. Following an EOD evaluation, induction chemotherapy, generally a methotrexate-based regimen, is started. Choice of sequential systemic agents for induction, as well as consolidation treatment strategies, are dependent on the patient's comorbidities and functional status, and often has institutional variability.

Clinical Pearls

1. The imaging differential diagnosis for an enhancing lesion consistent with CNS lymphoma includes CNS lymphoma, GBM, infections (i.e., abscess, toxoplasmosis, progressive multifocal leukoencephalopathy [PML], demyelinating disorders, or metastases).
2. Compared with malignant glioma, treatment response is considerable higher for patients with CNS lymphoma even without cytoreduction. Thus, stereotactic biopsy is favored.

CASE 6.4 MULTIFOCAL ENHANCING PARENCHYMAL LESIONS

Case. A 36-year-old female who first presented to medical attention after palpating a left breast mass. A breast ultrasound revealed a breast mass of mixed echogenicity; subsequent core needle biopsy revealed grade 3 invasive ductal carcinoma, estrogen receptor (ER)-positive, progesterone receptor (PR)-positive, and human epidermal growth factor (HER2)-positive. Staging scans revealed no sites of metastases. She subsequently received four cycles of neoadjuvant adriamycin and cyclophosphamide, followed by a mastectomy with sentinel lymph node biopsy showing complete response. She was maintained afterwards on trastuzumab and tamoxifen. About 1 year later, the patient presented to neurologic attention with worsening headaches, cognitive changes, and fatigue. A brain MRI revealed over 30 contrast enhancing lesions concerning for brain metastases (Fig. 6.4). Re-staging scans demonstrated continued extracranial complete response (CR). She was subsequently referred to radiation oncology for whole brain radiation.

Teaching Points: Imaging of Multifocal Brain Metastases. Brain metastases (BM) are the most common CNS malignancy. Although there is no epidemiological study that estimates incidence of BM in the modern era, population-level data estimate the incidence of BM at approximately 24,000 new cases annually in the United States.[26] BM is estimated to affect 10–30% of all adults with cancer, and up to 40% of patients with metastatic cancer.[27] Over the past decade, the incidence of BM has risen due to improved diagnostic testing that facilitate detection of asymptomatic BM and increased patient survival through better-tolerated and more effective treatment strategies. Lung (39–56%), breast cancer (13–30%), and melanoma (6–11%) are among the most likely systemic cancers to cross into the CNS.[28] Presenting symptoms are highly variable, and dependent on the compromised area within the brain.

Distribution of BM often parallels blood flow, and are frequently located in the juxta-cortical and vascular border-zone areas within the brain. Eighty percent of BM are located within the cerebral hemispheres, with the remainder in the posterior fossa.[28] On MRI, BM can have varied appearances. Almost all BM enhance, but there are many variable patterns (solid, heterogenous, cystic). Hemorrhagic metastases (characteristic of melanoma) can have intrinsically bright signal on T1 images and appear dark on SWI or GRE sequences. T2/FLAIR imaging typically depicts hyperintense lesions with adjacent vasogenic edema. There is usually no diffusion restriction with BM.

Imaging differential for multifocal brain lesions. Other diagnostic considerations include a GBM, abscess, or demyelinating disease. It can be challenging to distinguish a solitary BM from a GBM radiographically. History of a primary malignancy would obviously make it easier to distinguish. A GBM is generally within a deep location and may involve the corpus callosum, both of which are not stereotypical for BM. An abscess is usually associated with diffusion restriction. Demyelinating lesions more often occur in the subcortical white matter, and may have a "horseshoe-shaped" enhancement that opens toward the cortex.

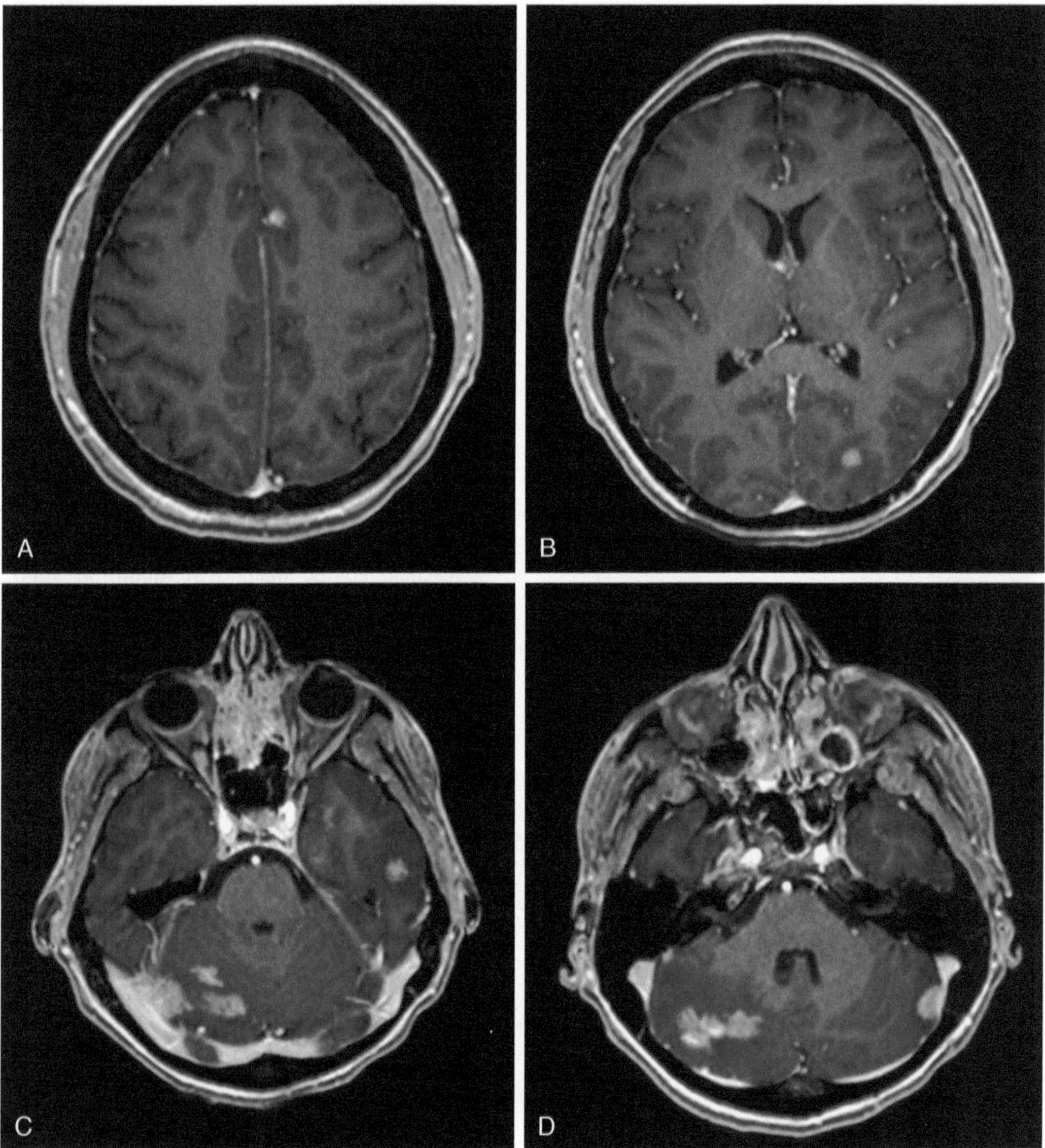

Fig. 6.4 Brain MRI for a patient with newly diagnosed brain metastases, with different axial slices of the T1 post-contrast sequence (A–D). This demonstrates areas of juxta-cortical contrast enhancement in multiple vascular distributions (A: left frontal, B: left occipital, C: left temporal and right cerebellum, D: bilateral cerebellar hemispheres) with surrounding edema.

Patient management. Treatment for BM is case-specific and evolving with the advent of targeted therapy and immunotherapy. In general, treatment usually entails a multi-disciplinary approach centered around surgical resection, radiotherapy, and systemic therapy. Treatment plans are dependent on many factors, such as performance status of patient, the number, location of, and primary tumor type of BM. Maximal safe surgical resection followed by radiotherapy is generally the standard of care for solitary or large symptomatic lesions.[29] Stereotactic radiosurgery alone is frequently used for small, asymptomatic BM and oligometastatic disease, which is commonly defined as up to four BM.[27,29] Finally, it may be recommended that patients with active extracranial disease receive systemic therapy after local brain therapy, as surgery and radiation alone are not curative.[27,29] Choice of systemic therapy is dependent on the patient's morbidities, genomic makeup of tumor, and CNS efficacy of systemic therapy.

Clinical Pearls

1. The imaging differential for multifocal brain metastasis includes multifocal GBM, abscess, demyelinating disease, or CNS lymphoma (in immunocompromised patient).
2. Multidisciplinary evaluation including radiology, neurosurgery, radiation oncology, medical oncology, and neuro-oncology help determine an optimal treatment plan.

Conclusion

Neuroimaging is a critical first step in the evaluation of patients with neurologic symptoms. This article presents radiographic patterns of several common brain tumors, differential diagnoses of such patterns, and initial workup. Brain tumors typically require multidisciplinary care, spanning neurosurgery, neuro-oncology, radiation oncology, and neuro-radiology. Open discussions with these care teams can assist in expanding differential diagnoses and directing care. Familiarity with presentation and imaging patterns will aid the neurologic clinician in optimal medical management (i.e., withholding steroids in cases of suspected lymphoma, dexamethasone for symptomatic edema in suspected glioma) and expeditious referrals to neurosurgery and neuro-oncology, which will facilitate better patient outcomes.

References

1. Louis DN, Perry A, Reifenberger G, et al. The 2016 World Health Organization classification of tumors of the central nervous system: a summary. *Acta Neuropathol.* 2016;131(6):803–820.
2. Klein JP, Dietrich J. Neuroradiologic pearls for neuro-oncology. *Continuum (Minneap Minn)*. 2017;23(6, Neuro-oncology):1619–1634.
3. Klatzo I. Pathophysiological aspects of brain edema. *Acta Neuropathol.* 1987;72(3):236–239.
4. Bitar R, Leung G, Perng R, et al. MR pulse sequences: what every radiologist wants to know but is afraid to ask. *Radiographics.* 2006;26(2):513–537.
5. Wen PY, Chang SM, van den Bent MJ, Vogelbaum MA, Macdonald DR, Lee EQ. Response assessment in neuro-oncology clinical trials. *J Clin Oncol.* 2017;35(21):2439–2449.
6. Okada H, Weller M, Huang R, et al. Immunotherapy response assessment in neuro-oncology: a report of the RANO working group. *Lancet Oncol.* 2015;16:e534–e542.
7. Verger A, Langen KJ. PET imaging in glioblastoma. In: De Vleeschouwer S, ed. *Glioblastoma.* Brisbane: Codon Publications; 2017. (Chapter 9).
8. Janvier L, Olivier P, Blonski M, et al. Correlation of SUV-derived indices with tumoral aggressiveness of gliomas in static 18F-FDOPA PET: use in clinical practice. *Clin Nucl Med.* 2015;40(9):e429–435.
9. Horska A, Barker PB. Imaging of brain tumors: MR spectroscopy and metabolic imaging. *Neuroimaging Clin N Am.* 2010;20(3):293–310.
10. Fussell D, Young RJ. Role of MRI perfusion in improving the treatment of brain tumors. *Imaging Med.* 2013;5(5):407–426.
11. de Robles P, Fiest KM, Folkis AD, et al. The worldwide incidence and prevalence of primary brain tumors: a systemic review and meta-analysis. *Neuro Oncol.* 2015;17:776–783.
12. Chang SM, Parney IF, Huang W, et al. Patterns of care for adults with newly diagnosed malignant glioma. *JAMA.* 2005;293(5):557–564.
13. Trifiletti DM, Alonso C, Grover S, Fadul CE, Sheehan JP, Showalter TN. Prognostic implications of extent of resection in glioblastoma: analysis from a large database. *World Neurosurg.* 2017;103:330–340.
14. Voorhies RM, Sundaresan N, Thaler HT. The single supratentorial lesion: an evaluation of pre-operative diagnostic tests. *J Neurosurg.* 1980;53(3):364–368.
15. Arrillaga-Romany I, Curry Jr WT, Jordan JT, et al. Performance of a hospital pathway for patients with a new single brain mass. *J Oncol Pract.* 2019;15(3):e211–e218.
16. Nabors LB, Portnow J, Ahluwalia M, et al. *NCCN Clinical Practice Guidelines in Oncology (NCCN Guidelines): Central Nervous System Cancers. Version 1*; 2019:2019.
17. Louis DN, Ohgaki H, Wiestler OD, et al. *WHO Classification of Tumors of the Central Nervous System.* 4th rev ed. Lyon: IARC; 2016.
18. Smith JS, Chang EF, Lamborn KR, et al. Role of extent of resection in the long-term outcome of low-grade hemispheric gliomas. *J Clin Oncol.* 2008;26(8):1338–1345.
19. Rubenstein JL, Gupta NK, Mannis GN, LaMarre AK, Treseler P. How I treat CNS lymphomas. *Blood.* 2003;122(14):2318–2320.
20. Han CH, Batchelor TT. Primary central nervous system lymphoma. *Continuum (Minneap Minn)*. 2017;23(6):1601–1618.
21. DeAngelis LM, Yahalom J, Heinemann MH, Cirrincione C, Thaler HT, Krol G. Primary CNS lymphoma: combined treatment with chemotherapy and radiotherapy. *Neurology.* 1990;40(1):80–86.
22. Bataille B, Delwail V, Menet E, et al. Primary intracerebral malignant lymphoma: report of 248 cases. *J Neurosurg.* 2000;92(2):261–266.
23. Grimm SA, Pulido JS, Jahnke K, et al. Primary intraocular lymphoma: an International primary central nervous system collaborative group report. *Ann Oncol.* 2007;18(11):1851–1855.
24. Batchelor T, Carson K, O'Neill A, et al. Treatment of primary CNS lymphoma with methotrexate and deferred radiotherapy: a report of NABTT 96–07. *J Clin Oncol.* 2003;21(6):1044–1049.
25. Rubenstein JL, Hsi ED, Johnson JL, et al. Intensive chemotherapy and immunotherapy in patients with newly diagnosed primary CNS lymphoma: CALGB 50202 (Alliance 50202). *J Clin Oncol.* 2013;31(25):3061–3068.

26. Cagney DN, Martin AM, Catalano PJ, et al. Incidence and prognosis of patients with brain metastases at diagnosis of systemic malignancy: a population-based study. *Neuro Oncol.* 2017;19(11):1511–1521.
27. Brastianos PK, Curry WT, Oh KS. Clinical discussion and review of the management of brain metastases. *J Natl Compr Canc Netw.* 2013;11:1153–1164.
28. Berghoff AS, Bartsch R, Wöhrer A, et al. Predictive molecular markers in metastases to the central nervous system: recent advances and future avenues. *Acta Neuropathol.* 2014;128(6):879–891.
29. Nayak L, Lee EQ, Wen PY. Epidemiology of brain metastases. *Curr Oncol Rep.* 2012;14(1):48–54.

Chapter 7

Evaluation of an infratentorial lesion

David E. Kram, Jacob J. Henderson, and Daniel E. Couture

CHAPTER OUTLINE

Introduction

The posterior fossa is the infratentorial compartment of the cranial vault, which houses the cerebellum and the bulk of the brainstem. Tumors that occur in this region can arise from, or spread to, any of the adjacent structures. The brainstem, which is composed of the midbrain, pons, and medulla, may develop or seed tumors that are intrinsic and contained within the brainstem, intrinsic with exophytic components, or extraaxial. Tumors in the posterior fossa may produce *general symptoms* caused by increased intracranial pressure, *localizing symptoms* due to compression of specific nerves or nuclei, or a combination of *both general and localizing symptoms*.

The posterior fossa is a small compartment compared with the supratentorium, and the cerebrospinal fluid (CSF) outflow tracts in this region are much smaller and less tolerant of compression. Even a small tumor in the midbrain region may produce significant aqueductal stenosis and obstructive hydrocephalus which may present with early morning awakening with headache, recumbent headaches, nausea, vomiting, and personality, mood, or mental capacity changes. Other tumors may produce symptoms specific to the tumor location. Tumors in the proximal brainstem commonly present with unilateral cranial nerve (CN) VI and VII palsies or with tectal involvement and Perinaud's syndrome. Tumors intrinsic to the pons typically present with a short clinical history, bilateral CN VI and VII dysfunction, ataxia, and long tract signs. Tumors in the medulla may cause deficits in cranial nerves VII, IX, and X early on, while obstructive symptoms including headaches or papilledema tend to occur later as the lesion compresses the fourth ventricle. Midline cerebellar tumors can cause truncal and gait ataxia, whereas lateral cerebellar hemispheric tumors tend to cause unilateral appendicular ataxia, commonly worse in the arm compared with the leg. Children with lateral cerebellar hemispheric tumors may be found tilting their heads away from the side of the tumor.[1]

Across all ages, brain tumors are predominantly located supratentorially. However, in children 3–18 years old, infratentorial tumors are more prevalent than supratentorial tumors, accounting for more than 60% of all CNS cancers in this age group.[2] The differential diagnosis for lesions found in the posterior fossa, therefore, is highly age-dependent. The index of suspicion for a tumor in an adult with a posterior fossa lesion on imaging, in whom the most common expansile lesion in this location is a subacute stroke followed by cerebellar metastasis, is different compared with children, in whom primary brain tumors are the most common solid tumor.[2]

General principles of posterior fossa imaging

CT and MRI are the primary neuroimaging techniques used to investigate posterior fossa lesions. For most posterior fossa tumors, gadolinium-enhanced MRI is the modality of choice because of its superior anatomic resolution and sensitivity in detecting pathologic alterations relative to normal brain architecture. The benefit of CT studies, however, is that they are quicker, less expensive, more widely available at small and medium-sized hospitals than MRI, and can more easily be obtained without sedation. Nonenhanced CT can rapidly exclude life-threatening emergencies such as hydrocephalus, hemorrhage, or significant mass effect. Although CT can be used to screen for hydrocephalus, MRI is superior at isolating a posterior fossa lesion that may be causing obstruction of the cerebral aqueduct or the fourth ventricle. Though an acute hemorrhage associated with a brain tumor can be visualized on CT as a hyperdense lesion, a subacute hemorrhage is more often isodense to normal brain and harder to detect by CT alone; subacute hemorrhage is visible on MRI as it produces a bright signal on both T1- and T2-weighted sequences. Additionally, whereas contrast-enhanced CT and MRI can localize a tumor that has disrupted the blood-brain barrier and is, thus, contrast-enhancing, non-enhancing tumors are often isodense to brain, making MRI scans significantly more sensitive for detecting such lesions. Finally, advanced MRI techniques, such as diffusion-weighted imaging (DWI), perfusion-weighted imaging (PWI), MR-PET, and dynamic contrast-enhanced studies increase diagnostic confidence and may be helpful in distinguishing different tumor types and histological grades.

Computed tomography. Certain characteristics of tumors imaged with CT can provide clues as to tumor type. Tumors with high cellularity, such as high-grade gliomas (HGGs), metastases, medulloblastoma, ependymoma, and atypical teratoid rhabdoid tumor (ATRT), may appear hyperdense or isodense compared with surrounding tissue, whereas tumors with low cellularity, such as low-grade gliomas (LGGs), are likely to appear hypodense. LGGs may be associated with intratumoral cysts that can be seen on CT, though cysts are not unique to LGGs, as medulloblastomas and hemangioblastomas can also have cystic components. Calcifications, which are better visualized with CT versus MRI, may be found up to 20% of cases of medulloblastoma and 50% of cases of ependymoma.[3]

Magnetic resonance imaging. MRI features can help differentiate posterior fossa tumor types, though there is significant heterogeneity of imaging characteristics of all tumors. The pattern of T1 hypointensity and T2 hyperintensity is common among LGG and HGG, ATRT, many medulloblastoma, hemangioblastoma, and gangliocytoma, whereas ependymoma tends to be T1 hyperintense and T2 hypointense. Contrast enhancement patterns can also be useful. Contrast enhancement is highly variable in medulloblastoma, with distinct molecular subgroups of medulloblastoma expressing variable levels of gadolinium enhancement.[4] Choroid plexus tumors tend to enhance brightly. Gliomas often enhance heterogeneously, with LGGs frequently enhancing at the cyst wall or the mural portion, and higher-grade gliomas showing more ring-like enhancement patterns. Importantly, DWI is becoming increasingly recognized as a method for differentiating different tumor types. Medulloblastoma, ATRT, and embryonal tumor with multilayered rosettes all typically show restricted diffusion, whereas ependymomas most often do not restrict diffusion (they appear darker on DWI imaging).[5,6] Other advanced MRI techniques, including PWI, diffusion tensor imaging, and MR spectroscopy, have been evaluated as a means to differentiate brain metastases and other lesions such as HGG, CNS lymphoma, and abscess. Although no one technique can completely accurately discriminate a brain metastasis from other lesions, differences in peritumoral edema characteristics (purely vasogenic with metastases versus vasogenic edema plus infiltrative neoplastic cells in HGGs) may provide helpful clues.[7]

Imaging differential of posterior fossa lesion. Non-malignant lesions of the posterior fossa can also be characterized with CT and/or MRI imaging. Demyelination, either from a post-infectious cause or due to an underlying progressive neurologic disorder, often appears as hyperintense lesions on T2-weighted imaging. These lesions may be focal or more diffuse, depending on the underlying pathophysiology. Similarly, inflammation of structures in the posterior fossa most frequently causes hyperintensity on fluid attenuated inversion recovery (FLAIR)/T2 weighted images, though MRI features can be incredibly heterogeneous depending on the underlying cause of inflammation, its chronicity, and other complications such as abscess, meningitis, or autoimmune disease.[8]

Clinical cases

CASE 7.1 MIDLINE FOURTH VENTRICULAR LESION

Case. A 4-year-old previously healthy male presented with 4 weeks of progressive headaches, nausea, and vomiting. The headaches were initially attributed to streptococcal pharyngitis diagnosed by throat culture; however, the headaches worsened in frequency and severity, and became progressively associated with emesis. Headaches and vomiting tended to worsen throughout the day. By history, he was not exhibiting any lack of coordination, nor did he have any weakness or reported tingling. Additionally, family denied fevers, chills, rashes, chest pain or palpitations, shortness of breath, abdominal discomfort, or change in vision. He did not have papilledema on examination, and the remainder of the neurological examination was grossly normal. Given the progressive nature of his symptoms, a head CT was obtained (Fig. 7.1A,B), which

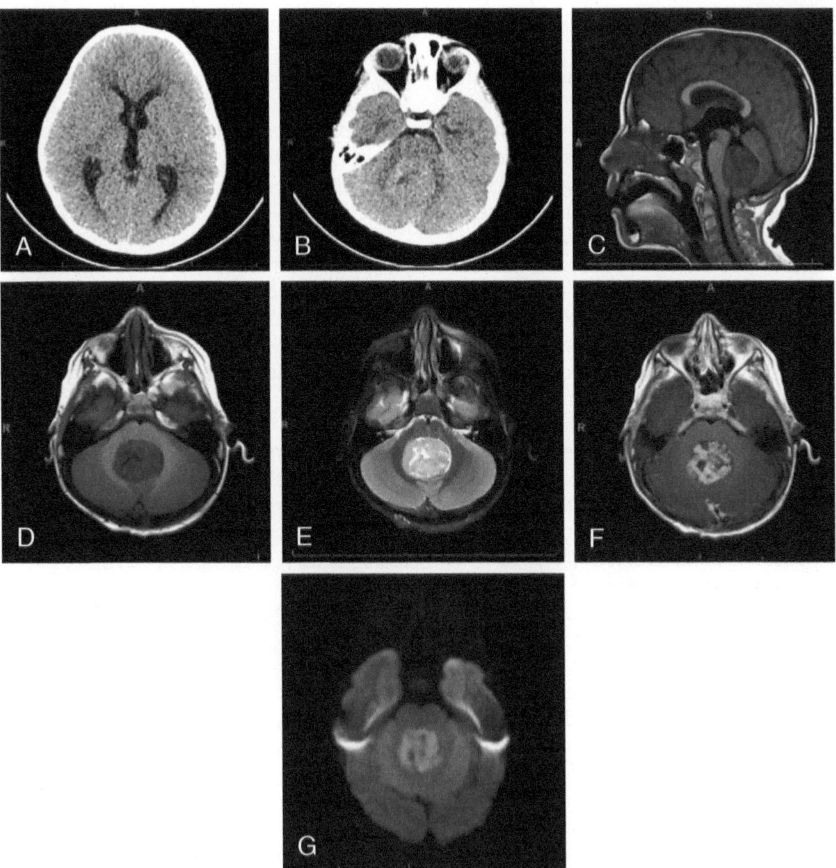

Fig. 7.1 (A) Axial CT head without contrast. Hydrocephalus involving lateral and third ventricles. (B) Axial CT head without contrast. Mildly hyperdense midline posterior fossa tumor with no definite calcifications. Tumor is expanding the fourth ventricle. 3.9 × 3.5 cm cross-section. (C) T1 sagittal MRI. T1 hypointense lesion centered in the fourth ventricle, appearing to arise from the inferior roof of the fourth ventricle, measuring 3.4 × 4.0 × 4.1 cm in AP, transverse, and craniocaudal dimensions, respectively. (D) T1 axial MRI. (E) T2 axial MRI. T2 mildly hyperintense (F) T1 axial FLAIR + contrast. The mass enhances heterogeneously. (G) Diffusion weight imaging (DWI). The mass demonstrates restricted diffusion, appearing white on DWI, suggesting increased cellularity. *AP*, Anterior-posterior; *FLAIR*, fluid attenuated inversion recovery.

revealed an isodense midline posterior fossa tumor, expanding into the fourth ventricle, and causing obstructive hydrocephalus of the lateral and third ventricles. There were no visible calcifications within the tumor. This prompted an urgent referral to a pediatric emergency department (ED), where brain MRI was obtained (Fig. 7.1C–G). MRI revealed a T1 hypointense, T2 mildly hyperintense, heterogeneously enhancing mass centered in the fourth ventricle, appearing to arise from the inferior roof of the fourth ventricle, measuring 3.4 × 4.0 × 4.1 cm in anterior-posterior, transverse, and craniocaudal dimensions, respectively. The mass demonstrated restricted diffusion.

Teaching Points: Differential Diagnosis for Midline Fourth Ventricular Lesion. The patient's young age and absence of systemic complaints immediately raises the suspicion for a primary brain tumor. The tumor's specific location within the posterior fossa—midline and arising from or within the fourth ventricle—is most consistent with medulloblastoma or ependymoma. Other possible tumors in this location include tumors arising from the choroid plexus (choroid plexus papilloma or choroid plexus carcinoma) and exophytic LGGs growing from the lower brainstem/medulla oblongata. In contrast, tumors arising just lateral to midline, at the cerebellopontine angle or at the Foramen of Luschka, are more likely to be ATRT or a favorable subtype of medulloblastoma called WNT subtype. The CT findings of an isodense lesion correlates with either medulloblastoma or ependymoma. MRI is helpful in differentiating between medulloblastoma and ependymoma here, with the T1 hypointense and T2 hyperintense pattern with heterogeneous contrast enhancement favoring medulloblastoma. Finally, the restricted diffusion also suggests medulloblastoma.

Ultimately, however, the diagnosis must be made pathologically, not radiographically.

Diagnostic workup. Urgent referral to a pediatric neurosurgeon should be made. Virtually all children with a posterior fossa mass will undergo a craniotomy, as opposed to stereotactic or open biopsy. The goal of this surgery is threefold: to relieve mass effect (including any obstructive hydrocephalus), to obtain tissue for pathologic diagnosis, and to debulk the tumor. Nearly all tumors in this region in children would benefit from maximal safe resection, though there are some nuances. Whereas the prognosis of medulloblastoma is unchanged if there remains less than 1.5 cm^2 of tissue, the prognosis of ependymoma is dismal in the absence of gross total resection.[9–11] LGGs are cured by gross total resection, but those that are partially resected to spare surgical morbidity may still have long-term survival, though often at the expense of needing recurrent surgeries or multiple courses of adjuvant chemotherapy and/or radiation therapy. In this particular case, with the most likely etiologies being medulloblastoma and ependymoma, an attempt at near total or gross total resection should be made. The patient successfully underwent gross total resection, and did not need any CSF diversion following tumor resection.

Following surgery of a posterior fossa tumor, there is time to wait for definitive pathologic diagnosis while the patient recovers. Staging and treatment planning entirely depend on the tumor type, so waiting for pathology while the patient recovers from craniotomy is reasonable. Approximately 10 days after surgery, a final pathologic diagnosis confirmed medulloblastoma, WHO grade IV, without nodular, desmoplastic, anaplastic, or large cell features. Over the past 15 years, integrative genomic and methylomic studies have shown that medulloblastoma is not a single entity, but rather a heterogeneous group of diseases with distinct clinical, radiographic, molecular, and prognostic features.[12–15] Testing, including immunohistochemistry for nuclear beta-catenin, p53, MYC, and NMYC, all confirmed that this patient had a non-WNT, non-Sonic Hedgehog (SHH), group 3/4 non-MYC amplified, non-p53-mutated, medulloblastoma. Of note, upward of 25% of patients with SHH medulloblastoma have a germline mutation in cancer predisposition genes including TP53 or BRCA, so patients with this medulloblastoma subtype benefit from genetic counseling.[16]

Staging of medulloblastoma. With the pathologic diagnosis in hand, staging workup can proceed. Typically, medulloblastoma only spreads within the CNS, and this workup is done with a full spine MRI and lumbar puncture. Ideally, both of those are done at least 2 weeks following surgery, as blood products in the subarachnoid space can be misinterpreted as metastatic tumor. The patient underwent sedated spine MRI and lumbar puncture, both of which were negative, confirming non-metastatic medulloblastoma. The combination of non-metastatic group 3/4 medulloblastoma that is non-MYC amplified is considered standard risk and is associated with an overall survival of 75–90%.[14]

Patient management. The mainstay of treatment for standard risk medulloblastoma is surgery, followed by craniospinal radiation with a posterior fossa boost along with concurrent vincristine, followed by multi-agent cytotoxic chemotherapy. Mainly for social reasons, this patient opted to undergo conventional photon intensity-modulated radiation therapy (as opposed to proton beam radiation, which is increasingly becoming standard-of-care for most children with medulloblastoma). The entire treatment course is long: from surgery through radiation and chemotherapy, the course takes over 1 year. Survivors of medulloblastoma will also often experience long-term sequelae of therapy, including neurocognitive deficits, endocrinopathies, hearing loss, and secondary malignancy risk. At last follow up, the patient is 2 years off-therapy, doing well overall but has an individualized education plan in school to accommodate for some neurocognitive deficits.

Clinical Pearls

1. The imaging differential of a midline posterior fossa lesion in a child should include medulloblastoma (e.g., "M" for midline) and ependymoma. Pilocytic astrocytomas tend to occur in the lateral cerebellum.

CASE 7.2 LATERAL CEREBELLAR CYSTIC LESION

Case. A 20-month-old female with no significant past medical history presented with a 1-month history of gait instability and emesis. The patient's mother reported a jerky, shaky, unstable body, most noticeable in the patient's arms, rendering her unable feed herself ("She just keeps missing her mouth."). Emesis began 3 days prior to presentation, which occurred most often while she was in a moving car, though not exclusively. She was born full-term and had been healthy since. No fevers, rashes, joint swelling, extremity injuries, abdominal discomfort, or changes in vision. To this point she had been developing normally and had not lost developmental milestones in her speech and language domains. In the ED, she was found to have appendicular ataxia when reaching for objects, as well as a waddling gait with frequent falls to her left side. Given these symptoms, a head CT was obtained, which revealed a right cerebellar cystic tumor measuring 5.6 × 6.4 × 4.6 cm in anterior-posterior, transverse, and craniocaudal dimensions, respectively, with mass effect and leftward displacement of the fourth ventricle and cerebellum (Fig. 7.2A). MRI was then obtained, which revealed a large, T1 hypointense right cerebellar cystic mass, with some T2 intensity adjacent to the cyst, and a thin peripheral enhancement; the mass did not demonstrate restricted diffusion (Fig. 7.2B–F).

Teaching Points: Differential Diagnosis of Lateral Cerebellar Cyst With Mural Nodule. In a young patient with a new large cerebellar cystic mass, a primary brain tumor should be highly suspected. Cerebellar hemispheric lesions in children have a relatively short differential diagnosis, including LGGs such as pilocytic astrocytomas, oligodendrogliomas, or mixed glial/neuronal tumors, higher-grade gliomas, and medulloblastoma, especially the SHH subtype. The cystic

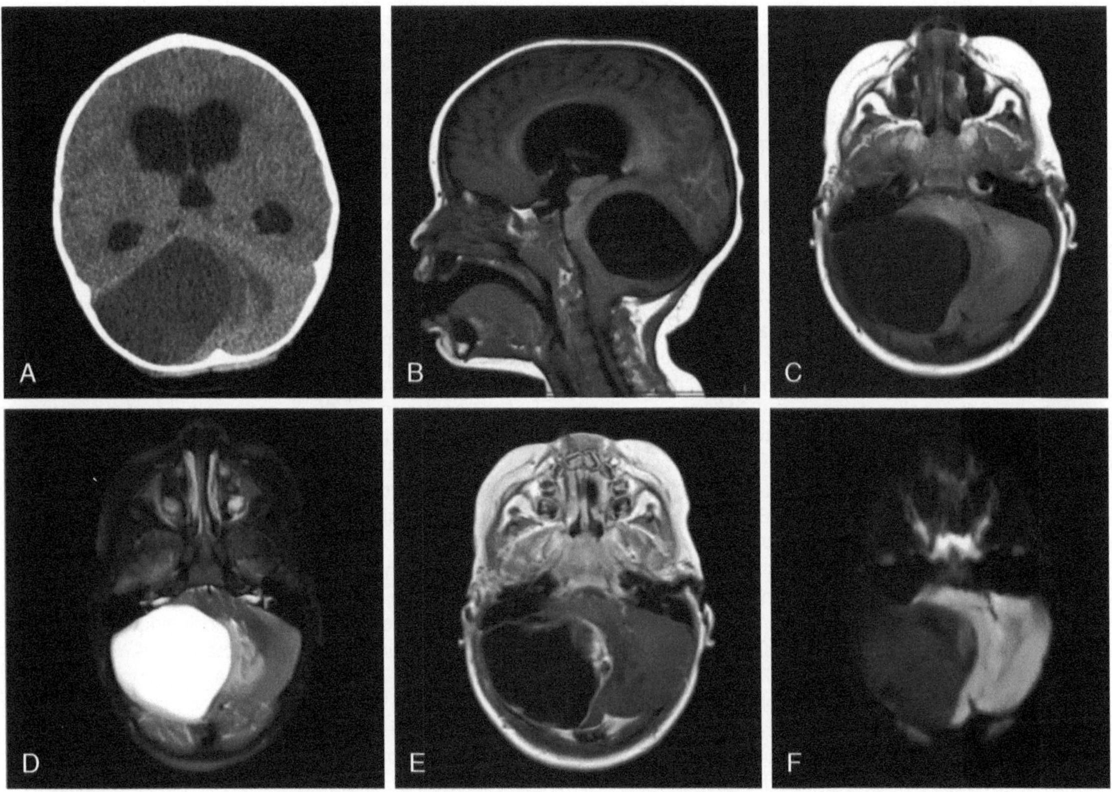

Fig. 7.2 (A) Axial CT head without contrast. Right cerebellar tumor measuring 5.6 × 6.4 × 4.6 cm (AP × TV × CC) with mass effect and leftward displacement of the fourth ventricle and cerebellum. (B) T1 sagittal MRI. T1 hypointense cystic mass with substantial compression of the midbrain and pons with obstructive hydrocephalus at the level of the aqueduct and fourth ventricle. (C) T1 axial MRI. T1 hypointense cystic mass. (D) T2 axial MRI. Some T2 hyperintensity adjacent to the cyst likely related to peritumoral edema. (E) T1 axial FLAIR MRI + contrast. There is a thin peripheral enhancement. Additionally, there is irregularly enhancing soft tissue at the medial/inferior aspects of the mass with a few enhancing septations traversing the cystic portion (not shown). (F) Diffusion weight imaging. The mass does not restrict diffusion. *AP*, Anterior-posterior; *CC*, craniocaudal; *FLAIR*, fluid attenuated inversion recovery; *TV*, transverse.

component, along with enhancement of the cystic wall, narrows the differential diagnosis even further: in children, cysts are most often associated with gliomas, predominantly LGGs. A cystic cerebellar tumor in adults should raise the suspicion for hemangioblastoma, a rare, WHO grade I, vascular tumor, which is generally sporadic in adults. Hemangioblastomas can rarely occur in children and are often associated with von Hippel–Lindau syndrome, a cancer predisposition syndrome. Hemangioblastoma usually appears as a cyst with an enhancing mural nodule. Unlike gliomas, in which the nodule often enhances, the cyst wall of a hemangioblastoma rarely enhances. Although medulloblastoma may be cystic, the lack of any significant solid portion in this patient's tumor would be very atypical for medulloblastoma.

Diagnostic workup. This tumor is causing obstructive hydrocephalus and, therefore, warrants immediate intervention by a pediatric neurosurgeon. Surgery would aim to achieve three objectives: (1) symptomatic relief of obstructive hydrocephalus, (2) obtain tissue for pathologic diagnosis, and (3) tumor debulking. Given the narrow differential diagnosis consisting mainly of gliomas, maximal safe resection should be the surgical goal. The prognosis for pediatric LGGs with gross total resection is excellent, with progression-free survival approaching 100%. For those that achieve subtotal resection, the prognosis remains quite high, and some pediatric LGGs may even spontaneously regress.[17] Gross total resection of a HGG, if achievable, improves overall survival; however, the infiltrative nature of these tumors often precludes this without also inflicting unacceptable morbidity.[18] Following a safe maximal resection, if the tumor is considered a higher grade or an unexpected diagnosis that would benefit from a more complete resection, a second-look surgery can be considered for any residual resectable tumor.

This patient's tumor was resected, and pathology returned WHO grade I juvenile pilocytic astrocytoma. Regarding staging, as pediatric LGGs carry an extremely low metastatic potential, no other CNS imaging was obtained at that time.

Patient management. The diagnosis of pilocytic astrocytoma is a histological diagnosis. As in most tumors, there is increasing understanding of the biology of these tumors, information that is relevant diagnostically, prognostically, and regarding treatment. It is now clear that the vast majority of pediatric LGGs are associated with or driven by alterations in the mitogen-activated protein kinase (MAPK) pathway, most prominently BRAF and NF1 mutations.[19] Some data suggest that certain recurrent mutations, such as BRAF V600E, may negatively impact prognosis, but other data refute this.[20,21] However, emerging data suggest that this entity, if present in pediatric LGGs, may be targetable with BRAF inhibitor drugs in cases in which the tumor is not completely resectable or in the rare instances in which it recurs.[22,23] Genomic testing by next-generation sequencing was obtained on the resected tumor tissue, which revealed a BRAF V600E mutation; there were no other identifiable mutations. With this in hand, and given the favorable prognosis associated with even subtotally resected pediatric LGG, observation with serial MRIs was proposed as treatment for this brain tumor.

The patient is now more than 2 years since resection, with no evidence of tumor growth. The small area of questionable residual tissue seen postoperatively resolved, suggesting that this finding represented postoperative changes as opposed to residual tumor tissue. In the event of tumor recurrence, first-line management is re-resection with the goal to achieve a gross total resection. If this is not possible, or if the tumor arose in an unresectable location, the standard-of-care would be cytotoxic chemotherapy. Several chemotherapy regimens have been studied, and all of them carry nearly the same event-free-survival: nearly 50% of tumors will progress on any one regimen. If one regimen fails, it is common to proceed to a second, then a third, and so on. Optimal timing to employ a new targeted agent, such as a BRAF inhibitor for tumors that harbor BRAF mutations, is unclear, but these agents are typically reserved for recurrent and/or refractory cases. Finally, although pediatric LGGs are somewhat radiosensitive, this mode of therapy is avoided for as long as possible to prevent the late effects of ionizing radiation.[24]

Clinical Pearls

1. Lateral cerebellar cystic lesion with a mural nodule should raise suspicion for a pilocytic astrocytoma in children and for a cerebellar hemangioblastoma in adults.

CASE 7.3 NON-ENHANCING PONTINE LESION

Case. A 9-year-old male with autism, who was non-verbal at baseline, presented to an ED with a 5-day history of balance issues, including falling while walking, vomiting, and increased sleepiness. Although he was unable to explicitly report symptoms, his teachers reported that he had been acting off-balance during the past few days. The ED providers found him to be lethargic but arousable, with left gaze preference and nystagmus, with mild right arm dysmetria, and prominent truncal ataxia, leaning/falling toward the left side. Given these symptoms and this examination, a head CT was obtained, which revealed a hypodense mass centered in the pons (Fig. 7.3A,B). MRI Brain was obtained, which revealed a large T1 hypointense, T2 hyperintense, non-enhancing lesion with ill-defined borders centered in the pons measuring 7 × 4.3 × 4.4 cm in anterior-posterior, transverse, and craniocaudal dimensions, respectively (Fig. 7.3C–G). There was mass effect on the fourth ventricle, which was incompletely effaced with encasement of the basilar artery. There was a T1 hyperintense area within the right posterior lateral portion of the mass, compatible with more cellular tumor, and the tumor did not restrict diffusion.

Teaching Points: Differential Diagnosis of an Intrinsic Brainstem Lesion. A large, ill-defined lesion, hypodense on CT, T2 hyperintense on MRI, and non-enhancing that is centered in the pons of a child is most likely a glioma. It is conceivable that other tumors could mimic this appearance, such as primitive neuroectodermal tumors including medulloblastoma and ATRT; however, although those tumors may expand into the pons, the T2 hyperintensity and lack of enhancement, along with the location entirely in the pons without any exophytic growth is highly specific for a pontine glioma. Pontine gliomas were previously classified as diffuse intrinsic pontine gliomas (DIPG), and spanned the WHO grading scale from grade II to IV. However, mounting data from biopsies and postmortem tissue analysis of intrinsic pontine tumors highlight that the majority of the grade IV pontine tumors harbor histone mutations, namely H3K27M. In fact, most HGGs in children that are midline, from the supratentorial space down to the brainstem, harbor this histone mutation. Because these tumors have much more in common with each other than lower-grade intrinsic pontine tumors, a new diagnostic entity was added to the 2016 WHO classification called diffuse midline gliomas (see Chapter 1 for molecular classification of glioma).[25] To date, pontine glioma is universally fatal. However, a patient with a WHO grade II astrocytoma in the pons may live longer than a patient with a WHO grade IV glioma.[26] Similarly, emerging data suggests that the two most common variants of the histone mutations found in diffuse midline gliomas, H3.1K27M and H3.3K27M, are associated with different life expectancies, with H3.3K27M-mutant tumors being less responsive to radiation, and quicker to recur and lead to a patient's death.[27]

Diagnostic workup. High-quality MRI imaging alone is usually enough to make the diagnosis of this fatal disease. However, whereas biopsy of an intrinsic pontine tumor (formerly DIPG) was previously thought unhelpful, unnecessary, and therefore rarely performed, practice is slowly shifting toward considering stereotactic biopsy to help inform prognosis (life expectancy) and eligibility for early-phase studies.

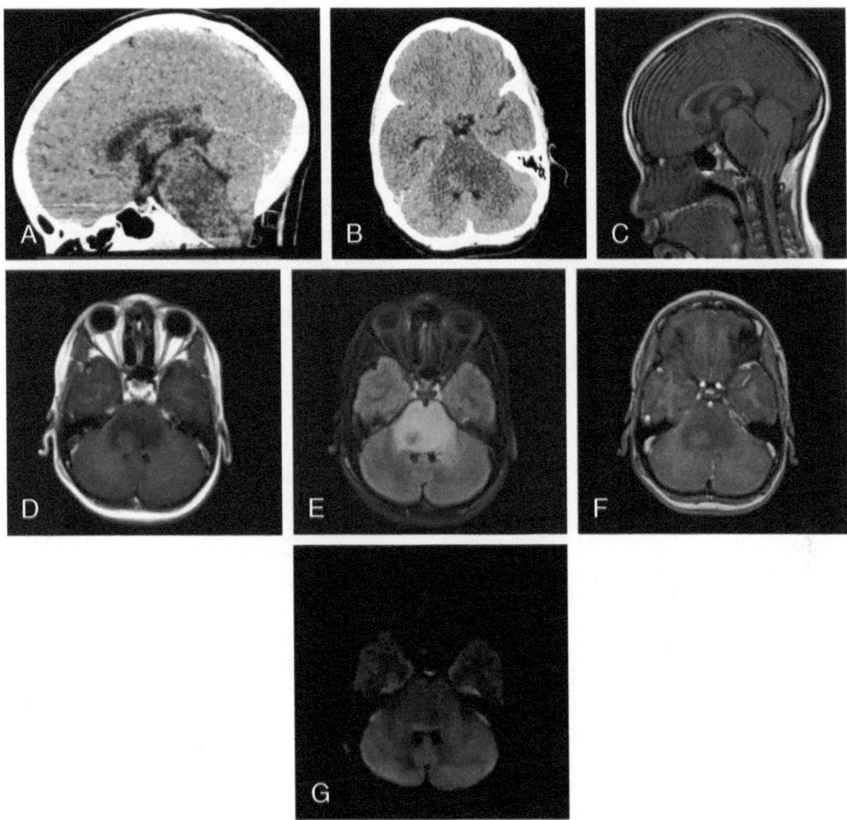

Fig. 7.3 (A) Sagittal CT head without contrast. Hypodense mass centered in the pons. No cysts or calcifications present. (B) Axial CT head without contrast. Hypodense mass in the pons. There is a small area of hyperdensity in the right posterior lateral portion of the mass, compatible with more cellular tumor. (C) T1 sagittal MRI. T1 hypointense lesion centered in the pons, measuring 3.7 × 4.3 × 4.4 cm in AP, transverse, and craniocaudal dimensions, respectively. There is mass effect on the fourth ventricle, which is incompletely effaced. (D) T1 axial MRI. Intrinsically T1 hyperintense area within the right posterior lateral portion of the mass, compatible with more cellular tumor. (E) T2 axial MRI. Heterogeneously T2 hyperintense mass centered in the pons. (F) T1 axial FLAIR MRI + contrast. There is no enhancement of the tumor. (G) Diffusion weight imaging. The mass does not demonstrate restricted diffusion. *AP*, Anterior-posterior; *FLAIR*, fluid attenuated inversion recovery.

This option was discussed with the family, and ultimately the family declined biopsy. Gliomas intrinsic to the pons have some metastatic potential; however, the poor prognosis makes staging futile, so spine imaging and CSF sampling are rarely done. Additionally, rare cases of atypical radiographic findings (e.g., exophytic component, cystic components, etc.) may warrant biopsy, as these findings may indicate an entity other than histone-mutated midline glioma.

Patient management. There is no known cure for pontine diffuse midline gliomas. The diffuse nature of this tumor, lackluster chemo- and radiation sensitivity, and the critical anatomic location make resection impossible and render this tumor universally fatal. Radiation is the standard of care, but this treatment is palliative in nature. It can be effective, as 70–80% of tumors will shrink on imaging, and the vast majority of patients will experience some temporary clinical improvement. However, nearly all intrinsic pontine tumors that are exposed to radiation therapy will recur locally and many have little if any clinically relevant response. There are different interventional strategies under active investigation, including small molecule inhibitors, vaccines against the histone mutations, chimeric antigen receptor T-cell therapy (CAR-T), and convection-enhanced delivery of drug, but all of these are in early-phase trials.

The patient presented in this case opted to receive focal radiation to the tumor. Each radiation dose had to be administered under sedation due to his age and developmental delay. The tumor caused considerable dysfunction of his gag reflex, and he required intubation to protect his airway during each of the first two sedation administrations for radiation. Given this undue burden and the goal to improve, not worsen, the quality of his life, radiation was ceased after just two doses. The patient ultimately died only 2.5 months after diagnosis.

Clinical Pearls

1. The imaging differential diagnosis for an intrinsic pontine brainstem glioma should include causes of rhombencephalitis (e.g., infectious, inflammatory, paraneoplastic) including *Listeria* infection, enterovirus, other viral encephalitis (e.g., HSV, EBV, HHV6), Behcet's disease, Erdheim-Chester disease, or other etiologies.
2. Pontine gliomas are typically expansile with enlargement of the central pons, often with the basilar artery displaced anteriorly or with the tumor appearing to engulf the artery.

CASE 7.4 ENHANCING CEREBELLAR LESION IN AN ADULT

Case. A 55-year-old female with a history of metastatic breast cancer to the lung, type 2 diabetes mellitus, and chronic obstructive pulmonary disease presented with a 3-week history of worsening dizziness and 1 day of emesis. She described the dizziness as feeling like she was walking sideways. Her dizziness improved when lying down, was worse when standing, and was associated with nausea. She also had morning headaches that improved shortly after rising out of bed. She denied fevers, chills, diplopia, blurred vision, and weakness. Brain MRI was obtained, which revealed a heterogeneously enhancing mass in the right cerebellar hemisphere measuring 2.8 cm that was associated with T2/FLAIR signal hyperintensity (Fig. 7.4A–C). The peritumoral region did not restrict diffusion, and the peritumoral FLAIR signal was thought most consistent with purely vasogenic edema (Fig. 7.4D).

Teaching Points: Differential Diagnosis of Enhancing Cerebellar Lesion in Adult. An isolated cerebellar lesion in an adult should raise the suspicion for brain metastasis as, in this demographic, metastatic tumors involving the brain are more common than primary brain tumors. Furthermore, metastases to the posterior fossa are not rare, with the infratentorium harboring between 15–25% of all brain metastases.[28] The peritumoral edema appearing largely vasogenic suggests that this is a brain metastasis, as opposed to a primary brain tumor such as a HGG, in which case the peritumoral FLAIR signal may represent mixed vasogenic edema with tumor infiltration. The known history of metastatic breast cancer makes this new lesion highly suspicious for metastatic breast cancer.

Basic awareness of incidences of primary malignancies that can metastasize to the brain can be helpful in guiding the workup of a patient who has imaging concerning for brain metastases. The most common primary malignancy that metastasizes to the brain is lung, followed by breast, melanoma, renal, colorectal, and gynecological.[29] With regards to primary tumors that are most likely to metastasize to the posterior fossa specifically, uterine, prostate, and gastrointestinal are the most common.[30] Whether and how to embark on a search for a primary malignancy in the event that an isolated posterior fossa mass is found in a patient without a known history of metastatic cancer is beyond the scope of this chapter; however, a thorough history and physical examination may prompt a neurologist seeing a patient with imaging concerning for possible brain metastases to make the appropriate referrals (oncology, gynecological oncology, surgical oncology, etc.).

Diagnostic workup. The edema and mass effect, along with the patient's noxious symptoms should trigger urgent evaluation by neurosurgery and oncology. Ultimately, diagnosis must be made with tissue biopsy and evaluation by pathology. This can sometimes be more safely obtained with extra-CNS tissue. Like most posterior fossa tumors, this tumor is amenable for resection in an effort to mitigate any developing increased intracranial pressure, to obtain tissue for diagnosis, and to debulk or fully resect the tumor. Stereotactic radiosurgery could be considered for small, asymptomatic tumors with clear diagnoses. Surgical resection was performed on this patient.

Gross total resection was achieved as confirmed on postoperative MRI. Pathology revealed poorly differentiated carcinoma, consistent with metastatic breast carcinoma. The finding of a new CNS metastasis in an already metastatic breast cancer may prompt a search for other sites of metastasis, with extra-CNS imaging.

Patient management. Surgical resection and radiation therapy remain the primary approaches for most brain metastases, particularly at the time of first diagnosis. These efforts are aimed at achieving local control of the disease. Various surgical techniques have been used, and more are being studied, including cryoablation and laser-heat ablation techniques (see Chapter 2, Case 2.3 for further discussion of surgical approaches including laser ablation for brain tumors). Similarly, various radiation techniques have been utilized and are being investigated, including whole brain radiation, stereotactic radiosurgery ("gamma knife"), and using prophylactic radiation as a preventative measure. Systemic therapies are typically employed at second and greater relapse. Conventional chemotherapies that have good CNS penetration are often used, but increasingly, targeted agents aimed at either intrinsic tumor characteristics or at properties associated with brain metastases biology are being studied, as are immunotherapies such as checkpoint inhibition.

Outcomes for brain metastases are often poor, with a survival of typically less than 6 months for most tumor types.[31] However, precise prognoses are difficult to estimate due to the heterogeneity of this disease, with different primary cancers, varying metastatic burden, and individuals undergoing a wide variety of treatments. The patient described recovered well from the cerebellar tumor resection, and she is now 9 months post-resection, receiving oral chemotherapies, and in remission without any evidence of recurrent tumors in the brain or elsewhere.

Clinical Pearls

1. The cerebellum is the second most common parenchymal location for brain metastasis.
2. Management of cerebellar metastasis should include definitive tumor treatment as well as a consideration for reducing brainstem compression, maintaining CSF flow, and providing a tissue diagnosis when there is no contributory systemic malignancy present.

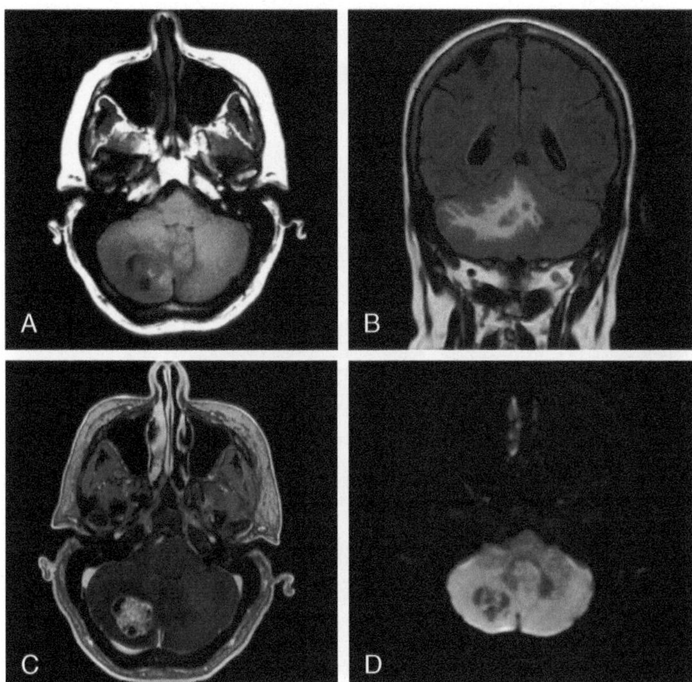

Fig. 7.4 (A) T1 axial MRI. Small amount of T1 hyperintensity, likely representing a tiny foci of hemorrhage. (B) T2/FLAIR coronal MRI. T2 hypointense with diffuse vasogenic edema in the right greater than left cerebellar hemispheres resulting in mass effect on adjacent structures. (C) T1 + contrast axial MRI. Heterogeneously enhancing mass in the right cerebellar hemisphere, measuring approximately 2.4 × 2.8 × 2.1 cm, (AP × TV × CC). (D) Diffusion weighted imaging: The mass does not demonstrate restricted diffusion. *AP*, Anterior-posterior; *CC*, craniocaudal; *FLAIR*, fluid attenuated inversion recovery; *TV*, transverse.

CASE 7.5 NON-ENHANCING CEREBELLAR LESION

Case. A 6-year-old female with no significant past medical history presented to the ED with 2 weeks of progressively worsening headaches and 1 week of nausea and vomiting. Three days after the onset of symptoms, she tested positive for streptococcal pharyngitis and was treated with intramuscular penicillin G due to vomiting. In the ED, she was dehydrated, but did not have ataxia or any other cerebellar symptoms or signs on examination. Given her progressive symptoms without any resolution from fluids, ondansetron, prednisolone, or acetaminophen, she underwent head CT, which revealed generalized cerebellar edema, with cerebellar tonsils extending into the foramen magnum, as well as hydrocephalus of the lateral and third ventricles (Fig. 7.5A–C). MRI was then obtained and showed a diffuse and nearly symmetric cerebellar edematous process, with caudal tonsillar displacement into the magnum, enlarged cerebellar hemispheres, effacement of cerebellar sulci, T2/FLAIR hyperintensity in the cortex and cerebellar white matter, diffuse enhancement along the surface of the cerebellum, and without any focal lesions that enhanced or restricted diffusion (Fig. 7.5D–G).

Teaching Points: Differential Diagnosis for Non-Enhancing Diffuse Cerebellitis. Symmetric and diffuse cerebellar edema that spares the cerebrum and is T2 hyperintense in a child with an acute presentation is suspicious for infectious or potentially post-infectious cerebellitis. Acute cerebellitis (AC) is a heterogeneous clinical syndrome characterized by cerebellar ataxia or dysfunction that is attributable to a recent or concurrent infection, a recent vaccination, or an ingestion of medication, and in which an MRI shows evidence of cerebellar inflammation.[32] This diagnosis has significant overlap with another clinical syndrome, acute cerebellar ataxia (ACA), in which there is necessarily ataxia and which is also often post-infectious. Other etiologies could mimic AC on CT and MRI, including a diffuse tumor with associated edema, metabolic diseases, demyelinative disorders, and meningitis.[33] Notably, when the cerebellitis is unilateral, sometimes referred as hemicerebellitis, there is a more complex differential diagnosis, which includes dysplastic cerebellar gangliocytoma (Lhermitte-Duclos), vasculitis, and inflammatory processes related to cytarabine or other toxicities.[34,35] However, the absence of a well-defined mass and serial imaging showing improvement or disappearance of the abnormalities can help solidify the diagnosis of AC.

Given the rarity of this finding on imaging, expert involvement by pediatric neurology, pediatric oncology, pediatric rheumatology, pediatric infectious disease, and certainly pediatric neurosurgery (to potentially alleviate obstructive hydrocephalus) should be considered.

Diagnostic workup. The posterior fossa in this patient, clinically and radiographically, was under pressure. In parallel with the diagnostic workup, a ventricular drain to relieve high-pressure CSF should be considered. Given the risk for herniation, lumbar puncture for diagnostic testing should be avoided. Instead, CSF should be obtained during the CSF diversion procedure.

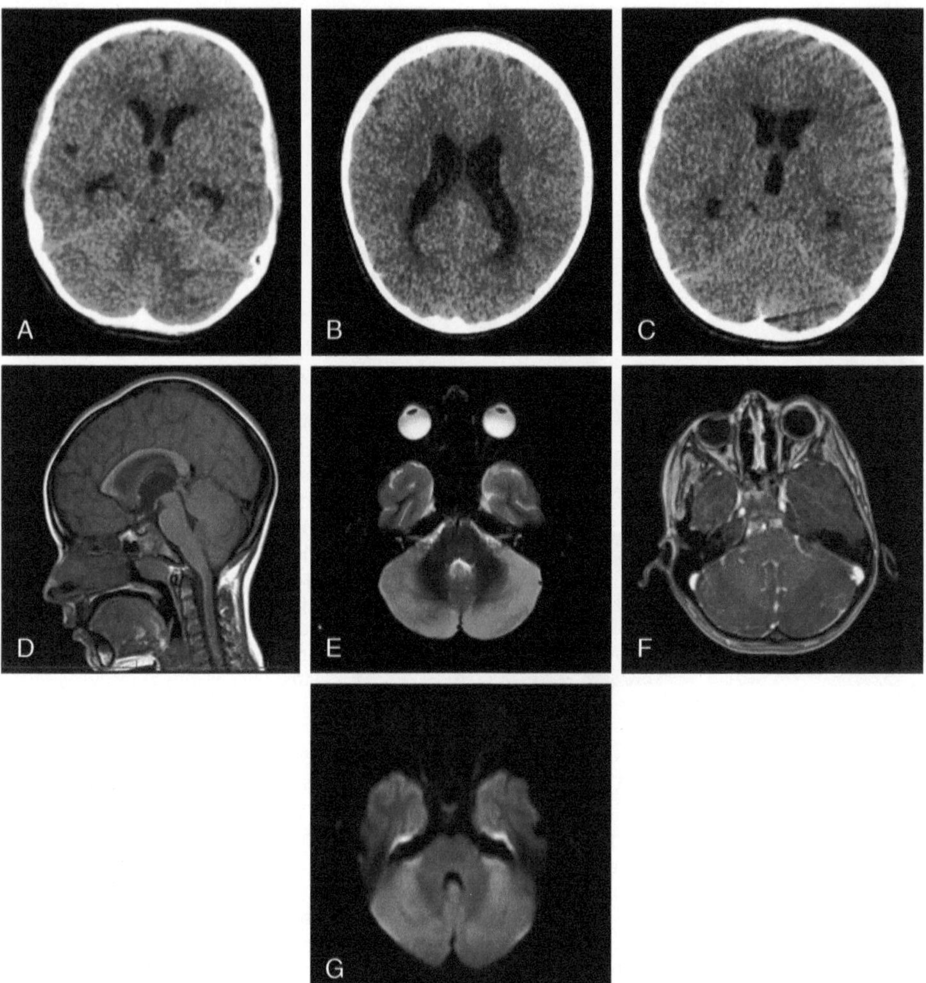

Fig. 7.5 (A) Axial CT head without contrast. Suggestion of edema within the bilateral cerebellum. Cerebellar tonsils extending into the foramen magnum (not shown). (B) Axial CT head without contrast. Temporal horns mildly rounded, and there is a mild degree of crowding of sulci. (C) Axial CT head without contrast. Enlarged third ventricle. (D) T1 sagittal MRI. No focal areas of T1 hyper- or hypointensity. Diffuse and nearly symmetric cerebellar edema with caudal tonsillar displacement into the foramen magnum. (E) T2/FLAIR axial MRI. Bilateral cerebellar hemispheres are enlarged with effacement of sulci and abnormal T2/FLAIR signal in the cortex and cerebellar white matter. (F) T1 axial MRI with contrast. Diffuse enhancement along the surface of the cerebellum. No focal enhancing mass-like lesion. (G) Diffusion weight imaging. No focal areas of restricted diffusion. *FLAIR*, Fluid attenuated inversion recovery.

Pediatric neurosurgery evaluated the patient and promptly placed an external ventricular drain. Given the broad differential, CSF and blood were tested for a wide range of potential infectious etiologies, including viruses, bacteria, and fungi; rheumatologic etiologies; autoimmune/inflammatory etiologies; and demyelinating disorders. Infectious pathogens are commonly implicated in AC. Those that have been associated with AC include the human herpes viruses (VZV, CMV, HSV), certain enteroviruses (Coxsackie, polio), mycoplasma pneumoniae, group A Streptococcus, and other viruses and bacteria. AC has also rarely been associated with certain vaccinations, including those against VZV and measles/mumps/rubella.

Patient management. Testing for anti-streptolysin antibodies was positive, suggesting this patient had been exposed to group A Streptococcus at some point. Additionally, titers for mycoplasma pneumonia were positive, whereas the remainder of the investigation was negative. Mycoplasma PCR was negative. Repeat MRI only 5 days after diagnosis showed marked improvement with methylprednisolone and CSF shunting. As there was no evidence of active infection of either of those two pathogens, no antimicrobials were administered. Taken together, this episode is most consistent with post-infectious (group A Streptococcus vs mycoplasma pneumoniae) AC. The patient made a rapid and complete recovery, which is consistent with the literature.[36] She has returned to baseline and has no ongoing needs for CSF shunting.

Clinical Pearls

1. Acute cerebellitis is a heterogeneous clinical syndrome characterized by cerebellar ataxia or dysfunction that is attributable to a recent or concurrent infection, a recent vaccination, or an ingestion of medication.
2. MRI imaging of typical acute bilateral cerebellitis includes metabolic diseases, demyelinative disorders, and meningitis.
3. In cases of hemicerebellitis when imaging findings are asymmetric, the imaging differential includes dysplastic cerebellar gangliocytoma (Lhermitte-Duclos), vasculitis, and inflammatory processes related to cytarabine or other toxicities.

Conclusion

Neuroimaging has been a cornerstone of diagnosis, prognosis, and surveillance of brain tumors and other posterior fossa lesions and pathologies for decades. The clinicians' knowledge of the basic imaging features of commonly seen pathologies, as well as an understanding of strengths and weaknesses of the various imaging modalities, is vital in establishing efficient and accurate diagnoses. MRI with contrast remains the gold standard for the majority of neuroimaging. It is important to note that in non-emergent situations, it is ideal to discuss specific MRI sequencing or other nuanced parameters with a neuroradiologist and/or neurosurgeon in order to optimize quality and quantity of data obtained. In facilities without MRI capabilities, or when trying to emergently evaluate for potential neurologic catastrophe such as severe hydrocephalus, acute hemorrhage, or impending herniation, a CT scan will provide rapid information.

Although MRI and CT scans account for the vast majority of neuroimaging obtained of the posterior fossa, it is notable that there is a host of developing technologies that will play increasingly important roles in future imaging assessments, including MR spectroscopy, CT-PET, perfusion-weighted imaging, and others. These technologies are beyond the scope of this chapter but may become vital tools in the imaging armamentarium of clinicians caring for patients with posterior fossa lesions.

Clinical pearls

1. MRI offers higher soft-tissue resolution with more qualitative data on posterior fossa lesions, though it is not available at all centers, requires a degree of technical expertise, is slower, may necessitate sedation for younger and unstable patients, and is more expensive than CT.
2. CT is fast, less expensive, and more widely available than MRI, and offers insights into calcifications and boney involvement of lesions though with limited resolution and narrow lesion characteristics. Additionally, CT can be used to rapidly assess potentially life-threatening complications of posterior fossa masses, including hydrocephalus, acute hemorrhage, or pending herniation.
3. In pediatric patients with space-occupying posterior fossa lesions, a primary brain tumor is by far the most likely diagnosis, with metastatic lesions in this population being exceedingly rare.
4. In older adults, a space-occupying lesion in the posterior fossa is more likely to be a metastatic tumor or acute hemorrhage, and should prompt a comprehensive history and physical examination and consideration of additional body imaging to evaluate for a primary tumor or risk factors for stroke.
5. Location and characteristics of pediatric tumors can guide the clinician regarding a most likely diagnosis, which may include low-grade glioma, high-grade glioma, medulloblastoma, ependymoma, ATRT, or others.

References

1. Louis DN, Cavenee WK, Devita H. *Rosenberg's Cancer: Principles & Practice of Oncology*. 10th ed. Philadelphia, PA: Wolters Kluwer; 2015.
2. Pollack IF. Brain tumors in children. *N Engl J Med.* 1994;331(22):1500–1507.
3. Eran A, Ozturk A, Aygun N, Izbudak I. Medulloblastoma: atypical CT and MRI findings in children. *Pediatr Radiol.* 2010;40(7):1254–1262.
4. Iv M, Zhou M, Shpanskaya K, et al. MR Imaging-based radiomic signatures of distinct molecular subgroups of medulloblastoma. *AJNR Am J Neuroradiol.* 2019;40(1):154–161.
5. Brandao LA, Young Poussaint T. Posterior fossa tumors. *Neuroimaging Clin N Am.* 2017;27(1):1–37.
6. D'Arco F, Khan F, Mankad K, Ganau M, Caro-Dominguez P, Bisdas S. Differential diagnosis of posterior fossa tumours in children: new insights. *Pediatr Radiol.* 2018;48(13):1955–1963.
7. Fink KR, Fink JR. Imaging of brain metastases. *Surg Neurol Int.* 2013;4(suppl 4):S209–S219.
8. Rath TJ, Hughes M, Arabi M, Shah GV. Imaging of cerebritis, encephalitis, and brain abscess. *Neuroimaging Clin N Am.* 2012;22(4):585–607.

9. Robertson PL, Zeltzer PM, Boyett JM, et al. Survival and prognostic factors following radiation therapy and chemotherapy for ependymomas in children: a report of the Children's Cancer Group. *J Neurosurg*. 1998;88(4):695–703.
10. Zeltzer PM, Boyett JM, Finlay JL, et al. Metastasis stage, adjuvant treatment, and residual tumor are prognostic factors for medulloblastoma in children: conclusions from the Children's Cancer Group 921 randomized phase III study. *J Clin Oncol*. 1999;17(3):832–845.
11. Thompson EM, Hielscher T, Bouffet E, et al. Prognostic value of medulloblastoma extent of resection after accounting for molecular subgroup: a retrospective integrated clinical and molecular analysis. *Lancet Oncol*. 2016;17(4):484–495.
12. Cho YJ, Tsherniak A, Tamayo P, et al. Integrative genomic analysis of medulloblastoma identifies a molecular subgroup that drives poor clinical outcome. *J Clin Oncol*. 2011;29(11):1424–1430.
13. Taylor MD, Northcott PA, Korshunov A, et al. Molecular subgroups of medulloblastoma: the current consensus. *Acta Neuropathol*. 2012;123(4):465–472.
14. Ramaswamy V, Remke M, Bouffet E, et al. Risk stratification of childhood medulloblastoma in the molecular era: the current consensus. *Acta Neuropathol*. 2016;131(6):821–831.
15. Kram DE, Henderson JJ, Baig M, et al. Embryonal tumors of the central nervous system in children: the era of targeted therapeutics. *Bioengineering (Basel, Switzerland)*. 2018;5(4).
16. Waszak SM, Northcott PA, Buchhalter I, et al. Spectrum and prevalence of genetic predisposition in medulloblastoma: a retrospective genetic study and prospective validation in a clinical trial cohort. *Lancet Oncol*. 2018;19(6):785–798.
17. Rozen WM, Joseph S, Lo PA. Spontaneous regression of low-grade gliomas in pediatric patients without neurofibromatosis. *Pediatric Neurosurg*. 2008;44(4):324–328.
18. Yang T, Temkin N, Barber J, et al. Gross total resection correlates with long-term survival in pediatric patients with glioblastoma. *World Neurosurgery*. 2013;79(3–4):537–544.
19. Packer RJ, Pfister S, Bouffet E, et al. Pediatric low-grade gliomas: implications of the biologic era. *Neuro Oncol*. 2017;19(6):750–761.
20. Lassaletta A, Zapotocky M, Mistry M, et al. Therapeutic and prognostic implications of BRAF V600E in pediatric low-grade gliomas. *J Clin Oncol*. 2017;35(25):2934–2941.
21. Jones DTW, Kieran MW, Bouffet E, et al. Pediatric low-grade gliomas: next biologically driven steps. *Neuro Oncol*. 2018;20(2):160–173.
22. Bavle A, Jones J, Lin FY, Malphrus A, Adesina A, Su J. Dramatic clinical and radiographic response to BRAF inhibition in a patient with progressive disseminated optic pathway glioma refractory to MEK inhibition. *Pediatr Hematol Oncol*. 2017;34(4):254–259.
23. Lassaletta A, Guerreiro Stucklin A, Ramaswamy V, et al. Profound clinical and radiological response to BRAF inhibition in a 2-month-old diencephalic child with hypothalamic/chiasmatic glioma. *Pediatr Blood Cancer*. 2016;63(11):2038–2041.
24. Bandopadhayay P, Bergthold G, London WB, et al. Long-term outcome of 4,040 children diagnosed with pediatric low-grade gliomas: an analysis of the Surveillance Epidemiology and End Results (SEER) database. *Pediatr Blood Cancer*. 2014;61(7):1173–1179.
25. Louis DN, Perry A, Reifenberger G, et al. The 2016 World Health Organization classification of tumors of the central nervous system: a summary. *Acta Neuropathol*. 2016;131(6):803–820.
26. Hoffman LM, Veldhuijzen van Zanten SEM, Colditz N, et al. Clinical, radiologic, pathologic, and molecular characteristics of long-term survivors of diffuse intrinsic pontine glioma (DIPG): a collaborative report from the International and European Society for Pediatric Oncology DIPG registries. *J Clin Oncol*. 2018;36(19):1963–1972.
27. Castel D, Philippe C, Calmon R, et al. Histone H3F3A and HIST1H3B K27M mutations define two subgroups of diffuse intrinsic pontine gliomas with different prognosis and phenotypes. *Acta Neuropathol*. 2015;130(6):815–827.
28. Roux A, Botella C, Still M, et al. Posterior fossa metastasis-associated obstructive hydrocephalus in adult patients: literature review and practical considerations from the neuro-oncology club of the French Society of Neurosurgery. *World Neurosurg*. 2018;117:271–279.
29. Zhang X, Zhang W, Cao WD, Cheng G, Liu B, Cheng J. A review of current management of brain metastases. *Ann Surg Oncol*. 2012;19(3):1043–1050.
30. Delattre JY, Krol G, Thaler HT, Posner JB. Distribution of brain metastases. *Arch Neurol*. 1988;45(7):741–744.
31. Stelzer KJ. Epidemiology and prognosis of brain metastases. *Surg Neurol Int*. 2013;4(suppl 4):S192–S202.
32. Emelifeonwu JA, Shetty J, Kaliaperumal C, et al. Acute cerebellitis in children: a variable clinical entity. *J Child Neurol*. 2018;33(10):675–684.
33. Steinlin M, Blaser S, Boltshauser E. Cerebellar involvement in metabolic disorders: a pattern-recognition approach. *Neuroradiology*. 1998;40(6):347–354.
34. Kornreich L, Shkalim-Zemer V, Levinsky Y, Abdallah W, Ganelin-Cohen E, Straussberg R. Acute cerebellitis in children: a many-faceted disease. *J Child Neurol*. 2016;31(8):991–997.
35. Carceller Lechon F, Duat Rodriguez A, Sirvent Cerda SI, et al. Hemicerebellitis: report of three paediatric cases and review of the literature. *Eur J Paediatr Neurol*. 2014;18(3):273–281.
36. Hennes E, Zotter S, Dorninger L, et al. Long-term outcome of children with acute cerebellitis. *Neuropediatrics*. 2012;43(5):240–248.

Chapter 8

Imaging of spinal lesions

Teddy E. Kim, Carl M. Nechtman, and Wesley Hsu

CHAPTER OUTLINE

Introduction

Spinal cord tumors are uncommon causes of back pain, radicular pain, and sensorimotor deficits in adults and pediatric patients.[1] Primary spinal tumors are less common than intracranial tumors and represent approximately 2–4% of primary central nervous system (CNS) tumors.[2]

Classification of spinal cord tumors

Spinal cord tumors are classified as either (1) intradural intramedullary, (2) intradural extramedullary, or (3) extradural depending on the relationship to the spinal cord and dura.[3]

Extradural tumors. The majority of spinal tumors are extradural, accounting for 60% of spinal cord tumors and are frequently compressive osseous metastatic lesions.[1] Intradural spine tumors can originate adjacent to the spinal cord (e.g., extramedullary) or within the cord (e.g., intramedullary).[1] The differential diagnosis can be narrowed by recognizing where the tumor is located relative to the thecal sac and spinal cord.

Intramedullary tumors. Intradural intramedullary spinal cord tumors (IMSCTs) comprise 8–10% of primary spinal cord tumors, of which 60–70% are ependymomas and 30–40% are astrocytomas.[4] The third most common IMSCT is hemangioblastoma, which represents 3–8% of all IMSCT.[5] Hemangioblastomas are associated with von Hippel-Lindau (VHL) syndrome in 15–25% of cases.[5] The clinical presentation of primary spinal cord tumors depends on the location of the lesion.[2] In a recent series of IMSCTs, pain was the most common presenting symptom (72%) and can manifest as back pain (27%), radicular pain (25%), or central pain (20%).[2] Motor disturbance was next most common (55%), followed by sensory problems (39%).[2]

Intradural extramedullary tumors. Intradural extramedullary spinal tumors are usually benign lesions with a few exceptions and can be cured with preserved neurologic function with surgery alone in the majority of cases.[1] Intradural extramedullary tumors comprise more than 70% of intradural spinal cord tumors in adults and are only slightly less common in pediatric patients.[1] The most common intradural extramedullary tumors are derived from nerve sheath cells (schwannomas and neurofibromas) or meningeal cells (meningiomas). Myxopapillary ependymoma is an extramedullary lesion arising from the conus medullaris and filum terminalis.[1] Other rare extramedullary tumors include hemangiopericytomas, paragangliomas, malignant peripheral nerve sheath tumors, epidermoid cysts, and dermoid cysts.

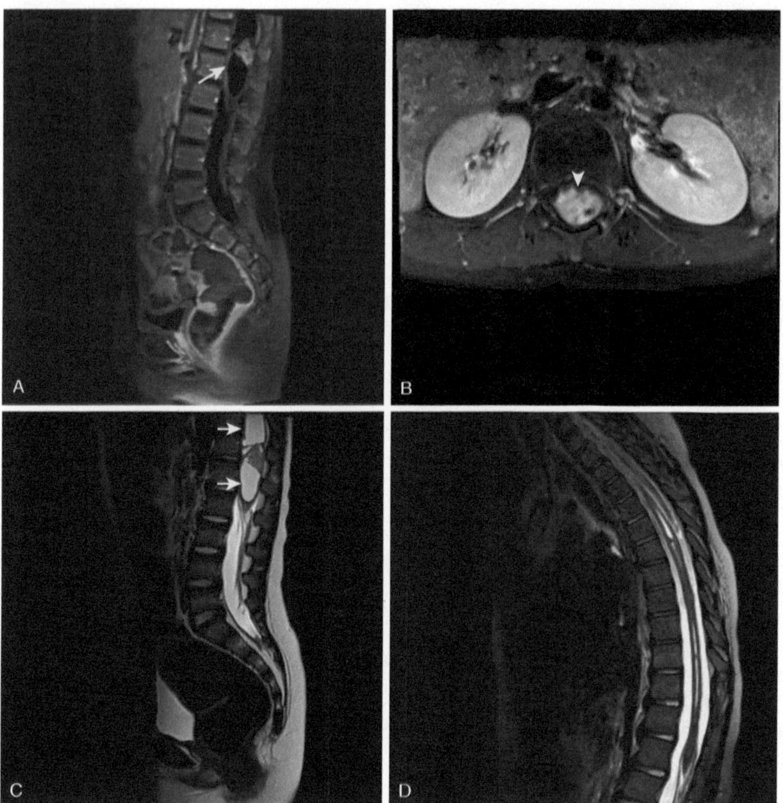

Fig. 8.1 Imaging of an intramedullary lesion consistent with astrocytoma as seen on the sagittal T1-weighted gadolinium-enhanced MRI (A, *small arrow*). This tumor consists of an enhancing mural nodule seen on the axial T1-weighted gadolinium-enhanced sequence (B, *arrowhead*) and a surrounding cystic area seen on the sagittal T2-weighted sequences (C, *arrows*). The lesion shows characteristic findings of an intramedullary tumor as it expands the conus medullaris and fills the canal at the level of T12–L1. Postoperative MRI (D) after gross total resection of tumor resulting in decreased size of the intramedullary cyst.

Clinical cases

CASE 8.1 SPINAL CORD ENHANCING MASS LESION IN A CHILD

Case. A 5-year-old boy presented to the pediatric orthopedic clinic with complaints of worsening back pain and scoliosis. He had been previously evaluated for his scoliosis with a plan to conservatively manage and observe clinical symptoms. Due to the progressive nature of his complaints, an MRI of the thoracic and lumbar spine were obtained, which demonstrated a 21-mm enhancing intramedullary lesion with a distal cystic component at the thoracolumbar region of the spinal cord with an associated syrinx proximally (Fig. 8.1). On examination, he maintained a kyphotic posture due to pain and had dysesthesias throughout his bilateral lower extremities but no appreciable strength deficits. Reflexes in the lower extremities were symmetrically absent. Surgical resection was recommended, and the patient underwent laminectomy and gross total resection of the tumor. The surgery and his postoperative course were uneventful, and he was discharged to a rehabilitation facility 1 week later. Final pathology was consistent with a pilocytic astrocytoma. His follow-up imaging demonstrated complete tumor removal without residual enhancement and improvement in his syrinx. He continues to do well without functional imitations on serial follow-up.

Teaching Points: Imaging of Spinal Cord Astrocytoma. Astrocytomas account for 80–90% of IMSCT in childhood and approximately 60% in adolescence.[6] The peak incidence of astrocytomas is in the third decade of life, but they are not as common as intramedullary ependymomas in this age group.[1] In adults, astrocytomas make up almost 25% of IMSCT with equal incidence in men and women.[1] Intramedullary astrocytomas are predominantly located in the cervicothoracic or thoracic region in pediatric patients, but cervical involvement is more common in the adult population.[1,6] Astrocytomas can span multiple vertebral levels and can have associated cyst formation.[1,3] Low-grade astrocytomas and fibrillary astrocytomas account for almost two-thirds of intramedullary astrocytomas in adults and almost 90% of intramedullary astrocytomas in children.[1] High-grade lesions are rarer and account for about 10% of intramedullary astrocytomas.[1]

Imaging and histology. MRI of low-grade spinal astrocytomas reveals an enlarged homogeneous mass with hypointense to isointense signal on T1-weighted images and hyperintense signal on T2-weighted images.[3] There is very little edema and no hemorrhage in low-grade astrocytomas. Most intramedullary astrocytomas enhance, and calcifications are rare.[7] While pilocytic astrocytomas can have well-defined borders, fibrillary astrocytomas are poorly defined with irregular tumor margins.[1] High-grade anaplastic astrocytoma or glioblastoma account for only about 10% of intramedullary astrocytomas.[1] These higher grade lesions display heterogeneous enhancement associated with necrosis, edema, and cyst formation.[1] Microscopically, low-grade astrocytomas show a low degree of cellularity, low mitotic activity, and absence of necrosis and microvascular proliferation.[1] Anaplastic astrocytoma and glioblastoma show moderate to high cellularity and an increased mitotic index.[1] Glioblastoma specifically exhibits a high degree of necrosis and microvascular proliferation.[1]

Clinical features. Presentation of intramedullary spinal cord astrocytoma is variable and typically progresses over months to years.[8] Pain is the earliest and most frequent presenting complaint and can be local or radicular.[8] Sensory disturbance is also common and may consist of dysesthesias or loss of sensation unilaterally or bilaterally.[8] Spasticity and weakness follow with loss of bowel and bladder function occurring late with the exception of tumors involving the conus medullaris.[9,10] Due to the centrally located nature of the tumor, motor deficits present with weakness in the upper extremities preceding the lower extremity.[8] In children, pain is the most common first symptom, but gait deterioration, motor regression, torticollis, and kyphoscoliosis are also significant presenting findings.[6] In malignant tumors, pain is followed by rapid neurological deterioration resulting in significant disability in 3 to 5 months.[11,12]

Patient management. Treatment is directed at total surgical resection, particularly for low-grade gliomas. There is no evidence that the degree of resection affects outcome in high-grade gliomas,[13] and the goal of surgery for these patients should be a less extensive resection in order to reduce post-surgical morbidity.[1]

Electrophysiologic monitoring is frequently used intraoperatively during the resection of IMSCT with motor-evoked and somatosensory-evoked potentials being the most common modalities.[1] Gross total resection is achievable with pilocytic astrocytomas due to its well-circumscribed nature.[1] However, the infiltrative nature of even low-grade astrocytomas make gross total resection difficult without risking postoperative morbidity. The rate of gross total resection is reported to be between 30% and 70%.[10,14,15]

Subtotal resection of fibrillary astrocytomas is appropriate in many cases, and there does not seem to be any significant difference in survival between total and subtotal resection techniques in long-term survival when controlled for tumor grades.[16–18] Intramedullary fibrillary astrocytomas have a high recurrence rate that ranges from 25% in low-grade tumors to almost 100% in high-grade tumors.[10,19] Adjuvant radiotherapy at diagnosis of high-grade astrocytoma or with tumor recurrence is frequently utilized.[1] The utility of concomitant chemotherapy is uncertain due to systemic toxicity and inability of large molecules to bypass the blood-spinal cord barrier.[20] In low-grade astrocytomas, 5-year survival ranges from 80–100%.[14] Patients with intramedullary anaplastic astrocytomas or glioblastoma have an average life expectancy of 15 months.[10,14]

Clinical Pearls

1. Intramedullary spinal cord tumors account for ~10% of primary spinal cord tumors and are most often ependymomas, which are slightly favored over astrocytomas.
2. Most intramedullary WHO grade 1 pilocytic astrocytomas enhance on neuroimaging and may be confused with higher-grade lesions without a tissue diagnosis.

CASE 8.2 SPINAL CORD ENHANCING INTRAMEDULLARY LESION IN ADULT

Case. A 53-year-old man was admitted after a cycling accident in which he sustained a displaced left C7 transverse process fracture in addition to a left clavicular fracture. He noted some numbness and mild weakness in his left hand. He was initially treated conservatively in a hard collar for his fractures and returned with plain x-rays at 3 months. He received an MRI to evaluate his persistent pain, which demonstrated an intramedullary enhancing lesion from C7 to T3 causing expansion of the cord and surrounding edema. There was susceptibility artifact associated with the lesion suggestive of microhemorrhage consistent with ependymoma (Fig. 8.2). Thoracic laminectomy for removal of the tumor was performed. The patient awoke with new-onset right greater than left leg weakness, of which the left leg improved more rapidly. He was discharged to a rehabilitation facility and continued to recover strength. His postoperative course was further complicated by a deep vein thrombosis managed with warfarin before developing a subdural hematoma, which required cessation of anticoagulation. His final pathology was consistent with grade II ependymoma. He was referred to radiation oncology. He underwent 50 Gy in 28 fractions of intensity modulated radiation therapy (IMRT) to the tumor bed. He continues to have some right lower extremity weakness on examination but was able to ambulate without assistance.

Teaching Points: Imaging Differential of Enhancing Spinal Cord Ependymoma. Clinical features of intramedul-

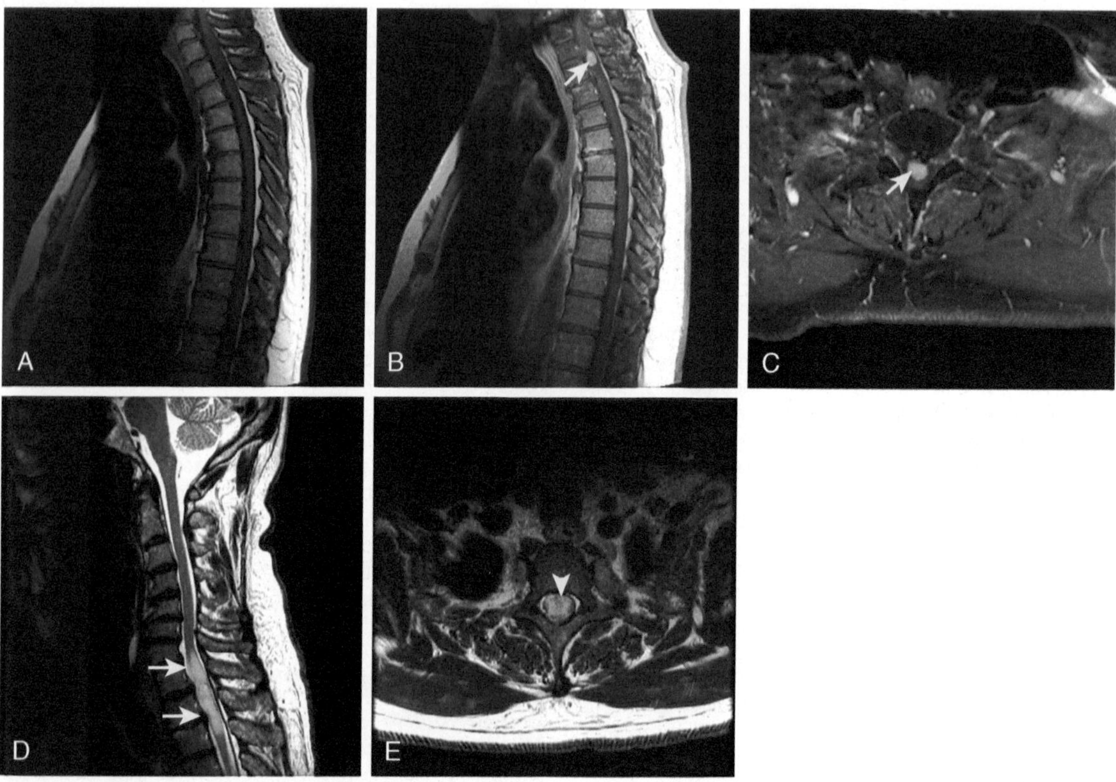

Fig. 8.2 Imaging of an ependymoma in the cervical spinal cord. T1-weighted pre- (A) and post-contrast (B) sequences demonstrate a discrete enhancing nodule at the cervicothoracic junction (B, *small arrow*) that is centrally located within the cord as seen on the axial T1-weighted post-contrast sequence (C, *small arrow*). There is marked cord signal change appearing hyperintense on the T2-weighted image (D, *large arrows*). This lesion shows characteristics of an intramedullary tumor on the T2-weighted axial sequence with expansion of the cord that fills the spinal canal (E, *arrowhead*).

lary ependymomas are variable.[21] The classic central cord syndrome with suspended sensory loss with descending progression, symmetric upper extremity mixed upper and lower motor neuron weakness, and bilateral spastic lower extremities is infrequently seen.[22] Early symptoms are usually nonspecific and may only subtly progress.[21] Time of onset to symptoms ranges from 3–4 years, although intratumoral hemorrhage may precipitate a rapid decline.[17,23] Sensory symptoms, particularly dysesthesias, are the earliest to present in upward of 70% of patients.[17,24–28] Painful aching sensation at the level of the tumor is rarely radicular and can occur early in disease progression.[22] Symptoms mainly depend on the location of the tumor. Upper extremity symptoms predominate in patients with cervical lesions, while lower extremity spasticity and sensory disturbances predominate with thoracic lesions.[21,22] Numbness is also a common complaint and typically begins distally in the legs, with proximal progression.[21] Tumors in the lumbar spinal cord/conus can present with back pain and leg pain, with leg pain being radicular in nature.[21] Urogenital and anorectal dysfunction occurs earlier with conus lesions.[21]

Imaging and histology. MRI shows a lesion hypointense on T1-weighted imaging and hyperintense on T2-weighed imaging.[3] Intramedullary ependymomas enhance homogeneously with contrast.[3] Although not encapsulated, intramedullary ependymomas often have a distinct plane between the tumor and adjacent spinal cord, despite its frequent association with cysts, syrinxes, and hemorrhage.[1]

Intramedullary ependymomas are circumscribed lesions of modest vascularity.[23] The tumor is usually soft and somewhat friable, but a firmer, more nodular appearance is occasionally encountered.[23] Hemorrhage is more frequent in intramedullary ependymomas compared to astrocytomas. Microscopically, spinal ependymomas might display ependymal rosettes, but perivascular pseudorosettes are more prominent.[1]

Features and management. Intramedullary ependymomas represent 40–60% of adults with IMSCT, with peak incidence in the fourth to fifth decade of life.[15,19,29] Intramedullary ependymomas account for only 16–35% of IMSCT in the pediatric population.[18,29] Most intramedullary ependymomas arise from the cervical or cervicothoracic region.[18,23,30] Intramedullary ependymomas are mostly well circumscribed,

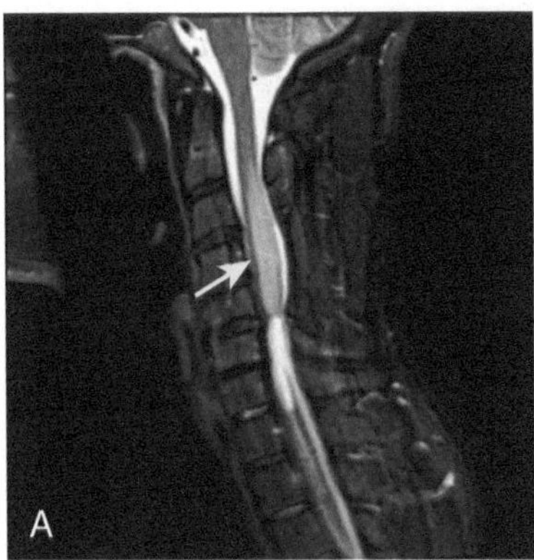

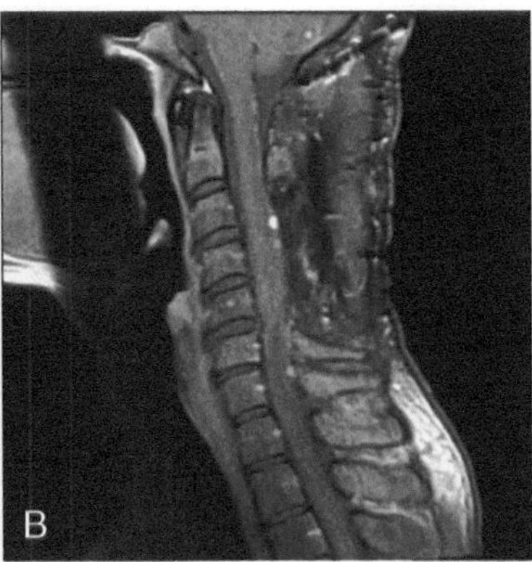

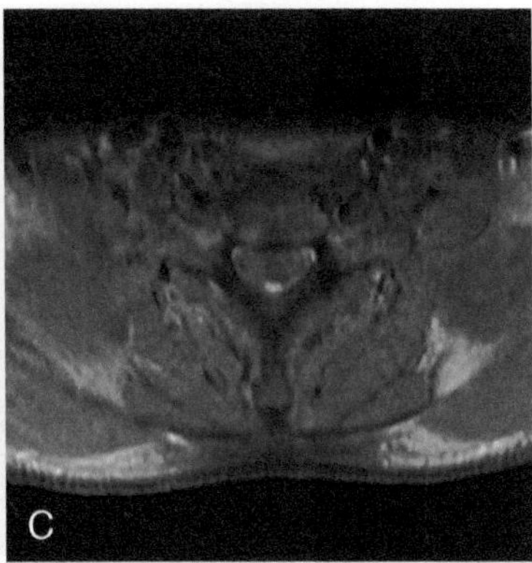

Fig. 8.3 (A) Sagittal T2-weighted MRI image and (B) axial T1-weighted post-contrast image demonstrating a biopsy-proven spinal cord hemangioblastoma in a patient with Von-Hippel Lindau (VHL) disease. These lesions expand the cord (A, *arrow*) and faintly enhances with contrast (B, *arrow*). Axial imaging (C) shows cord expansion at the level of the enhancement.

which helps with total surgical resection in 70–100% of cases.[18,31,32] Tumor recurrence is reported to be less than 10% but can be unrecognized secondary to the slow growth rate of ependymomas.[1] Tumor recurrence is significantly higher with subtotal resection, with reported rates from 50–70%.[31,33] Therefore, prognosis for patients with intramedullary ependymomas is dependent upon the extent of surgical resection.[1] Postoperative radiation is controversial but can increase tumor-free survival rates of adult patients with high-grade or subtotally resected tumors.[33–35] Radiation is debated in children due to radiation-induced damage to the CNS.[10] In addition, both adult and pediatric patients may have increased postoperative neurological morbidity with prior adjuvant radiotherapy.[1] The 5-year survival rate for low-grade intramedullary ependymoma ranges from 83% to 100% but decline rapidly with higher-grade ependymomas, only reaching 20% 5-year overall survival.[23,31,34,36]

Clinical Pearls

1. Enhancing spinal cord tumors can mimic inflammatory and infectious lesions in the spinal cord including transverse myelitis, multiple sclerosis, neuromyelitis optic spectrum disorder, infectious myelitis, and other related conditions.

CASE 8.3 SPINAL CORD LESIONS IN A PATIENT WITH VON HIPPEL-LINDAU DISEASE

Case. A 36-year-old man with a known family history of VHL and multiple cerebellar mass resections presented for evaluation of increasing cervical pain. On examination, he had mild left-handed weakness and numbness, which had worsened recently. His MRI demonstrated multiple small enhancing lesions throughout the cervical spinal cord, with one associated with an enlarging cyst (Fig. 8.3). Given the progression of symptoms and dorsal location of the cystic lesion, he underwent cervical laminectomy for removal of the dorsal mass and cyst decompression. He did well with no additional postoperative deficits and went home on postoperative day 2. He continues to be followed for his VHL and multiple lesions.

Teaching Points: Imaging Differential for Spinal Cord Hemangioblastoma. *Hemangioblastomas* of the spinal cord are predominantly intramedullary, but these tumors can be extramedullary and extradural. Presenting symptoms depend on the location of the lesion, although most patients present with symptoms of compressive myelopathy.[37] Intramedullary hemangioblastomas represent about 4% of spinal tumors and occur sporadically or in association with VHL (see Chapter 18, Case 18.1 for further discussion of approach to managing VHL).[1] Of the people diagnosed with intramedullary hemangioblastoma, almost 25% are found to have VHL.[38] Sporadic intramedullary hemangioblastomas have a peak incidence in the third or fourth decade, and men are more commonly affected than women.[1] Hemangioblastoma associated with VHL have earlier onset of disease.[39] Most hemangioblastomas are solitary, but multiple lesions are not uncommon.[39]

Imaging. On MRI, intramedullary hemangioblastomas often appear as cysts with enhancing mural nodules. Associated syringobulbia and syringomyelia are common. Gadolinium provides homogeneous enhancement of smaller tumors and heterogeneous enhancement of larger tumors.[1,3] Due to the vascular nature of the tumor, feeding arteries and draining veins may be visible with contrasted MRI.[1] Spinal angiography can also be useful in diagnosis and surgical planning.[1]

Histology. Microscopically, hemangioblastoma display a reticular pattern of small capillary and foamy stromal cells.[1] There is a highly vascular solid portion with small arteries, capillaries, and large dilated draining veins. The tumor nidus consists mainly of endothelial cells and interspersed stromal

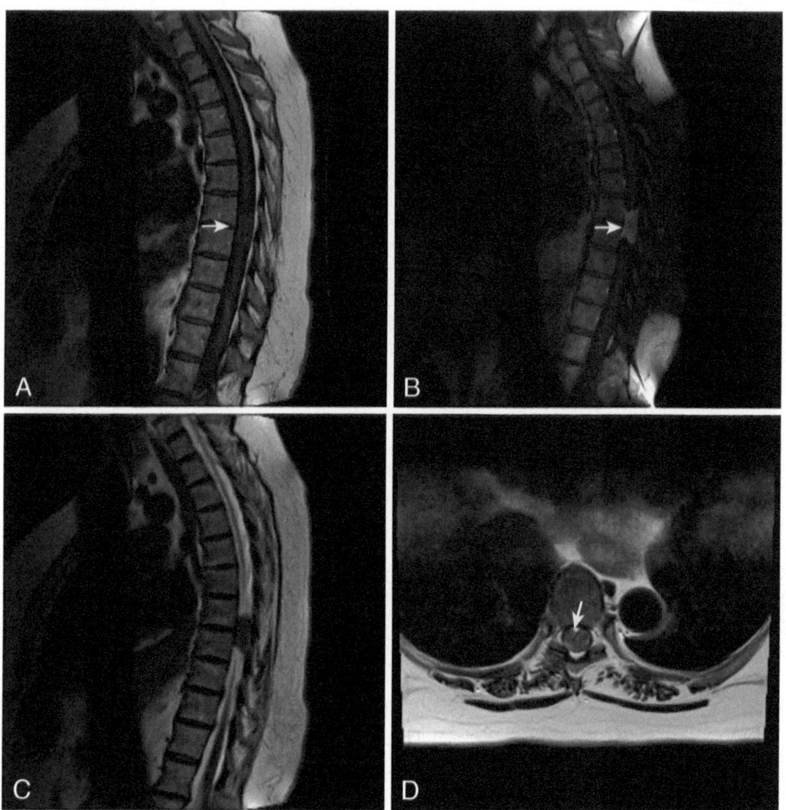

Fig. 8.4 Imaging of an intradural extramedullary lesion consistent with meningioma in the mid-thoracic spinal canal. Sagittal T1-weighted pre- (A) and post-contrast (B) imaging shows avid homogeneous enhancement *(large arrows)*, which is characteristic. Note that the sagittal and axial T2-weighted image (C, D) reveals that the spinal cord is not expanded as is expected with intramedullary lesions, but is displaced to the right side (D, *arrow*), indicating an intradural extramedullary location on the left side.

cells. Accompanying the solid portion are large cysts lined by fibrillary astrocytes.

Patient management. (See Chapter 18, Case 18.1) Gross total resection of symptomatic intramedullary hemangioblastoma is preferred and is associated with low morbidity.[37,40] When there are multiple lesions in the spinal cord, surgical management should be directed toward the symptomatic lesion. There have been no reports of adjuvant chemotherapy or radiotherapy in the treatment of intramedullary hemangioblastomas of sporadic origin or in associated with VHL. However, there are a few published works on treating intracranial hemangioblastomas with antiangiogenic drugs like thalidomide, interferon-alpha, and SU5416.[1]

Clinical Pearls

1. Spinal hemangioblastomas are the prototypical tumor associated with von-Hippel Lindau disease.
2. Hemangioblastomas associated with VHL have earlier onset of disease, and are often solitary but can be multiple including the cerebellum.

CASE 8.4 INTRADURAL EXTRAMEDULLARY SPINAL MENINGIOMA

Case. A 59-year-old woman presented to her primary care physician with increasing bilateral leg numbness. She also noted increasing leg heaviness, difficulty ambulating, and balance problems. She was referred to a neurologist, and an MRI of the spine was ordered, which demonstrated a homogenously enhancing intradural extramedullary dural-based lesion within the thoracic spinal canal (Fig. 8.4). Although she had no weakness on examination, she demonstrated decreased vibratory sensation and proprioception. Surgery was recommended given the size of the mass, evidence of ongoing compression, and proximity to the spinal cord. She underwent a thoracic laminectomy for intradural decompression of the spinal cord, which proceeded uneventfully. Final pathology demonstrated a grade I meningioma. She was discharged to a rehabilitation facility 1 week later with full strength in her lower extremities.

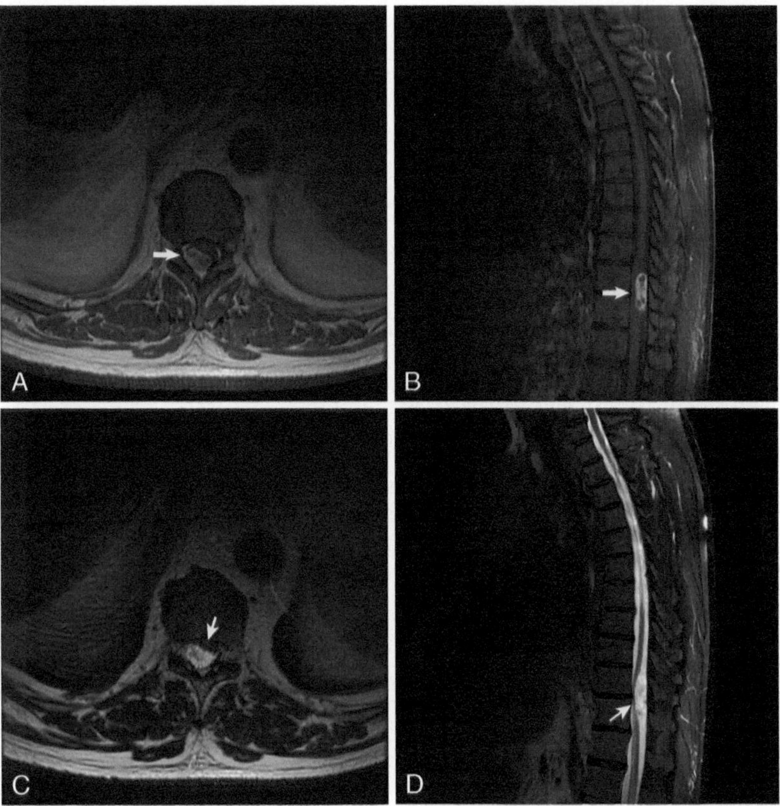

Fig. 8.5 Imaging of an intradural, extramedullary schwannoma of the spinal cord. The axial (A) and sagittal (B) T1-weighted gadolinium enhanced images reveal a variably enhancing mass in the lower thoracic spinal canal *(large arrows)*. There is displacement of the cord anteriorly *(small arrows)* and compression of the spinal cord as evident on the axial (C) and sagittal (D) T2-weighted images.

Teaching Points: Imaging Differential for Spinal Cord Meningioma. Spinal meningiomas account for up to 46% of spinal neoplasms and are more common intradurally than extradurally.[41] The small percentage of spinal meningiomas that are extradural commonly extend into the intradural space.[1] The thoracic level is the most common location for spinal meningiomas, and there is a predilection for women in their fifth to seventh decade of life.[1] Intradural meningiomas are mostly located laterally and posterior to the spinal cord, with anterior location being less frequent.[41,42] Although intradural meningiomas are usually solitary lesions, there can be multiple lesions usually associated with neurofibromatosis (NF) type 2 (see Chapter 16 for further discussion of approach to managing NF2).[1]

Imaging. On MRI, spinal meningiomas have a hypointense to isointense signal on T1-weighted images and hyperintense signal on T2-weighted images.[1] Addition of gadolinium contrast results in strong homogeneous enhancement, although calcifications are common and may preclude gadolinium enhancement.[1,3]

Histology. Histologically, meningothelial and psammomatous meningiomas are the most common histologic subtypes of spinal meningioma. Intradural clear-cell meningioma is less frequent and associated with worse prognosis.[43] Atypical and anaplastic variants are rare. Meningiomas stain positive for vimentin and epithelial membrane antigen.

Patient management. Most intradural meningiomas are noninvasive, benign neoplasms and can be cured with gross total resection.[1] Even considering the technical challenges of ventrally located lesions, total surgical resection is attainable in 90% of patients.[44] Tumor recurrence rate with total or subtotal resection is between 3% and 7%.[41,42,45] Atypical and anaplastic spinal meningiomas have a higher recurrence rate but rarely metastasize.[1] Radiotherapy can be considered after subtotal resection or with recurrence, which is analogous to the management of intracranial meningiomas.[1]

Clinical Pearls

Meningiomas are common spinal neoplasms which frequently benefit from surgical decompression if symptomatic.

CASE 8.5 INTRADURAL EXTRAMEDULLARY SPINAL CORD SCHWANNOMA

Case. A 64-year-old man presented to a local orthopedic surgeon for evaluation of chronic back pain. An MRI Lumbar Spine was ordered, which was unremarkable except for a T10–11 enhancing intradural mass. MRI Thoracic Spine confirmed the presence of a heterogeneously enhancing, 4 cm extramedullary lesion with areas of bright T2 signal causing spinal cord compression at T10–11 (Fig. 8.5). He was referred to our institution for management, and resection was recommended. He underwent thoracic laminectomy with intradural tumor resection, which was uneventful. He recovered well with full strength in his lower extremities and was discharged home after 3 days.

Teaching Points: Imaging Differential for Spinal Cord Schwannoma. Schwannomas and neurofibromas account for up to a third of intradural spinal cord tumors in the adult population but are less common in children. Peak incidence of nerve sheath tumors are in the fourth to fifth decade of life, with equal incidence in men and women.[1] Schwannomas are more common than neurofibromas, and occasionally multiple schwannomas are seen with schwannomatosis or NF2 (Chapter 16).[1] Neurofibromas often show multiplicity, especially in NF1. Intradural nerve sheath tumors most commonly affect the lumbosacral region, likely secondary to the long intradural course of the caudal spinal nerve roots in the neuraxis.[45]

Imaging. About 60–80% of nerve sheath tumors arise from nerve roots before leaving the dural sac.[1] An additional 10% arises from the nerve root as it leaves the dural sac and becomes surrounded by the dural root sleeve.[1] These tumors, therefore, display both intradural and extradural components and are referred to as dumbbell tumors.[1] It is difficult to distinguish between a schwannoma and neurofibroma on MRI findings alone. Nerve sheath tumors are isointense on T1-weighted images and hyperintense on T2-weighted images.[1] Gadolinium adds variable enhancement ranging from homogeneous to a peripheral ring-like enhancement.[1,41] It is important to note that an irregular enhancement pattern is associated with malignant tumors but must be correlated with clinical findings.[1]

Histology. Histologically, schwannomas display neoplastic Schwann cells without nerve fibers. Verocay bodies (e.g., palisading nuclei pattern seen in Antoni B areas) are characteristic. Loose Antoni A areas and dense Antoni B areas are seen on hematoxylin and eosin staining. Neurofibromas more frequently invade the nerve root and display Schwann cells, nerve fibers, and fibroblasts. When involving the main peripheral nerve trunk, neurofibromas cause fusiform expansion with the typical wavy nuclei and "shredded carrot" type collagen.[46] Both schwannoma and neurofibroma stain positive for S100.[46]

Patient management. Nerve sheath tumors are generally benign neoplasms, although tumors rarely undergo malignant transformation and become malignant peripheral nerve sheath tumors (MPNSTs). Most MPNSTs are associated with NF1. Schwannomas tend to arise from the dorsal nerve root, whereas neurofibromas tend to arise from the ventral nerve root.

Primary treatment of nerve sheath tumors is directed at total surgical resection.[1] However, this is not always attainable, and a subtotal resection may need to be performed when the tumor is attached to the spinal cord or when the extradural component is attached to vital structures.[45] In order to obtain complete surgical resection, the ventral or dorsal root may need to be sacrificed. Interestingly, sacrifice of nerve roots in these situations may not be associated with a postoperative neurological deficit.[45] Schwannomas arise from the dorsal nerve root and are less invasive than neurofibromas. Therefore, surgical resection is less often associated with pronounced motor deficits compared to resection of neurofibromas.[1]

Radiotherapy and chemotherapy are reserved for tumors that have malignant characteristics or with recurrence.[1] One must note that radiation should not be performed in NF1 patients, as this increases further tumor formation and malignant transformation due to loss of heterozygosity (see Chapter 16).[2]

Clinical Pearls

1. Schwannomas and neurofibromas account for up to one-third of intradural spinal cord tumors and appear as homogeneously enhancing extramedullary masses.

CASE 8.6 EXTRADULAR SPINAL VERTEBRAL METASTASIS

Case. A 60-year-old man with known metastatic prostate cancer presented to an outside hospital with worsening back pain and difficulty ambulating over 1 month. MRI demonstrated circumferential spinal canal involvement of an enhancing, extradural mass with severe canal stenosis. Given his disease burden, he was treated initially with radiation therapy. After a failure to improve, he presented to our hospital for evaluation for surgical decompression. On examination, he had mild weakness and hyperreflexia with difficulty sustaining resistance in his bilateral lower extremities consistent with compressive myelopathy of the thoracic spine. He underwent thoracic laminectomy for tumor debulking and decompression of the spinal cord. The patient noted an improvement in his leg strength and sensation postoperatively and was able to regain his ambulatory status. He resumed and completed his radiation to the tumor bed with continued good local control on follow up.

Teaching Points: Differential Diagnosis and Management of Epidural Spinal Metastasis. Many types of cancers can metastasize to the spine, with lung cancer, breast cancer, and prostate cancer being the most frequent.[47] Epidural metastases originate in either the vertebral column (85%), paravertebral tissues (10–15%), or epidural space itself.[48] The vertebral body is a very common site of bony metastases from cancer, and 80% of vertebral epidural metastases are localized to the vertebral body, with fewer in the posterior arch.[49]

It is thought that the high propensity for malignancy to metastasize to the vertebral body is secondary to the highly vascular nature of the bone marrow.[48] As the tumor grows in the epidural space, it encroaches on the thecal sac, compresses the spinal cord or spinal nerve roots, and compresses the epidural venous plexus that may lead to vasogenic edema and infarction of the spinal cord.[48] The majority of epidural metastases develop in the thoracic spine (60%), followed by the lumbosacral area and cervical spine.[48] Involvement of multiple spinal levels is not uncommon and occurs in 20–35% of cases.

Imaging and histology. Although the clinical picture can raise suspicion, the definitive diagnosis of metastatic epidural spinal cord compression (MESCC) is made radiographically with MRI of the spine with and without contrast.[48] Because metastatic disease can be multifocal, it is important to obtain imaging of the entire spine.[48] MRI can be useful in demonstrating the extent and configuration of epidural disease involvement of the bony structures and adjacent soft tissue as well, which helps guide further treatment planning.[48]

Patient management. The most important prognostic factor to regain ambulation after treatment of MESCC is prior neurological status.[50–53] Once the patient loses their ability to ambulate, it is uncommon to regain the ability to walk.[54] The objective of treatment of MESCC is prevention of or reversal of neurological deficits and pain control.[48] The three mainstays of treatment are medical management, radiation, and surgical intervention.[48] Corticosteroids continue to be used in patients with neurological signs or symptoms of epidural compression despite limited documented evidence of benefit.[55] The optimal dosage of dexamethasone in MESCC is not well established, ranging from 10–100 mg, followed by progressive tapering.[48] Typically, a higher dose is recommended for patients with neurological deficits.[55] In patients with minimal neurological symptoms or signs, a bolus dose of dexamethasone 10 mg followed by 16 mg daily with subsequent tapering is a reasonable approach.[48]

Laufer et al. describes the NOMS framework for the decision making-process in the management of spinal metastatic tumors.[56] The NOMS framework consists of neurologic, oncologic, mechanical, and systemic considerations.[56] Neurologic assessment is considered in conjunction with radiographic assessment.[56] The degree of MESCC is graded by the six-point grading system validated by Spine Oncology Study Group.[56] Oncologic assessment is determining the responsiveness of the tumor to available treatment modalities.[56] Mechanical assessment represents independent indication for surgical stabilization or percutaneous cement augmentation, regardless of the degree of MESCC or grade and radiosensitivity of the tumor (see also Chapter 23, Case 23.3 for management of epidural metastasis in patients with hematologic malignancies).[56] Mechanical instability, regardless of the degree of MESCC or radiosensitivity of the tumor, is an indication for surgical intervention. Systemic assessment reflects the fact that all treatment decisions are predicated on the patients' ability to tolerate the proposed intervention. Consideration of these factors emphasizes durable tumor control while minimizing treatment-related morbidity and optimizing patient care.

Clinical Pearls

1. As patient survival increases, spinal metastasis is becoming increasingly common.
2. Literature has demonstrated a clear functional and survival benefit to patients with compressive metastatic lesions who undergo surgical decompression if life expectancy is greater than 3 months.[57]

Conclusion

When evaluating patients with new presentation of myelopathy and imaging evidence of a spinal cord lesion, the first step is to localize the presentation and lesion into one of three categories: (1) extradural; (2) intradural, extramedullary; and (3) intramedullary. This can aid in the diagnostic investigation, differential diagnosis formation, and approach to treatment.

References

1. Traul DE, Shaffrey ME, Schiff D. Part I: spinal-cord neoplasms-intradural neoplasms. *Lancet Oncol*. 2007;8:35–45. https://doi.org/10.1016/S1470-2045(06)71009-9.
2. Chamberlain MC, Tredway TL. Adult primary intradural spinal cord tumors: a review. *Curr Neurol Neurosci Rep*. 2011;11:320–328. https://doi.org/10.1007/s11910-011-0190-2.
3. Esiashvili N, Nanda R, Khan M, Eaton B. Spinal tumors. *Radiat Oncol Pediatr CNS Tumors*. 2017;50:335–351.
4. Parsa AT, Chi JH, Acosta FL, Ames CP, McCormick PC. Intramedullary spinal cord tumors: molecular insights and surgical innovation. *Clin Neurosurg*. 2005;52:76–84.
5. Lonser RR, Weil RJ, Wanebo JE, Devroom HL, Oldfield EH. Surgical management of spinal cord hemangioblastomas in patients with von Hippel-Lindau disease. *J Neurosurg*. 2003;98:106–116. https://doi.org/10.3171/jns.2003.98.1.0106.
6. Constantini S, Houten J, Miller DC, et al. Intramedullary spinal cord tumors in children under the age of 3 years. *J Neurosurg*. 1996;85:1036–1043. https://doi.org/10.3171/jns.1996.85.6.1036.
7. Runge VM, Muroff LR, Jinkins JR. Central nervous system: review of clinical use of contrast media. *Top Magn Reson Imaging*. 2001;12:231–263. https://doi.org/10.1097/00002142-200108000-00003.
8. Roonprapunt C, Houten JK. Spinal cord astrocytomas: presentation, management, and outcome. *Neurosurg Clin N Am*. 2006;17:29–36.

9. Reimer R, Onofrio BM. Astrocytomas of the spinal cord in children and adolescents. *J Neurosurg*. 2009;63: 669–675.
10. Myseros JS. Intramedullary spinal tumors in children. In: Tonn JC, Reardon DA, Rutka JT, Westphal M, eds. *Oncology of CNS Tumors*. 2010.
11. Cohen AR, Wisoff JH, Allen JC, Epstein F. Malignant astrocytomas of the spinal cord. *J Neurosurg*. 2009;70:50–54. https://doi.org/10.3171/jns.1989.70.1.0050.
12. Epstein FJ, Farmer JP, Freed D. Adult intramedullary astrocytomas of the spinal cord. *J Neurosurg*. 2009;77(3):355–359. https://doi.org/10.3171/jns.1992.77.3.0355.
13. Liu A, Sankey EW, Bettegowda C, Burger PC, Jallo GI, Groves ML. Poor prognosis despite aggressive treatment in adults with intramedullary spinal cord glioblastoma. *J Clin Neurosci*. 2015;22(10):1628–1631. https://doi.org/10.1016/j.jocn.2015.05.008.
14. Rossitch Jr E, Zeidman SM, Burger PC, et al. Clinical and pathological analysis of spinal cord astrocytomas in children. *Neurosurgery*. 1990;27:193–196. https://doi.org/10.1097/00006123-199008000-00003.
15. Kane PJ, el-Mahdy W, Singh A, Powell MP, Crockard HA. Spinal intradural tumours: part II—Intramedullary. *Br J Neurosurg*. 1999;13:558–563. https://doi.org/10.1080/02688699943051.
16. Minehan KJ, Shaw EG, Scheithauer BW, Davis DL, Onofrio BM. Spinal cord astrocytoma: pathological and treatment considerations. *J Neurosurg*. 1995;83:590–595.
17. Cristante L, Herrmann HD. Surgical management of intramedullary spinal cord tumors: functional outcome and sources of morbidity. *Neurosurgery*. 1994;35:69–74. https://doi.org/10.1227/00006123-199407000-00011.
18. Innocenzi G, Raco A, Cantore G, Raimondi AJ. Intramedullary astrocytomas and ependymonas in the pediatric age group: a retrospective study. *Childs Nerv Syst*. 1996;12:776–780. https://doi.org/10.1007/bf00261597.
19. Stein BM, McCormick PC. Intramedullary neoplasms and vascular malformations. *Clinical Neurosurg*. 1992;39:361–387.
20. Tobin MK, Geraghty JR, Engelhard HH, Linninger AA, Mehta AI. Intramedullary spinal cord tumors: a review of current and future treatment strategies 2015;39:E14.
21. Schwartz TH, McCormick PC. Intramedullary ependymomas: clinical presentation, surgical treatment strategies and prognosis. *J Neuro Oncol*. 2000;47:211–218. https://doi.org/10.1023/A:1006414405305.
22. McCormick PC, Stein BM. Intramedullary tumors in adults. *Neurosurg Clin N Am*. 1990;1:609–630. https://doi.org/10.1016/s1042-3680(18)30793-9.
23. McCormick PC, Torres R, Post KD, Stein BM. Intramedullary ependymoma of the spinal cord. *J Neurosurg*. 2009;72:523–532. https://doi.org/10.3171/jns.1990.72.4.0523.
24. McCormick PC, Post KD, Stein BM. Intradural extramedullary tumors in adults. *Neurosurg Clin N Am*. 1990;1:591–608. https://doi.org/10.1016/s1042-3680(18)30792-7.
25. Hoshimaru M, Koyama T, Hashimoto N, Kikuchi H. Results of microsurgical treatment for intramedullary spinal cord ependymomas: analysis of 36 cases. *Neurosurgery*. 1999;44:264–269. https://doi.org/10.1097/00006123-199902000-00012.
26. Sandler HM, Papadopoulos SM, Thornton Jr AF, Ross DA. Spinal cord astrocytomas: results of therapy. *Neurosurgery*. 1992;30:490–493. https://doi.org/10.1227/00006123-199204000-00003.
27. Epstein FJ, Farmer JP, Freed D. Adult intramedullary spinal cord ependymomas: the result of surgery in 38 patients. *J Neurosurg*. 1993;79(2):204–209. https://doi.org/10.3171/jns.1993.79.2.0204.
28. Cooper PR. Outcome after operative treatment of intramedullary spinal cord tumors in adults: intermediate and long-term results in 51 patients. *Neurosurgery*. 1989;25:855–859. https://doi.org/10.1097/00006123-198912000-00001.
29. Miller DC. Surgical pathology of intramedullary spinal cord neoplasms. *J Neuro Oncol*. 2000;47:189–194. https://doi.org/10.1023/A:1006496204396.
30. Ferrante L, Mastronardi L, Celli P, Lunardi P, Acqui M, Fortuna A. Intramedullary spinal cord ependymomas—a study of 45 cases with long-term follow-up. *Acta Neurochir*. 1992;119:74–79. https://doi.org/10.1007/BF01541785.
31. Raco A, Esposito V, Lenzi J, Piccirilli M, Delfini R, Cantore G. Long-term follow-up of intramedullary spinal cord tumors: a series of 202 cases. *Neurosurgery*. 2005;56:972–981. https://doi.org/10.1227/01.NEU.0000158318.66568.CC.
32. Epstein FJ, Farmer JP. Pediatric spinal cord tumor surgery. *Neurosurg Clin N Am*. 1990;1:569–590. https://doi.org/10.1016/s1042-3680(18)30791-5.
33. Chang UK, Choe WJ, Chung SK, Chung CK, Kim HJ. Surgical outcome and prognostic factors of spinal intramedullary ependymomas in adults. *J Neuro Oncol*. 2002;57:133–139. https://doi.org/10.1023/A:1015789009058.
34. Stüben G, Stuschke M, Kroll M, Havers W, Sack H. Postoperative radiotherapy of spinal and intracranial ependymomas: analysis of prognostic factors. *Radiother Oncol*. 1997;45:3–10. https://doi.org/10.1016/S0167-8140(97)00138-2.
35. Lin YH, Huang CI, Wong TT, et al. Treatment of spinal cord ependymomas by surgery with or without postoperative radiotherapy. *J Neuro Oncol*. 2005;71:205–210. https://doi.org/10.1007/s11060-004-1386-y.
36. Lee TT, Gromelski EB, Green BA. Surgical treatment of spinal ependymoma and post-operative radiotherapy. *Acta Neurochir*. 1998;140:309–313. https://doi.org/10.1007/s007010050103.
37. Cristante L, Herrmann HD. Surgical management of intramedullary hemangioblastoma of the spinal cord. *Acta Neurochir*. 1999;141:333–339. https://doi.org/10.1007/s007010050308.
38. Neumann HP, Eggert HR, Scheremet R, et al. Central nervous system lesions in von Hippel-Lindau syndrome. *J Neurol Neurosurg Psychiatry*. 1992;55:898–901. https://doi.org/10.1136/jnnp.55.10.898.
39. Murota T, Symon L. Surgical management of hemangioblastoma of the spinal cord: a report of 18 cases. *Neurosurgery*. 1989;25:699–707. https://doi.org/10.1097/00006123-198911000-00003.
40. Spetzler RF, Detwiler PW, Riina HA, Porter RW. Modified classification of spinal cord vascular lesions. *J Neurosurg*. 2002;96:145–156. https://doi.org/10.3171/spi.2002.96.2.0145.
41. Roux FX, Nataf F, Pinaudeau M, Borne G, Devaux B, Meder JF. Intraspinal meningiomas: review of 54 cases with discussion of poor prognosis factors and modern therapeutic management. *Surg Neurol*. 1996;46:458–463. https://doi.org/10.1016/S0090-3019(96)00199-1.
42. Gezen F, Kahraman S, Çanakci Z, Bedük A. Review of 36 cases of spinal cord meningioma. *Spine*. 2000;25:727–731. https://doi.org/10.1097/00007632-200003150-00013.
43. Oviedo A, Pang D, Zovickian J, Smith M. Clear cell meningioma: case report and review of the literature. *Pediatr Dev Pathol*. 2005;8:386–390. https://doi.org/10.1007/s10024-005-0119-3.
44. Solero CL, Fornari M, Giomnini S, et al. Spinal meningiomas: review of 174 operated cases. *Neurosurgery*. 1989;25:153–160. https://doi.org/10.1097/00006123-198908000-00001.

45. Jinnai T, Koyama T. Clinical characteristics of spinal nerve sheath tumors: analysis of 149 cases. *Neurosurgery*. 2005;56:510–515. https://doi.org/10.1227/01.NEU.0000153752.59565. (BB).
46. Rodriguez FJ, Folpe AL, Giannini C, Perry A. Pathology of peripheral nerve sheath tumors: diagnostic overview and update on selected diagnostic problems. *Acta Neuropathol*. 2012;123:295–319. https://doi.org/10.1007/s00401-012-0954-z.
47. Bilsky MH, Lis E, Raizer J, Lee H, Boland P. The diagnosis and treatment of metastatic spinal tumor. *Oncol*. 1999;4:459–469. https://doi.org/10.1634/theoncologist.4-6-459.
48. Yáñez ML, Miller JJ, Batchelor TT. Diagnosis and treatment of epidural metastases. *Cancer*. 2017;123:1106–1114. https://doi.org/10.1002/cncr.30521.
49. Chamberlain MC. Neoplastic meningitis and metastatic epidural spinal cord compression. *Hematol Oncol Clin North Am*. 2012;26:917–931. https://doi.org/10.1016/j.hoc.2012.04.004.
50. Maranzano E, Latini P. Effectiveness of radiation therapy without surgery in metastatic spinal cord compression: final results from a prospective trial. *Int J Radiat Oncol Biol Phys*. 1995;32:959–967. https://doi.org/10.1016/0360-3016(95)00572-G.
51. Maranzano E, Latini P, Checcaglini F, et al. Radiation therapy of spinal cord compression caused by breast cancer: report of a prospective trial. *Int J Radiat Oncol Biol Phys*. 1992;24:301–306. https://doi.org/10.1016/0360-3016(92)90685-B.
52. Maranzano E, Latini P, Checcaglini F, et al. Radiation therapy in metastatic spinal cord compression. A prospective analysis of 105 consecutive patients. *Cancer*. 1991;67:1311–1317. https://doi.org/10.1002/1097-0142(19910301)67:5<1311::AID-CNCR2820670507>3.0. CO;2-R.
53. Martenson JA, Evans RG, Lie MR, et al. Treatment outcome and complications in patients treated for malignant epidural spinal cord compression (SCC). *J Neuro Oncol*. 1985;3:77–84. https://doi.org/10.1007/BF00165175.
54. O'Phelan KH. Emergency neurologic life support: spinal cord compression. *Neurocrit Care*. 2017;27:144–151. https://doi.org/10.1007/s12028-017-0459-7.
55. Loblaw DA, Mitera G, Ford M, Laperriere NJ. A 2011 updated systematic review and clinical practice guideline for the management of malignant extradural spinal cord compression. *Int J Radiat Oncol Biol Phys*. 2012;84:312–317. https://doi.org/10.1016/j.ijrobp.2012.01.014.
56. Laufer I, Rubin DG, Lis E, et al. The NOMS framework: approach to the treatment of spinal metastatic tumors. *Oncol*. 2013;18:744–751. https://doi.org/10.1634/theoncologist.2012-0293.
57. Patchell et al. Direct decompressive surgical resection in the treatment ofspinal cord compression caused by metastatic cancer: a randomised trial. *Lancet* 2005;366.

Chapter 9

Evaluation of peripheral nerve lesions

K. Ina Ly and Justin T. Jordan

CHAPTER OUTLINE

Disclosures

Dr. Ly has no disclosures.
Dr. Jordan has research funding from the Department of Defense, the National Institutes of Health, and the Burke Foundation. He receives royalties from Elsevier and has received honoraria from the American Academy of Neurology. He performs paid consultation for CereXis Pharmaceuticals, Navio Theragnostics, Health2047 Inc., and the Neurofibromatosis Network.

Introduction

Peripheral nerve lesions encompass a broad differential diagnosis and may be manifestations of an underlying autoimmune, infectious, benign, or malignant neoplastic process. Benign neoplasms include neurofibromas or schwannomas, which frequently arise sporadically but may also occur in the context of tumor predisposition syndromes such as neurofibromatosis type 1 (NF1), neurofibromatosis type 2 (NF2), or schwannomatosis (SWN). These diseases are autosomal dominant genetic syndromes that, among other manifestations, predispose to benign and malignant tumors of the central and peripheral nervous system (also see Chapter 16 for further discussion of approach to NF1, NF2, and SWN). Malignant peripheral nerve sheath tumor is the most common primary malignancy associated with the nerve sheaths and often arises in preexisting plexiform neurofibromas. Other malignant etiologies include direct extension or metastatic disease from various cancers such as lymphoma and leukemia.

In this chapter, we discuss typical presentations of peripheral nerve sheath tumors that arise sporadically and in the context of genetic syndromes. We first provide an overview of NF1, NF2, and SWN, followed by case presentations and a discussion of characteristic imaging features that can be used to guide the evaluation of patients presenting with peripheral nerve sheath lesions.

Neurofibromatosis type 1

NF1 is the most common nerve sheath tumor predisposition syndrome, with an estimated birth incidence of 1:2600 to 1:3000.[1,2] It is caused by a germline mutation in the *NF1* gene on chromosome 17q11.2.[3,4] The hallmark tumor type in NF1 are neurofibromas. In addition, NF1 is characterized by numerous cutaneous manifestations, such as hyperpigmented patches known as café-au-lait macules, abnormal freckling in the axillary, inguinal, and inframammary regions, and cutaneous neurofibromas. Other distinct features include certain ophthalmologic and skeletal abnormalities. In addition to nerve sheath tumors,

NF1 patients carry a higher risk for other tumor types, including gliomas, pheochromocytomas, gastrointestinal stromal tumors (GISTs), and breast cancer. The diagnosis of NF1 is based on the National Institutes of Health clinical criteria[5,6] (Table 9.1), which are highly sensitive and specific in the majority of patients.

Neurofibromatosis type 2

NF2 is an autosomal dominant tumor predisposition syndrome caused by a germline loss-of-function mutation of the

Table 9.1 Clinical diagnostic criteria for neurofibromatosis type 1, neurofibromatosis type 2, and schwannomatosis[a]

Neurofibromatosis type 1[1]	Neurofibromatosis type 2[2]	Schwannomatosis[3]
Presence of ≥2 of the following: 1. ≥6 café-au-lait macules >5 mm in diameter in prepubertal individuals and >15 mm in postpubertal individuals 2. ≥2 neurofibromas of any type or 1 plexiform neurofibroma 3. Freckling in the axillary or inguinal regions 4. ≥2 Lisch nodules 5. Optic glioma 6. A distinctive osseous lesion such as sphenoid wing dysplasia or thinning of long bone cortex, with or without pseudarthrosis 7. First-degree relative (parents, sibling, or offspring) with NF1 based on above criteria	Any 1 of the following: 1. Bilateral vestibular schwannomas (VS) before age 70[4] 2. Unilateral VS before age 70 AND first-degree relative with NF2 3 Any 2 of the following: meningioma, non-vestibular schwannoma, neurofibroma, glioma, cerebral calcification, cataract AND • First-degree relative with NF2 OR • Unilateral VS AND negative LZTR1 testing[b] 4 Multiple meningiomas AND • Unilateral VS OR • Any 2 of the following: non-vestibular schwannoma, neurofibroma, glioma, cerebral calcification, cataract 5. Constitutional or mosaic pathogenic NF2 mutation from blood or by identification of an identical mutation from 2 separate tumors in the same individual	**Definite** Age >30 years and ALL of the following: • ≥2 non-intradermal schwannomas (at least one with histologic confirmation) • Diagnostic criteria for NF2 not fulfilled • No evidence of vestibular tumor on high-quality MRI scan • No first-degree relative with NF2 • No known constitutional NF2 mutation OR Age >30 years AND one pathologically confirmed non-vestibular schwannoma AND a first-degree relative who meets above criteria **Possible** Age <30 years and ALL the following: • ≥2 non-intradermal schwannomas (at least one with histologic confirmation) • Diagnostic criteria for NF2 not fulfilled • No evidence of vestibular tumor on high-quality MRI scan • No first-degree relative with NF2 • No known constitutional NF2 mutation OR Age >45 years and ALL of the following: • ≥2 non-intradermal schwannomas (at least one with histologic confirmation) • No symptoms of 8th cranial nerve dysfunction • No first-degree relative with NF2 • No known constitutional NF2 mutation OR Radiographic evidence of a non-vestibular schwannoma AND first-degree relative meeting criteria for definite schwannomatosis

[a]See also Chapter 16 for clinical review of neurofibromatosis type 1, neurofibromatosis type 2, and schwannomatosis.
[b]If qualifying tumors include ≥2 non-intradermal schwannomas.
[1]From Gutmann DH, et al. The diagnostic evaluation and multidisciplinary management of neurofibromatosis 1 and neurofibromatosis 2. *JAMA*. 1997, 278:51–57; National Institutes of Health Consensus Development Conference Statement: neurofibromatosis. Bethesda, MD, July 13–15, 1987. *Neurofibromatosis*. 1988;1(3):172–178.
[2]From National Institutes of Health Consensus Development Conference (1988). Neurofibromatosis. Consensus Statement. *Arch Neurol*. 1988;45(5): 575–578; Evans DG, et al. A clinical study of type 2 neurofibromatosis. *Q J Med*. 1992;84:603–618; Gutmann DH, et al. The diagnostic evaluation and multidisciplinary management of neurofibromatosis 1 and neurofibromatosis 2. *JAMA*. 1997, 278:51–57; Smith MJ, Bowers NL, Bulman M, et al. Revisiting neurofibromatosis type 2 diagnostic criteria to exclude LZTR1-related schwannomatosis. *Neurology*. 2017;88(1):87–92.
[3]From MacCollin M, Chiocca EA, Evans DG, et al. Diagnostic criteria for schwannomatosis. *Neurology*. 2005;64(11):1838–1845; Baser ME, Friedman JM, Evans DG. Increasing the specificity of diagnostic criteria for schwannomatosis. *Neurology*. 2006;66(5):730–732; Plotkin SR, Blakeley JO, Evans DG, et al. Update from the 2011 International Schwannomatosis Workshop: From genetics to diagnostic criteria. *Am J Med Genet A*. 2013;161A(3):405–416.
[4]Some clinicians will use an age cutoff of 30 years as bilateral vestibular schwannomas will be present by the age of 30 years in the vast majority of people with NF2 (See Chapter 16).

NF2 gene on chromosome 22q11.2. The estimated incidence is 1:25,000 to 1:33,000.[1,7] More than 95% of patients with NF2 have bilateral vestibular schwannomas.[8] These frequently cause bilateral sensorineural hearing loss, tinnitus, and imbalance, and may progress to deafness, brainstem compression, and other cranial nerve deficits.[9] Other tumors frequently seen in NF2 include meningiomas, spinal ependymomas, and schwannomas of the non-vestibular cranial, spinal, and peripheral nerves (Table 9.1). Unlike plexiform neurofibromas in NF1, NF2-associated schwannomas rarely undergo malignant transformation, although it has been reported after radiation.[10–12]

Schwannomatosis

SWN is the least common nerve sheath tumor predisposition syndrome, with an estimated incidence of 1:40,000 to 1:100,000.[8] It is also autosomal dominant in inheritance but the median age of symptom onset is 30 years and diagnosis is often delayed by up to 10 years.[13] To date, two genes—*SMARCB1* and *LZTR1*—have been linked to SWN, although these do not account for all cases and there is ongoing research to identify other associated genes. *SMARCB1* mutations are found in approximately 40–50% of familial and 10% of sporadic cases,[14–18] and *LZTR1* mutations have been reported in 38% of familial and 22% of sporadic cases.[19] There is substantial phenotypic overlap between NF2 and SWN and, unless a *SMARCB1* or *LZTR1* mutation is identified, the diagnosis of SWN is typically made after NF2 has been excluded (Table 9.1). As opposed to NF2, SWN is characterized by multiple *non-vestibular* and non-intradermal schwannomas (although a small proportion of LZTR1-mutant schwannomatosis patients have been reported to have unilateral vestibular schwannomas). Meningiomas are found in approximately 5% of SWN patients,[13] compared to about 50% of NF2 patients.[20] Schwannomas most commonly involve the spinal (74%) and peripheral nerves (89%); cranial nerve schwannomas (8%) and meningiomas (5%) are rare.[13] Patients with SWN may also develop subcutaneous schwannomas.[13,21] Malignant transformation of schwannomas has been reported but is exceedingly rare.[22–24]

Clinical cases

CASE 9.1 SPORADIC SOLITARY PERIPHERAL NERVE SHEATH TUMOR DIAGNOSED AS NEUROFIBROMA

Case. A 27-year-old otherwise healthy woman presented for evaluation of a left neck mass that she discovered when palpating her neck. She did not have any associated pain or neurologic symptoms. Her clinical examination was unremarkable except for the presence of one café-au-lait macule. An MRI of the neck demonstrated a mass involving the left brachial plexus (Fig. 9.1). An initial needle biopsy was non-diagnostic. Subsequent surgical resection revealed a neurofibroma. MRIs of the brain and spine did not show any additional nerve sheath tumors. Genetic testing of blood and tumor tissue was negative for mutations in the NF1, NF2, SMARCB1, or LZTR1 genes. Taken together, this case is consistent with a diagnosis of sporadic neurofibroma.

Teaching Points: Evaluation and Management of Sporadic Solitary Neurofibroma. Up to 90% of neurofibromas are sporadic (i.e., not associated with NF1). Most patients present in their third to fourth decade.[25] Histologically, neurofibromas are composed of Schwann cells, perineural-like cells, fibroblasts, and inflammatory cells such as mast cells and lymphocytes.[26] Morphologically, they can be classified into localized (as seen in this case), diffuse, and plexiform types (Table 9.2).[26] Nearly all plexiform neurofibromas occur in NF1 patients, although rare cases of solitary plexiform neurofibromas in patients without NF1 have been reported.[27] Plexiform neurofibromas also have the potential for transformation into malignant peripheral nerve sheath tumors (MPNSTs). The vast majority of neurofibromas are benign, but a small proportion can display atypical histologic features, including nuclear atypia, loss of neurofibroma architecture, and increased mitotic activity. These tumors, known as "atypical neurofibromatous neoplasm of uncertain biologic potential," may carry an increased risk of malignant transformation.[28]

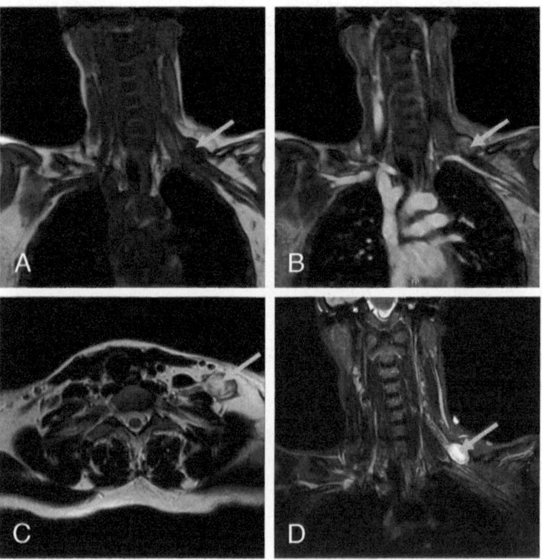

Fig. 9.1 Coronal (A, B, D) and axial (C) MRI of a neurofibroma (arrows) of the left brachial plexus. It is hypointense on T1-weighted pre-contrast sequences (A) and enhances heterogeneously after contrast administration (B). In addition, it is hyperintense on T2-weighted (C) and STIR sequences (D). *STIR*, Short tau inversion recovery.

Table 9.2 Morphologic subtypes of neurofibromas

Localized (intraneural)	Diffuse	Plexiform
• Fusiform expansion of the nerve roots, nerve trunks, nerve plexuses, or peripheral nerves • Focal lesions • Well-circumscribed borders • Located deeper than cutaneous and subcutaneous tissue	• Plaque-like enlargement of a nerve • Typically occur in head and neck region	• Involvement of multiple nerve fascicles or multiple components of nerve plexus • Can undergo malignant transformation into malignant peripheral nerve sheath tumor

Note that these neurofibromas are different from the cutaneous neurofibromas typically seen in NF1 patients.

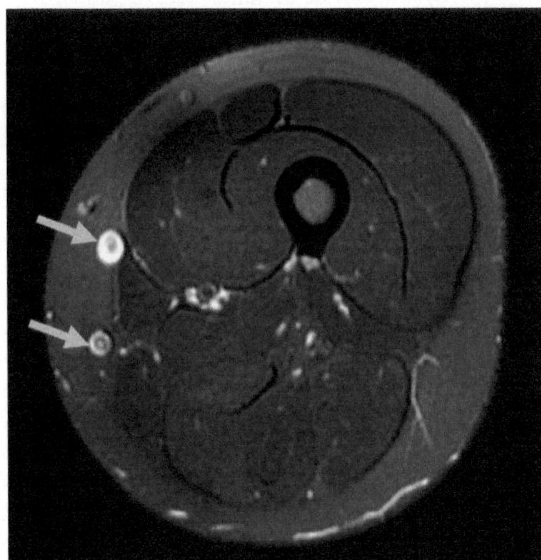

Fig. 9.2 Axial T2-weighted MR image of the left femur in a patient with multiple neurofibromas, demonstrating hyperintense lesions with a central hypointense area *(arrows)*. This "target sign" can be seen in benign neurofibromas and schwannomas.

Imaging characteristics. MRI is the gold standard for imaging of peripheral nerve sheath tumors. On MRI, benign neurofibromas are typically clearly demarcated, un-encapsulated, fusiform or round lesions.[25,29] They are hypo- to isointense (to muscle) on T1-weighted and hyperintense on T2-weighted sequences. Enhancement is variable and can demonstrate a heterogeneous or homogeneous pattern (Fig. 9.1).[25] Short tau inversion recovery (STIR) sequences are particularly helpful to visualize peripheral nerve sheath tumors and display a hyperintense mass (Fig. 9.1D). A characteristic "target sign," defined as a hyperintense rim with a central hypointense region on T2-weighted sequences (Fig. 9.2), is seen with some benign neurofibromas. Histologically, the hyperintense region reflects myxoid tissue with high water content, whereas the hypointense region in the center contains dense collagenous and fibrous tissue.[25,30] Notably, the target sign is not specific to neurofibromas, as it may also be seen with schwannomas.[29] In addition, a "split-fat" sign may be seen on T1-weighted images, which reflects a rim of fat surrounding an intramuscular tumor at the proximal and distal ends.[25,29]

Recommendations for patient management. Evaluation of a patient with an apparently isolated neurofibroma should include a detailed history and neurologic and skin examination, with particular attention to any neurologic dysfunction (e.g., focal weakness or paresthesias) and cutaneous stigmata of NF1 (e.g., café-au-lait macules, skinfold freckling, or cutaneous neurofibromas). Patients should undergo a slit-lamp examination for evaluation of Lisch nodules and MRI of the brain and spine to assess for additional neurofibromas, since the presence of these features supports an underlying NF1 diagnosis. Surgical referral should be considered if the neurofibroma is causing neurologic or functional compromise or if imaging is concerning for a malignant lesion. In the absence of these features, clinical and radiographic monitoring is a reasonable strategy.

Clinical Pearls

1. The vast majority of neurofibromas are sporadic and not associated with NF1.
2. Characteristic MRI features include heterogeneous enhancement on T1-weighted post-contrast and hyperintensity on T2-weighted and STIR sequences. A target and/or split-fat sign may be seen.
3. The main differential diagnosis for a neurofibroma is schwannoma, and these two entities may be difficult to distinguish based on MRI alone.

CASE 9.2 BENIGN PLEXIFORM NEUROFIBROMA IN NEUROFIBROMATOSIS TYPE 1

Case. A 29-year-old woman with NF1 presented to clinic for evaluation, reporting left leg weakness without pain or a growing, palpable tumor. A lumbar spine MRI revealed enhancing, T2- and STIR-hyperintense lesions of the ganglionic and post-ganglionic nerve roots at all lumbar and sacral levels, suggestive of plexiform neurofibromas. The patient also underwent a whole-body MRI (Fig. 9.3), which demonstrated extensive neurofibroma bur-

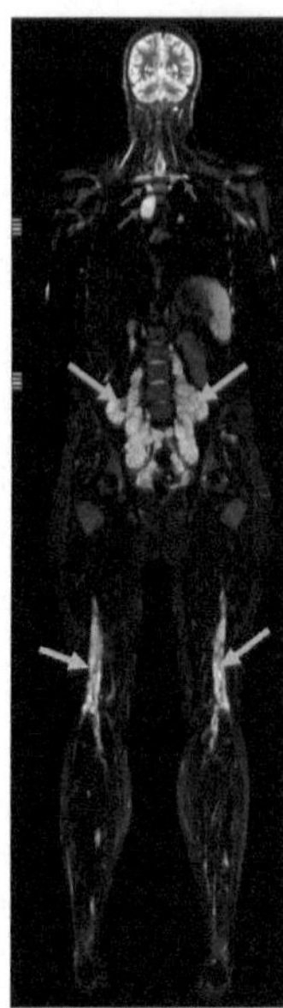

Fig. 9.3 Coronal STIR image from a whole-body MRI scan, demonstrating multiple STIR-hyperintense neurofibromas along the lumbosacral plexus *(blue arrows)* and bilateral sciatic nerves *(yellow arrows)*, giving rise to the appearance of a bunch of grapes or ropes, respectively. In addition, there are neurofibromas arising from the thoracic neuroforamina *(red arrows)*. *STIR*, Short tau inversion recovery.

den involving the spinal, intercostal, and sciatic nerves. She has been monitored clinically and radiographically since, without any changes in her symptoms or tumor appearance.

Teaching Points: Diagnosis and Management of Plexiform Neurofibromas in Patients With NF1. Plexiform neurofibromas (pNFs) are histologically benign tumors of the peripheral nerve sheath that involve multiple nerve fascicles or components of a nerve plexus.[26] They are thought to be congenital lesions[31] and can be superficial or deep. Superficial pNFs diffusely involve the cutaneous tissues and may be associated with skin overgrowth and hyperpigmentation. Deep pNFs are located internally and frequently asymptomatic. They can only be detected with imaging and affect 40–50% of NF1 patients.[21,32,33] Some deep pNFs can grow together as multiple masses, giving them the appearance of a rope or "bag of worms" (Fig. 9.3).[25] pNFs tend to grow slowly if at all over a patient's lifetime but appear to grow most rapidly during childhood and adolescence.[32,34] Despite their benign histology, they can cause significant disfigurement and morbidity due to pain, compression of adjacent anatomical structures, and loss of function of nerves, vessels, and airways.[35] pNFs can transform into MPNSTs, which are associated with high mortality.

Imaging characteristics. Like solitary neurofibromas, pNFs are hypointense on T1-weighted and hyperintense on T2-weighted and STIR sequences. Enhancement is common and a target sign may be seen. Whole-body MRI is used at some centers to assess a patient's baseline internal tumor burden and may gain increasing importance as a tool to monitor tumor response and progression with the emergence of effective therapeutic agents.[36]

Clinical Pearls

1. Plexiform neurofibromas (pNFs) affect 40–50 of patients with NF1.
2. Although histologically benign and typically slow growing, pNFs can cause significant morbidity due to local mass effect and infiltration of vital anatomical structures. A small proportion of pNFs can transform into malignant peripheral nerve sheath tumors.
3. A regional MRI with contrast-enhanced and STIR sequences of the affected region should be obtained. Whole-body MRI may be useful to assess a patient's baseline tumor burden.

CASE 9.3 MALIGNANT PERIPHERAL NERVE SHEATH TUMOR

Case. A 30-year-old man with known NF1 presented to his neuro-oncologist for a routine follow-up visit. At age 13, he was diagnosed with a plexiform neurofibroma that extended from the left buttock to the left calf (Fig. 9.4). He underwent partial resection of the inferior part of the lesion at age 21 and was monitored clinically thereafter. At the current visit, the patient reported a new mass along the left calf which developed 3 months prior and had grown to the size of a golf ball. It was associated with significant new pain, which was only minimally relieved with hydrocodone/acetaminophen. MRI of the leg revealed an 8.5 × 7 cm heterogeneously enhancing soft tissue mass within the lateral gastrocnemius muscle (Fig. 9.5). The patient underwent resection of the mass. Pathology revealed a high-grade MPNST with negative margins. He successfully completed adjuvant radiation therapy and was monitored clinically and radiographically for signs of tumor recurrence. Fourteen months later, a chest CT demonstrated a new 3.9 × 3.7 cm mass in the right lower lobe. Pathology revealed metastatic sarcoma. While being evaluated for adjuvant chemotherapy, a chest CT demonstrated multiple new lung nodules. He received six cycles of adjuvant MAID (mesna, doxorubicin, ifosfamide, and dacarbazine) chemotherapy but developed disease progression and was transitioned to single-agent doxorubicin. Despite this, he continued to decline clinically and passed away from progressive disease 28 months after the initial diagnosis of MPNST.

Teaching Points: Clinical and Imaging Features of Malignant Peripheral Nerve Sheath Tumors. MPNSTs are aggressive soft tissue sarcomas arising from the Schwann cells of peripheral nerves. Fifty percent of MPNSTs are associated with NF1 and 8–16% of NF1 patients develop an MPNST in their lifetime.[37,38] Risk factors for MPNST in individuals with NF1 include a higher number and volume of internal pNFs,[33,39,40] presence of subcutaneous neurofibromas,[33,40] presence of pain,[41] *NF1* gene microdeletion,[42] family/personal history of MPNST,[43] and

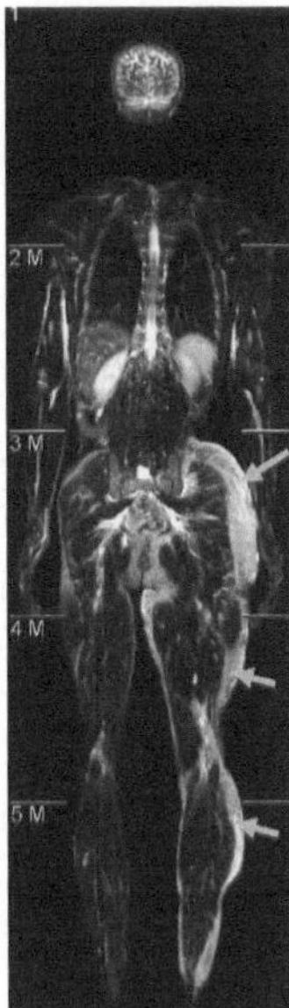

Fig. 9.4 Coronal STIR image from a whole-body MRI scan, demonstrating an extensive plexiform neurofibroma *(arows)* involving the left buttock and lateral aspect of the entire left leg. *STIR*, Short tau inversion recovery.

presence of atypical neurofibromas.[44,45] As in this case, MPNSTs most often develop within a preexisting pNFs,[45,46] although they may also arise *de novo*. The presence of rapid tumor growth, new or worsening pain, or neurologic dysfunction in an NF1 patient should prompt evaluation for MPNST, which should include a contrast-enhanced regional MRI of the involved body area.

Imaging characteristics. MRI signs of malignancy include large tumor size (>5 cm), peripheral enhancement, the presence of a perilesional edema-like zone on T2-weighted images, intratumoral cystic lesions, infiltrative tumor margins, and heterogeneous signal intensity.[47,48] Physiologic MRI techniques such as diffusion-weighted imaging (DWI) and dynamic contrast-enhanced (DCE) imaging (which probes the vascular state of tumors, including vascular permeability) can increase the sensitivity to detect malignancy and are used at some centers.[29] For instance, lower minimum apparent diffusion coefficient (ADC) values (ADC_{min}) on DWI and the presence of early arterial enhancement on DCE imaging have been shown to discriminate between benign neurofibromas and MPNSTs.[48] If the MRI or clinical history is suggestive of an MPNST, a ^{18}F-fluorodeoxyglucose (^{18}F-FDG) PET/CT should also be obtained to confirm the presence of malignancy and identify FDG-avid areas suitable for biopsy. ^{18}F-FDG PET/CT has high sensitivity (89–95%) to detect NF1-associated MPNSTs but lower specificity (72–95%).[29]

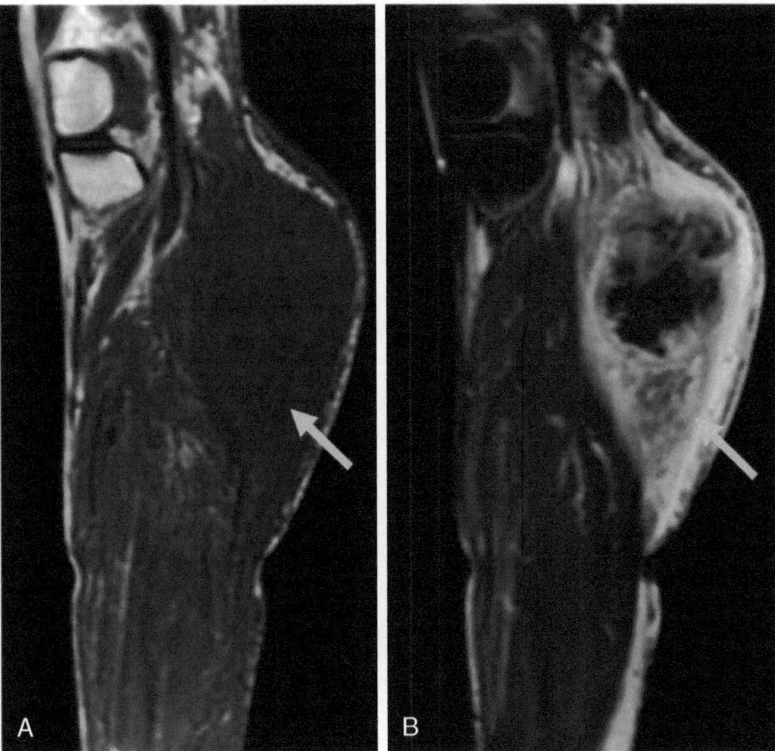

Fig. 9.5 Coronal T1-weighted pre- (A) and post-contrast (B) images of an NF1 patient who developed an MPNST within a preexisting plexiform neurofibroma. The MPNST demonstrates heterogeneous contrast enhancement *(arrows)* and a central area of necrosis after contrast administration (B). *MPNST*, Malignant peripheral nerve sheath tumor; *NF1*, neurofibromatosis type 1.

Recommendations for patient management. Patients with biopsy-confirmed MPNST should be managed by a multidisciplinary team, including a surgeon, radiation oncologist, and medical oncologist. For localized disease, complete resection with wide negative margins is potentially curative, although this may be limited by the degree of tumor infiltration into adjacent nervous and soft tissue structures. Adjuvant radiotherapy is often used to reduce the risk of local recurrence[49,50] and help eliminate the need for limb amputation. Adjuvant chemotherapy is typically provided for advanced and metastatic disease. Even with treatment, however, prognosis is generally poor, with 5-year survival rates ranging from 15% to 50%.[51] Poor prognostic factors include tumor size >5 cm, higher tumor grade, more advanced age, presence of distant metastases at the time of diagnosis, and inability to achieve wide negative tumor margins.[52]

Clinical Pearls

1. Rapid development or changes of symptoms (e.g., tumor growth, pain, or neurologic dysfunction) in a patient with NF1 should prompt evaluation for MPNST.
2. Initial workup should include a contrast-enhanced regional MRI of the affected body region. DWI with ADC mapping may aid in the detection of malignant foci. If the history or MRI is suggestive of malignancy, a ^{18}F-FDG PET/CT should be obtained to identify metabolically active areas suitable for biopsy and histologic confirmation of malignancy.
3. Patients should be referred to a surgeon for an image-guided biopsy and managed by an experienced multidisciplinary team including a surgeon, radiation oncologist, and medical oncologist.
4. Prognosis is poor even with treatment, particularly for patients with advanced or metastatic disease.

CASE 9.4 DIFFUSE LUMBOSACRAL NERVE ROOT THICKENING

Case. A 25-year-old man with relapsing-remitting multiple sclerosis (MS) was referred to the neurofibromatosis clinic for evaluation of an abnormal MRI. The patient had undergone screening procedures for an MS clinical trial, which included a spine MRI. This demonstrated diffuse thickening and enhancement of the lumbar nerve roots without significant nodularity (Fig. 9.6). Clinical examination did not reveal Lisch nodules, typical café-au-lait macules, skinfold freckling, or cutaneous neurofibromas. Electromyography (EMG) and nerve conduction studies (NCS) demonstrated findings consistent with a chronic demyelinating polyneuropathy such as chronic inflammatory demyelinating polyneuropathy (CIDP) or Charcot–Marie–Tooth disease.

Teaching Points: Differential Diagnosis and Management of Patients With Diffuse Lumbosacral Nerve Thickening. Nerve root thickening and enhancement on MRI encompass a broad differential diagnosis (Table 9.3).[53,54] Nerve root thickening in NF1 usually reflects the presence of a neurofibroma, typically displays variable enhancement, and has a more nodular appearance (Fig. 9.7). Nodular nerve roots can also be seen in neurosarcoidosis.[54,55] Nerve root enhancement without significant nerve hypertrophy is frequently observed in leptomeningeal carcinomatosis and neurosyphilis.[54] CIDP and hereditary motor and sensory neuropathies (HSMN, e.g., Charcot-Marie-Tooth disease and Dejerine Sottas disease) may be distinguished on MRI based on the degree of enhancement: it is common in CIDP due to breakdown of the blood–brain barrier and occurs less often in HSMN.[53]

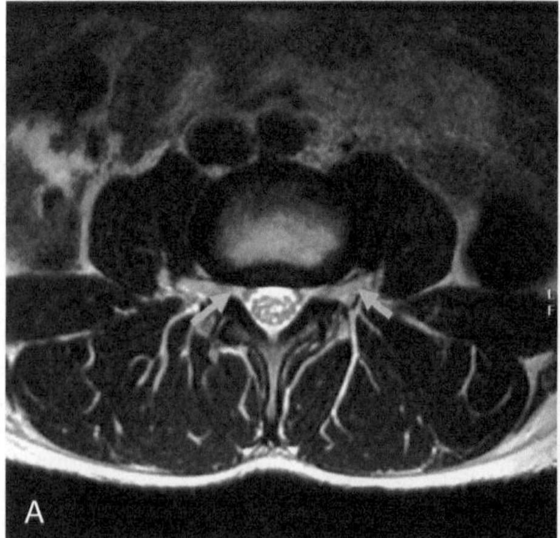

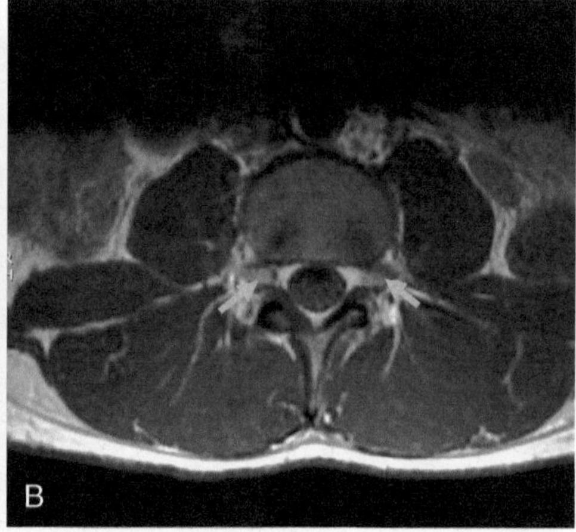

Fig. 9.6 Axial MR images of the lumbar nerve roots from a patient with chronic demyelinating polyneuropathy, demonstrating diffuse thickening of the nerve roots *(arrows)* with concomitant high signal on T2-weighted sequences (A) and contrast enhancement on T1-weighted post-contrast sequences (B).

Recommendations for patient management. The clinical history should particularly focus on the timeline of symptoms (e.g., malignancy typically presents with rapid onset of symptoms, whereas patients with hereditary causes tend to report an insidious onset), family history (given the association of nerve root thickening/enhancement with multiple familial disorders), as well as infectious and constitutional symptoms (given the association with infectious, neoplastic, and autoimmune disorders). Examination should include a thorough dermatologic, neurologic, and musculoskeletal assessment. Workup should be tailored toward each individual depending on the clinical suspicion for a certain disease and, in addition to a whole-spine MRI, may include brain MRI, CT of the chest/abdomen/pelvis (e.g., if systemic malignancy is suspected), EMG/NCS (to characterize the degree and type of neuropathy/radiculopathy), and cerebrospinal fluid analysis (including cytology and flow cytometry).

Table 9.3 Differential diagnosis for nerve root thickening and enhancement on MRI.

Etiology	Example
Inflammatory/ Autoimmune	• Guillain-Barré syndrome • Chronic inflammatory demyelinating polyneuropathy • Sarcoidosis
Hereditary	• Charcot-Marie-Tooth disease • Dejerine-Sottas syndrome
Infectious	• Cytomegalovirus polyradiculomyelopathy • Neurosyphilis
Neoplastic[a]	• Lymphoma • Leukemia • Leptomeningeal disease
Other	• Amyloidosis

[a]Also see Chapter 5 for imaging evaluation and clinical management of leptomeningeal disease and Chapter 23 for clinical management of patients with CNS-involving hematologic malignancies.

Clinical Pearls

1. The etiology of nerve root thickening and enhancement on spine MRI includes inflammatory/autoimmune, hereditary, infectious, and neoplastic causes.
2. The degree of nerve root thickening, presence of significant nodularity, degree of enhancement, and clinical and family history can help narrow down the differential diagnosis.
3. Additional studies should be patient-specific and may include brain MRI, systemic body imaging, EMG/NCS, and cerebrospinal fluid analysis.

CASE 9.5 PERIPHERAL NERVE SCHWANNOMA IN A PATIENT WITH NF2

Case. A 36-year-old woman presented for evaluation of multiple schwannomas. At age 29, a spine MRI was performed after she reported a history of "jolting" electrical back pain. This demonstrated thoracic lesions, which were resected and diagnosed as schwannomas. Her sensory symptoms resolved after surgery but recurred 2 years later. A repeat MRI revealed two new lesions in the lumbar spine, which were again confirmed to be schwannomas after resection. She denied hearing loss, tinnitus, or balance difficulties. There was no family history of

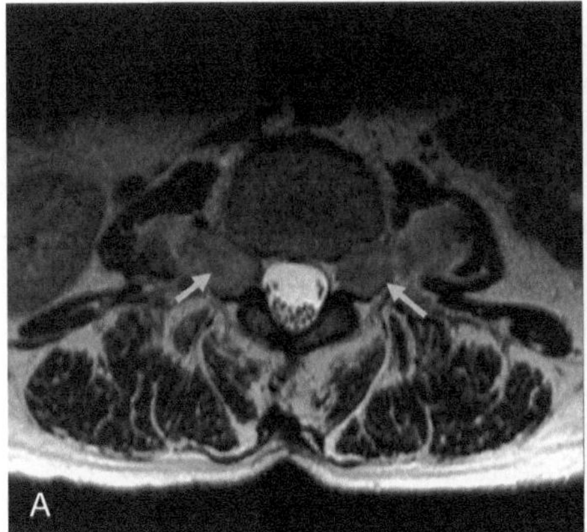

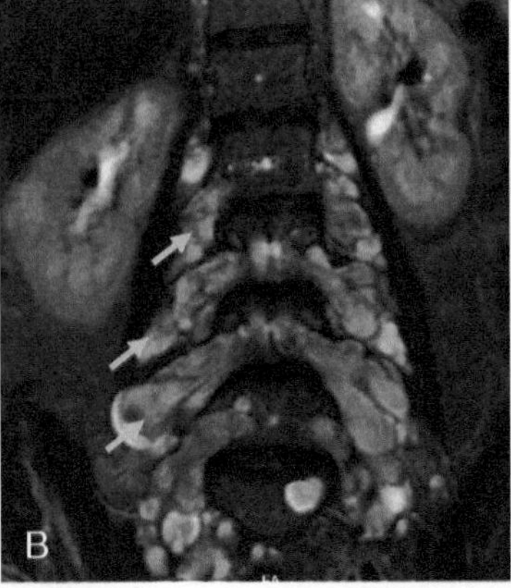

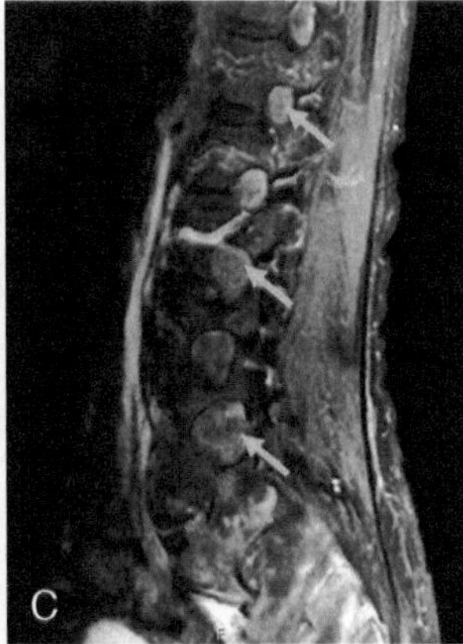

Fig. 9.7 MR images of lumbar neurofibromas on axial T2-weighted (A), coronal STIR (B), and sagittal T1-weighted fat-saturated post-contrast sequences (C) from a patient with NF1. All lumbar levels are involved and the nerve roots appear significantly enlarged and nodular *(arrows)*, which contrasts the non-nodular thickening in the case of chronic demyelinating polyneuropathy (Fig. 9.6). *STIR*, Short tau inversion recovery.

NF2 or SWN. She underwent a brain MRI with thin cuts through the internal auditory canal, which revealed enhancing lesions of the bilateral vestibular nerves, consistent with vestibular schwannomas. Repeat spine MRI demonstrated enhancing extramedullary lesions at the right L1–L2 and L3–L4 levels and an enhancing intramedullary lesion at T4–T5, most suggestive of spinal schwannomas (Fig. 9.8) and an ependymoma (Fig. 9.9), respectively. Based on these imaging findings, the patient fulfilled the diagnostic criteria for NF2 (Table 9.1).

Teaching Points: Evaluation and Management of Peripheral Nerve Schwannomas in Patients With NF2. The majority of schwannomas are solitary and arise sporadically,[25] and the presence of multiple schwannomas should prompt evaluation for a genetic syndrome such as NF2 or SWN (Table 9.1). In fact, bilateral vestibular schwannomas are pathognomonic for NF2 (Table 9.1). Schwannomas are iso- to hypointense (compared to muscle) on T1-weighted images and hyperintense on T2-weighted and STIR sequences, and enhance after contrast administration.[56] Oftentimes, schwannomas cannot be distinguished from neurofibromas based on MRI alone.[25] For instance, fusiform shape and the target sign can be seen in both types of tumors.[25,56] However, heterogeneous signal intensity and contrast enhancement are more commonly seen in schwannomas than neurofibromas due to underlying cystic degeneration.[25,56]

Imaging characteristics. Imaging workup for a patient presenting with a schwannoma should include a high-resolution contrast-enhanced brain MRI with axial and thin cuts (1–3 mm) through the internal auditory meatus to detect small vestibular tumors. A spine MRI with and without contrast should be obtained to evaluate for spinal schwannomas, ependymomas, or meningiomas. Spinal schwannomas arise from the dorsal root and often assume a characteristic dumbbell shape.[57] Ependymomas are expansile, T2-hyperintense, and enhancing intramedullary lesions, whereas spinal meningiomas arise in the extramedullary space. NF2 patients may also develop schwannomas of the peripheral nerves and present with focal neurologic symptoms and pain. If indicated, a regional MRI of the involved body part should be obtained.

Recommendations for patient management. Management of NF2-associated schwannomas is different from their sporadic counterparts and requires a multidisciplinary approach. The goal is to preserve function and maximize quality of life. For vestibular schwannomas, watchful monitoring may be appropriate, given the risk of iatrogenic hearing loss with surgery, in addition to the risk of bilateral hearing loss from tumors alone.[58] Patients with brainstem or spinal cord compression or with obstructive hydrocephalus should be referred for surgery. Monitoring is generally also indicated for non-vestibular cranial and peripheral schwannomas, as they are typically slow growing and rarely symptomatic. Radiation is usually reserved for surgically inaccessible tumors or those that recur after surgery, although the long-term risk of malignant transformation should be considered in younger patients.[10–12,59] Lastly, bevacizumab, an anti-vascular endothelial growth factor antibody, has been shown to improve hearing and produce durable radiographic responses in NF2 patients with progressive vestibular schwannomas.[60]

Clinical Pearls

1. Most schwannomas are solitary and occur sporadically. The presence of multiple schwannomas should prompt evaluation for an underlying genetic syndrome such as NF2 or SWN.
2. A contrast-enhanced MRI of the entire brain and with thin cuts through the internal auditory canals to evaluate for vestibular schwannomas should be obtained. Similarly, a spine MRI with and without contrast is required to assess for the presence of spinal schwannomas, ependymomas, and meningiomas.
3. Non-vestibular schwannomas may be difficult to distinguish from neurofibromas on MRI, but the patient's history and examination can help establish the diagnosis.

CASE 9.6 PERIPHERAL NERVE SCHWANNOMAS IN SCHWANNOMATOSIS

Case. A 38-year-old man presented for evaluation of multiple nerve sheath tumors. At age 22, he developed pain in the left medial thigh, leading to an MRI that revealed a mass in the vastus intermedius. Resection was performed, and pathology demonstrated a schwannoma. At age 24, he developed an aching sensation in the right foot and leg. MRI showed an enhancing mass of the right posterior tibial nerve, again pathologically confirmed to be a schwannoma. A year later, he developed identical symptoms in the left leg and was found to have a schwannoma of the left posterior tibial nerve. A subsequent spine MRI revealed multiple mass lesions of the cervical and thoracic nerve roots (Fig. 9.10). A brain MRI with thin cuts through the internal auditory canal did not reveal any vestibular schwannomas. There was no family history of NF2 or early hearing loss. In addition, physical examination revealed pea-sized, hard, and exquisitely tender subcutaneous masses in the left hip and left chest. He underwent genetic testing which revealed a germline mutation in the *LZTR1* gene, and a definite diagnosis of SWN was made. Over the subsequent years, he underwent multiple surgeries for cervical and thoracic spinal tumors. On whole-body MRI, additional asymptomatic tumors were detected, involving the left anterior chest wall, right thoracic paraspinous region, and left sciatic nerve (Fig. 9.11). Notably, the patient developed chronic pain related to his SWN, which required a complex regimen of opiates and neuropathic pain medications.

Teaching Points: Evaluation and Management of Peripheral Nerve Schwannomas in Schwannomatosis. This patient with SWN developed spinal, peripheral, and subcutaneous schwannomas. As is typical for SWN, there was a long delay between initial symptom onset and the time of diagnosis. Pain is a prominent symptom in SWN patients.

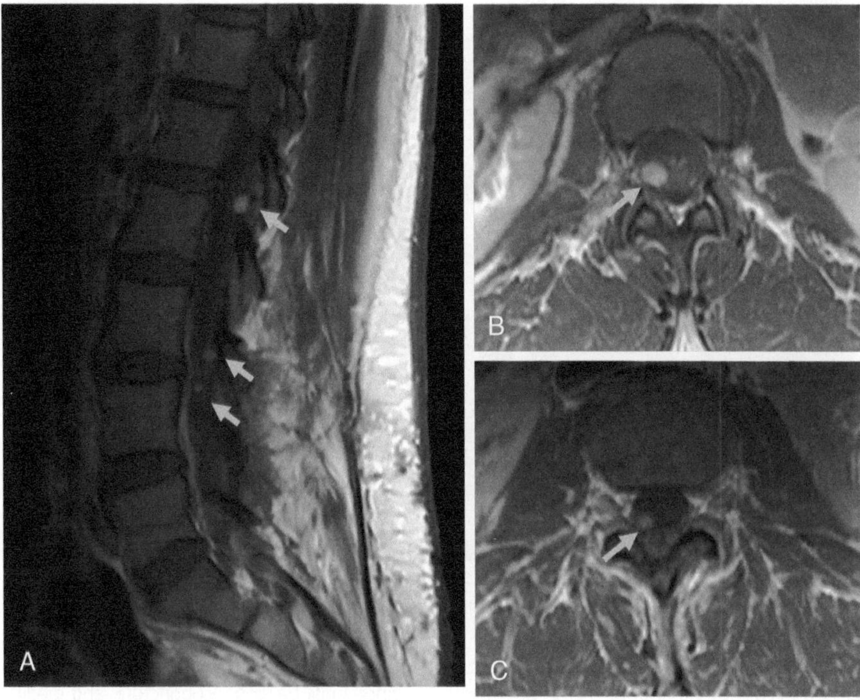

Fig. 9.8 Sagittal (A) and corresponding axial (B, C) T1-weighted post-contrast images of enhancing extramedullary lesions *(arrows)* at the right L1 (A, B) and right L3–L4 (A, C) levels in a patient with NF2, consistent with spinal schwannomas.

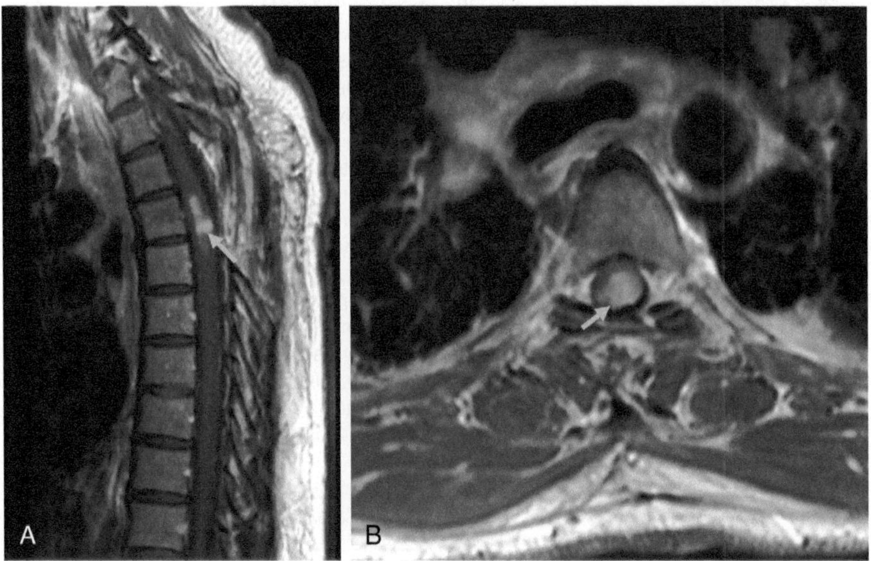

Fig. 9.9 Sagittal (A) and axial (B) T1-weighted post-contrast images of an enhancing intramedullary lesion *(arrows)* centered at the level of T4. In the setting of neurofibromatosis type 2; this most likely represents an ependymoma.

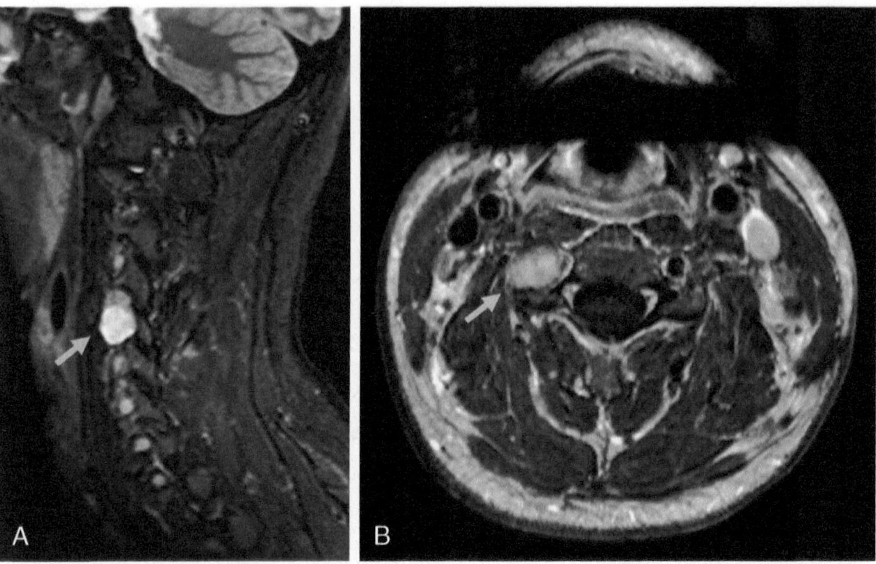

Fig. 9.10 Sagittal T2-weighted (A) and axial post-contrast (B) sequences of a cervical schwannoma (arrows) at the C5–C6 level. The tumor is T2-hyperintense (A) and homogeneously enhancing (B) and displays a dumbbell-like shape.

Up to 68% of SWN patients have chronic pain,[13] and patients with *LZTR1*-associated SWN may experience higher pain levels and worse pain-associated quality of life than those with *SMARCB1*-associated SWN.[61] Patients with suspected SWN should undergo MRI of the entire neuraxis, including a brain MRI with thin cuts through the internal auditory canal to exclude the presence of *bilateral* vestibular schwannomas (which would be diagnostic of NF2). Of note, a small proportion of patients with *LZTR1*-associated SWN may develop *unilateral* vestibular schwannomas,[62,63] and the presence of a unilateral tumor therefore does not rule out a diagnosis of SWN.

Imaging characteristics. A baseline whole-body MRI at the time of diagnosis may be helpful to assess tumor burden, although is not considered standard of care at this time.[64] Similar to solitary schwannomas in non-SWN patients, SWN-associated schwannomas are typically isointense on T1-weighted and heterogeneously hyperintense on STIR sequences and enhance heterogeneously on T1-weighted post-contrast images.[23] Notably, despite their benign histology, schwannomas can be FDG-avid on PET imaging and display SUV values that are typically seen in MPNSTs.[65] Many experts currently recommend routine genetic testing for mutations in the *NF2*, *SMARCB1*, and *LZTR1* genes to differentiate between NF2 and SWN, given the significant phenotypic overlap between these two disorders, particularly between mosaic NF2 (a condition where a somatic mutation in the *NF2* gene occurs later in embryonic development, as opposed to a germline *NF2* mutation) and SWN.

Recommendations for patient management. Pain management is an integral part of patient care in SWN. A combination of pharmacologic agents may be necessary, including neuropathic pain medications such as pregabalin, gabapentin, duloxetine, and tricyclic antidepressants, opioids, and nonsteroidal antiinflammatory drugs. Non-pharmacologic approaches including mindfulness training, acupuncture, and meditation may also be useful. Surgical resection of tumors is usually reserved for patients with medically refractory pain and who have evidence of compression of the spinal cord or other vital organs. However, even with surgery, many patients continue to experience pain.[13,66]

Clinical Pearls

1. Schwannomas in SWN patients most commonly involve the spinal and peripheral nerves.
2. Evaluation of a patient presenting with possible NF2 or SWN should include a brain MRI with thin cuts through the internal auditory canal to evaluate for the presence of bilateral vestibular schwannomas as well as a spine MRI.
3. Benign schwannomas can display FDG avidity on PET/CT and mimic malignancy.
4. Genetic testing for mutations in the *NF2*, *SMARCB1*, and *LZTR1* genes is recommended given the significant phenotypic overlap between NF2 and SWN.
5. Management should focus on pharmacologic and non-pharmacologic treatment of pain and, if medically refractory, surgical resection of symptomatic or compressive tumors. Even with surgery, however, some patients may continue to experience pain.

Conclusion

The etiology of peripheral nerve lesions is broad and, among other causes, includes various neoplastic causes such as neurofibromas and schwannomas. The majority

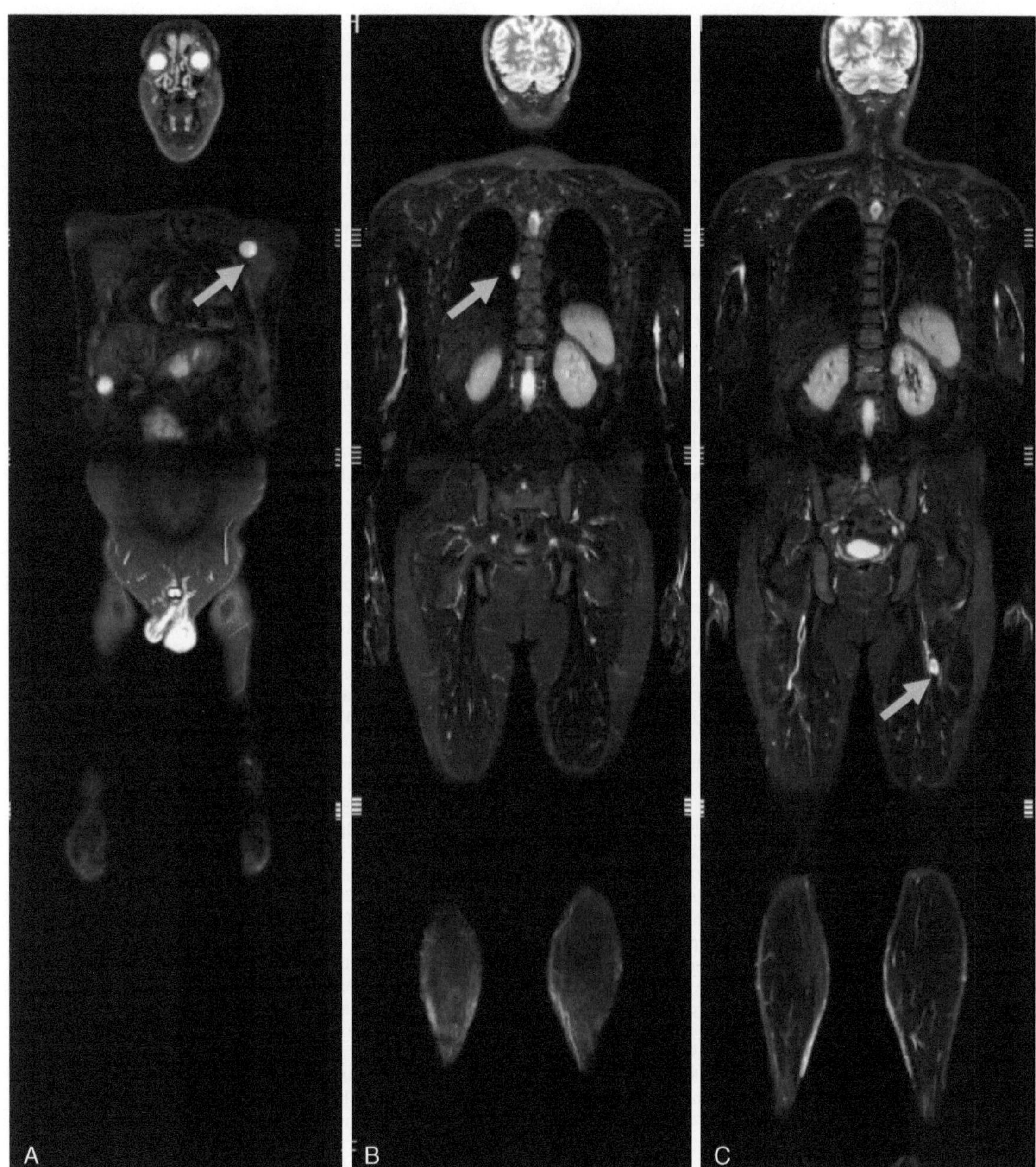

Fig. 9.11 Coronal STIR sequences from a whole-body MRI demonstrate STIR-hyperintense schwannomas *(arrows)* involving the left anterior chest wall (A), left thoracic paraspinous region (B), and left sciatic nerve (C). *STIR*, Short tau inversion recovery.

of neurofibromas and schwannomas occur sporadically, but some arise in the context of NF1, NF2, and SWN. The diagnosis rests upon the patient's clinical history, a detailed physical examination (with particular attention to neurologic, dermatologic, and ophthalmologic features), and MRI of the brain, spine, and other symptomatic body areas. Genetic testing is indicated in some patients.

References

1. Evans DG, Howard E, Giblin C, et al. Birth incidence and prevalence of tumor-prone syndromes: estimates from a UK family genetic register service. *Am J Med Genet A.* 2010;152A(2):327–332.
2. Lammert M, Friedman JM, Kluwe L, Mautner VF. Prevalence of neurofibromatosis 1 in German children at elementary school enrollment. *Arch Dermatol.* 2005;141(1):71–74.
3. Messiaen LM, Callens T, Mortier G, et al. Exhaustive mutation analysis of the NF1 gene allows identification of 95% of mutations and reveals a high frequency of unusual splicing defects. *Hum Mutat.* 2000;15(6):541–555.
4. Skuse GR, Kosciolek BA, Rowley PT. Molecular genetic analysis of tumors in von Recklinghausen neurofibromatosis: loss of heterozygosity for chromosome 17. *Gene Chromosome Canc.* 1989;1(1):36–41.
5. Gutmann DH, Aylsworth A, Carey JC, et al. The diagnostic evaluation and multidisciplinary management of neurofibromatosis 1 and neurofibromatosis 2. *JAMA.* 1997;278(1):51–57.
6. National Institutes of Health consensus development conference statement: neurofibromatosis. Bethesda, Md., USA, July 13–15, 1987. *Neurofibromatosis.* 1988;1(3):172–178.
7. Evans DG, Moran A, King A, Saeed S, Gurusinghe N, Ramsden R. Incidence of vestibular schwannoma and neurofibromatosis 2 in the North West of England over a 10-year period: higher incidence than previously thought. *Otol Neurotol.* 2005;26(1):93–97.
8. Plotkin SR, Wick A. Neurofibromatosis and Schwannomatosis. *Semin Neurol.* 2018;38(1):73–85.
9. Blakeley JO, Plotkin SR. Therapeutic advances for the tumors associated with neurofibromatosis type 1, type 2, and schwannomatosis. *Neuro Oncol.* 2016;18(5):624–638.
10. Baser ME, Evans DG, Jackler RK, Sujansky E, Rubenstein A. Neurofibromatosis 2, radiosurgery and malignant nervous system tumours. *Br J Cancer.* 2000;82(4):998.
11. Balasubramaniam A, Shannon P, Hodaie M, Laperriere N, Michaels H, Guha A. Glioblastoma multiforme after stereotactic radiotherapy for acoustic neuroma: case report and review of the literature. *Neuro Oncol.* 2007;9(4):447–453.
12. Thomsen J, Mirz F, Wetke R, Astrup J, Bojsen-Møller M, Nielsen E. Intracranial sarcoma in a patient with neurofibromatosis type 2 treated with gamma knife radiosurgery for vestibular schwannoma. *Am J Otol.* 2000;21(3):364–370.
13. Merker VL, Esparza S, Smith MJ, Stemmer-Rachamimov A, Plotkin SR. Clinical features of schwannomatosis: a retrospective analysis of 87 patients. *Oncologist.* 2012;17(10):1317–1322.
14. Smith MJ, Wallace AJ, Bowers NL, et al. Frequency of SMARCB1 mutations in familial and sporadic schwannomatosis. *Neurogenetics.* 2012;13(2):141–145.
15. Sestini R, Bacci C, Provenzano A, Genuardi M, Papi L. Evidence of a four-hit mechanism involving SMARCB1 and NF2 in schwannomatosis-associated schwannomas. *Hum Mutat.* 2008;29(2):227–231.
16. Rousseau G, Noguchi T, Bourdon V, Sobol H, Olschwang S. SMARCB1/INI1 germline mutations contribute to 10% of sporadic schwannomatosis. *BMC Neurol.* 2011;11:9.
17. Hadfield KD, Newman WG, Bowers NL, et al. Molecular characterisation of SMARCB1 and NF2 in familial and sporadic schwannomatosis. *J Med Genet.* 2008;45(6):332–339.
18. Boyd C, Smith MJ, Kluwe L, Balogh A, Maccollin M, Plotkin SR. Alterations in the SMARCB1 (INI1) tumor suppressor gene in familial schwannomatosis. *Clin Genet.* 2008;74(4):358–366.
19. Smith MJ, Isidor B, Beetz C, et al. Mutations in LZTR1 add to the complex heterogeneity of schwannomatosis. *Neurology.* 2015;84(2):141–147.
20. Evans DG, Huson SM, Donnai D, et al. A clinical study of type 2 neurofibromatosis. *Q J Med.* 1992;84(304):603–618.
21. Plotkin SR, Bredella MA, Cai W, et al. Quantitative assessment of whole-body tumor burden in adult patients with neurofibromatosis. *PLoS One.* 2012;7(4):e35711.
22. Carter JM, O'Hara C, Dundas G, et al. Epithelioid malignant peripheral nerve sheath tumor arising in a schwannoma, in a patient with "neuroblastoma-like" schwannomatosis and a novel germline SMARCB1 mutation. *Am J Surg Pathol.* 2012;36(1):154–160.
23. Ahlawat S, Baig A, Blakeley JO, Jacobs MA, Fayad LM. Multiparametric whole-body anatomic, functional, and metabolic imaging characteristics of peripheral lesions in patients with schwannomatosis. *J Magn Reson Imaging.* 2016;44(4):794–803.
24. Gonzalvo A, Fowler A, Cook RJ, et al. Schwannomatosis, sporadic schwannomatosis, and familial schwannomatosis: a surgical series with long-term follow-up. Clinical article. *J Neurosurg.* 2011;114(3):756–762.
25. Pilavaki M, Chourmouzi D, Kiziridou A, Skordalaki A, Zarampoukas T, Drevelengas A. Imaging of peripheral nerve sheath tumors with pathologic correlation: pictorial review. *Eur J Radiol.* 2004;52(3):229–239.
26. Rodriguez FJ, Folpe AL, Giannini C, Perry A. Pathology of peripheral nerve sheath tumors: diagnostic overview and update on selected diagnostic problems. *Acta Neuropathol.* 2012;123(3):295–319.
27. Lin V, Daniel S, Forte V. Is a plexiform neurofibroma pathognomonic of neurofibromatosis type I? *Laryngoscope.* 2004;114(8):1410–1414.
28. Miettinen MM, Antonescu CR, Fletcher CDM, et al. Histopathologic evaluation of atypical neurofibromatous tumors and their transformation into malignant peripheral nerve sheath tumor in patients with neurofibromatosis 1–a consensus overview. *Hum Pathol.* 2017;67:1–10.
29. Ahlawat S, Blakeley JO, Langmead S, Belzberg AJ, Fayad LM. Current status and recommendations for imaging in neurofibromatosis type 1, neurofibromatosis type 2, and schwannomatosis. *Skeletal Radiol.* 2019;49:199–219.
30. Bhargava R, Parham DM, Lasater OE, Chari RS, Chen G, Fletcher BD. MR imaging differentiation of benign and malignant peripheral nerve sheath tumors: use of the target sign. *Pediatr Radiol.* 1997;27(2):124–129.
31. Waggoner DJ, Towbin J, Gottesman G, Gutmann DH. Clinic-based study of plexiform neurofibromas in neurofibromatosis 1. *Am J Med Genet.* 2000;92(2):132–135.
32. Nguyen R, Dombi E, Widemann BC, et al. Growth dynamics of plexiform neurofibromas: a retrospective cohort study of

201 patients with neurofibromatosis 1. *Orphanet J Rare Dis.* 2012;7:75.

33. Mautner VF, Asuagbor FA, Dombi E, et al. Assessment of benign tumor burden by whole-body MRI in patients with neurofibromatosis 1. *Neuro Oncol.* 2008;10(4):593–598.
34. Dombi E, Solomon J, Gillespie AJ, et al. NF1 plexiform neurofibroma growth rate by volumetric MRI: relationship to age and body weight. *Neurology.* 2007;68(9):643–647.
35. Mautner VF, Hartmann M, Kluwe L, Friedrich RE, Fünsterer C. MRI growth patterns of plexiform neurofibromas in patients with neurofibromatosis type 1. *Neuroradiology.* 2006;48(3):160–165.
36. Dombi E, Baldwin A, Marcus LJ, et al. Activity of selumetinib in neurofibromatosis type 1-related plexiform neurofibromas. *N Engl J Med.* 2016;375(26):2550–2560.
37. Evans DG, Baser ME, McGaughran J, Sharif S, Howard E, Moran A. Malignant peripheral nerve sheath tumours in neurofibromatosis 1. *J Med Genet.* 2002;39(5):311–314.
38. Uusitalo E, Rantanen M, Kallionpää RA, et al. Distinctive cancer associations in patients with neurofibromatosis type 1. *J Clin Oncol.* 2016;34(17):1978–1986.
39. Nguyen R, Jett K, Harris GJ, Cai W, Friedman JM, Mautner VF. Benign whole body tumor volume is a risk factor for malignant peripheral nerve sheath tumors in neurofibromatosis type 1. *J Neurooncol.* 2014;116(2):307–313.
40. Tucker T, Wolkenstein P, Revuz J, Zeller J, Friedman JM. Association between benign and malignant peripheral nerve sheath tumors in NF1. *Neurology.* 2005;65(2):205–211.
41. King AA, Debaun MR, Riccardi VM, Gutmann DH. Malignant peripheral nerve sheath tumors in neurofibromatosis 1. *Am J Med Genet.* 2000;93(5):388–392.
42. De Raedt T, Brems H, Wolkenstein P, et al. Elevated risk for MPNST in NF1 microdeletion patients. *Am J Hum Genet.* 2003;72(5):1288–1292.
43. Malbari F, Spira M, Knight P B, et al. Malignant peripheral nerve sheath tumors in neurofibromatosis: impact of family history. *J Pediatr Hematol Oncol.* 2018;40(6):e359–e363.
44. Reilly KM, Kim A, Blakely J, et al. Neurofibromatosis type 1-associated MPNST state of the science: outlining a research agenda for the future. *J Natl Cancer Inst.* 2017;109(8).
45. Beert E, Brems H, Daniëls B, et al. Atypical neurofibromas in neurofibromatosis type 1 are premalignant tumors. *Gene Chromosome Canc.* 2011;50(12):1021–1032.
46. Woodruff JM. Pathology of tumors of the peripheral nerve sheath in type 1 neurofibromatosis. *Am J Med Genet.* 1999;89(1):23–30.
47. Wasa J, Nishida Y, Tsukushi S, et al. MRI features in the differentiation of malignant peripheral nerve sheath tumors and neurofibromas. *AJR Am J Roentgenol.* 2010;194(6):1568–1574.
48. Demehri S, Belzberg A, Blakeley J, Fayad LM. Conventional and functional MR imaging of peripheral nerve sheath tumors: initial experience. *AJNR Am J Neuroradiol.* 2014;35(8):1615–1620.
49. Wong WW, Hirose T, Scheithauer BW, Schild SE, Gunderson LL. Malignant peripheral nerve sheath tumor: analysis of treatment outcome. *Int J Radiat Oncol Biol Phys.* 1998;42(2):351–360.
50. Carli M, Ferrari A, Mattke A, et al. Pediatric malignant peripheral nerve sheath tumor: the Italian and German soft tissue sarcoma cooperative group. *J Clin Oncol.* 2005;23(33):8422–8430.
51. Farid M, Demicco EG, Garcia R, et al. Malignant peripheral nerve sheath tumors. *Oncologist.* 2014;19(2):193–201.
52. Dunn GP, Spiliopoulos K, Plotkin SR, et al. Role of resection of malignant peripheral nerve sheath tumors in patients with neurofibromatosis type 1. *J Neurosurg.* 2013;118(1):142–148.
53. Kale HA, Sklar E. Magnetic resonance imaging findings in chronic inflammatory demyelinating polyneuropathy with intracranial findings and enhancing, thickened cranial and spinal nerves. *Australas Radiol.* 2007;51. Spec No.:B21–24.
54. Aho TR, Wallace RC, Pitt AM, Sivakumar K. Charcot-Marie-Tooth disease: extensive cranial nerve involvement on CT and MR imaging. *AJNR Am J Neuroradiol.* 2004;25(3):494–497.
55. Ginat DT, Dhillon G, Almast J. Magnetic resonance imaging of neurosarcoidosis. *J Clin Imaging Sci.* 2011;1:15.
56. Crist J, Hodge JR, Frick M, et al. Magnetic resonance imaging appearance of Schwannomas from head to toe: a pictorial review. *J Clin Imaging Sci.* 2017;7:38.
57. Abul-Kasim K, Thurnher MM, McKeever P, Sundgren PC. Intradural spinal tumors: current classification and MRI features. *Neuroradiology.* 2008;50(4):301–314.
58. Liu R, Fagan P. Facial nerve schwannoma: surgical excision versus conservative management. *Ann Otol Rhinol Laryngol.* 2001;110(11):1025–1029.
59. Evans DG, Birch JM, Ramsden RT, Sharif S, Baser ME. Malignant transformation and new primary tumours after therapeutic radiation for benign disease: substantial risks in certain tumour prone syndromes. *J Med Genet.* 2006;43(4):289–294.
60. Plotkin SR, Merker VL, Halpin C, et al. Bevacizumab for progressive vestibular schwannoma in neurofibromatosis type 2: a retrospective review of 31 patients. *Otol Neurotol.* 2012;33(6):1046–1052.
61. Jordan JT, Smith MJ, Walker JA, et al. Pain correlates with germline mutation in schwannomatosis. *Medicine (Baltimore).* 2018;97(5):e9717.
62. Smith MJ, Bowers NL, Bulman M, et al. Revisiting neurofibromatosis type 2 diagnostic criteria to exclude LZTR1-related schwannomatosis. *Neurology.* 2017;88(1):87–92.
63. Pathmanaban ON, Sadler KV, Kamaly-Asl ID, et al. Association of genetic predisposition with solitary schwannoma or meningioma in children and young adults. *JAMA Neurol.* 2017;74(9):1123–1129.
64. Evans DGR, Salvador H, Chang VY, et al. Cancer and central nervous system tumor surveillance in pediatric neurofibromatosis 2 and related disorders. *Clin Cancer Res.* 2017;23(12):e54–e61.
65. Lieber B, Han B, Allen J, et al. Utility of positron emission tomography in schwannomatosis. *J Clin Neurosci.* 2016;30:138–140.
66. Li P, Zhao F, Zhang J, et al. Clinical features of spinal schwannomas in 65 patients with schwannomatosis compared with 831 with solitary schwannomas and 102 with neurofibromatosis type 2: a retrospective study at a single institution. *J Neurosurg Spine.* 2016;24(1):145–154.

Chapter | 10 |

Approach to the meningioma patient

Jennifer L. Franke, Christina Jackson and Michael Lim

CHAPTER OUTLINE

Introduction

Meningiomas are slow-growing extraaxial tumors that account for about 25% of all intracranial tumors. The World Health Organization (WHO) classifies meningiomas as grade I, II, or III based upon morphologic criteria with higher grades correlating with more aggressive behavior such as local invasion, recurrence, and shortened survival. The main options for the management of meningiomas include surgery, radiation, and observation. The management of these patients varies depending on a combination of clinical factors including the patient's clinical symptoms, radiographic characteristic of the tumor, grade of the tumor, and extent of prior resections. Grade I meningiomas in asymptomatic patients can typically be managed conservatively with clinical observation and serial imaging. For symptomatic patients or patients with more aggressive tumors, surgical resection with potential adjuvant radiation are favored depending on the grade and extent of resection. Unfortunately, medical therapy for recurrent meningiomas is lacking, although several clinical trials are underway to assess the efficacy of various adjuvant therapies.

The goal of this chapter is to help guide clinicians in providing the best clinical care for patients with meningiomas. Case-based presentations are used to discuss the management approaches to patients presenting with different clinical symptoms and grades of meningiomas. Although general guidelines to the management of these patients are proposed, the decision for treatment should be made on an individualized basis carefully weighing the risks and benefits of each treatment option.

Epidemiology

Meningiomas are extraaxial brain tumors that typically present as slowly growing dural-based masses, most of which (98.2%) are nonmalignant.[1] They are the most common of all primary central nervous system tumors (37.1%) with an incidence rate of 8.33 per 100,000 people.[1] There were 145,916 new cases diagnosed between 2011 and 2015, and 31,990 new cases are projected for 2019 according to the

Central Brain Tumor Registry in the United States.[1] The incidence of meningiomas increases significantly with age, as they occur most frequently in adults over the age of 65 and are rare in children ages 0–14. The median age of diagnosis is 66 years. Women are twice as likely to develop meningiomas as men, and thus an etiologic role for hormones in the development of meningiomas has been hypothesized.[1]

The etiology for the majority of meningiomas is unknown. These tumors are often benign, slow-growing, and solitary.[2] However, several potential risk factors have been shown to be associated with the development of meningiomas, including prior exposure to ionizing radiation and particular genetic conditions. Radiation-induced meningiomas are the most common brain neoplasm resulting from ionizing radiation.[3] These meningiomas are clinically and biologically more aggressive than sporadic meningiomas; they have more frequent mitoses, are often atypical and multifocal, and have higher recurrence rates.[4,5] In many cases, there can be a latency period of more than 20 years between radiation exposure and meningioma occurance.[6] In terms of genetic predispositions, 50 to 70% of individuals with neurofibromatosis type 2 (NF2), an autosomal dominant disorder characterized by mutations in the *NF2* gene, develop one or more meningiomas (see Chapter 16 for further discussion of NF2).[7] This gene is a tumor suppressor gene on chromosome 22 that encodes for the protein merlin, which regulates meningioma cell proliferation and tumor formation.[7] Meningiomas arising from this condition are phenotypically more aggressive and develop earlier in life than their sporadic counterparts.[8] The other broad class of genetically-driven meningiomas consists of those with mutations in other genes such as *Smoothened (SMO)*, *TRAF7*, *AKT1*, and *PI3KA*.[9] No genetic alterations are detected in 20% of meningiomas. In these meningiomas, epigenomic mutations may play a crucial role in tumor formation.[7]

Meningiomas arise from neoplastic arachnoid cap cells in the meningeal coverings of the brain and spinal cord. They can arise anywhere along the dura and are commonly found in the parasagittal and convexity regions. They may also arise in the skull base or at sites of dural reflection, including the falx cerebri, tentorium cerebelli, and venous sinuses. Meningiomas arising from the cerebral meninges account for 79.8%, and 4.2% arise from the spinal meninges.[1] Spinal meningiomas are most often found in the thoracic spine, followed by the cervical spine and the craniocervical junction. They may also arise in the optic nerve sheath and choroid plexus, but these locations are less common.[10]

Clinical presentation

Many meningiomas are asymptomatic and are discovered incidentally during neuroimaging for unrelated symptoms or at autopsy. One study showed that meningiomas are found in about 1% of brain magnetic resonance imaging (MRI) scans of the general adult population (ages 45 to 97).[11] Many meningiomas remain the same size or grow very slowly over a long period of time without the patient noticing symptoms.[12] These incidentally discovered tumors are usually treated conservatively with observation rather than surgical intervention. However, meningiomas may become symptomatic due to compression of nearby brain structures, blockage of cerebrospinal fluid (CSF) flow and venous sinuses, or even invasion into brain tissue. About 30% of patients with intracranial meningiomas present with seizures, but the pathogenesis of this is poorly understood.[13]

Symptomatic focal deficits are linked to the tumor location. As the tumors grow at a slow rate, symptom onset is typically gradual, and patients often do not notice these changes immediately. Patients may experience visual changes with tumors disrupting the optic pathway. Cerebellopontine angle meningiomas can lead to cranial nerve deficits including hearing loss and facial pain. Olfactory groove or sphenoid ridge meningiomas can compress the olfactory tract and interfere with smell. Large subfrontal meningiomas can cause behavioral changes such as inattention and apathy. Meningiomas in proximity to the motor strip can lead to focal weakness. In addition to symptoms caused by direct compression of adjacent neural structures, meningiomas can also cause symptoms related to increased intracranial pressure or obstruction of the ventricular system leading to obstructive hydrocephalus. These patients can present with headaches, gait difficulties, and even mental status deterioration.[10]

Classification

Meningiomas are usually lobular, well-circumscribed masses. Tumors that grow diffusely over the dura are referred to as meningioma *en plaque*. Although they often appear similar on imaging and macroscopically, meningiomas can exhibit heterogeneity on histopathology. The WHO classifies meningiomas into three groups based upon morphologic criteria (see Chapter 1, Case 1.5 for further discussion of histologic classification of meningioma).[14] These classifications have been shown to correlate with clinical outcomes. Most meningiomas are WHO grade I and carry an excellent prognosis, whereas rarer WHO grade II and III meningiomas are more likely to be invasive, recur locally following treatment, and have shorten overall survival. Due to these factors, treatment planning favors more aggressive approaches with increasing WHO grade.[15] The characteristics of each grade of meningioma are summarized below.

- WHO grade I: Account for 80.6% of meningiomas.[1] They are benign and subdivided into nine subtypes, including meningothelial, fibrous (fibroblastic),

transitional (mixed), psammomatous, angiomatous, microcystic, lymphoplasmacyte-rich, metaplastic, and secretory. Their histology includes occasional mitotic figures. The rate of recurrence is 7–25%.[16]
- WHO grade II: Account for 17.6% of meningiomas.[1] They include atypical, clear-cell, and choroid meningiomas. In contrast to grade I meningiomas, grade II tumors have histologic features including more mitotic activity (4 or more mitoses per 10 high-powered fields), brain invasion, or three or more of the following: prominent nucleoli, increased cellularity, small cells with high nuclear-to-cytoplasmic ratio, sheet-like growth, and localized spontaneous necrosis. The rate of recurrence is 29–59%.[16]
- WHO grade III: Account for 1.7% of meningiomas.[1] These tumors are malignant and include papillary, anaplastic, and rhabdoid meningiomas. Histologic features of these meningiomas include significantly increased mitotic activity (20 or more mitoses per 10 high-powered fields), loss of typical growth patterns, infiltration of the brain, atypical mitoses, and multifocal spontaneous necrosis. The rate of recurrence is very high at 60–94%.[16]

Nonmalignant meningiomas have a 5-year survival rate of 86.7% and a 10-year survival rate of 81.5% for all ages, and malignant meningiomas have a 5-year survival rate of 63.8% and a 10-year survival rate of 56.1% for all ages.[1]

Due to their slow growth rate and a majority of tumors being asymptomatic, incidental meningiomas can be managed conservatively with observation and serial imaging. For most cases of symptomatic meningioma, surgical resection is the preferred treatment. The 5-tier Simpson scale grades the extent of surgical resection and strongly correlates with risk of meningioma recurrence (Table 10.1).[17] The dural tail is the site of thickening and enhancement of the dura is seen adjacent to meningiomas. Whereas evidence on whether the dural tail harbors neoplastic cells continues to be controversial, with some studies suggesting that it is an imaging correlate of dilated meningeal vessels,[18] many still advocate for the removal of the dural tail during surgery, as it has been shown to affect the timing of tumor recurrence.[19–21] Bone involvement is common and can lead to hyperostosis and osteolysis. Hyperostosis occurs in 20% of cases and varies in appearance unrelated to tumor size.[15] It is often associated with bony invasion of tumor but may also represent a reactive phenomenon. The presence of strong, homogeneous enhancement within hyperostotic bone suggests tumor infiltration.[15] Malignant meningiomas typically invade the brain and can cause osteolysis of the adjacent calvarium with extension into the scalp.[15,22] This osteolytic activity results in sequestration of the tumor within bone.[23] Additionally, primary intraosseous meningiomas that cause osteolysis are more likely to behave in a malignant manner and have anaplastic or malignant hisopathology.[24,25]

Imaging characteristics

(Also see Chapter 5 for approach to the imaging of dural-based lesions.) MRI is currently the main diagnostic method of choice in the evaluation of meningiomas. Meningiomas typically appear as an isointense to slightly hypointense unilobular mass relative to grey matter with associated displacement of cortical grey matter on T1-weighted sequences pre-contrast. On post-contrast imaging, meningiomas demonstrate strong homogenous enhancement often seen with a dural tail, a peripheral dural thickening adjacent to the tumor. Areas of necrosis or calcifications within the tumor do not enhance and will give the tumor a patchy, heterogeneous appearance.[26] On T2-weighted images, meningiomas can demonstrate more heterogeneous intensity which may be indicative of particular tumor characteristics. Hyperintensity on T2-weighted images suggests softer tumor texture, whereas hypointensity suggests firmer texture or even calcification.[26,27] Hyperintense tumors are often accompanied by increased likelihood and

Table 10.1 Simpson scale of surgical meningioma removal and risk of tumor recurrence

	Extent of resection	Recurrence risk (10-year interval)
Grade I	Macroscopically complete removal of tumor, involved bones, venous sinuses, and dural tail.	9%
Grade II	Macroscopically complete removal of tumor, coagulation of dural tail.	19%
Grade III	Macroscopically complete removal of tumor, no resection of dural tail.	29%
Grade IV	Partial tumor removal, no resection of dural tail.	44%
Grade V	Simple decompression, no resection of dural tail.	100%

(Modified from Hortobágyi et al. Meningioma recurrence. *Open Med.* 2016;11(1):168–173.)

severity of brain edema. This is thought to be due to the elevated water content of these tumors that allows water diffusion into surrounding brain.[28] T2-weighted MRI can also provide an indication to the extent of brain invasion. Extraaxial tumors can exhibit a crescent-shaped cleft of CSF between the mass and brain, although this cleft can be absent in the setting when higher-grade meningiomas invade the brain.[29] An ambiguous brain-tumor border on T2-weighted MRI has been shown to be correlated with a greater degree of tumor proliferation.[30] Magnetic resonance venography (MRV) and magnetic resonance angiogram (MRA) are useful in determining a tumor's relation to surrounding vasculature. MRV can be used to evaluate the presence of local venous sinus invasion, interrupted blood flow, and the presence of collateral venous drainage. MRA and digital subtraction angiograph (DSA) can aid in identifying the arterial branches supplying the tumor and the extent of tumor vascularization. As meningiomas arise from the dura, arterial blood supply of the tumor is typically from the dural arteries that supply the dura adjacent to the tumor. In the setting of significant tumor vascularization, preoperative embolization of vessels supplying the tumor can significantly reduce blood loss during surgery. Meningiomas may grow near or even be in contact with eloquent regions of the brain, so surgical management of meningioma patients must balance extent of resection with preservation of eloquent function. Functional MRI (fMRI) can be used alongside intraoperative cortical mapping to inform the optimal degree of tumor resection for clinical outcome.[31]

CT images are often less useful in the evaluation of tumor characteristics and relationship to surrounding

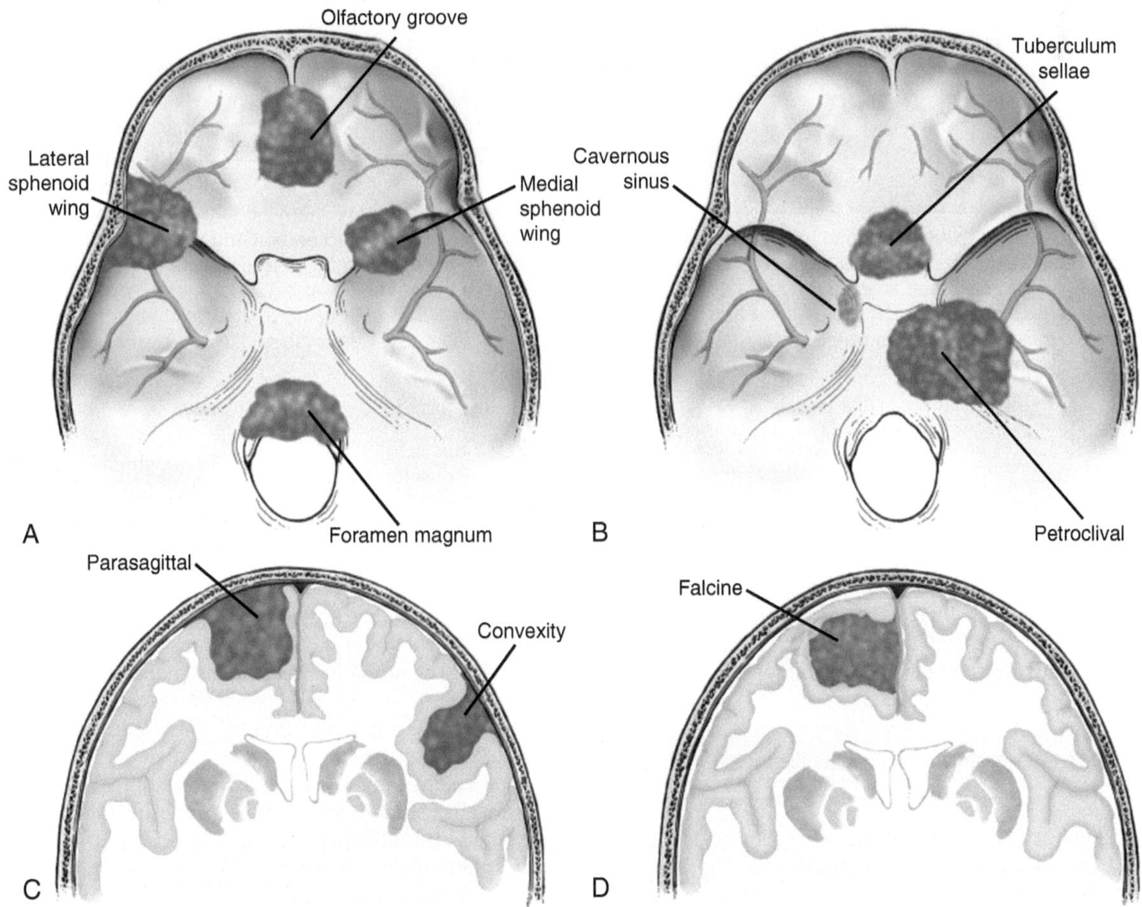

Fig. 10.1 Locations of intracranial meningiomas with relation to neighboring skull (A,B) and dural reflections and brain (C,D). (Reprinted from Perry A. Meningiomas. In: Perry A, Brat D, eds. *Practical Surgical Neuropathology: A Diagnostic Approach.* 2nd ed. Philadelphia, PA: Elsevier; 2018:259-298. Copyright 2018, with permission from Elsevier.)

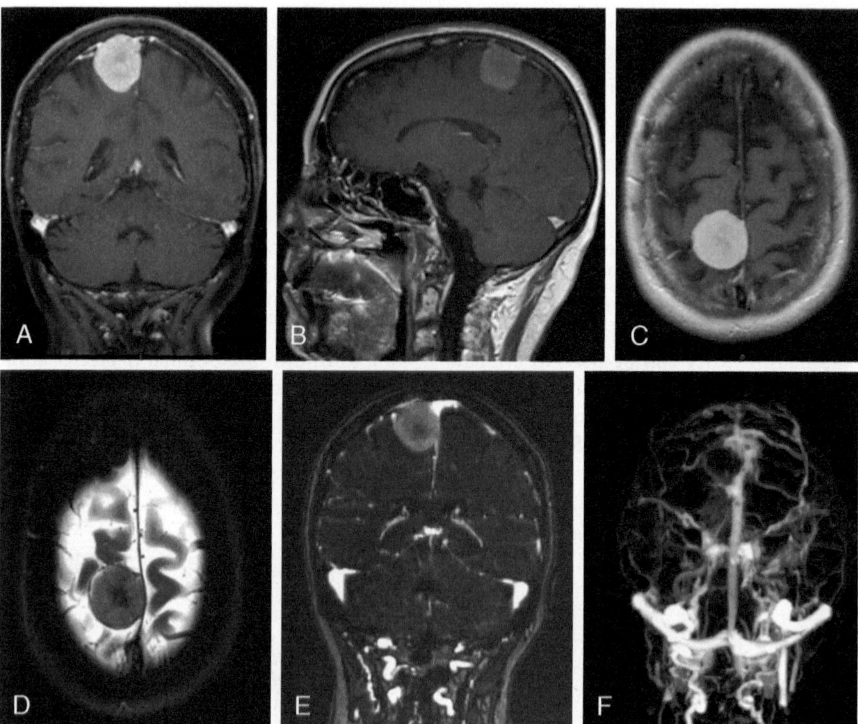

Fig. 10.2 An elderly patient found to have parasagittal mass during workup for sinus headaches. (A–C) T1-weighted MRI with contrast demonstrating parasagittal homogenously enhancing mass displacing the neighboring parietal white and grey matter. The dural tail is visualized as an enhancing area of dura above and adjacent to the tumor. (D) Axial T2-weighted MRI demonstrates minimal surrounding tumor associated edema and a CSF cleft around the tumor. (E, F) MRV demonstrates that tumor is causing local mass effect on the adjacent superior sagittal sinus without signs of occlusion. *CSF*, Cerebrospinal fluid; *MRV*, magnetic resonance venography.

neural structures and vasculature compared to MRI. However, CT scans can be useful in the evaluation of surrounding bony involvement. In addition to thickening of the adjacent dura, meningiomas can also extend locally into the surrounding bone, with localized hyperostosis or erosion. The effect of the tumor on the bony anatomy is best appreciated on a CT image. Calcifications of the tumor are also more evident on CT scan, shown as patchy areas of hyperdensity within the hypodense tumor.

Common sites of occurrence

Meningiomas can arise from any dura (Fig. 10.1).[32] Common sites of meningiomas are parasagittal (Fig. 10.2) and within the cerebral convexity (Fig. 10.3), with each location accounting for about 20% of meningiomas.[33]

With tumors in proximity to the superior sagittal sinus (SSS), evaluation of the extent of SSS involvement through MRV is critical for management decisions, surgical planning, and developing goals of SSS reconstruction.[34] Sindou classified parasagittal tumors based on the level of SSS involvement and invasion into six types (Fig. 10.4).[35,36]

- Type I: Tumor is attached to the outer surface of the SSS lateral wall.
- Type II: Tumor has invaded the lateral recess.
- Type III: The tumor has invaded the lateral wall.
- Type IV: The tumor has invaded the lateral wall and roof of the SSS.
- Type V: The tumor has invaded the whole SSS except one lateral wall.
- Type VI: The tumor has invaded the whole SSS.

Parasellar meningiomas arise from the tuberculum sellae and clinoid processes and can extend to the planum sphenoidale, olfactory groove, or sphenoid wing (Fig. 10.5). Very rarely, they can arise from the optic chiasm and spread anteriorly to the optic nerves and posteriorly through the optic tracts to the lateral geniculate bodies.[37]

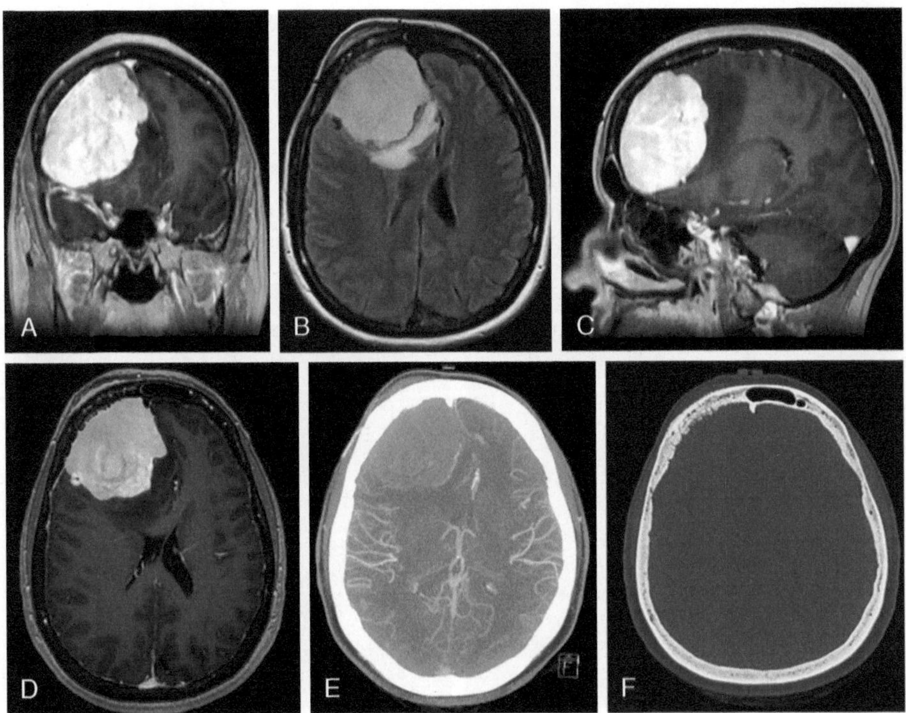

Fig. 10.3 A middle-aged patient presents with nausea and confusion. (A–C) T1-weighted MRI with contrast demonstrates a large, homogenously enhancing, extraaxial lesion in the left frontal convexity. The mass is causing significant mass effect on the surrounding brain parenchyma with midline shift and compression of the ventricular system. (D) T2 FLAIR sequence demonstrates significant tumor-associated vasogenic edema. (E). CTA shows displacement of the anterior cerebral artery branches from the tumor mass effect. (F) There is evidence of tumor invasion into the overlying bony calvarium with irregular and osseous infiltration on CT. *CTA*, Computed tomography angiography; *FLAIR*, fluid attenuated inversion recovery.

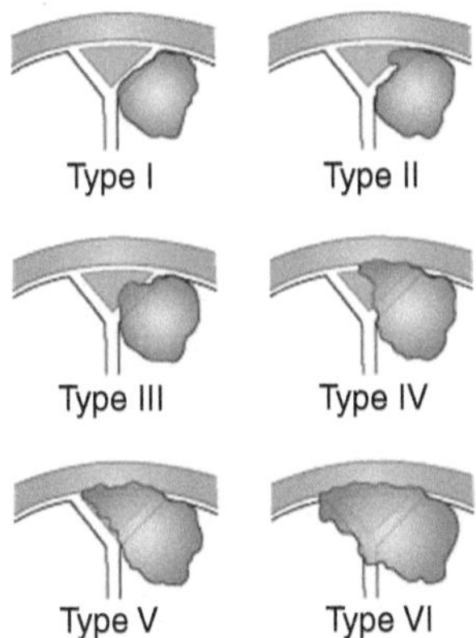

Fig. 10.4 Classification of meningiomas according to SSS invasion. (Reprinted from Sindou MP, Alvernia JE. Dural sinus invasion in meningiomas and repair. In: Necmettin PM, ed. *Meningiomas*. Philadelphia, PA: Elsevier/Saunders; 2010:355-364, with permission from Elsevier.)

Meningiomas can also occur at other, less common locations, including the tentorium (Fig. 10.6). Tentorial meningiomas account for about 5% of meningiomas and can extend supratentorially or infratentorially (Fig. 10.6).[26] Falcine meningiomas arise from the falx cerebri and account for 5 to 9% of meningiomas.[26] The remaining locations include the greater or lesser sphenoid wing, olfactory groove, and less commonly, the optic nerve sheath, choroid plexus, and spine. In about 1% of cases, meningiomas will arise outside of the dura, in sites including the temporal bone, mandible, mediastinum, and lung.[26]

Clinical cases

CASE 10.1 APPROACH TO THE PATIENT WITHOUT A TISSUE DIAGNOSIS

Case. An elderly patient presents with 2 years of intermittent sinus headaches without other associated symptoms. The patient has no other significant past medical history or history of

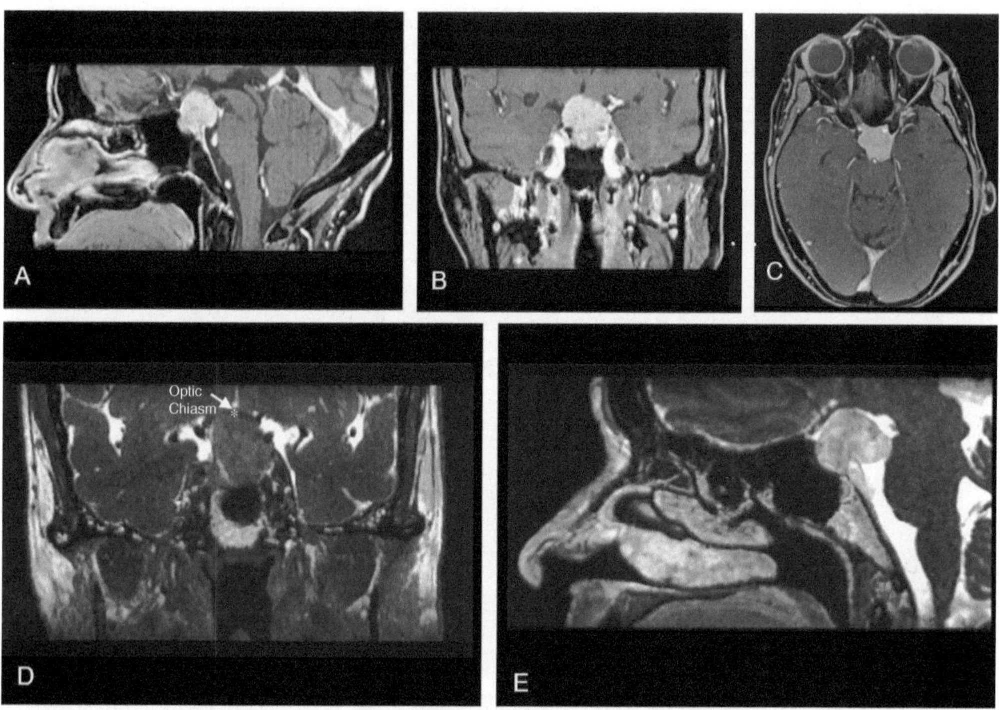

Fig. 10.5 A middle-aged patient found to have diminished peripheral vision during annual vision examination. T1-weighted MRI with contrast of suprasellar meningioma. (A) Sagittal view. (B) Coronal view. (C) Axial view. T1-weighted MRI sequences demonstrate a sellar-based mass extending into the suprasellar space superiorly and into the prepontine cistern posterior-inferiorly. (D, E) Superiorly, the mass displaces the optic chiasm with splaying of bilateral optic tracts. The posterior extension of the mass into the prepontine cistern exerts mass effect and deformity of the ventral pons.

other malignancies. Head CT demonstrates a partially calcified parasagittal mass.

Teaching Points: Evaluation and Management of a Parasagittal Meningioma. As with any patient who presents with a new chief complaint, the management of a patient presenting with a new mass suspicious for meningioma begins with a detailed clinical history including the onset, duration, and quality of symptoms. A clinical examination should include a full neurological assessment of mental status, cranial nerve, motor, sensory, and cerebellar function with emphasis on particular neurological systems depending on the location of the mass. Any deficits found on the neurological assessment should be correlated with tumor location, associated peritumoral edema, and vascular involvement.

Signs and symptoms of parasagittal and parafalcine meningiomas depend on their location along the SSS. Tumors arising in the anterior aspect of the falx and SSS often present with symptoms of personality changes and headaches. Meningiomas located along the middle third of the SSS can present with seizures and focal motor or sensory deficits. Masses in the posterior aspect of the falx and SSS can cause visual symptoms and compression of the ventricular system leading to headaches and papilledema. CT is the most common imaging modality to assess any new neurological complaints; therefore, patients often will present with CT findings suspicious for meningioma. An MRI should be obtained to further evaluate the location and characteristics of the tumor, including its relationship to surrounding neural structures, vasculature, and amount of peritumoral edema. An MRI with contrast was obtained for the patient which demonstrated a parasagittal homogenously enhancing mass with minimal surrounding T2 fluid attenuated inversion recovery (FLAIR) signal (Fig. 10.2). MRV demonstrated the tumor abutting the SSS without occlusion (Fig. 10.2E,F).

Because of the slow-growing nature of meningiomas, most of these tumors are discovered incidentally and can be observed without surgical intervention. In patients who present with a newly diagnosed mass suspicious for meningioma without prior tissue diagnosis, the management options depend vastly on the patient's symptoms. In the asymptomatic patient, observation is generally favored, especially in elderly patients (>85 years of age), as with the patient presented in this case. Conservative management consists of surveillance imaging and symptom monitoring. MRI scans are performed at 3-month intervals after initial diagnosis of the tumor. If the tumor demonstrates stable size, then MRI scans can be spaced out to 6 months, then yearly to ensure

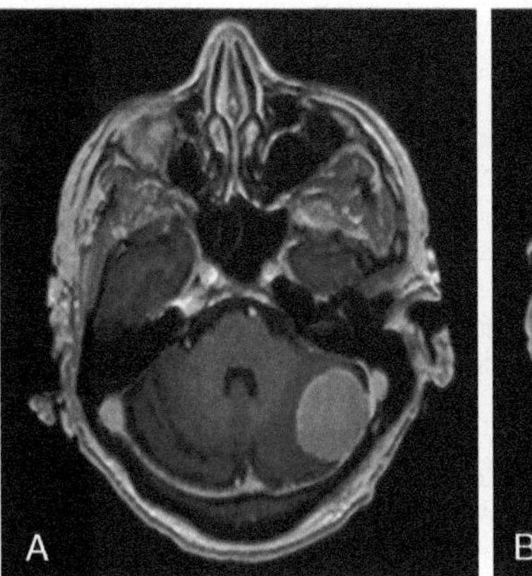

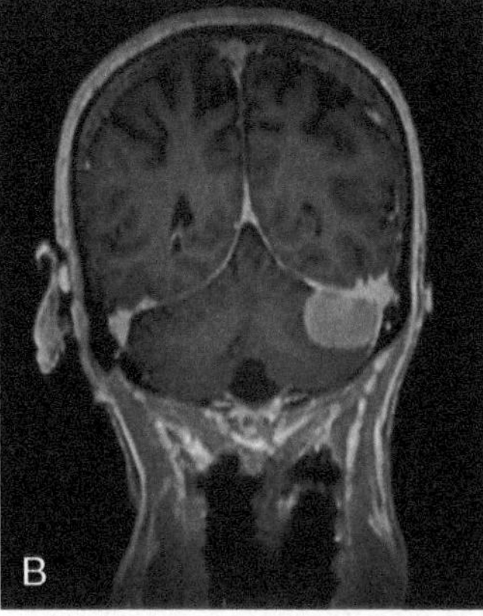

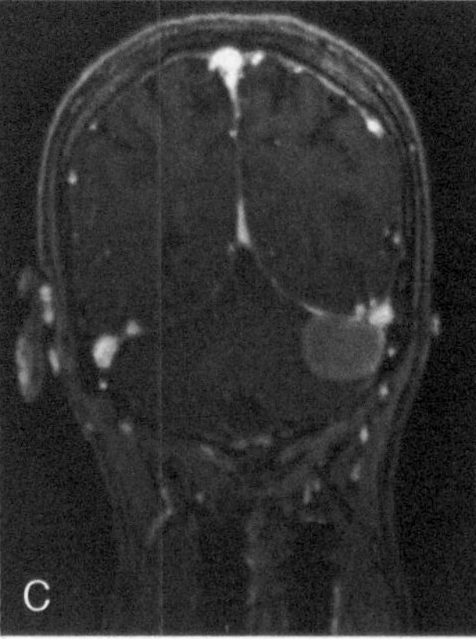

Fig. 10.6 A middle-aged patient presents with headaches and dizziness. (A, B) T1-weighted MRI with contrast demonstrates a homogenously enhancing tentorial meningioma. The mass is attached to the left tentorial leaflet inferiorly and displaces the cerebellum. The dural tail is visible superior to the mass in A as a thickened area of enhancing dura. (C) MRV demonstrates patency of the adjacent dural venous sinuses. *MRV,* Magnetic resonance venography.

the tumor remains stable. If the tumor demonstrates evidence of growth, then more frequent imaging is performed, and treatment options are discussed with the patient. Observation is also preferred in younger patients with asymptomatic meningiomas located in non-eloquent regions without peritumoral edema and mass effect. The authors' practice is to follow patients with serial imaging for life, as the tumor's growth pattern can change over time. As is the case with this patient, who is above the age of 85 with no prior history of cancer, presenting with an asymptomatic parasagittal meningioma without significant peritumor edema or mass effect, conservative observation with serial imaging was the elected management.

There are cases, however, where surgical intervention may be recommended in asymptomatic patients. A tissue diagnosis through biopsy or resection, if feasible, may be necessary if the diagnosis of meningioma is not certain, such as in patients with history of prior malignancy with concerns for metastatic disease. Additionally, there are certain imaging and clinical characteristics of the tumor that may suggest a more aggressive growth pattern or a higher-grade meningioma. These tumors would prompt early tissue diagnosis to further dictate postoperative adjuvant treatment. Tumors that display significant T2 signal on MRI that lack calcification are more likely to have an aggressive growth pattern. Meningiomas in younger patients that are greater than 3 cm in size are more likely to have continued growth. In young patients with consistent tumor growth over the span of a year or two, surgical resection may be preferred given the natural history of the disease. Surgery at this time may be more beneficial with its smaller size. Furthermore, in tumors with close proximity to vital vascular structures or eloquent regions, early surgical intervention may be preferred to prevent potential invasion into these structures with subsequent growth and to minimize surgical risk.

Clinical Pearls

1. The decision for observation or surgery of a meningioma should be made on an individual basis after discussions with the patient, taking into account the patient's clinical presentation, imaging characteristics, tumor growth patterns, and other medical history and comorbidities.
2. In symptomatic patients or patients with rapidly enlarging tumors without tissue diagnosis, surgery is the main treatment modality for both symptomatic relief and pathologic diagnosis.

CASE 10.2 APPROACH TO THE PATIENT WITH A WHO GRADE I MENINGIOMA

Case. While on a trip out of state, a middle-aged patient experienced nausea, diarrhea, headaches, and disorientation. Upon arrival at a local hospital, they were noted to have an episode of speech difficulty concerning for seizure activity. CT and MRI scans show a large right frontal extraaxial mass with significant T2 FLAIR intensity and mass effect (Fig. 10.3). The patient also noted an expanding, tender lump on the right side of their forehead over the last year.

Teaching Points: Management of Meningioma of the Convexity. The patient's physical and neurological examination was normal, with the exception of a bony, tender protrusion on their right forehead. The MRI was most consistent with a right frontal convexity meningioma. In contrast to the MRI findings from the previous patient, this patient's tumor is significantly larger (>3 cm) with significant peritumoral edema and associated mass effect on the surrounding normal brain. Tumors with significant edema also increase the risk of seizure activity. Given the patient's relatively young age, large tumor size, significant cerebral edema associated with the tumor, mass effect of the tumor on the adjacent brain, and the fact that they are symptomatic, surgery was recommended for diagnosis, to decrease mass effect, and for symptomatic relief.

Patients who present with seizures should be placed on antiepileptic drug therapy (AED). In patients who have significant peritumoral edema leading to focal neurological deficits or symptoms of increased intracranial pressure, corticosteroids can be administered to decrease cerebral edema prior to surgery. However, many patients with meningioma have very little to no vasogenic edema, even in cases of large tumors. When indicated, dexamethasone can be started on doses up to 16 mg/day divided over four doses and tapered down to a minimal effective dose or discontinued in the postoperative period.[15] The patient was started on levetiracetam and dexamethasone.

Gross total resection (GTR) of tumor is the goal for any surgical resection of meningioma if feasible. The estimated 10-year progression-free survival rates are about 60–80% for GTR of WHO grade I meningiomas and about 50% for those with subtotal resection (STR).[7] Once surgical intervention is decided, further preoperative evaluation of the tumor's relationship to neighboring structures is needed for safe surgical planning. Given the tumor's proximity to the anterior cerebral arteries, MRA and CTA were obtained to further evaluate the tumor's relationship to the vasculature. The patient's CTA demonstrated that the anterior cerebral arteries were displaced medially by the tumor and showed an incidental right anterior cerebral artery aneurysm (Fig. 10.3E). The patient's MRI further demonstrated enhancement in the subgaleal space and the skull adjacent to the tumor (Fig. 10.3B). A CT was performed to better evaluate the extent of bone involvement, which showed osseous infiltration of the tumor (Fig. 10.3F). The patient underwent surgical resection of the meningioma and involved calvarium in conjunction with plastic surgery with subsequent cranioplasty. With the advent of modern surgical navigation and techniques, combined with the favorable location of this patient's frontal convexity meningioma, it was possible to achieve a GTR including the involved dura and bone. Reported surgical complication rates are low for convexity meningiomas between 8–10%.[38] A study found that less than 2% of patients with large (>4 cm) convexity tumors experienced new neurological deficits postoperatively.[38]

The patient's pathologic diagnosis returned as a WHO grade I meningioma. Grade I meningiomas are the most common and are benign, with a recurrence rate of 7–25%.[9] Aggressiveness and recurrence of WHO grade I meningiomas depends largely on extent of surgical resection and tumor location. The extent of resection, graded on the Simpson Scale, predicts the probability of recurrence and therefore determines treatment course. For grade I meningiomas, the overall tumor recurrence rate for Simpson grades I, II, III, and IV resections are 5%, 22%, 31%, and 35%, respectively.[39] Grade I meningioma resections with Simpson grades I–III (indicating total/near total resection of tumor) generally only require observation with serial MRI scans following surgery as the risk of tumor recurrence is low. Resections with Simpson grades IV–V (indicating partial/minimal resection of tumor) have a higher recurrence rate. In those cases, planning for a combination of STR followed by adjuvant high precision stereotactic radiosurgery (SRS) or intensity modulated radiotherapy can be considered to maximize complete tumor treatment while minimizing the risk of adverse events, especially in tumors in critical areas such as the skull base.[40] Tumors located in the skull base have significantly reduced recurrence-free survival and overall survival likely due to the inability to achieve gross total or near total resection.[41]

In grade I meningiomas that are not conducive to complete surgical resection or near total resection due to high surgical risks to surrounding neural structures, such as those of the skull base, SRS can be used as first-line therapy.[7] SRS consists of extremely precise, high dose per fraction radiotherapy delivered with a 3D localization system in a single session usually to small, well-defined targets (see Chapter 3, Case 3.2 for stereotactic radiotherapy in neuro-oncology). This option is typically feasible for tumors less than 3–4 cm in diameter that are at least 2 mm away from critical structures such as the optic nerve and chiasm. A retrospective study found a 5-year progression-free survival of 87% for grade I, 56% for grade II, and 47% for grade III meningiomas treated with SRS.[42] Tumors involving the skull base can be challenging to target in one radiosurgery session due to variable contours, ambiguous margins, and proximity to critical structures. Fractionated SRS may be used in these cases to deliver ablative doses over several treatments. Intensity-modulated radiation therapy refers to external beam radiation therapy from distinct beam orientations. This treatment can be optimized to provide a desired dose distribution in the patient.[43]

Following the successful GTR of the meningioma, the patient was followed with surveillance imaging to monitor for tumor recurrence initially at 3-month and 6-month intervals followed by yearly intervals. They remain well with no evidence of tumor recurrence.

Clinical Pearls

1. GTR is the goal of any meningioma surgery.
2. Extent of resection after meningioma surgery is determined by the Simpson grading scale with Simpson grades I–III indicating total/near total resection of tumor and Simpson grades IV–V indicating partial/minimal resection of tumor.
3. For WHO grade I meningiomas, tumors can be monitored with serial imaging after GTR if the patient remains asymptomatic.

CASE 10.3 APPROACH TO THE PATIENT WITH WHO GRADE II MENINGIOMA

Case. A middle-aged patient was found to have diminished peripheral vision during a routine vision examination. A skull base MRI showed an enhancing suprasellar mass with displacement of the pituitary gland anteriorly (Fig. 10.5). Neurological examination was notable for bitemporal hemianopsia. Endocrine laboratory tests were within normal limits.

Teaching Points: Evaluation and Management of a Suprasellar Meningioma. Skull-based tumors such as the one in this case are more challenging to achieve GTR surgically, especially if there is invasion into the cavernous sinus. However, studies have suggested that skull-base meningiomas may have a less aggressive biology than non–skull-base cranial tumors.[44–46] The most common symptoms of sellar and suprasellar meningiomas are visual disturbance (58%) and headache (16%), with a mean symptom duration of 13 months. Endocrinopathy can also be present. Hyperprolactinemia is present in about one-third of patients.[47]

The options for the treatment of this lesion include observation, surgery, or radiation. The patient is symptomatic from the lesion and there is evidence of optic chiasm compression on imaging. These factors, especially the proximity of the mass to the optic chiasm, make surgical intervention the more preferred option. Both endonasal and craniotomy approaches were considered, and a craniotomy was performed due to the anterior displacement of the pituitary gland.

The complex anatomy of the skull base and the proximity of tumor to critical neurovascular structures often make complete GTR less feasible, which may necessitate careful surgical debulking followed by adjuvant therapy. During surgery, the optic chiasm, optic nerves, and carotid arteries were visualized. Surgical resection was carried out until the bulk of the tumor had been removed. The infundibulum was noted to be adherent to the surface of the tumor anteriorly and manipulation of the tumor tissue began to cause tension on the optic chiasm despite careful dissection. The residual tumor was unable to be safely dissected from the infundibulum and the optic chiasm; therefore, resection was halted at that time. Studies on sellar and suprasellar meningiomas have reported visual impairment improvement in 80% of patients and headaches improvement in in 7% of patients postoperatively. Postoperative complications have been reported in about one-third of cases at 3 months.[47]

Postoperatively, the patient had significant improvement in their vision. The patient was placed on levetiracetam for seizure prophylaxis and dexamethasone for cerebral edema management. It is common in the authors' practice to place the patient on seizure prophylaxis postsurgery even if there was not history of seizures preoperatively, as the risk of postoperative seizure following meningioma resection can be significant, with reported rates as high as 20%.[48]

Pathologic diagnosis revealed a WHO grade II meningioma. The initial management for grade II meningiomas is surgical resection with the goal of maximal safe resection. Several studies have demonstrated the importance of maximal surgical resection in the natural history of grade II meningiomas. The progression-free survival at 5 years is 59–90% after GTR but is only 30–70% after STR.[49] This grade of tumor implies that risk of recurrence is greater. At this point, a decision between observation and adjuvant radiotherapy was made by the clinician based on tumor size, proximity to critical structures, and patient history of radiation exposure. In this case, the tumor's location among both the optic nerve and pituitary infundibulum made radiation less ideal, and the physician and patient opted for close observation through MRI scans and neurological examinations at 3 months, 6 months, and then annually.

Based on retrospective data, there has been a trend toward adjuvant radiation following resection of WHO grade II meningiomas in favorable locations. However, the strength of radiation as an effective adjuvant therapy is still unclear due to lack of outcome data.[50] Several trials are currently evaluating differences in outcomes of radiation delivery modalities and techniques (Table 10.2).[43,51–55] Molecular features have not been included in clinical trial design to date. This will be necessary in the future to individualize therapy to subgroups who will benefit most from adjuvant therapy.[43]

Adjuvant SRS and external beam radiation therapy following STR have resulted in equivalent rates of tumor control in the long term.[49] However, prior external beam radiation therapy is a negative predictor of outcome in patients undergoing SRS for WHO grade II meningioma. Thus the radiation exposure of patients should be considered when deciding whether to use SRS.[49] Currently, treatment of grade II and grade III meningiomas typically begins with surgery, followed by observation, radiosurgery, or repeated surgery depending on the tumor's characteristics, patient age and symptoms, and the judgement of the patient's neurosurgical team. Walcott et al. developed a general treatment plan based on the National Comprehensive Cancer Network Clinical Practice Guidelines in Oncology (Fig. 10.7).[51,56]

Clinical Pearls

1. Evidence supports safe GTR of WHO grade II meningiomas as the first-line treatment for surgically resectable lesions.
2. Retrospective data supports a trend toward adjuvant radiation following resection of WHO grade II meningiomas in favorable locations; however, the strength of radiation as an effective adjuvant therapy in these patients is still unclear.
3. At 5 years, 60–90% of patients will be free of meningioma recurrence after GTR and 30–70% of patients will be recurrence free after STR.

CASE 10.4 APPROACH TO THE PATIENT WITH WHO GRADE II MENINGIOMA WITH RESIDUAL POSTOPERATIVE DISEAS

Case. A middle-aged patient with known history of meningioma is referred by neuro-ophthalmology with proptosis, chemosis, vision loss, and ophthalmoplegia of their right eye. MRI demonstrates significant growth of the patient's known

Table 10.2 Clinical trials evaluating radiotherapy in the treatment of atypical and malignant meningiomas[51–54]

Clinical trial	Name	Objective
NCT03180268	Observation or radiation therapy in treating patients with newly diagnosed grade II meningioma that has been completely removed by surgery	To determine, in terms of progression-free survival, the extent of clinical benefit of the addition of adjuvant radiotherapy to gross total resection for patients with newly diagnosed WHO grade II meningioma.
NCT00626730	Radiation therapy in treating patients who have undergone surgery for newly diagnosed grade II or grade III meningioma	To assess the impact of high-dose radiotherapy on progression-free survival, treatment tolerance, and posttreatment global cognitive functioning in patients with atypical (WHO grade II) or malignant (WHO grade III) meningioma.
NCT00895622	Observation or radiation therapy in treating patients with grade I, grade II, or grade III meningioma	To compare observation and radiation therapy in treating patients with grade I, grade II, or grade III meningioma.
ISRCTN71702099	Radiation versus observation following surgical resection of atypical meningioma: a randomized control trial	To determine whether early adjuvant fractionated radiotherapy reduces the risk of tumor recurrence or death due to any cause compared to active monitoring in newly diagnosed atypical meningioma.

meningioma, now representing a large orbital, right sphenoid wing mass with extension into the cavernous sinus and displacement of optic nerve medially.

Teaching Points: Evaluation and Management of Orbital, Sphenoid Wing Meningioma. Due to the tumor's proximity to critical neurovascular structures, the patient underwent STR of the tumor with decompression of the orbit in conjunction with neuro-ophthalmology. Postoperative MRI showed residual tumor in the medial and posterior portions of their right orbit, cavernous sinus, interior greater sphenoid wing, and the pterygopalatine fossa. The pathology of their tumor demonstrated severely atypical meningioma, WHO grade II. Postoperatively, the patient had improvement in the ptosis of their right eye but had persistent poor vision. At this time, following STR and persistent symptoms, the patient's treatment options included repeat surgery, radiotherapy, and observation. Given the unfavorable location of their residual tumor, additional surgical debulking carried high neurological risks. Given the extent of their disease, significant symptoms, WHO grade II histology, and the likelihood of additional deficits if their residual disease continues to grow, conventionally fractionated radiotherapy was recommended.

In contrast to the patient presented in Case 10.3, this patient's persistent visual symptoms and significant residual tumor burden influenced the decision to pursue adjuvant radiation therapy after surgical debulking. A complex balance between clinical benefit and treatment risk must be reached for each individual patient when deciding whether to pursue radiation therapy for meningiomas near critical structures.

Atypical meningioma may result in metastatic spread in rare cases. Staging CT scans were performed on the patient to rule out metastatic disease. The patient was treated with 180 cGy per fraction delivered once per day over 33 days. Following treatment, MRI scans demonstrated stable tumor size without continued growth. They were recommended to follow up with serial MRI scans. Should the tumor show significant recurrence or progression, their treatment options would include repeat surgery, radiotherapy, or more conservative observation.

Clinical Pearls

1. If GTR is not feasible for a WHO grade II meningioma, STR with adjuvant radiotherapy should be considered.

CASE 10.5 APPROACH TO THE PATIENT WITH WHO GRADE III MENINGIOMA

Case. A middle-aged patient presents with a newly diagnosed brain tumor. For the last month, they have experienced worsening headaches when they sneeze and cough, accompanied

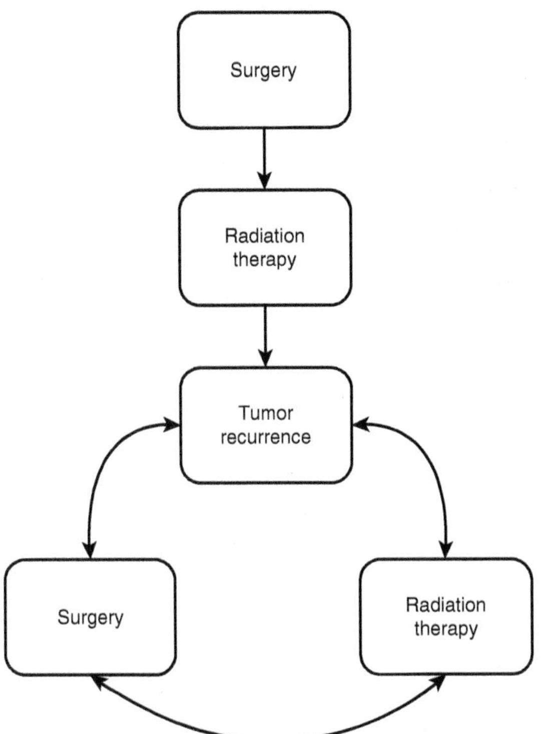

Fig. 10.7 Management strategy for WHO grade II and III meningioma. Diagnosis is made based on tissue biopsy taken during surgery, followed by radiation for many subtotal resections. Should recurrence occur, the patient and physician decide among repeat surgery, radiation, or observation. (Modified from Walcott BP, et al. Radiation treatment for WHO grade II and III meningiomas. *Front Oncol*. 2013;3:227.)

by lightheadedness in the last week. CT scan at the local emergency department revealed a brain tumor. MRI scan is consistent with tentorial meningioma.

Teaching Points: Management of a Grade III Tentorial Meningioma. The MRI scan (Fig. 10.6) demonstrated a tentorial meningioma arising from the tentorium cerebelli causing mass effect on the adjacent cerebellar hemisphere. MRV demonstrated that, although the tumor abuts the transverse and sigmoid sinus, the venous sinuses remain patent (Fig. 10.6C).

The most common symptoms of tentorial meningiomas include headache, cerebellar ataxia, psychiatric disturbances, and impaired cranial nerve function. The location of the tentorium near the brainstem and draining sinuses can complicate surgical efforts toward complete resection.

The patient's options for treatment included surgery, radiation, and observation. Surgery was favored due to the growing size of the tumor and recent onset of symptoms that would likely worsen over time. A suboccipital craniectomy was performed with GTR of the tumor. Histologic diagnosis returned as a WHO grade III anaplastic meningioma due to a presence of over 20 mitotic figures per 10 high-powered fields.

Even after macroscopic GTR, the recurrence rate is high in malignant meningiomas. Thus, adjuvant radiation therapy is a standard component of clinical management of WHO grade III meningiomas following any extent of safe maximal resection.[49] The tumor's proximity to critical structures and the desire to protect nearby healthy brain from high radiation doses made intensity modulated radiotherapy the most promising treatment option. Beginning a month after surgery, the patient received 33 fractions of radiotherapy administered over 47 days. Short-term side effects of radiotherapy can include fatigue, nausea, and headaches, and long-term side effects can include cognitive issues, radiation necrosis, and edema.

The patient had MRI scans at 3, 6, and 10 months after surgery, then every 6 to 12 months for 5 years to evaluate for tumor recurrence or progression. After this time, MRI scans were spaced out to every 3 years for surveillance. Most recurrences of atypical meningiomas are local to the original site of the tumor, but rarely metastases can appear in the spinal cord.[57]

There is a subset of patients with highly aggressive meningiomas who develop recurrent disease after surgery and radiation therapy. Treatment options for these individuals are currently inadequate, but there is increasing interest in developing systemic treatments. Patients with surgery- and radiation-refractory grade II and III meningiomas treated with medical therapies have an average 6-month progression-free survival of 26%.[49] Although no phase II clinical trials for chemotherapeutic agents have proven their effectiveness so far, there are several ongoing clinical trials for systemic therapeutic agents (Table 10.3).[58–63]

Small molecule inhibitors of vascular endothelial growth factor are the most promising for systemic treatment for malignant meningiomas but are pending phase III trials.[64] Although thoroughly studied, tyrosine kinase inhibitors and hydroxyurea (ribonucleotide reductase inhibitor) have not shown a significant impact on progression-free survival so far.[65,66] The higher incidence of meningioma in women suggests a potential hormonal involvement in the development and growth of these tumors.[1] Studies have explored the effectiveness of hormone receptor targeting agents in meningioma treatment, but at this time, estrogen and progesterone receptor inhibitors have not shown activity against these tumors.[58] Additionally, although recombinant interferon alpha inhibits the growth of meningioma cells in vitro, clinical trials only suggest limited activity.[67,68] In terms of immunotherapy, a promising future investigational endeavor lies in PD-1/PD-L1 pathway inhibition, as recent studies have shown upregulation of PD-L1 expression in anaplastic meningiomas.[69] One study reported incidental decrease in the size of a patient's meningioma after treatment with nivolumab, an anti-PD1 antibody therapy, for concurrent lung cancer, suggesting that PD-1 antibodies may be a potential therapeutic option for the treatment of meningiomas.[70] There are currently two clinical trials (NCT01892397 and NCT02847559) utilizing delivery of alternating electrical current to tumor with and without bevacizumab for recurrent WHO grades II and III meningiomas.[7,71,72]

Table 10.3 Ongoing clinical trials for systemic treatment of refractory or recurrent meningioma[58–62]

Agent	Phase	Mechanism of action	Clinical trial identifier
Alpelisib and trametinib	II	Pi3Kα and MEK inhibitor	NCT03631953
Bevacizumab	II	VEGF antibody	NCT01125046
Nivolumab	II	PD-1 antibody	NCT02648997
Pembrolizumab	II	PD-1 antibody	NCT03279692
Vistusertib	II	mTOR inhibitor	NCT03071874

VEGF, Vascular endothelial growth factor.

Clinical Pearls

1. WHO grade III meningiomas are aggressive malignant neoplasms.
2. Safe maximal resection should be pursued for WHO grade III meningiomas followed by radiotherapy.
3. Even with maximal aggressive therapy, rates of recurrence are as high as 60–90%.

CASE 10.6 APPROACH TO RECURRENT MENINGIOMA

Case. A middle-aged patient with a history of grade II atypical meningioma with multiple recurrences following resections, repeated radiation, and immunotherapy trial, presents with worsening headaches and right homonymous hemianopsia. Repeat MRI demonstrated growth of their aggressive meningioma. The patient underwent repeat surgical resection of the recurrent tumor and pathology returned as grade III meningioma.

Teaching Points: Clinical Approach to Recurrent Meningioma. About 3 months after their most recent surgery, the patient noted some decline in their reading and cognition. MRI demonstrated new contrast enhancement involving the surface of the posterior left hemisphere and edema within the posterior left hemisphere that has developed since their postoperative MRI. Due to their recent functional decline in combination with new enhancement, the decision was made to begin bevacizumab treatment. A recent update on a phase II clinical trial evaluating bevacizumab treatment for recurrent meningioma stated that 82% of patients with grade III malignant meningioma achieved stable disease following treatment, and 18% experienced progressive disease.[73]

Unfortunately, after three cycles of bevacizumab, the patient's MRI showed continued growth of the posterior left hemisphere meningioma. It also demonstrated compression and potential tumor invasion into the SSS. Due to progression of their disease, bevacizumab was discontinued. The patient was then enrolled in a clinical trial of nivolumab for the treatment of malignant meningiomas. After three sets of infusions, the patient was noted to have worsening symptoms, and repeat MRI showed significant interval increase in the extension of the patient's tumor, with growth across the falx into the right parafalcine region. At this point, the patient had nearly exhausted adjuvant therapies, having progressed despite multiple prior surgeries, radiotherapy, and systemic therapies. The decision was made to pursue repeat surgical debulking for relief of mass effect and symptom management. Postoperatively, the patient noticed improvement in their vision and headaches. They will be followed with serial imaging and symptom monitoring. Should they exhibit evidence of tumor progression in the future, further surgical resection and radiation may be potential options.

Clinical Pearls

1. If recurrent meningioma is detected that poses a significant risk to neighboring brain structures or patient quality of life, the patient and clinician can choose between repeated surgery or radiation therapy (Fig. 10.7).
2. Systemic therapies have not been shown to improve outcomes in newly diagnosed meningiomas but are often considered in multiply recurrent, treatment-refractory, or metastatic meningiomas.
3. In recent years, several clinical trials of systemic therapies have become available for patients with grade II and III meningiomas refractory to surgery and radiation.

Clinical approach to symptomatic management in meningioma patients

Seizures. Seizures are a very common symptom; they have been observed in about 30% of all patients with supratentorial meningiomas. They are more typical among patients with parasagittal and convexity tumors and less common in those with skull-based tumors. Out of patients who experience preoperative seizures, 70% achieved seizure freedom following tumor resection, while the remaining 30% continue to experience seizures. Twelve percent of patients without preoperative seizures will have new onset of seizures following tumor resection. The presence of peritumoral edema, younger age, male gender, and increasing midline shift are some factors associated with preoperative seizure occurrence. Uncontrolled preoperative seizures are associated with decreased seizure control following tumor resection.[13,74] Currently, the use of AEDs is usually prompted in the preoperative period if a patient has evidence of seizure activity related to the tumor. The choice of AED is based on clinician preference. Additional AEDs can be added to a patient's medication regimen if their current regimen does not function adequately to control their seizures.

Antiepileptic drug therapy. There are no standard guidelines for the use of AEDs to prevent postoperative seizures. Several studies have not found evidence of reduced seizure burden following administration of AEDs, and randomized control trials are likely needed to define the role of AEDs in postsurgery management.[74–76] In patients without seizures, AEDs are generally given immediately before surgery and after surgery for prophylaxis. For patients without preoperative seizures, weaning of the AEDs typically occurs 1 to 2 weeks after surgery. Patients with a history of preoperative seizures or who experience postoperative seizures typically remain on their AED regimen for 1–2 months after surgery or indefinitely if evidence of seizure activity persists. A study found that the most common AEDs administered at the time of surgery are phenytoin, levetiracetam, divalproex, and carbamazepine. These were given in combination in about 40% of cases.[74]

Site-specific meningioma management

Cavernous sinus meningiomas. Meningiomas of the cavernous sinus pose a challenge for resection due to their close association with cranial nerves II–VI and the internal carotid artery. They can compress or invade these structures and present with neurological deficits. Due to the proximity of these tumors to critical neural structures, GTR of these tumors is often not feasible and carries significant surgical risks. There has been a paradigm shift in treatment from a single-treatment modality with radical surgery to a multimodal therapy consisting of surgical resection followed by radiosurgery. The goal of this treatment regimen is to debulk portions of the tumor while creating a plane of separation between the tumor and surrounding structures that would allow for precise radiosurgical targeting of the residual tumor.[77,78] Reports have shown that the percentage of patients experiencing postoperative ocular nerve dysfunction has decreased from 55 to 16% using this approach.[79]

Optic sheath meningiomas. Many patients with orbit-associated and optic sheath meningioma present with optic disturbance, much of which remains or worsens during treatment due to the complicated nature of surgical resection of tumors in this region. Recent studies have found that the use of radiotherapy following or instead of surgical resection improves visual acuity postoperatively. Thus, use of early radiation therapy may be advantageous in treating meningiomas in these locations.[80,81]

Olfactory groove and anterior skull-base meningiomas. Meningiomas of the olfactory groove are rare but are very strongly associated with postoperative ipsilateral and bilateral anosmia. Meningiomas causing a midline shift across the frontal base are often associated with preoperative anosmia. Preoperative lateralized olfactory testing influences the neurosurgeon in choosing a suitable surgical route to preserve the remaining olfactory functioning.[82] Anterior skull-base meningiomas are often associated with abnormal personality and behavior that varies depending on the precise location of the tumor. For example, patients with damage to the ventromedial prefrontal cortex experienced a specific deficit in value-based decision making. As decline of adaptive function was found to continue to decline postoperatively, early detection and resection of meningiomas of the anterior skull base is the best way to halt worsening personality and behavior deficits as the tumor grows.[83]

Complications of radiation therapy for meningioma treatment

(See also Chapter 24 for approach to radiation necrosis.) As discussed earlier, gamma knife radiosurgery is a treatment option for tumors that cannot be completely resected. Radiation-induced intratumoral necrosis (RIN) is a sign of treatment response but is associated with peritumoral edema that can worsen mass effect of tumors adjacent to critical structures. A study found that new RIN developed in about one-third of meningioma tumors at a median time of 6.5 months following gamma knife radiosurgery. RIN development is associated with high radiation target volumes (above 4.5 cc) and the maximum dose (above 25 Gy). Out of the patients who developed RIN, about 40% developed symptoms including dizziness, headache, and seizure.[84] The unwanted effects of RIN can require steroid administration or decompressive surgery to resolve. Other side effects of radiation include nausea, vomiting, headaches, focal alopecia, and focal skin erythema. Patients may also experience systemic fatigue or permanent damage to the optic nerve.[15]

Conclusion

Main treatment options for meningioma consist of observation, radiation, and surgery. Observation through serial MRI is typically chosen for benign tumors that show slow growth and do not cause symptoms. More aggressive strategies including radiation and surgery are favored for tumors causing symptoms, cerebral edema, and of a higher-grade histologically. GTR is the goal of any meningioma surgery. For WHO grade I meningiomas, tumors can be monitored with serial imaging after GTR if the patient remains asymptomatic. Evidence supports safe GTR of grade II meningiomas as the first-line treatment for surgically resectable lesions. If GTR is not feasible, STR with adjuvant radiotherapy should be pursued. Similarly, safe maximal resection should be pursued for WHO grade III meningiomas followed by radiotherapy.[49] Following treatment, patients should be monitored over time with repeated MRI scans to monitor for tumor recurrence or progression. If substantial tumor is detected that poses a significant risk to neighboring brain structures or patient quality of life, the patient and clinician may choose between repeated surgery or radiation therapy. Although clinical trials of systemic therapies are increasingly available to patients with grade II and III meningiomas refractory to surgery and radiation, larger randomized trials are needed to determine the efficacy of systemic therapies in the treatment of atypical and malignant meningiomas. Goldbrunner et al. established an algorithm for recommended treatment based on assessments by the meningioma task force of the European Association of Neuro-Oncology (Fig. 10.8).[40]

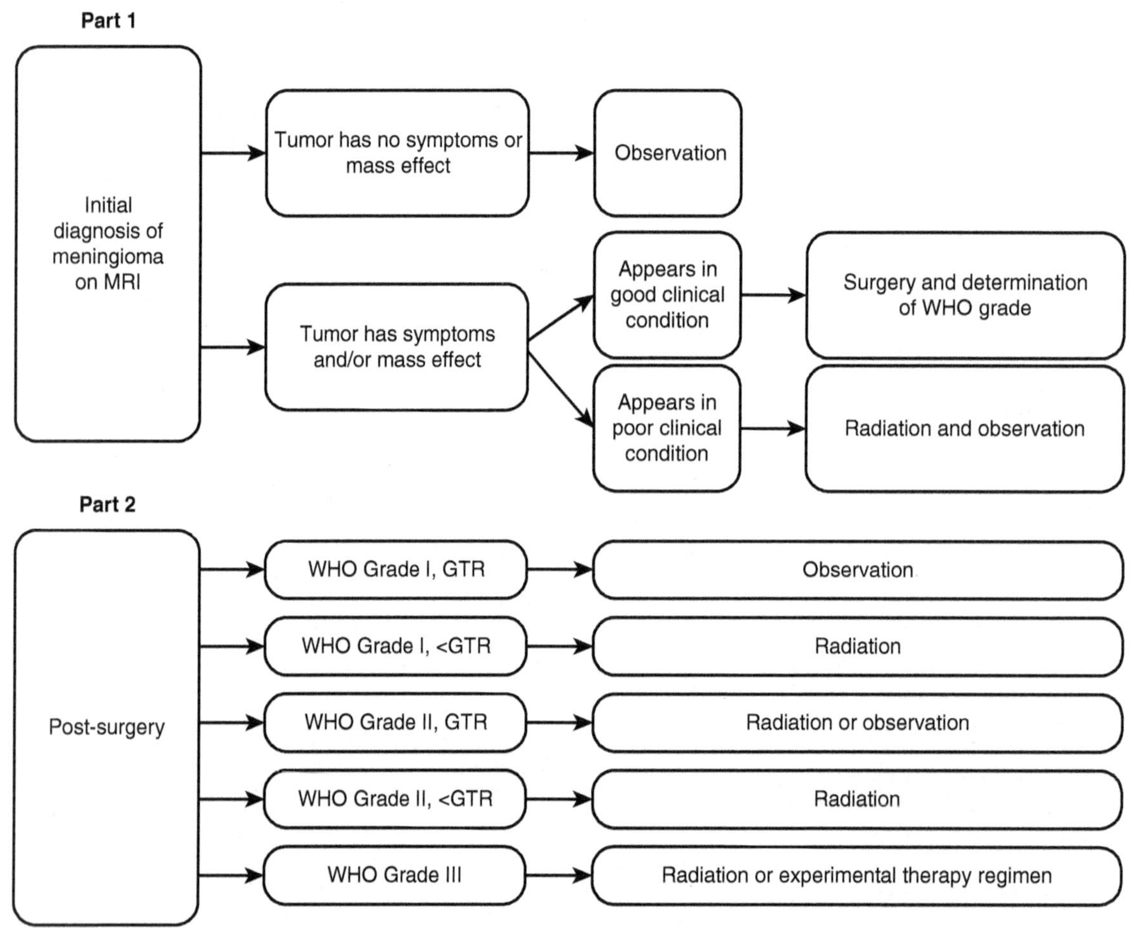

Fig. 10.8 Recommendation for management of WHO grades I–III meningiomas. *GTR,* Gross total resection. (Modified from Goldbrunner R, et al. EANO guidelines for the diagnosis and treatment of meningiomas. *Lancet Oncol.* 2016;17(9):e383-e391.)

References

1. Ostrom QT, Gittleman H, Truitt G, Boscia A, Kruchko C, Barnholtz-Sloan JS. CBTRUS Statistical Report: primary brain and other central nervous system tumors diagnosed in the United States in 2011–2015. *Neuro Oncol.* 2018;20(suppl 4):iv1–iv86. https://doi.org/10.1093/neuonc/noy131.
2. Hansson CM, Buckley PG, Grigelioniene G, et al. Comprehensive genetic and epigenetic analysis of sporadic meningioma for macro-mutations on 22q and micro-mutations within the NF2 locus. *BMC Genom.* 2007;8:16. https://doi.org/10.1186/1471-2164-8-16.
3. Agnihotri S, Suppiah S, Tonge PD, et al. Therapeutic radiation for childhood cancer drives structural aberrations of NF2 in meningiomas. *Nat Commun.* 2017;8(1):186. https://doi.org/10.1038/s41467-017-00174-7.
4. Morgenstern PF, Shah K, Dunkel IJ, et al. Meningioma after radiotherapy for malignancy. *J Clin Neurosci.* 2016;30:93–97. https://doi.org/10.1016/j.jocn.2016.02.002.
5. Neglia JP, Robison LL, Stovall M, et al. New primary neoplasms of the central nervous system in survivors of childhood cancer: a report from the childhood cancer survivor study. *J Natl Cancer Inst.* 2006;98(21):1528–1537. https://doi.org/10.1093/jnci/djj411.
6. Braganza MZ, Kitahara CM, Berrington de González A, Inskip PD, Johnson KJ, Rajaraman P. Ionizing radiation and the risk of brain and central nervous system tumors: a systematic review. *Neuro Oncol.* 2012;14(11):1316–1324. https://doi.org/10.1093/neuonc/nos208.
7. Shaikh N, Dixit K, Raizer J. Recent advances in managing/understanding meningioma. *F1000Res.* 2018;7. https://doi.org/10.12688/f1000research.13674.1.
8. Perry A, Giannini C, Raghavan R, et al. Aggressive phenotypic and genotypic features in pediatric and NF2-associated meningiomas: a clinicopathologic study of 53 cases. *J Neuropathol Exp Neurol.* 2001;60(10):994–1003. https://doi.org/10.1093/jnen/60.10.994.
9. Yuzawa S, Nishihara H, Tanaka S. Genetic landscape of meningioma. *Brain Tumor Pathol.* 2016;33(4):237–247. https://doi.org/10.1007/s10014-016-0271-7.
10. Whittle IR, Smith C, Navoo P, Collie D. Meningiomas. *Lancet.* 2004;363(9420):1535–1543. https://doi.org/10.1016/S0140-6736(04)16153-9.
11. Vernooij MW, Ikram MA, Tanghe HL, et al. Incidental findings on brain MRI in the general population. *N Engl J Med.* 2007;357(18):1821–1828. https://doi.org/10.1056/NEJMoa070972.
12. Niiro M, Yatsushiro K, Nakamura K, Kawahara Y, Kuratsu J. Natural history of elderly patients with asymptomatic meningiomas. *J Neurol Neurosurg Psychiatry.* 2000;68(1):25–28. https://doi.org/10.1136/jnnp.68.1.25.
13. Englot DJ, Magill ST, Han SJ, Chang EF, Berger MS, McDermott MW. Seizures in supratentorial meningioma: a systematic review and meta-analysis. *J Neurosurg.* 2016;124(6):1552–1561. https://doi.org/10.3171/2015.4.JNS142742.
14. Louis DN, Perry A, Reifenberger G, et al. The 2016 World Health Organization classification of tumors of the central nervous system: a summary. *Acta Neuropathol.* 2016;131(6):803–820. https://doi.org/10.1007/s00401-016-1545-1.
15. Fogh SE, Johnson DR, Barker FG, et al. Case-based review: meningioma. *Neuro Oncol Pract.* 2016;3(2):120–134. https://doi.org/10.1093/nop/npv063.
16. Marciscano AE, Stemmer-Rachamimov AO, Niemierko A, et al. Benign meningiomas (WHO grade I) with atypical histological features: correlation of histopathological features with clinical outcomes. *J Neurosurg.* 2016;124(1):106–114. https://doi.org/10.3171/2015.1.JNS142228.
17. Hortobágyi T, Bencze J, Varkoly G, Kouhsari MC, Klekner Á. Meningioma recurrence. *Open Med.* 2016;11(1):168–173. https://doi.org/10.1515/med-2016-0032.
18. Kawahara Y, Niiro M, Yokoyama S, Kuratsu J. Dural congestion accompanying meningioma invasion into vessels: the dural tail sign. *Neuroradiology.* 2001;43(6):462–465.
19. Tokumaru A, O'uchi T, Eguchi T, et al. Prominent meningeal enhancement adjacent to meningioma on Gd-DTPA-enhanced MR images: histopathologic correlation. *Radiology.* 1990;175(2):431–433. https://doi.org/10.1148/radiology.175.2.2326470.
20. Nakau H, Miyazawa T, Tamai S, et al. Pathologic significance of meningeal enhancement ("flare sign") of meningiomas on MRI. *Surg Neurol.* 1997;48(6):584–590. discussion 590–591.
21. Ildan F, Erman T, Göçer AI, et al. Predicting the probability of meningioma recurrence in the preoperative and early postoperative period: a multivariate analysis in the midterm follow-up. *Skull Base.* 2007;17(3):157–171. https://doi.org/10.1055/s-2007-970554.
22. Younis G, Sawaya R. Intracranial osteolytic malignant meningiomas appearing as extracranial soft-tissue masses. *Neurosurgery.* 1992;30(6):932–935. https://doi.org/10.1227/00006123-199206000-00022.
23. Rosahl SK, Mirzayan MJ, Samii M. Osteolytic intra-osseous meningiomas: illustrated review. *Acta Neurochir.* 2004;146(11):1245–1249. https://doi.org/10.1007/s00701-004-0380-7.
24. Yun JH, Lee SK. Primary osteolytic intraosseous atypical meningioma with soft tissue and dural invasion: report of a case and review of literatures. *J Korean Neurosurg Soc.* 2014;56(6):509–512. https://doi.org/10.3340/jkns.2014.56.6.509.
25. Elder JB, Atkinson R, Zee CS, Chen TC. Primary intraosseous meningioma. *Neurosurg Focus.* 2007;23(4):E13. https://doi.org/10.3171/FOC-07/10/E13.
26. Watts J, Box G, Galvin A, Brotchie P, Trost N, Sutherland T. Magnetic resonance imaging of meningiomas: a pictorial review. *Insights Imaging.* 2014;5(1):113–122. https://doi.org/10.1007/s13244-013-0302-4.
27. Hoover JM, Morris JM, Meyer FB. Use of preoperative magnetic resonance imaging T1 and T2 sequences to determine intraoperative meningioma consistency. *Surg Neurol Int.* 2011;2:142. https://doi.org/10.4103/2152-7806.85983.
28. Nakano T, Asano K, Miura H, Itoh S, Suzuki S. Meningiomas with brain edema: radiological characteristics on MRI and review of the literature. *Clin Imaging.* 2002;26(4):243–249.
29. Huang RY, Bi WL, Griffith B, et al. Imaging and diagnostic advances for intracranial meningiomas. *Neuro Oncol.* 2019;21(suppl 1):i44–i61. https://doi.org/10.1093/neuonc/noy143.
30. Hashiba T, Hashimoto N, Maruno M, et al. Scoring radiologic characteristics to predict proliferative potential in meningi-

omas. *Brain Tumor Pathol*. 2006;23(1):49–54. https://doi.org/10.1007/s10014-006-0199-4.
31. Villanueva-Meyer JE, Mabray MC, Cha S. Current clinical brain tumor imaging. *Neurosurgery*. 2017;81(3):397–415. https://doi.org/10.1093/neuros/nyx103.
32. Perry A. Meningiomas. In: Perry A, Brat D, eds. *Practical Surgical Neuropathology: A Diagnostic Approach*. 2nd ed. Philadelphia, PA: Elsevier; 2018:259–298. Available at: https://www.clinicalkey.com/#!/content/book/3-s2.0-B9780323449410000138. Accessed August 12, 2019.
33. Magill ST, Young JS, Chae R, Aghi MK, Theodosopoulos PV, McDermott MW. Relationship between tumor location, size, and WHO grade in meningioma. *Neurosurg Focus*. 2018;44(4):E4. https://doi.org/10.3171/2018.1.FOCUS17752.
34. Ricci A, Di Vitantonio H, De Paulis D, et al. Parasagittal meningiomas: our surgical experience and the reconstruction technique of the superior sagittal sinus. *Surg Neurol Int*. 2017;8:1. https://doi.org/10.4103/2152-7806.198728.
35. Sindou M, Hallacq P. Venous reconstruction in surgery of meningiomas invading the sagittal and transverse sinuses. *Skull Base Surg*. 1998;8(2):57–64.
36. Sindou MP, Alvernia JE. Dural sinus invasion in meningiomas and repair. In: Necmettin PM, ed. *Meningiomas*. Philadelphia, PA: Elsevier/Saunders; 2010:355–364. https://doi.org/10.1016/B978-1-4160-5654-6.00025-8. Accessed August 12, 2019.
37. Hershey BL. Suprasellar masses: diagnosis and differential diagnosis. *Semin Ultrasound CT MR*. 1993;14(3):215–231. https://doi.org/10.1016/S0887-2171(05)80082-4.
38. Morokoff AP, Zauberman J, Black PM. Surgery for convexity meningiomas. *Neurosurgery*. 2008;63(3):427–434. https://doi.org/10.1227/01.NEU.0000310692.80289.28.
39. Nanda A, Bir SC, Maiti TK, Konar SK, Missios S, Guthikonda B. Relevance of Simpson grading system and recurrence-free survival after surgery for World Health Organization grade I meningioma. *J Neurosurg*. 2017;126(1):201–211. https://doi.org/10.3171/2016.1.JNS151842.
40. Goldbrunner R, Minniti G, Preusser M, et al. EANO guidelines for the diagnosis and treatment of meningiomas. *Lancet Oncol*. 2016;17(9):e383–e391. https://doi.org/10.1016/S1470-2045(16)30321-7.
41. Mendenhall WM, Friedman WA, Amdur RJ, Foote KD. Management of benign skull base meningiomas: a review. *Skull Base*. 2004;14(1):53–60. https://doi.org/10.1055/s-2004-821364.
42. Kaprealian T, Raleigh DR, Sneed PK, Nabavizadeh N, Nakamura JL, McDermott MW. Parameters influencing local control of meningiomas treated with radiosurgery. *J Neuro Oncol*. 2016;128(2):357–364. https://doi.org/10.1007/s11060-016-2121-1.
43. Brastianos PK, Galanis E, Butowski N, et al. Advances in multidisciplinary therapy for meningiomas. *Neuro Oncol*. 2019;21(suppl 1):i18–i31. https://doi.org/10.1093/neuonc/noy136.
44. McGovern SL, Aldape KD, Munsell MF, Mahajan A, DeMonte F, Woo SY. A comparison of World Health Organization tumor grades at recurrence in patients with non–skull base and skull base meningiomas: clinical article. *J Neurosurg*. 2010;112(5):925–933. https://doi.org/10.3171/2009.9.JNS09617.
45. Hashimoto N, Rabo CS, Okita Y, et al. Slower growth of skull base meningiomas compared with non–skull base meningiomas based on volumetric and biological studies: clinical article. *J Neurosurg*. 2012;116(3):574–580. https://doi.org/10.3171/2011.11.JNS11999.
46. Kane AJ, Sughrue ME, Rutkowski MJ, et al. Anatomic location is a risk factor for atypical and malignant meningiomas. *Cancer*. 2011;117(6):1272–1278. https://doi.org/10.1002/cncr.25591.
47. Kwancharoen R, Blitz AM, Tavares F, Caturegli P, Gallia GL, Salvatori R. Clinical features of sellar and suprasellar meningiomas. *Pituitary*. 2014;17(4):342–348. https://doi.org/10.1007/s11102-013-0507-z.
48. Wirsching HG, Morel C, Gmür C, et al. Predicting outcome of epilepsy after meningioma resection. *Neuro Oncol*. 2016;18(7):1002–1010. https://doi.org/10.1093/neuonc/nov303.
49. Sun SQ, Hawasli AH, Huang J, Chicoine MR, Kim AH. An evidence-based treatment algorithm for the management of WHO grade II and III meningiomas. *Neurosurg Focus*. 2015;38(3):E3. https://doi.org/10.3171/2015.1.FOCUS14757.
50. Kaur G, Sayegh ET, Larson A, et al. Adjuvant radiotherapy for atypical and malignant meningiomas: a systematic review. *Neuro Oncol*. 2014;16(5):628–636. https://doi.org/10.1093/neuonc/nou025.
51. Walcott BP, Nahed BV, Brastianos PK, Loeffler JS. Radiation treatment for WHO grade II and III meningiomas. *Front Oncol*. 2013;3:227. https://doi.org/10.3389/fonc.2013.00227.
52. Observation or Radiation Therapy in Treating Patients with Newly Diagnosed Grade II Meningioma That Has Been Completely Removed by Surgery. *ClinicalTrials.gov*. Available at: https://clinicaltrials.gov/ct2/show/NCT03180268. Accessed June 13, 2019.
53. Radiation Therapy in Treating Patients Who Have Undergone Surgery for Newly Diagnosed Grade II or Grade III Meningioma. *ClinicalTrials.gov*. Available at: https://clinicaltrials.gov/ct2/show/NCT00626730. Accessed June 13, 2019.
54. Observation or Radiation Therapy in Treating Patients with Grade I, Grade II, or Grade III Meningioma. *ClinicalTrials.gov*. Available at: https://clinicaltrials.gov/ct2/show/NCT00895622. Accessed June 13, 2019.
55. Jenkinson MD, Javadpour M, Haylock BJ, et al. The ROAM/EORTC-1308 trial: radiation versus observation following surgical resection of atypical meningioma: study protocol for a randomised controlled trial. *Trials*. 2015;16(1):519. https://doi.org/10.1186/s13063-015-1040-3.
56. Brem SS, Bierman PJ, Brem H, et al. Central nervous system cancers. *J Natl Compr Canc Netw*. 2011;9(4):352–400.
57. Chuang HC, Lee HC, Cho DY. Intracranial malignant meningioma with multiple spinal metastases—a case report and literature review: case report. *Spine*. 2006;31(26):E1006–E1010. https://doi.org/10.1097/01.brs.0000245952.71265.9b.
58. Wen PY, Quant E, Drappatz J, Beroukhim R, Norden AD. Medical therapies for meningiomas. *J Neuro Oncol*. 2010;99(3):365–378. https://doi.org/10.1007/s11060-010-0349-8.
59. Bevacizumab in Treating Patients with Recurrent or Progressive Meningiomas. *ClinicalTrials.gov*. Available at: https://clinicaltrials.gov/ct2/show/NCT01125046. Accessed June 18, 2019.
60. An Open-Label Phase II Study of Nivolumab in Adult Participants with Recurrent High-Grade Meningioma. *ClinicalTrials.gov*. Available at: https://clinicaltrials.gov/ct2/show/NCT02648997. Accessed June 18, 2019.
61. Phase II Trial of Pembrolizumab in Recurrent or Residual High-Grade Meningioma. *ClinicalTrials.gov*. Available at: https://clinicaltrials.gov/ct2/show/NCT03279692. Accessed June 18, 2019.

62. Combination of Alpelisib and Trametinib in Progressive Refractory Meningiomas. *ClinicalTrials.gov*. Available at: https://clinicaltrials.gov/ct2/show/NCT03631953. Accessed June 18, 2019.
63. Vistusertib (AZD2014) For Recurrent Grade II-III Meningiomas. *ClinicalTrials.gov*. Available at: https://clinicaltrials.gov/ct2/show/NCT03071874. Accessed June 18, 2019.
64. Raizer JJ, Grimm SA, Rademaker A, et al. A phase II trial of PTK787/ZK 222584 in recurrent or progressive radiation and surgery refractory meningiomas. *J Neuro Oncol*. 2014;117(1):93–101. https://doi.org/10.1007/s11060-014-1358-9.
65. Swinnen LJ, Rankin C, Rushing EJ, Laura HF, Damek DM, Barger GR. Phase II study of hydroxyurea for unresectable meningioma (Southwest Oncology Group S9811). *J Clin Oncol*. 2009;27(suppl 15):2063–2063. https://doi.org/10.1200/jco.2009.27.15_suppl.2063.
66. Norden AD, Raizer JJ, Abrey LE, et al. Phase II trials of erlotinib or gefitinib in patients with recurrent meningioma. *J Neuro Oncol*. 2010;96(2):211–217. https://doi.org/10.1007/s11060-009-9948-7.
67. Koper JW, Zwarthoff EC, Hagemeijer A, et al. Inhibition of the growth of cultured human meningioma cells by recombinant interferon-alpha. *Eur J Cancer*. 1991;27(4):416–419.
68. Chamberlain MC. IFN-α for recurrent surgery- and radiation-refractory high-grade meningioma: a retrospective case series. *CNS Oncol*. 2013;2(3):227–235. https://doi.org/10.2217/cns.13.17.
69. Du Z, Abedalthagafi M, Aizer AA, et al. Increased expression of the immune modulatory molecule PD-L1 (CD274) in anaplastic meningioma. *Oncotarget*. 2015;6(7):4704–4716. https://doi.org/10.18632/oncotarget.3082.
70. Gelerstein E, Berger A, Jonas-Kimchi T, et al. Regression of intracranial meningioma following treatment with nivolumab: case report and review of the literature. *J Clin Neurosci*. 2017;37:51–53. https://doi.org/10.1016/j.jocn.2016.11.011.
71. Pilot Study of Optune (NovoTTF-100A) for Recurrent Atypical and Anaplastic Meningioma. *ClinicalTrials.gov*. Available at: https://clinicaltrials.gov/ct2/show/NCT01892397. Accessed July 24, 2019.
72. Optune Delivered Electric Field Therapy and Bevacizumab in Treating Patients with Recurrent or Progressive Grade 2 or 3 Meningioma. *ClinicalTrials.gov*. Available at: https://clinicaltrials.gov/ct2/show/NCT02847559. Accessed July 24, 2019.
73. Grimm SA, Kumthekar P, Chamberlain MC, et al. Phase II trial of bevacizumab in patients with surgery and radiation refractory progressive meningioma. *J Clin Oncol*. 2015;33(suppl 15):2055–2055. https://doi.org/10.1200/jco.2015.33.15_suppl.2055.
74. Chaichana KL, Pendleton C, Zaidi H, et al. Seizure control for patients undergoing meningioma surgery. *World Neurosurg*. 2013;79(3–4):515–524. https://doi.org/10.1016/j.wneu.2012.02.051.
75. Islim AI, McKeever S, Kusu-Orkar TE, Jenkinson MD. The role of prophylactic antiepileptic drugs for seizure prophylaxis in meningioma surgery: a systematic review. *J Clin Neurosci*. 2017;43:47–53. https://doi.org/10.1016/j.jocn.2017.05.020.
76. Komotar RJ, Raper DMS, Starke RM, Iorgulescu JB, Gutin PH. Prophylactic antiepileptic drug therapy in patients undergoing supratentorial meningioma resection: a systematic analysis of efficacy. *J Neurosurg*. 2011;115(3):483–490. https://doi.org/10.3171/2011.4.JNS101585.
77. Maruyama K, Shin M, Kurita H, Kawahara N, Morita A, Kirino T. Proposed treatment strategy for cavernous sinus meningiomas: a prospective study. *Neurosurgery*. 2004;55(5):1068–1075. https://doi.org/10.1227/01.NEU.0000140839.47922.5A.
78. Couldwell WT, Kan P, Liu JK, Apfelbaum RI. Decompression of cavernous sinus meningioma for preservation and improvement of cranial nerve function: technical note. *J Neurosurg*. 2006;105(1):148–152. https://doi.org/10.3171/jns.2006.105.1.148.
79. Abdel Aziz KM, Froelich SC, Dagnew E, et al. Large sphenoid wing meningiomas involving the cavernous sinus: conservative surgical strategies for better functional outcomes. *Neurosurgery*. 2004;54(6):1375–1384. https://doi.org/10.1227/01.NEU.0000125542.00834.6D.
80. Pandit R, Paris L, Rudich DS, Lesser RL, Kupersmith MJ, Miller NR. Long-term efficacy of fractionated conformal radiotherapy for the management of primary optic nerve sheath meningioma. *Br J Ophthalmol*. 2019;103:1436–1440. https://doi.org/10.1136/bjophthalmol-2018-313135.
81. Terpolilli NA, Ueberschaer M, Niyazi M, et al. Long-term outcome in orbital meningiomas: progression-free survival after targeted resection combined with early or postponed postoperative radiotherapy. *J Neurosurg*. 2019:1–11. https://doi.org/10.3171/2019.3.JNS181760.
82. Hendrix P, Fischer G, Linnebach AC, et al. Perioperative olfactory dysfunction in patients with meningiomas of the anteromedial skull base. *Clin Anat*. 2019;32(4):524–533. https://doi.org/10.1002/ca.23346.
83. Abel TJ, Manzel K, Bruss J, Belfi AM, Howard MA, Tranel D. The cognitive and behavioral effects of meningioma lesions involving ventromedial prefrontal cortex. *J Neurosurg*. 2016;124(6):1568–1577. https://doi.org/10.3171/2015.5.JNS142788.
84. Lee SR, Yang KA, Kim SK, Kim SH. Radiation-induced intratumoral necrosis and peritumoral edema after gamma knife radiosurgery for intracranial meningiomas. *J Korean Neurosurg Soc*. 2012;52(2):98–102. https://doi.org/10.3340/jkns.2012.52.2.98.

Chapter 11

Approach to the low-grade glioma patient

Carlos G. Romo, Ananyaa Sivakumar, and Matthias Holdhoff

CHAPTER OUTLINE

Introduction

The understanding of low-grade gliomas has significantly changed over the past 10 years. Genomic and epigenetic discoveries have revolutionized our understanding of these cancers. For the first time, the 2016 WHO classification of central nervous system tumors integrated molecular information with histologic classification to more precisely differentiate types of brain and spinal cord tumors. Previous histologic systems classified low-grade gliomas as astrocytomas, oligodendrogliomas, or mixed oligoastrocytomas based on their histologic appearance. Now, molecular classification has allowed for a more precise characterization of tumor biology (see Chapter 1 for further discussion of molecularly defined classification of gliomas).

Most diffuse low-grade gliomas can be separated into three molecularly, prognostically, and clinically distinct groups: (1) *Isocitrate dehydrogenase (IDH)*-gene mutated tumors with co-deletion of chromosomes 1p and 19q (e.g., *IDH*-mutated, co-deleted low-grade gliomas), (2) *IDH*-mutant non–co-deleted diffuse gliomas, and (3) *IDH* wild-type diffuse gliomas. This first group of *IDH*-mutant, co-deleted tumors are molecularly the pure oligodendrogliomas that are associated with a prolonged survival and an excellent response to chemotherapy. *IDH*-mutant, non–co-deleted tumors do not possess loss of chromosomes 1p and 19q (e.g., non–co-deleted) and are molecularly astrocytomas. They have an intermediate prognosis; compared to the *IDH*-wild-type gliomas, they have better survival rates and response to chemotherapy. *IDH* wild-type gliomas have the worst prognosis of the three groups and behave similarly to glioblastoma despite their lower grade.

Molecular characterization now not only influences our classification of gliomas but also guides molecularly driven clinical management decisions. Compared to treatment of high-grade gliomas, the decision for treatment of low-grade gliomas is more complex. Available data do not address all clinical questions that confront treating clinicians. One of the common challenges in clinical management of patients with low-grade gliomas is whether to initiate treatment at the time of first diagnosis or to wait until tumor growth is evident (e.g., timing of therapy). Another challenge is choosing which chemotherapeutic regimen is most optimal. Common regimens include temozolomide or lomustine, procarbazine, and vincristine (PCV) (see Chapter 4 for an evidence-based review of chemotherapy for glioma).

In this chapter, we present a single clinical case of a patient presenting with a low-grade glioma and walk through key data that guides the increasingly complex algorithms for managing patients with low-grade gliomas.

Clinical case

CASE 11.1 NEWLY DIAGNOSED LOW-GRADE GLIOMA PATIENT

Case. A 51-year-old woman without contributory medical history acutely developed word-finding difficulties. A few minutes later she lost consciousness, collapsed to the ground, and had generalized involuntary jerking movements consistent with a generalized tonic-clonic seizure. The episode lasted for approximately 2 minutes before she regained consciousness. She was evaluated in the emergency room where her physical examination was significant for lethargy and disorientation to place and situation. Her Karnofsky performance status (KPS) was 90%. A CT scan of the head revealed an area of hypodensity in the right parietal lobe; there were no signs concerning for intracranial hemorrhage.

Brain magnetic resonance imaging (MRI) with and without contrast was requested to better characterize the lesion (Fig. 11.1). The images showed an infiltrative lesion that involved the cortex and the subcortical white matter. The mass had a significant amount of perilesional T2/fluid attenuated inversion recovery (FLAIR) hyperintensity with minimal punctate contrast enhancement. The patient gradually recovered over the next 4 hours and was back to her baseline status without residual deficits on examination. She was started on levetiracetam 500 mg orally twice daily and dexamethasone 4 mg every 6 hours.

The patient was evaluated by a neurosurgeon who recommended performing an open biopsy through an awake craniotomy. The surgeon achieved a subtotal resection a few days after her initial presentation, while preserving eloquent brain regions. Histologic appearance was consistent with a low-grade oligodendroglioma, WHO grade II. The Ki-67 proliferation index was low and molecular studies revealed deletions of the entire short arm of chromosome 1 and the entire long arm of chromosome 19 (e.g., 1p/19q co-deletion), as well as an *IDH1* R132H gene mutation. Her seizures were controlled medically and she was tapered off corticosteroids quickly after surgery. Once the pathology results were available, neuro-oncology and radiation oncology consults were requested.

Key clinical questions for consideration by consultants:

1. What final diagnosis integrates the histopathologic analysis with molecular characterization?
2. Is this patient at high or low risk of early tumor progression?
3. Should active therapy be recommended now or is initial observation an option?
4. If treatment is recommended, which treatment should the patient receive?

Key points

Teaching point #1: How to determine an integrated histologic and molecular diagnosis of low-grade glioma

The tumor in this case was found to be a WHO grade II diffuse glioma with an *IDH1* gene mutation and whole arm loss of chromosomes 1p and 19q, which is consistent with a diagnosis of *IDH*-mutated, co-deleted low-grade glioma. Historically, the diagnosis of low-grade gliomas was based on histopathologic analysis showing a glial-based tumor that infiltrated brain tissue and was low-grade with no or low mitotic activity, no endothelial proliferation, and no pseudopallisading necrosis (representative examples shown in Fig. 11.2). Over the past decade, landmark discoveries, including genome-wide studies, have shown that profiling molecular characteristics of cancer provides a more accurate way to predict treatment response and risk of recurrence. Molecular features are now a major component in the diagnosis and subgrouping of tumors and trump histopathologic interpretation and provide a more precise description of the tumor's biology, as well as prognostic and treatment implications (Fig. 11.3). Occasionally, histopathologic findings in low-grade gliomas can be difficult to distinguish from a reactive process or other brain tumors. Pilocytic astrocytomas can have a morphology that resembles oligodendrogliomas. Some tumors have features of both oligodendrogliomas and astrocytomas, historically described as oligoastrocytomas or "mixed" gliomas. In these instances, molecular characterization can guide the diagnosis. In fact, in the most recent WHO classification of gliomas, this entity of "mixed" gliomas virtually ceases to exist and these tumors are classified as oligodendrogliomas (e.g., *IDH*-mutant, 1p19q co-deleted) or astrocytomas (e.g., *IDH*-mutant, non–co-deleted) based on molecular characteristics.

Integrated glioma diagnoses

Oligodendrogliomas are characterized by the presence of an *IDH1* or *IDH2* mutation and synchronous whole arm

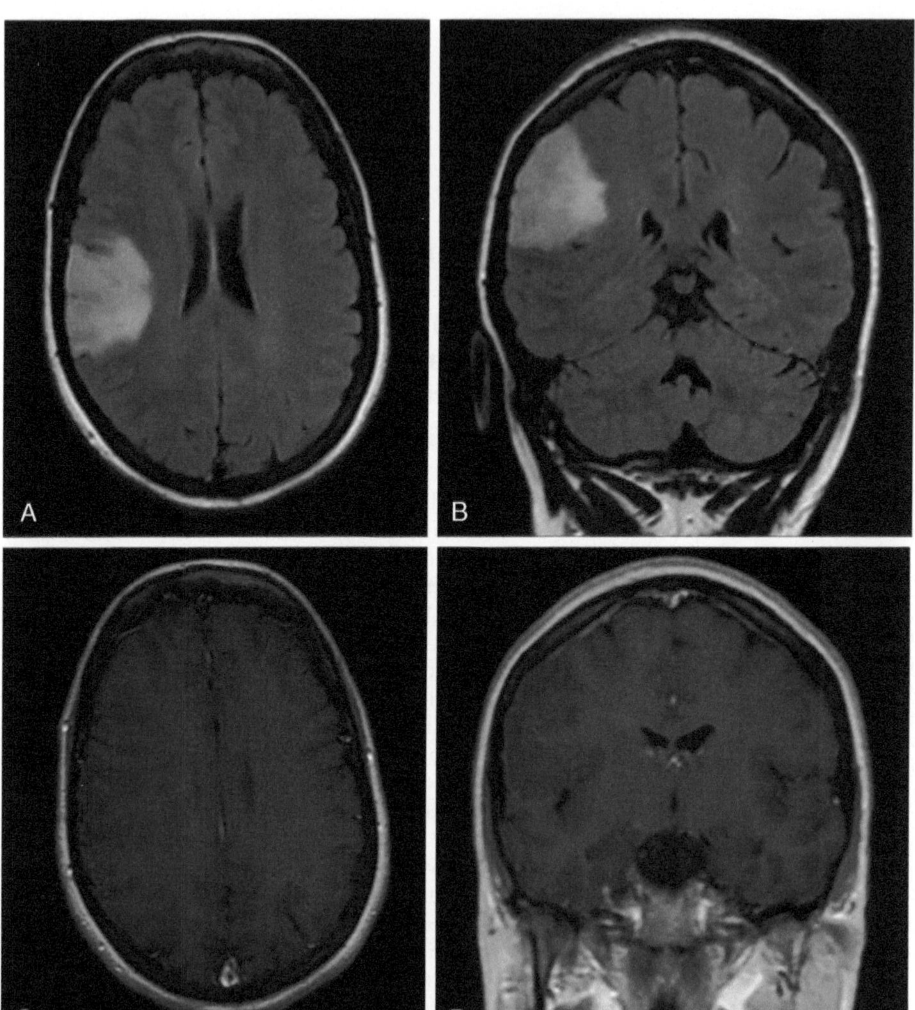

Fig. 11.1 Magnetic resonance images of the brain at the time of diagnosis. (A, B) FLAIR, axial and coronal sections demonstrating a right frontoparietal infiltrative lesion with perilesional edema affecting the cortex and subcortical white matter. (C, D) Axial and coronal T1 images after administration of gadolinium with small areas of faint contrast enhancement within the lesion. *FLAIR*, Fluid attenuated inversion recovery.

deletions of chromosomes 1p and 19q. Partial deletions of 1p and 19q do occur and are not associated with the oligodendroglial phenotype; they are frequently associated with tumors of astrocytic lineage, which carry a worse prognosis.[1,2] Oligodendrogliomas frequently have an activating mutation of the *TERT* promoter region[3–5] and mutations of the *CIC* and *FUBP1* genes.[5,6–8] Astrocytic tumors may also demonstrate *IDH1* or *IDH2* mutation but lack co-deletion of 1p/19q and *TERT* promoter mutations, and instead are characterized by a loss of *ATRX* and mutations in the *TP53* gene.[9]

Gliomas have a similar histologic appearance in adult and pediatric populations; however, the molecular signatures of low-grade gliomas differ by age. Approximately 80–90% of low-grade tumors in adult patients harbor a mutation in the *IDH1* or *IDH2* genes. By contrast, low-grade gliomas in children rarely have these mutations.[10] Adult patients with *IDH* wild-type diffuse astrocytomas carry a worse prognosis, especially those with a *TERT* promoter mutation, *EGFR* amplification, or a concurrent whole chromosome 10 loss and whole chromosome 7 gain.[11–14] Due to the more aggressive nature of these tumors, it has been

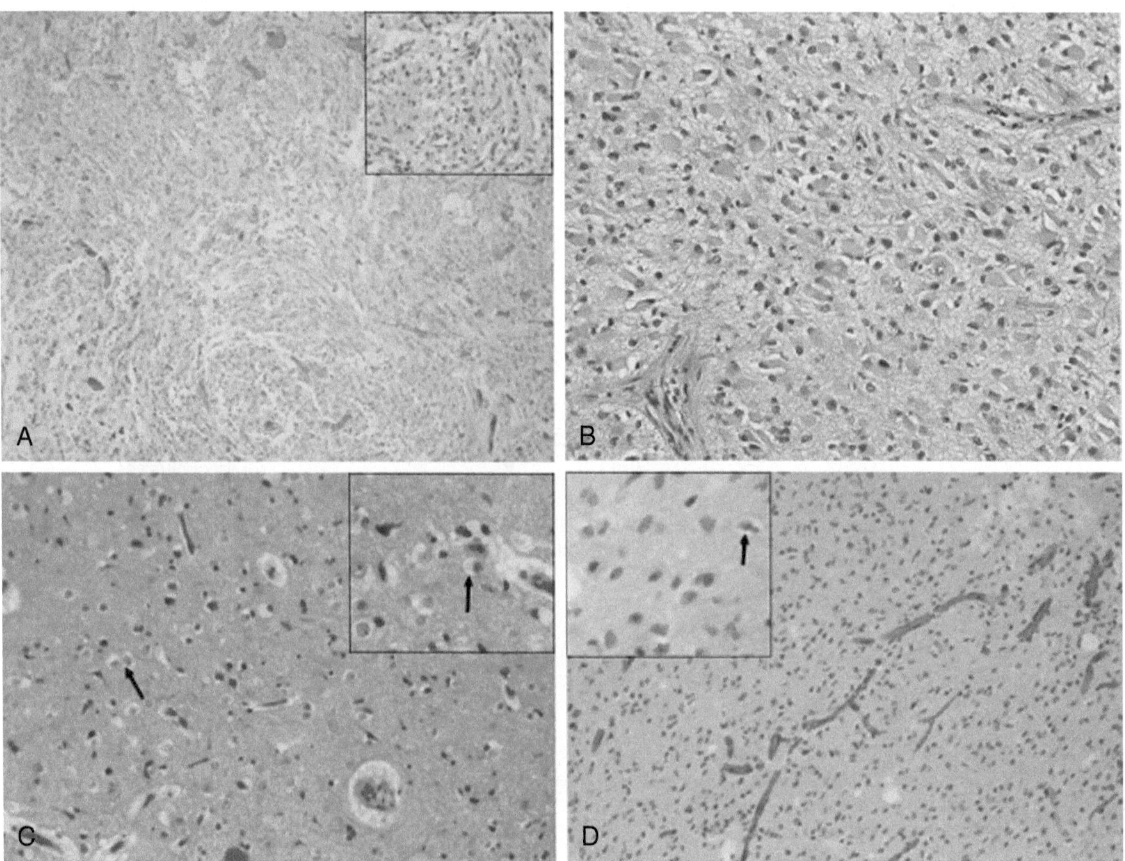

Fig. 11.2 Photomicrographs. (A) Pilocytic astrocytoma (WHO grade I) with low to moderate cellularity and a biphasic pattern of dense fibrillary regions alternating with loosely textured areas. (B) Diffuse astrocytoma (WHO grade II) is an infiltrating tumor with increased cellular density and nuclear atypia and a fibrillary background. The elongated processes are a hallmark of glial neoplasms and can aid in the diagnosis. Mitotic figures and vascular proliferation are absent. (C, D) Oligodendroglioma (WHO grade II) with monomorphic neoplastic cells and perinuclear clearing giving the typical "fried egg" appearance *(black arrows)*. The chromatin is loosely organized. Branching capillaries are frequently present and may form a network that resembles a "chicken wire".

suggested that they be classified as grade IV neoplasms, irrespective of their histologic appearance.[15]

In addition to low-grade diffuse oligodendrogliomas and diffuse astrocytomas, both of which are classified as WHO grade II tumors, there are a myriad of other low-grade gliomas. These include several histologic subtypes of tumors with an astrocytic lineage such as pilocytic astrocytoma (WHO grade I), pilomyxoid astrocytoma, gemistocytic astrocytoma, subependymal giant cell astrocytoma (SEGA), pleomorphic xanthoastrocytoma, and astroblastoma among others. Some of these tumors are exclusively seen in young adults and in the pediatric population. Other low-grade tumors arise from ependymal surfaces; these include subependymomas and ependymomas of different subtypes (myxopapillary, clear cell, tanacytic, and papillary).

Teaching point #2: How to differentiate high-risk from low-risk low-grade glioma

The patient in this case had both favorable and concerning clinical prognostic features at presentation. On the one hand, the patient was considered to be at high risk for early disease progression due to her age (i.e., >40 years), subtotal resection (instead of complete resection of the tumor), and the proximity of the tumor to eloquent brain areas. On the other hand, several favorable prognostic factors were also identified, including her good performance status, and favorable molecular features including the presence of 1p/19q co-deletion and *IDH*-gene mutation.

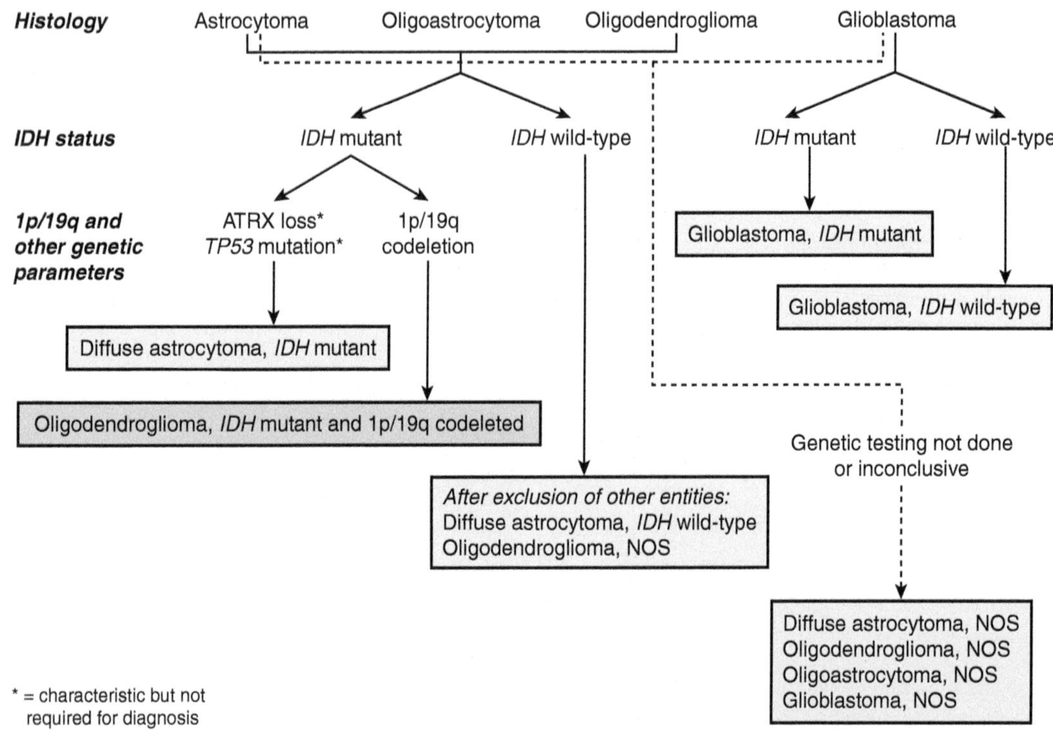

Fig. 11.3 A simplified algorithm for the classification of gliomas based on histologic and genetic features. Profiling the molecular characteristics of cancers allows for a more accurate classification of tumors; in some instances, genetic features may supersede morphologic characteristics in achieving an "integrated" diagnosis. *NOS*, Not otherwise specified. (From Louis DN, Perry A, Reifenberger G, et al. The 2016 World Health Organization of tumors of the central nervous system: a summary. *Acta Neuropathol.* 2016;131(6):803–820.)

Clinical presentation and prognostic risk factors

The clinical presentation of a low-grade glioma varies depending on the tumor location. Signs and symptoms may include seizures, headaches, changes in mental status, and other symptoms associated with intracranial hypertension. Imaging findings can suggest the etiology, but in most cases, pathologic examination of a tissue sample from a biopsy or resection is needed to confirm the diagnosis. A lumbar puncture for analysis of cerebrospinal fluid has low diagnostic yield and could lead to severe complications in cases where there is risk of herniation. Patients who present with seizures are managed with antiepileptics and, when focal neurologic deficits or symptoms of increased intracranial pressure are evidenced, corticosteroids are initiated.

The natural history and prognosis of low-grade gliomas is highly variable, and assessment of risk in newly diagnosed patients is complex. There are currently no uniformly agreed-upon validated criteria to assess risk factors for early progression and poor prognosis. However, several clinical risk factors have been identified that can be used in clinical decision-making. These include tumor-related symptoms, poor performance status, preoperative tumor size (worse if ≥5 cm), incomplete resection, age (high-risk is >40 years of age), astrocytic histology, and high proliferative index (poor if MIB-1 is >3%). In addition, the absence of *IDH* mutation and co-deletion of 1p/19q are adverse risk factors. Many of these factors represent a continuum (for example, age), and the interplay of the different factors needs to be carefully considered on an individual basis. The best possible risk assessment relies on a personalized evaluation of clinical, molecular, and treatment factors to determine those patients who may benefit from early postoperative treatment and those for whom initial observation may be appropriate.

Teaching point #3: How to determine whether to observe the tumor or initiate treatment at diagnosis

The treatment options in this case included (1) close observation and initiation of treatment at first evidence of tumor progression or (2) initiation of treatment now. Careful consideration of these options is best conducted by a multidisciplinary team that engages the patient and caregiver in shared decision-making. After careful deliberation, the patient and her multidisciplinary team opted to proceed with treatment.

Treatment of low-grade gliomas

When treated, low-grade gliomas are managed with maximal safe resection. Radiation therapy is recommended when residual tumor is present after surgical treatment or when patients are considered to be high-risk. The randomized European Organization for Research and Treatment of Cancer (EORTC) trial 22845 compared treatment with radiation at initial diagnosis versus deferring radiation to the time of progression in patients with low-grade gliomas.[16] This trial showed that early treatment did not affect overall survival. Median survival was 7.4 years in patients treated with immediate radiotherapy of 54 Gy in 6 weeks and 7.2 years in patients who were treated at progression. However, early treatment was associated with prolonged progression-free survival (median 5.4 versus 3.7 years) and reduced seizure burden at 1 year. The lack of an overall survival benefit from early treatment with radiation has served as a rationale for postponing adjuvant radiation in patients with low-grade gliomas who are appropriate for initial observation, thereby delaying radiation-related toxicity. This must be weighed against the potential benefit of delaying tumor progression and controlling seizures.

A select group of low-grade gliomas may be treated with targeted therapies. That is the case for the subependymal giant cell astrocytomas (SEGAs) that occur in tuberous sclerosis complex (see Chapter 17, Case 17.4 for the approach to SEGA in tuberous sclerosis) for which treatment with an inhibitor of the mammalian target of rapamycin (mTOR) pathway (e.g., everolimus or sirolimus) has been shown to be effective. Patients with pleomorphic xanthoastrocytomas, and to a lesser extent those with pilocytic astrocytomas, commonly harbor a *BRAF* V600E gene mutation and have shown responses to treatment with the combination of BRAF and MEK inhibitors. To minimize the risk of adverse effects, these therapies require specific screening studies before their administration and patients should be monitored closely while on treatment for signs of complications and tumor progression.

Teaching point #4: How to determine a patient-specific treatment plan

The patient in this case was treated with radiation therapy followed by six cycles of adjuvant chemotherapy with PCV. The patient required dose reductions of her chemotherapy due to myelosuppression, and vincristine was discontinued after two cycles due to early signs of neuropathy that later resolved. After treatment, she was closely monitored with MRI images every 3 months for 2 years and then every 6 months. She continues to be observed with serial MR scans 7 years after her initial diagnosis, with no evidence of tumor recurrence.

The role of surgery

Diffuse low-grade gliomas (with the exception of *IDH* wild-type gliomas) typically grow slower than the high-grade malignant gliomas (e.g., WHO grade III and grade IV gliomas). They follow a more indolent disease course. Nonetheless, these tumors are not considered curable, and the majority of patients eventually die from their disease or disease-related complications. The goal of treating these cancers is to not only prolong survival and time to tumor recurrence but to also carefully consider treatment-related morbidity, as patients often live for several years and sometimes decades with their disease. Treatment decisions are best made with a multidisciplinary team including neurosurgeons, medical or neuro-oncologists, and radiation oncologists. Surgery is usually the first step in management of low-grade gliomas (see Chapter 2 for further discussion of surgical approaches to glioma). Surgery helps to establish the diagnosis and provides cytoreduction through debulking of the tumor. The extent of surgery is location-dependent, and some patients are candidates for biopsy only. In rare situations, such as in some brainstem locations, even a biopsy is not feasible.

The benefit of greater extents of resection has been a controversial topic. Immediate best possible surgical resection is most commonly pursued. In select cases of small, asymptomatic, or minimally symptomatic tumors (including in patients with controlled seizures), initial observation can be considered, with more aggressive resection reserved for time of progression or worsening symptoms. Arguments for early diagnosis and best possible resection include (1) maximizing reduction of tumor burden; (2) allowing for accurate risk assessment based on histological features, tumor grade, and molecular markers at the time of diagnosis; and (3) improved assessment of prognosis, treatment choice, and timing of postoperative therapy.

The role of chemotherapy

To date, the largest clinical trial that has addressed the question of a potential benefit from adding chemotherapy to radiation is the Radiation Therapy in Oncology Group study RTOG 9802[17] (also see Chapter 4 for review of evidence-based approaches to chemotherapy for glioma). In this study, 251 adult patients with supratentorial low-grade gliomas were randomized to receive either radiation alone or radiation followed by chemotherapy with lomustine, procarbazine, and vincristine (PCV, planned six cycles). Patients with oligodendrogliomas, astrocytomas, and oligoastrocytomas were included. As this study was designed prior to the discovery of the role of *IDH* mutations and co-deletion of 1p/19q, these molecular markers could not be factored into the analysis. Also, this study started prior to the introduction of temozolomide as a treatment option for patients with gliomas. RTOG 9802 showed an overall survival benefit from the addition of PCV chemotherapy to radiation compared to radiation alone of 13.3 versus 7.8 years, which was statistically significant. Separated by histology, there were clear differences in magnitude of benefit from chemotherapy in association with histology. Patients with oligodendrogliomas derived the most overall benefit, followed by oligoastrocytomas, followed by astrocytomas; although there was a separation in survival curves also in patients with astrocytomas, the benefit from the addition of PCV was not statistically significant in this subgroup (Fig. 11.4)[17]. In tumors for which *IDH* mutation data were available, a clear overall benefit from the addition of chemotherapy was observed. As this study did not include information on 1p/19q co-deletion, and only incomplete *IDH* mutation data, these data need to be interpreted with great caution. In patients with low-grade astrocytomas, the benefit of the addition of chemotherapy to radiation has not yet fully been elucidated and remains controversial.[18]

Teaching point #5: How to select a patient-specific chemotherapy regimen

The patient in this case was treated with PCV—procarbazine, CCNU or lomustine, and vincristine. The choice of chemotherapy for low-grade gliomas remains controversial and many clinicians consider either temozolomide or PCV (see Chapter 4 for evidence-based approach to chemotherapy for glioma); however, head-to-head data are not available; and it is not currently known whether these regimens are interchangeable or whether one is more effective.

In 1p/19q co-deleted oligodendrogliomas with *IDH* mutation, the highest level of evidence exists for the use of radiation and PCV based on data extrapolated from several clinical trials in patients with anaplastic oligodendroglioma (i.e., EORTC 26951 and RTOG 9402) and in low-grade gliomas (i.e., RTOG 9802). Temozolomide is the standard chemotherapy used in the treatment of glioblastoma and other malignant gliomas (i.e., WHO grade III and grade IV gliomas). Importantly, PCV was not shown to have comparable benefit to temozolomide in treating glioblastoma or anaplastic astrocytoma, and these two chemotherapy regimens cannot be considered interchangeable. Chemoradiation with temozolomide followed by adjuvant temozolomide is the standard of care for treatment of glioblastoma and tends to be tolerated better than PCV with lower adverse event rates. Temozolomide may also have the advantage of functioning as a radiation sensitizer when administered during the concurrent radiation treatment phase. However, these two regimens have not been prospectively compared in patients with low-grade gliomas, and controversy remains.

Low-grade gliomas with co-deletion of 1p/19q are markedly more sensitive to chemotherapy than gliomas without co-deletion. In select patients with co-deleted oligodendrogliomas for whom treatment is needed but there is concern for radiation-related side effects (e.g., due to tumor size, age, and frailty), treatment with chemotherapy alone with deferred radiation may be considered. Data on long-term outcomes with this approach are limited. This approach should therefore only be considered with great caution. A multidisciplinary evaluation may be helpful to carefully weigh the short- and long-term risks and benefits and select a patient-specific approach to treatment.

Patient-specific treatment using molecularly defined algorithm for low-grade gliomas

Approach to *IDH*-mutant low-grade gliomas

In general, newly diagnosed *IDH*-mutant low-grade gliomas can be divided into co-deleted and non–co-deleted tumors. The prognosis for tumors that are *IDH*-mutant and 1p/19q co-deleted ("true" oligodendrogliomas) is more favorable than for patients without co-deletion (i.e., mostly astrocytomas). Some patients may have had prior brain imaging, which can be helpful in assessing tumor aggressiveness based on growth over time. In patients who do not have prior imaging data available, risk assessment is based on clinical, histopathologic, and molecular factors alone.

Observation with deferred treatment

Based on data from the study EORTC 22845, observation of low-risk asymptomatic patients, including patients with controlled seizures, is reasonable and typically includes magnetic resonance imaging every 3 months, which is gradually lengthened in patients whose gliomas show stability. If rapid tumor growth is detected, new symptoms occur, or if there is concern for malignant degeneration to a higher grade (e.g., new contrast enhancement), treatment is initiated. In select cases, if there is concern for progression to a higher grade or more aggressive biology, repeat neurosurgical biopsy or resection may be considered.

Treatment approach

Once a patient is considered appropriate for postoperative therapy (either immediately, or after observation), a

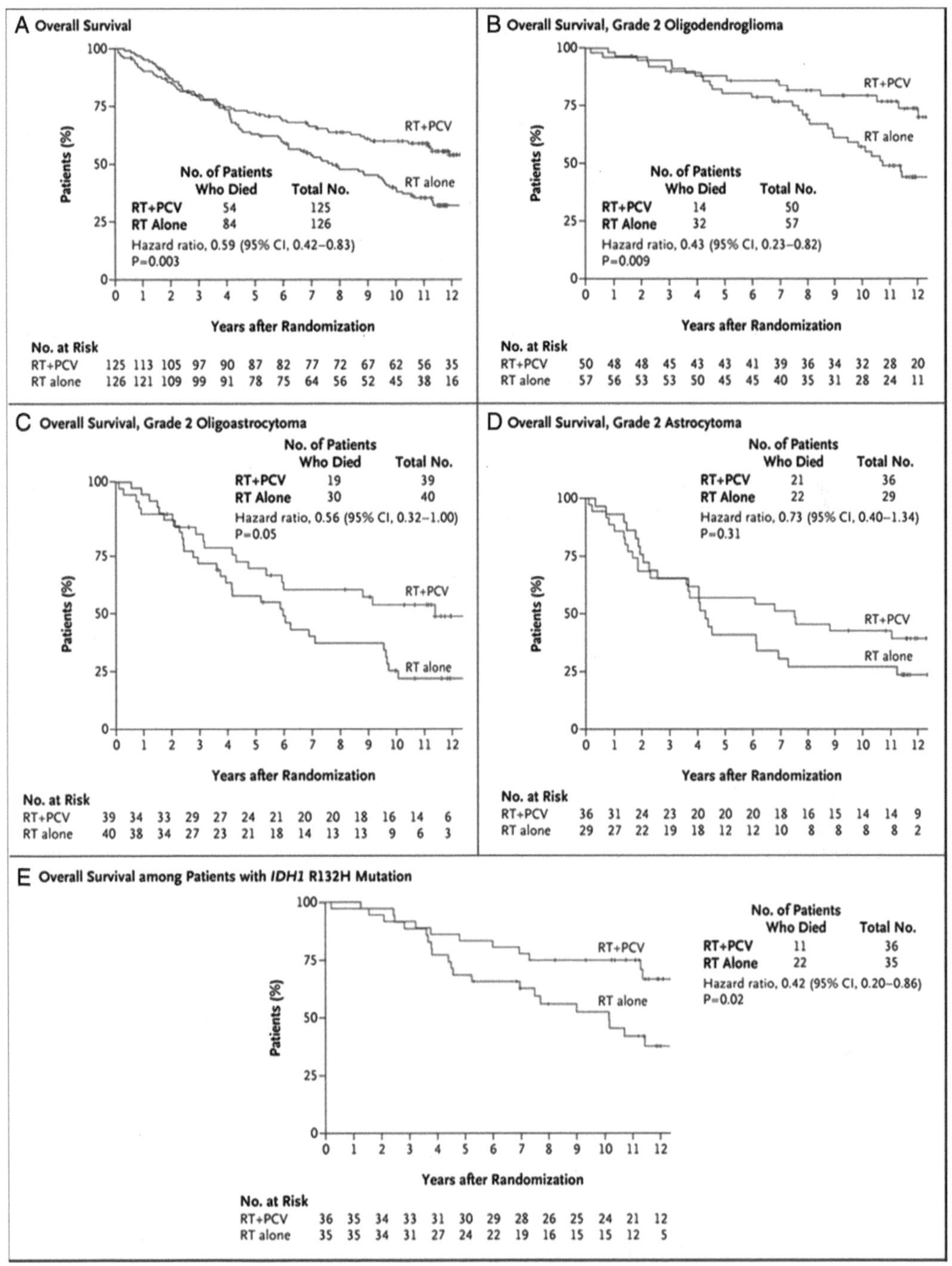

Fig. 11.4 Overall survival according to tumor type and treatment group. Treatment included radiation as monotherapy vs radiation in combination with a chemotherapy combination regimen (*PCV*: procarbazine, lomustine, and vincristine). A. Overall survival for the total number of patients in the study; B. Overall survival for patients with grade 2 oligodendroglioma; C. Overall survival for those with a grade 2 oligoastrocytoma; D. Overall survival for patients with a grade 2 astrocytoma; and E. Overall survival in the cohort of patients with an *IDH1* R132H mutation. All hazard ratios in the analyses of overall survival are for death, and all *P* values are two-sided. *CI*, Confidence interval; *RT*, radiotherapy. (From Buckner JC, Shaw EG, Pugh SL, et al. Radiation plus procarbazine, CCNU, and vincristine in low-grade glioma. *N Engl J Med.* 2016;374(14):1344–1355.)

decision should be made regarding a treatment regimen. Options include radiation followed by PCV or concurrent chemoradiation with temozolomide followed by adjuvant temozolomide. In select cases, chemotherapy alone with deferred radiation may be carefully considered.

- For 1p/19q co-deleted oligodendrogliomas, randomized phase 3 data from RTOG 9802 indicates that the most evidence-based treatment is radiation plus PCV. Many clinicians also consider chemoradiation with temozolomide followed by temozolomide an effective therapy for these patients. To date, these two regimens have never been prospectively compared in this population. A large ongoing clinical trial (i.e., CODEL study, NCT00887146), is comparing the two regimens in 1p/19q co-deleted gliomas and will eventually answer this question.
- For *IDH*-mutant non–co-deleted astrocytomas, the optimal treatment regimen is not as clear. The benefit from chemotherapy with PCV in these tumors has remained controversial (see Fig. 11.3). Data from the randomized phase 3 RTOG 9802 study provides the highest level of published evidence and shows a modest benefit from adding PCV to radiation therapy in patients with histologically defined astrocytomas. This study was not designed to prospectively compare outcomes by molecular subgroup and did not compare chemotherapy regimens. Low-grade astrocytomas will eventually progress to become anaplastic astrocytomas (WHO grade III) and/or glioblastomas (WHO grade IV), for which the most evidence-based therapy is temozolomide. Thus, some clinicians will extrapolate data from WHO grade III and grade IV gliomas, which favor the use of temozolomide over PCV in *IDH*-mutant non–co-deleted tumors. Further prospective data are needed to more definitively address this question.

Approach to *IDH* wild-type low-grade gliomas

A fraction of tumors with morphologic characteristics suggestive of a low-grade glioma carry molecular signatures that more resemble higher-grade neoplasms. The biology of these tumors is frequently more aggressive and patients tend to have worse outcomes.[9,12,19,20] This group is heterogeneous but, in general, these gliomas do not harbor mutations in the *IDH1* or *IDH2* genes and are *IDH* wild-type. Some *IDH* wild-type diffuse gliomas will develop in midline structures including the pons, thalamus, spinal cord, and parasagittal cortex. These tumors are considered diffuse midline gliomas and may harbor mutations in histone coding genes. Mutation of the *H3F3A* gene at the K27 position (i.e., H3 K27M mutation) is the most common of these alterations and confers a high-grade WHO grade IV classification even when routine pathologic criteria such as proliferation index may suggest lower-grade histology. Diffuse midline gliomas and the H3 K27M-mutant glioma are more frequently diagnosed in children and adolescents, but can present at any age and carry a dismal prognosis.

Additional molecular findings can aid in prognosticating patients with *IDH* wild-type low-grade gliomas. The presence of an *EGFR* amplification, *TERT* promoter mutation, or combined gain of chromosome 7 and loss of chromosome 10 (+7/−10) have been associated with an aggressive clinical course.[15,21] Patients with *IDH* wild-type diffuse gliomas are monitored closely with serial physical examinations and MRI studies. The optimal approach to treatment for these patients is not well established and should be individualized. Early treatment including radiation and chemotherapy may be offered. Participation in a clinical trial should be encouraged when possible; however, classification of these tumors as high-grade gliomas has not yet been widely adopted, and most clinical trials currently exclude patients with tumors that have a low-grade diagnosis by histology.

Approach to seizure management in low-grade gliomas

Seizures are common at initial presentation in patients with low-grade gliomas.[22] This patient population has a higher incidence of seizures when compared to patients with higher-grade neoplasms or metastatic central nervous system (CNS) disease. The overall frequency has been reported between 53% and 90%.[23–26] The majority of seizures are focal, but secondary generalization can occur. As with other forms of focal epilepsy, the semiology of the events depends on the location of the lesion. Tumors involving the frontal, temporal, and parietal cortex have a higher frequency of epileptic activity, especially if they are located in eloquent areas.[23,27] Other factors associated with the development of seizures include tumor burden and cortical involvement.[28] Interestingly, tumor progression, rate of growth, or mass effect have not been strongly associated with a higher frequency of seizures.[23,28,29] Conversely, gross total resection of the tumor correlates with improved seizure freedom.[30]

In patients with primary brain tumors, including low-grade gliomas, who have never experienced a seizure, the use of prophylactic anticonvulsants is not recommended.[31] Randomized studies evaluating seizure prophylaxis have failed to show a significant improvement in seizure-free survival.[32–35] If used, perioperative prophylactic anticonvulsants may be tapered 1 week after craniotomy to avoid the potential deleterious effects of these medications and their interactions with other drugs.[31,34,36]

Well-established treatment options for tumor-related epilepsy primarily include anticonvulsant medications and resection of the epileptic focus. The basic tenets of treatment for epilepsy in patients with brain tumors is not significantly different from those with other types of symptomatic focal seizures. Although no evidence-based guidelines are available for this patient population, a few considerations are important when choosing an anticonvulsant regimen. When possible, monotherapy is preferable to decrease the risk of adverse effects and to avoid interactions with other medications. Unfortunately, refractory seizures are common, and a combination of drugs might be necessary. Several anticonvulsants have been studied (Table 11.1). Levetiracetam is commonly prescribed as a first-line therapy due to its favorable efficacy, tolerability, and few interactions with other medications.[37–39] The efficacy of lacosamide as an adjunctive agent has been evaluated in patients with gliomas and metastatic tumors with focal seizures with or without secondary generalization. A 50% reduction in seizure frequency was reported in 40–50% of patients, and seizure-freedom was reported to be as high as 43%.[40–42] Lacosamide is generally well tolerated and does not have significant drug-to-drug interactions.

Anticonvulsants that induce cytochrome P450 (CYP) and glucuronyl transferase (GT) should be used with caution, as they have the potential of decreasing the concentrations and efficacy of other medications including chemotherapy and corticosteroids.[67] For this reason, phenytoin, phenobarbital, carbamazepine, and primidone are often not favored as long-term anticonvulsants but can be helpful for acute management. Topiramate may also induce hepatic enzymes when prescribed at doses higher than 200 mg per day.

Valproic acid is an effective antiepileptic agent in patients with gliomas and has been studied, with little success, as an adjunctive antineoplastic agent due to its histone deacetylase activity.[48,68–70] It is an inhibitor of several isoenzymes of the CYP enzymatic system and can lead to increased concentrations of chemotherapy.[67] Hematologic complications, including neutropenia and thrombocytopenia, can be exacerbated when valproic acid is administered concurrently with chemotherapy agents metabolized by this CYP system.[51]

Additional therapies have been explored with different degrees of success, including ketogenic and modified Atkins diets, laser interstitial thermal therapy (LITT), as well as interstitial and stereotactic radiosurgery of the epileptic focus.[71–76] Studies have shown an improvement in seizure control in patients with low-grade gliomas treated with early radiation therapy, even those with medically intractable seizures.[16,77] It is important to note that radiation did not improve the performance status of these patients and that it may lead to cognitive dysfunction.

Approach to the diagnosis and management of neurological complications of treatment for low-grade gliomas

As the survival of patients with primary brain tumors improves, so does the prevalence of adverse effects associated with their treatments. These can present acutely, subacutely, or as chronic sequelae of therapy. Neurologic deficits that result from surgical interventions are typically acute and may decrease overall survival.[78] For this reason, a more aggressive surgical approach with greater cytoreduction may not be ideal, and a maximal safe resection should be attempted. To minimize the risk of surgically induced deficits, functional and intraoperative MRI, preoperative cortical mapping, awake craniotomies, and neurophysiological intraoperative monitoring have been used.

Acute neurological complications of radiation (during treatment)

Neurologic complications from radiotherapy that occur during treatment and up to 1 month after its completion are considered acute. They include headache, nausea, and vomiting. Injury to capillaries can exacerbate edema and cause worsening neurologic deficits.[79] Additionally, nonspecific side effects may occur in the acute phase, such as fatigue, changes in the sense of taste, decreased salivation, loss of appetite, and alopecia. Several risk factors for developing these complications have been identified and include large treatment volumes, high total doses of radiation (>5000 cGy), higher dose per fraction (>200 cGy), longer periods of treatment, repeat courses of radiotherapy, and stereotactic radiosurgery. Certain chemotherapy agents may have radiosensitizing properties and increase the risk of complications such as taxanes, irinotecan, and methotrexate. Their concurrent use with radiation should be avoided. Patients at the extremes of life tend to be more sensitive to radiation and have a higher incidence of side effects, especially children under 5 years of age and adults over 60 years.[80]

Subacute neurological complications of radiation (within 1–6 months of treatment)

Subacute complications from radiation therapy occur between 1 and 6 months after completion of treatment. These may include worsening fatigue, cognitive deficits, and drowsiness. Pseudoprogression is frequently encountered during this period of time. It is characterized by changes on imaging studies that mimic tumor progression including an increase of contrast enhancement and T2/FLAIR hyperintensities. These abnormalities are often accompanied by deterioration of focal neurologic deficits, headaches, and somnolence. Changes on clinical exam and imaging due to pseudoprogression tend to be reversible and improve with corticosteroids and bevacizumab. On the other hand, adverse effects from radiation that present more than 6 months after therapy are typically permanent deficits. Cognitive deficits can develop in an insidious pattern and can range in severity from minor memory deficits to severe dementia.

Table 11.1 Anticonvulsants studied in patients with tumor-related epilepsy

Anticonvulsant	Initial dose	Maintenance dose	Common side effects	Mechanism of action	Other considerations	Ref
Levetiracetam	500 mg BID	500–1500 mg BID	Somnolence, irritability, asthenia	Proposed mechanisms include inhibition of Ca^{+} channels and binding to synaptic vesicle protein 2 (SV2A)	Dose adjustments might be necessary in patients with renal impairment.	Lim et al., 2009[43]; Maschio et al., 2011b[37]; Dinapoli et al., 2009[44]
Lacosamide	50–100 mg BID	150–200 mg BID	Dizziness, blurred vision, nausea	Slow inactivation of ionotropic voltage-gated Na^{+} channels	Risk of bradycardia and AV block. EKG prior to therapy in patients with cardiac conduction abnormalities.	Ruda et al., 2018[45]; Villanueva et al., 2016[42]; Sepulveda-Sanchez et al., 2017[46]
Zonisamide	50 mg at bedtime	400 mg at bedtime	Dizziness, ataxia, somnolence	Na^{+} and Ca^{+} channel inhibitor	Monitor kidney function periodically, adjustments might be necessary in patients with renal impairment.	Maschio et al., 2017[47]; Maschio et al., 2009b[48]
Lamotrigine	12.5–25 mg daily	100–300 mg BID	Nausea, ataxia, tremor, vivid dreams	Ionotropic voltage-gated Na^{+} channel inhibitor	Slow titration to a therapeutic dose is critical. SJS/TEN, DRESS and HLH are rare but potentially fatal.	Cacho-Diaz, San-Juan, Salmeron, Boyzo, & Lorenzana-Mendoza, 2018[49]; van Breemen, Wilms, & Vecht, 2007[50]
Valproic acid	10–15 mg/kg per day	Max 60 mg/kg per day	Tremor, weight gain, hair loss, dizziness	Acts as a GABA receptor agonist and possibly inhibits glutamate transmission at NMDA receptors	Life-threatening hepatotoxicity and pancreatitis may occur. Highly teratogenic.	Kerkhof et al., 2013[39]; Bourg, Lebrun, Chichmanian, Thomas, & Frenay, 2001[51]

Table 11.1 Anticonvulsants studied in patients with tumor-related epilepsy.—cont'd

Anticonvulsant	Initial dose	Maintenance dose	Common side effects	Mechanism of action	Other considerations	Ref
Pregabalin	50–75 mg BID	75–300 mg BID	Dizziness, somnolence, peripheral edema	Modulates activity at Ca^+ channels	Use with caution in patients with heart failure.	Rossetti et al., 2014[52]; Novy, Stupp, & Rossetti, 2009[53]; Maschio et al., 2012b[54]
Topiramate	25 mg BID	50–200 mg BID	Impaired cognition, fatigue, paresthesia, weight loss	Acts as a GABA receptor agonist, inhibits ionotropic voltage-gated Na^+ channels and NMDA receptors	Nephrolithiasis may occur. Concurrent use with valproate may increase the risk of adverse effects.	Maschio et al., 2008a[55]; Maschio et al., 2008b[56]
Clobazam	5 mg BID	20 mg BID	Sedation, ataxia, irritability	GABA-A receptor agonist with a half-life of 36 hours.	Risk of respiratory depression increases when used with other sedatives or narcotics.	Jennesson, van Eeghen, Caruso, Paolini, & Thiele, 2013[57]; Thome-Souza et al., 2016[58]; Vecht, Royer-Perron, Houillier, & Huberfeld, 2017b[59]
Oxcarbazepine	300 mg BID	600 mg BID	Somnolence, ataxia, diplopia, tremor, rash	Ionotropic voltage-gated Na^+ channel inhibitor	Periodic monitoring of sodium levels. May cause pancytopenia, monitor closely especially if used concurrently with chemotherapy.	Mauro et al., 2007[60]; Maschio et al., 2012a[61]; Maschio et al., 2009a[62]
Perampanel	2 mg at bedtime	8–12 mg at bedtime	Somnolence, vertigo, irritability, lethargy	AMPA receptor inhibition	Serious psychiatric events have been reported.	Vecht et al., 2017a[63]; Maschio et al., 2019[64]; Dunn-Pirio et al., 2018[65]
Vigabatrin	500 mg BID	1000–1500 mg BID	Irreversible visual field defects, lethargy	Inhibits GABA transaminase	Risk of vision loss; vision assessment at baseline.	Overwater et al., 2015[66]

AMPA, Alpha-amino-3-hydroxy-5-methyl-4-isoxazolepropionic acid; *AV*, atrioventricular; *BID*, twice daily; *Ca+*, calcium; *DRESS*, drug rash with eosinophilia and systemic symptoms; *EKG*, electrocardiogram; *GABA*, gamma aminobutyric acid; *HLH*, hemophagocytic lymphohistiocytosis; *Na+*, sodium; *NMDA*, *N*-methyl-D-aspartate; *SJS*, Stevens-Johnson syndrome; *TEN*, toxic epidermal necrolysis.

Chronic neurological complications from radiation (late events)

The treatment of cognitive deficits associated with radiation therapy is challenging (see Chapter 25 for further discussion of managing radiation-induced neurocognitive decline), and potential neuroprotective agents have largely been unsuccessful in preventing their development. Deteriorating cognition including inattention and slow processing is frequently multifactorial. Its evaluation should include anamnesis of sleeping patterns, a review of medications, particularly sedative and anticholinergic drugs, as well as screening for depression and anxiety. Radiation-induced endocrine dysfunction including central hypothyroidism, hypogonadism, and adrenal insufficiency should also be ruled out and treated if present, as it may contribute to cognitive deficits. Imaging of the brain may aid in identifying other potentially reversible causes of cognitive decline, including a chronic subdural hematoma or hydrocephalus. Lesions in the frontal lobes may lead to personality changes, apathy, and abulia; these signs should be distinguished from cognitive decline, as their management is different.

Limited data is available to guide the treatment of cognitive dysfunction, especially in patients with low-grade gliomas. The use of stimulants including methylphenidate and modafinil has been evaluated in patients with primary or metastatic tumors to both prevent and treat memory loss, with modest to no benefit in quality of life.[81–83] When successful, they improve attention deficit, depressed mood, and ameliorate fatigue. Donepezil is an acetylcholinesterase inhibitor used off label for the treatment of radiation-induced cognitive deficits. Available data regarding its benefits are conflicting. A phase III randomized, placebo-controlled study showed no benefit on its primary endpoint, a composite score of eight individual cognitive assessment tools[84]; on the other hand, a phase 2 study of 35 patients reported improvement in cognitive functioning, mood, and quality of life as measured by performance status and patient responses to a functional assessment questionnaire (FACT-Br).[85] Memantine, an *N*-methyl-D-aspartate (NMDA) receptor antagonist, was studied in a randomized, double-blind, placebo-controlled trial with 149 analyzable patients. The study showed a trend toward improvement in time to cognitive decline, but the difference from placebo was not statistically significant.[86] Memantine is generally well tolerated, but its cost may be prohibitive. In addition to these medications, seizure control in tumor-associated epilepsy may improve cognition and functional status.[87,88]

Neurological complications of chemotherapy

Complications from chemotherapy agents used in the treatment of low-grade gliomas may affect the central and peripheral nervous systems. Vincristine, a vinca alkaloid that inhibits microtubule formation, may be administered to patients with oligodendrogliomas as part of the "PCV" regimen along with procarbazine and lomustine. Neurologic side effects from vincristine include encephalopathy, cranial nerve dysfunction, and, more frequently, peripheral neuropathy. Due to concerns for poor CNS distribution as a result of its low penetration through the blood-brain barrier, vincristine is commonly discontinued when adverse reactions occur without compromising the efficacy of treatment. Procarbazine may also cause acute encephalopathy, headache, and delirium. The risk for these adverse effects is greater if there is concurrent use of sympathomimetic agents or consumption of tyramine-containing foods due to its minor activity as a monoamine oxidase inhibitor. Patients are instructed to follow a tyramine-free diet during procarbazine treatment to avoid such reactions. Lomustine is considered to be the most active component of the PCV regimen. A common toxicity is myelosuppression. Neurologic complications are rare, but ataxia, encephalopathy, dysarthria, and lethargy have been reported with an unclear association to the drug. Temozolomide has also shown activity against low-grade gliomas, as previously described, and its role in patients with 1p/19q co-deleted oligodendrogliomas is currently being studied in the CODEL trial (NCT00887146).[89–93] Temozolomide is generally well tolerated with no significant neurologic side effects. Fatigue is a common nonspecific complaint. Headache and ataxia have been reported, as well as a potential flare-up of focal neurologic deficits upon initiation of treatment.[94] These adverse events tend to be self-limited over time.

References

1. Vogazianou AP, Chan R, Backlund LM, et al. Distinct patterns of 1p and 19q alterations identify subtypes of human gliomas that have different prognoses. *Neuro Oncol*. 2010;12(7):664–678. https://doi.org/10.1093/neuonc/nop075.
2. Romo CG, Palsgrove DN, Sivakumar A, et al. Widely metastatic IDH1-mutant glioblastoma with oligodendroglial features and atypical molecular findings: a case report and review of current challenges in molecular diagnostics. *Diagn Pathol*. 2019;14(1):1–5. https://doi.org/10.1186/s13000-019-0793-5.
3. Arita H, Narita Y, Fukushima S, et al. Upregulating mutations in the TERT promoter commonly occur in adult malignant gliomas and are strongly associated with total 1p19q loss. *Acta Neuropathol*. 2013;126(2):267–276. https://doi.org/10.1007/s00401-013-1141-6.

4. Killela PJ, Reitman ZJ, Jiao Y, et al. TERT promoter mutations occur frequently in gliomas and a subset of tumors derived from cells with low rates of self-renewal. *Proc Natl Acad Sci U S A*. 2013;110(15):6021–6026. https://doi.org/10.1073/pnas.1303607110.
5. Suzuki H, Aoki K, Chiba K, et al. Mutational landscape and clonal architecture in grade II and III gliomas. *Nat Genet*. 2015;47(5):458–468. https://doi.org/10.1038/ng.3273.
6. Yip S, Butterfield YS, Morozova O, et al. Concurrent CIC mutations, IDH mutations, and 1p/19q loss distinguish oligodendrogliomas from other cancers. *J Pathol*. 2012;226(1):7–16. https://doi.org/10.1002/path.2995.
7. Bettegowda C, Agrawal N, Jiao Y, et al. Mutations in CIC and FUBP1 contribute to human oligodendroglioma. *Science*. 2011;333(6048):1453–1455. https://doi.org/10.1126/science.1210557.
8. Sahm F, Koelsche C, Meyer J, et al. CIC and FUBP1 mutations in oligodendrogliomas, oligoastrocytomas and astrocytomas. *Acta Neuropathol*. 2012;123(6):853–860. https://doi.org/10.1007/s00401-012-0993-5.
9. Cancer Genome Atlas Research Network, Brat DJ, Verhaak RG, Aldape KD, et al. Comprehensive, integrative genomic analysis of diffuse lower-grade gliomas. *N Engl J Med*. 2015;372(26):2481–2498. https://doi.org/10.1056/NEJMoa1402121.
10. Chiang JC, Ellison DW. Molecular pathology of paediatric central nervous system tumours. *J Pathol*. 2017;241(2):159–172. https://doi.org/10.1002/path.4813.
11. Yan H, Parsons DW, Jin G, et al. IDH1 and IDH2 mutations in gliomas. *N Engl J Med*. 2009;360(8):765–773. https://doi.org/10.1056/NEJMoa0808710.
12. Eckel-Passow JE, Lachance DH, Molinaro AM, et al. Glioma groups based on 1p/19q, IDH, and TERT promoter mutations in tumors. *N Engl J Med*. 2015;372(26):2499–2508. https://doi.org/10.1056/NEJMoa1407279.
13. Hartmann C, Hentschel B, Wick W, et al. Patients with IDH1 wild type anaplastic astrocytomas exhibit worse prognosis than IDH1-mutated glioblastomas, and IDH1 mutation status accounts for the unfavorable prognostic effect of higher age: implications for classification of gliomas. *Acta Neuropathol*. 2010;120(6):707–718. https://doi.org/10.1007/s00401-010-0781-z.
14. Weller M, Weber RG, Willscher E, et al. Molecular classification of diffuse cerebral WHO grade II/III gliomas using genome- and transcriptome-wide profiling improves stratification of prognostically distinct patient groups. *Acta Neuropathol*. 2015;129(5):679–693. https://doi.org/10.1007/s00401-015-1409-0.
15. Brat DJ, Aldape K, Colman H, et al. cIMPACT-NOW update 3: recommended diagnostic criteria for "diffuse astrocytic glioma, IDH-wildtype, with molecular features of glioblastoma, WHO grade IV". *Acta Neuropathol*. 2018;136(5):805–810. https://doi.org/10.1007/s00401-018-1913-0.
16. van den Bent MJ, Afra D, de Witte O, et al. Long-term efficacy of early versus delayed radiotherapy for low-grade astrocytoma and oligodendroglioma in adults: the EORTC 22845 randomised trial. *Lancet*. 2005;366(9490):985–990. https://doi.org/10.1016/S0140-6736(05)67070-5.
17. Buckner JC, Shaw EG, Pugh SL, et al. Radiation plus procarbazine, CCNU, and vincristine in low-grade glioma. *N Engl J Med*. 2016;374(14):1344–1355. https://doi.org/10.1056/NEJMoa1500925.
18. Strowd RE, Holdhoff M, Grossman SA. Chemotherapy for treatment of grade II gliomas. *Oncology (Williston Park)*. 2014;28(12):1036–1043.
19. Ceccarelli M, Barthel FP, Malta TM, et al. Molecular profiling reveals biologically discrete subsets and pathways of progression in diffuse glioma. *Cell*. 2016;164(3):550–563. https://doi.org/10.1016/j.cell.2015.12.028.
20. Leu S, von Felten S, Frank S, et al. IDH/MGMT-driven molecular classification of low-grade glioma is a strong predictor for long-term survival. *Neuro Oncol*. 2013;15(4):469–479. https://doi.org/10.1093/neuonc/nos317.
21. Hasselblatt M, Jaber M, Reuss D, et al. Diffuse astrocytoma, IDH-wildtype: a dissolving diagnosis. *J Neuropathol Exp Neurol*. 2018;77(6):422–425. https://doi.org/10.1093/jnen/nly012.
22. Ruda R, Bello L, Duffau H, Soffietti R. Seizures in low-grade gliomas: natural history, pathogenesis, and outcome after treatments. *Neuro Oncol*. 2012;14(suppl 4). https://doi.org/10.1093/neuonc/nos199. iv55–64.
23. Pallud J, Audureau E, Blonski M, et al. Epileptic seizures in diffuse low-grade gliomas in adults. *Brain*. 2014;137(Pt 2):449–462. https://doi.org/10.1093/brain/awt345.
24. Vecht CJ, Wilms EB. Seizures in low- and high-grade gliomas: current management and future outlook. *Expert Rev Anticancer Ther*. 2010;10(5):663–669. https://doi.org/10.1586/era.10.48.
25. Vertosick FT, Selker RG, Arena VC. Survival of patients with well-differentiated astrocytomas diagnosed in the era of computed tomography. *Neurosurgery*. 1991;28(4):496–501. https://doi.org/10.1097/00006123-199104000-00002.
26. Telfeian AE, Philips MF, Crino PB, Judy KD. Postoperative epilepsy in patients undergoing craniotomy for glioblastoma multiforme. *J Exp Clin Cancer Res*. 2001;20(1):5–10.
27. Sperling MR, Ko J. Seizures and brain tumors. *Semin Oncol*. 2006;33(3):333–341. doi:S0093-7754(06)00116-3.
28. Hildebrand J, Lecaille C, Perennes J, Delattre JY. Epileptic seizures during follow-up of patients treated for primary brain tumors. *Neurology*. 2005;65(2):212–215. https://doi.org/10.1212/01.wnl.0000168903.09277.8f.
29. Beaumont A, Whittle IR. The pathogenesis of tumour associated epilepsy. *Acta Neurochir (Wien)*. 2000;142(1):1–15. https://doi.org/10.1007/s007010050001.
30. Englot DJ, Berger MS, Barbaro NM, Chang EF. Predictors of seizure freedom after resection of supratentorial low-grade gliomas. A review. *J Neurosurg*. 2011;115(2):240–244. https://doi.org/10.3171/2011.3.JNS1153.
31. Glantz MJ, Cole BF, Forsyth PA, et al. Practice parameter: anticonvulsant prophylaxis in patients with newly diagnosed brain tumors. Report of the quality standards subcommittee of the American Academy of Neurology. *Neurology*. 2000;54(10):1886–1893. https://doi.org/10.1212/wnl.54.10.1886.
32. Forsyth PA, Weaver S, Fulton D, et al. Prophylactic anticonvulsants in patients with brain tumour. *Can J Neurol Sci*. 2003;30(2):106–112.
33. Glantz MJ, Cole BF, Friedberg MH, et al. A randomized, blinded, placebo-controlled trial of divalproex sodium prophylaxis in adults with newly diagnosed brain tumors. *Neurology*. 1996;46(4):985–991. https://doi.org/10.1212/wnl.46.4.985.
34. Franceschetti S, Binelli S, Casazza M, et al. Influence of surgery and antiepileptic drugs on seizures symptomatic of cerebral tumours. *Acta Neurochir (Wien)*. 1990;103(1–2):47–51.

35. North JB, Penhall RK, Hanieh A, Frewin DB, Taylor WB. Phenytoin and postoperative epilepsy. A double-blind study. *J Neurosurg*. 1983;58(5):672–677. https://doi.org/10.3171/jns.1983.58.5.0672.
36. Kuijlen JM, Teernstra OP, Kessels AG, Herpers MJ, Beuls EA. Effectiveness of antiepileptic prophylaxis used with supratentorial craniotomies: a meta-analysis. *Seizure*. 1996;5(4):291–298. https://doi.org/10.1016/S1059-1311(96)80023-9.
37. Maschio M, Dinapoli L, Sperati F, et al. Levetiracetam monotherapy in patients with brain tumor-related epilepsy: seizure control, safety, and quality of life. *J Neurooncol*. 2011b;104(1):205–214. https://doi.org/10.1007/s11060-010-0460-x.
38. Newton HB, Goldlust SA, Pearl D. Retrospective analysis of the efficacy and tolerability of levetiracetam in brain tumor patients. *J Neurooncol*. 2006;78(1):99–102. https://doi.org/10.1007/s11060-005-9070-4.
39. Kerkhof M, Dielemans JC, van Breemen MS, et al. Effect of valproic acid on seizure control and on survival in patients with glioblastoma multiforme. *Neuro Oncol*. 2013;15(7):961–967. https://doi.org/10.1093/neuonc/not057.
40. Saria MG, Corle C, Hu J, et al. Retrospective analysis of the tolerability and activity of lacosamide in patients with brain tumors: clinical article. *J Neurosurg*. 2013;118(6):1183–1187. https://doi.org/10.3171/2013.1.JNS12397.
41. Maschio M, Dinapoli L, Mingoia M, et al. Lacosamide as add-on in brain tumor-related epilepsy: preliminary report on efficacy and tolerability. *J Neurol*. 2011a;258(11):2100–2104. https://doi.org/10.1007/s00415-011-6132-8.
42. Villanueva V, Saiz-Diaz R, Toledo M, et al. NEOPLASM study: real-life use of lacosamide in patients with brain tumor-related epilepsy. *Epilepsy Behav*. 2016;65:25–32. https://doi.org/10.1016/j.yebeh.2016.09.033.
43. Lim DA, Tarapore P, Chang E, et al. Safety and feasibility of switching from phenytoin to levetiracetam monotherapy for glioma-related seizure control following craniotomy: a randomized phase II pilot study. *J Neurooncol*. 2009;93(3):349–354. https://doi.org/10.1007/s11060-008-9781-4.
44. Dinapoli L, Maschio M, Jandolo B, et al. Quality of life and seizure control in patients with brain tumor-related epilepsy treated with levetiracetam monotherapy: preliminary data of an open-label study. *Neurol Sci*. 2009;30(4):353–359. https://doi.org/10.1007/s10072-009-0087-x.
45. Ruda R, Pellerino A, Franchino F, et al. Lacosamide in patients with gliomas and uncontrolled seizures: results from an observational study. *J Neurooncol*. 2018;136(1):105–114. https://doi.org/10.1007/s11060-017-2628-0.
46. Sepulveda-Sánchez JM, Conde-Moreno A, Baron M, Pardo J, Reynes G, Belenguer A. Efficacy and tolerability of lacosamide for secondary epileptic seizures in patients with brain tumor: a multicenter, observational retrospective study. *Oncol Letters*. 2017;13(6):4093–4100. https://doi.org/10.3892/ol.2017.5988.
47. Maschio M, Dinapoli L, Zarabla A, et al. Zonisamide in brain tumor-related epilepsy: an observational pilot study. *Clin Neuropharmacol*. 2017;40(3):113–119. https://doi.org/10.1097/WNF.0000000000000218.
48. Maschio M, Dinapoli L, Saveriano F, et al. Efficacy and tolerability of zonisamide as add-on in brain tumor-related epilepsy: preliminary report. *Acta Neurol Scand*. 2009b;120(3):210–212. https://doi.org/10.1111/j.1600-0404.2009.01226.x.
49. Cacho-Diaz B, San-Juan D, Salmeron K, Boyzo C, Lorenzana-Mendoza N. Choice of antiepileptic drugs affects the outcome in cancer patients with seizures. *Clin Transl Oncol*. 2018;20(12):1571–1576. https://doi.org/10.1007/s12094-018-1892-6.
50. van Breemen MS, Wilms EB, Vecht CJ. Epilepsy in patients with brain tumours: epidemiology, mechanisms, and management. *Lancet Neurol*. 2007;6(5):421–430. https://doi.org/10.1016/S1474-4422(07)70103-5.
51. Bourg V, Lebrun C, Chichmanian RM, Thomas P, Frenay M. Nitroso-urea-cisplatin-based chemotherapy associated with valproate: increase of haematologic toxicity. *Ann Oncol*. 2001;12(2):217–219. https://doi.org/10.1023/a:1008331708395.
52. Rossetti AO, Jeckelmann S, Novy J, Roth P, Weller M, Stupp R. Levetiracetam and pregabalin for antiepileptic monotherapy in patients with primary brain tumors: a phase II randomized study. *Neuro Oncol*. 2014;16(4):584–588. https://doi.org/10.1093/neuonc/not170.
53. Novy J, Stupp R, Rossetti AO. Pregabalin in patients with primary brain tumors and seizures: a preliminary observation. *Clin Neurol Neurosurg*. 2009;111(2):171–173. https://doi.org/10.1016/j.clineuro.2008.09.009.
54. Maschio M, Dinapoli L, Sperati F, et al. Effect of pregabalin add-on treatment on seizure control, quality of life, and anxiety in patients with brain tumour-related epilepsy: a pilot study. *Epileptic Disord*. 2012b;14(4):388–397. https://doi.org/10.1684/epd.2012.0542.
55. Maschio M, Albani F, Jandolo B, et al. Temozolomide treatment does not affect topiramate and oxcarbazepine plasma concentrations in chronically treated patients with brain tumor-related epilepsy. *J Neurooncol*. 2008a;90(2):217–221. https://doi.org/10.1007/s11060-008-9651-0.
56. Maschio M, Dinapoli L, Zarabla A, et al. Outcome and tolerability of topiramate in brain tumor associated epilepsy. *J Neurooncol*. 2008b;86(1):61–70. https://doi.org/10.1007/s11060-007-9430-3.
57. Jennesson M, van Eeghen AM, Caruso PA, Paolini JL, Thiele EA. Clobazam therapy of refractory epilepsy in tuberous sclerosis complex. *Epilepsy Res*. 2013;104(3):269–274. https://doi.org/10.1016/j.eplepsyres.2012.10.010.
58. Thome-Souza S, Klehm J, Jackson M, et al. Clobazam higher-evening differential dosing as an add-on therapy in refractory epilepsy. *Seizure*. 2016;40:1–6. https://doi.org/10.1016/j.seizure.2016.05.014.
59. Vecht C, Royer-Perron L, Houillier C, Huberfeld G. Seizures and anticonvulsants in brain tumours: frequency, mechanisms and anti-epileptic management. *Curr Pharm Des*. 2017b;23(42):6464–6487. https://doi.org/10.2174/1381612823666171027130003.
60. Mauro AM, Bomprezzi C, Morresi S, et al. Prevention of early postoperative seizures in patients with primary brain tumors: preliminary experience with oxcarbazepine. *J Neurooncol*. 2007;81(3):279–285. https://doi.org/10.1007/s11060-006-9229-7.
61. Maschio M, Dinapoli L, Sperati F, et al. Oxcarbazepine monotherapy in patients with brain tumor-related epilepsy: open-label pilot study for assessing the efficacy, tolerability and impact on quality of life. *J Neurooncol*. 2012a;106(3):651–656. https://doi.org/10.1007/s11060-011-0689-z.
62. Maschio M, Dinapoli L, Vidiri A, et al. The role side effects play in the choice of antiepileptic therapy in brain tumor-related epilepsy: a comparative study on traditional antiepileptic drugs versus oxcarbazepine. *J Exp Clinl Cancer Res*. 2009a;28:6–60. https://doi.org/10.1186/1756-9966-28-60.

63. Vecht C, Duran-Peña A, Houillier C, Durand T, Capelle L, Huberfeld G. Seizure response to perampanel in drug-resistant epilepsy with gliomas: early observations. *J Neurooncol*. 2017a;133(3):603–607. https://doi.org/10.1007/s11060-017-2473-1.
64. Maschio M, Pauletto G, Zarabla A, et al. Perampanel in patients with brain tumor-related epilepsy in real-life clinical practice: a retrospective analysis. *Int J Neurosci*. 2019;129(6):593–597. https://doi.org/10.1080/00207454.2018.1555160.
65. Dunn-Pirio AM, Woodring S, Lipp E, et al. Adjunctive perampanel for glioma-associated epilepsy. *Epilepsy Behav Case Rep*. 2018;10:114–117. https://doi.org/10.1016/j.ebcr.2018.09.003.
66. Overwater IE, Bindels-de Heus K, Rietman AB, et al. Epilepsy in children with tuberous sclerosis complex: chance of remission and response to antiepileptic drugs. *Epilepsia*. 2015;56(8):1239–1245. https://doi.org/10.1111/epi.13050.
67. Oberndorfer S, Piribauer M, Marosi C, Lahrmann H, Hitzenberger P, Grisold W. P450 enzyme inducing and non-enzyme inducing antiepileptics in glioblastoma patients treated with standard chemotherapy. *J Neurooncol*. 2005;72(3):255–260. https://doi.org/10.1007/s11060-004-2338-2.
68. Eyal S, Yagen B, Sobol E, Altschuler Y, Shmuel M, Bialer M. The activity of antiepileptic drugs as histone deacetylase inhibitors. *Epilepsia*. 2004;45(7):737–744. https://doi.org/10.1111/j.0013-9580.2004.00104.x.
69. Li XN, Shu Q, Su JM, Perlaky L, Blaney SM, Lau CC. Valproic acid induces growth arrest, apoptosis, and senescence in medulloblastomas by increasing histone hyperacetylation and regulating expression of p21Cip1, CDK4, and CMYC. *Mol Cancer Ther*. 2005;4(12):1912–1922. https://doi.org/10.1158/1535-7163.MCT-05-0184.
70. Happold C, Gorlia T, Chinot O, et al. Does valproic acid or levetiracetam improve survival in glioblastoma? A pooled analysis of prospective clinical trials in newly diagnosed glioblastoma. *J Clin Oncol*. 2016;34(7):731–739. https://doi.org/10.1200/JCO.2015.63.6563.
71. Strowd RE, Cervenka MC, Henry BJ, Kossoff EH, Hartman AL, Blakeley JO. Glycemic modulation in neuro-oncology: experience and future directions using a modified Atkins diet for high-grade brain tumors. *Neurooncol Pract*. 2015;2(3):127–136. https://doi.org/10.1093/nop/npv010.
72. Scheck AC, Abdelwahab MG, Fenton KE, Stafford P. The ketogenic diet for the treatment of glioma: insights from genetic profiling. *Epilepsy Res*. 2012;100(3):327–337. https://doi.org/10.1016/j.eplepsyres.2011.09.022.
73. Pisipati S, Smith KA, Shah K, Ebersole K, Chamoun RB, Camarata PJ. Intracerebral laser interstitial thermal therapy followed by tumor resection to minimize cerebral edema. *Neurosurg Focus*. 2016;41(4):E13. https://doi.org/10.3171/2016.7.FOCUS16224.
74. Warnke PC, Berlis A, Weyerbrock A, Ostertag CB. Significant reduction of seizure incidence and increase of benzodiazepine receptor density after interstitial radiosurgery in low-grade gliomas. *Acta Neurochir Suppl*. 1997;68:90–92.
75. Scerrati M, Montemaggi P, Iacoangeli M, Roselli R, Rossi GF. Interstitial brachytherapy for low-grade cerebral gliomas: analysis of results in a series of 36 cases. *Acta Neurochir (Wien)*. 1994;131(1–2):97–105.
76. Schrottner O, Eder HG, Unger F, Feichtinger K, Pendl G. Radiosurgery in lesional epilepsy: brain tumors. *Stereotact Funct Neurosurg*. 1998;70(suppl 1):50–56. https://doi.org/10.1159/000056406.
77. Ruda R, Magliola U, Bertero L, et al. Seizure control following radiotherapy in patients with diffuse gliomas: a retrospective study. *Neuro-Oncology*. 2013;15(12):1739–1749. https://doi.org/10.1093/neuonc/not109.
78. McGirt MJ, Mukherjee D, Chaichana KL, Than KD, Weingart JD, Quinones-Hinojosa A. Association of surgically acquired motor and language deficits on overall survival after resection of glioblastoma multiforme. *Neurosurgery*. 2009;65(3):46–70. https://doi.org/10.1227/01.NEU.0000349763.42238.E9.
79. Giglio P, Gilbert MR. Neurologic complications of cancer and its treatment. *Curr Oncol Rep*. 2010;12(1):50–59. https://doi.org/10.1007/s11912-009-0071-x.
80. Cross NE, Glantz MJ. Neurologic complications of radiation therapy. *Neurol Clin*. 2003;21(1):249–277. https://doi.org/10.1016/S0733-8619(02)00031-2.
81. Butler JM, Case LD, Atkins J, et al. A phase III, double-blind, placebo-controlled prospective randomized clinical trial of d-threo-methylphenidate HCl in brain tumor patients receiving radiation therapy. *Int J Radiat Oncol Biol Phys*. 2007;69(5):1496–1501. https://doi.org/10.1016/j.ijrobp.2007.05.076.
82. Meyers CA, Weitzner MA, Valentine AD, Levin VA. Methylphenidate therapy improves cognition, mood, and function of brain tumor patients. *J Clin Oncol*. 1998;16(7):2522–2527. https://doi.org/10.1200/JCO.1998.16.7.2522.
83. Gehring K, Patwardhan SY, Collins R, et al. A randomized trial on the efficacy of methylphenidate and modafinil for improving cognitive functioning and symptoms in patients with a primary brain tumor. *J Neurooncol*. 2012;107(1):165–174. https://doi.org/10.1007/s11060-011-0723-1.
84. Rapp SR, Case LD, Peiffer A, et al. Donepezil for irradiated brain tumor survivors: a phase III randomized placebo-controlled clinical trial. *J Clin Oncol*. 2015;33(15):1653–1659. https://doi.org/10.1200/JCO.2014.58.4508.
85. Shaw EG, Rosdhal R, D'Agostino RB, et al. Phase II study of donepezil in irradiated brain tumor patients: effect on cognitive function, mood, and quality of life. *J Clin Oncol*. 2006;24(9):1415–1420. https://doi.org/10.1200/JCO.2005.03.3001.
86. Brown PD, Pugh S, Laack NN, et al. Memantine for the prevention of cognitive dysfunction in patients receiving whole-brain radiotherapy: a randomized, double-blind, placebo-controlled trial. *Neuro Oncol*. 2013;15(10):1429–1437. https://doi.org/10.1093/neuonc/not114.
87. de Groot M, Douw L, Sizoo EM, et al. Levetiracetam improves verbal memory in high-grade glioma patients. *Neuro Oncol*. 2013;15(2):216–223. https://doi.org/10.1093/neuonc/nos288.
88. Chaichana KL, Halthore AN, Parker SL, et al. Factors involved in maintaining prolonged functional independence following supratentorial glioblastoma resection. Clinical article. *J Neurosurg*. 2011;114(3):604–612. https://doi.org/10.3171/2010.4.JNS091340.
89. Baumert BG, Hegi ME, van den Bent MJ, et al. Temozolomide chemotherapy versus radiotherapy in high-risk low-grade glioma (EORTC 22033-26033): a randomised, open-label, phase 3 intergroup study. *Lancet Oncol*. 2016;17(11):1521–1532. https://doi.org/10.1016/S1470-2045(16)30313-8.
90. Fisher BJ, Hu C, Macdonald DR, et al. Phase 2 study of temozolomide-based chemoradiation therapy for high-risk low-grade gliomas: preliminary results of radiation therapy oncology group 0424. *Int J Radiat Oncol Biol Phys*. 2015;91(3):497–504. https://doi.org/10.1016/j.ijrobp.2014.11.012.

91. Wahl M, Phillips JJ, Molinaro AM, et al. Chemotherapy for adult low-grade gliomas: clinical outcomes by molecular subtype in a phase II study of adjuvant temozolomide. *Neuro Oncol*. 2017;19(2):242–251. https://doi.org/10.1093/neuonc/now176.
92. Quinn JA, Reardon DA, Friedman AH, et al. Phase II trial of temozolomide in patients with progressive low-grade glioma. *J Clin Oncol*. 2003;21(4):646–651. https://doi.org/10.1200/JCO.2003.01.009.
93. Pace A, Vidiri A, Galiè E, et al. Temozolomide chemotherapy for progressive low-grade glioma: clinical benefits and radiological response. *Ann Oncol*. 2003;14(12):1722–1726. https://doi.org/10.1093/annonc/mdg502.
94. Rosenthal MA, Ashley DL, Cher L. Temozolomide-induced flare in high-grade gliomas: a new clinical entity. *Intern Med J*. 2002;32(7):346–348.

Chapter 12

Approach to the high-grade glioma patient

David Olayinka Kamson and Stuart Grossman

CHAPTER OUTLINE

Introduction

The broad definition of high-grade glioma encompasses all central nervous system neoplasms that are derived from glial components of the brain and show anaplasia (i.e., poor cellular differentiation, atypia, pleomorphism, and loss of normal cellular organization). This chapter focuses on the high-grade diffuse gliomas including anaplastic oligodendrogliomas and astrocytomas, glioblastomas, and the recently added histone-3 K27M mutated diffuse midline gliomas. These tumors were classically labeled WHO grade III or IV based on histopathologic features suggestive of malignant behavior and are considered malignant gliomas. Since 2016, the WHO classification also considers molecular markers. Many of these markers are powerful predictors of survival and, in certain cases, override the histopathologic findings. Beyond the microscopic level, the prognosis is influenced by a myriad of anatomical, clinical, and socioeconomic factors. Consequently, there is a wide range of survival, from months in an untreated elderly person with glioblastoma to decades in a young patient with anaplastic oligodendroglioma. Regardless of which end of the survival spectrum patients are situated, the common denominator is the lack of curative treatment to date. High-grade gliomas almost inevitably recur causing the demise of those affected.

This chapter provides a case-based approach to the management of high-grade gliomas. Case 12.1 presents a patient with anaplastic oligodendroglioma and provides a summary of the clinical presentation and management considerations for these patients. Case 12.2 presents a patient with anaplastic astrocytoma. Case 12.3 provides a multi-step review of the care for patients with glioblastoma including: (1) the initial presentation, (2) management of neurological complications, (3) recognition and treatment of non-neurological complications, and (4) surveillance recommendations and treatment options at recurrence. The chapter ends with a brief summary of H3K27M-mutated diffuse midline gliomas, which is discussed in greater detail in Chapter 7 (Case 7.3).

Pathology and molecular classification of high-grade gliomas

The field of neuro-oncology is undergoing a major transformation where pathologists and clinicians struggle to

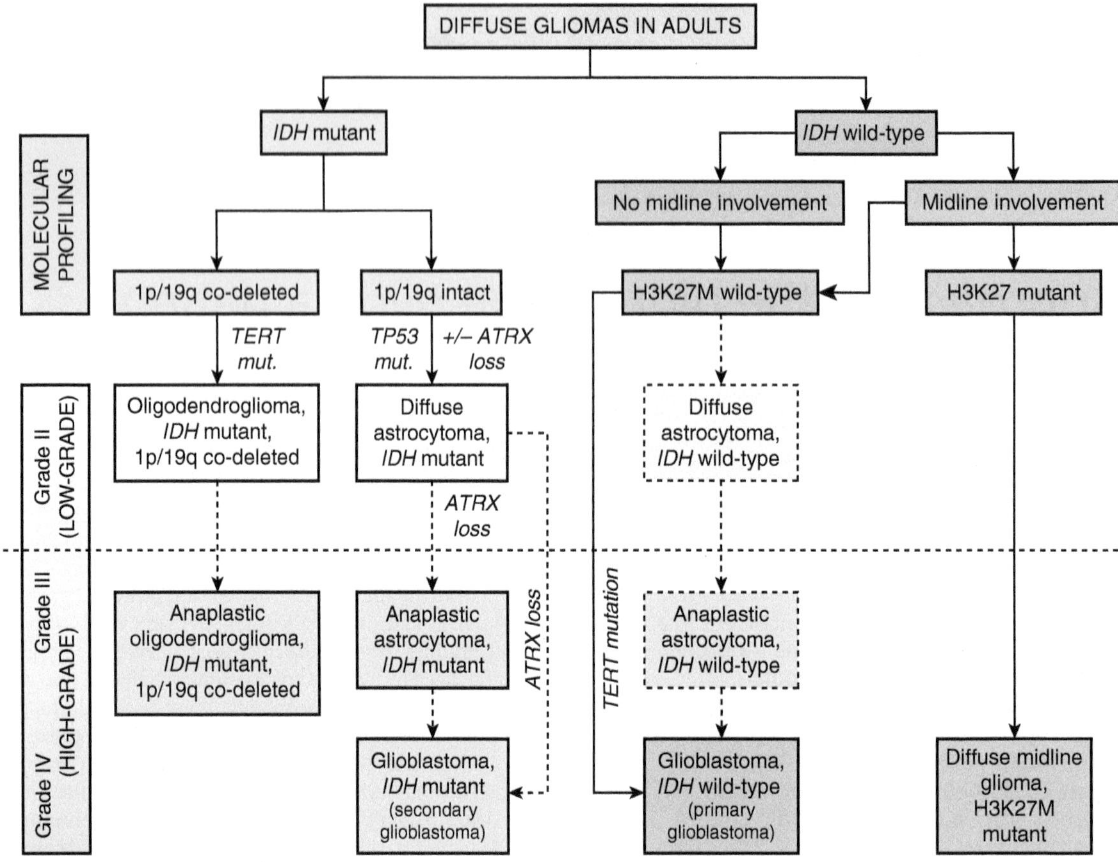

Fig. 12.1 Classification of diffuse gliomas in adults.

incorporate novel molecular data into day-to-day practice. Although there have been a number of incremental updates since its inception, this chapter relies on the 2016 WHO classification (Chapter 1).[1,2] According to these criteria, the determination of the type of malignant glioma is first established under the microscope based on the presence of astrocytic or oligodendroglial morphologic features. High-grade is primarily determined by the presence of malignant characteristics. Grade III tumors have anaplastic features, such as nuclear atypia with diffuse or regionally increased cellularity and mitotic activity (Ki-67 proliferative index 5–10%). Grade IV glioblastomas are characterized by microvascular proliferation and/or necrosis and brisk proliferation (Ki-67 >10%) though these may also be seen in anaplastic oligodendrogliomas in the appropriate molecular context.

Following histologic assessment, molecular confirmation is now part of routine diagnostics (Fig. 12.1). *Isocitrate dehydrogenase (IDH)* gene mutational status separates two major pathways of glioma genesis. Mutant *IDH* leads to the production of the oncometabolite 2-hydroxyglutarate (2HG). 2HG instigates a series of genetic and epigenetic alterations that result in slowly growing, lower-grade gliomas that eventually progress into high-grade tumors. *IDH* mutant gliomas have better prognosis and respond favorably to treatment. *IDH* mutant gliomas are further divided into oligodendrogliomas and astrocytomas, which are mutually exclusive based on the status of chromosomal arms 1p and 19q (Table 12.1). Oligodendrogliomas are defined by loss or co-deletion of chromosomes 1p/19q, which is also predictive of treatment response. They are virtually always *IDH* mutated, and typically have concurrent *TERT* promoter alterations. Conversely, *IDH* mutant astrocytomas (and "secondary glioblastomas") have intact 1p/19q and are characterized by *TP53* and *ATRX* gene mutations.

IDH wild-type astrocytomas are best represented by glioblastomas, which are responsible for 90–95% of this group. These are also referred to as "primary glioblastomas," as they typically present *de novo* without a preceding low-grade glioma that gave rise to malignant degeneration. *IDH* wild-type

Table 12.1 Incidence and molecular characteristics of *IDH* mutant and wild-type high-grade diffuse gliomas.

IDH MUTANT HIGH-GRADE GLIOMAS		*IDH* WILD-TYPE HIGH-GRADE GLIOMAS		
Anaplastic Oligodendroglioma	**Anaplastic Astrocytoma and Glioblastoma**	**Anaplastic Astrocytoma and Glioblastoma**	**Diffuse Midline Glioma, H3K27M mutant**	**Other Anaplastic Glial Neoplasms**
0.1 in 100K/year	*0.4 in 100K/year (AA)* *0.3 in 100K/year (GB)*	*~0.15 in 100K/year (AA)* *3–4 in 100K/year (GB)*	*<0.1 in 100K/year*	*<0.3 in 100K/year*
• *IDH1/2* mutation (100%) • 1p/19q co-deletion (100%) • *TERT* mutation (>95%) • MGMT*p* methylation (>90%) • *CIC* mutation (60%) • *FUBP*1 mutation (30%) • Polyploidy more common than in low-grade	• *IDH1* R132H mutation (>90%) • *ATRX* loss (100%) • *TP53* mutation (74%) • MGMT*p* methylation (70–80%) • Frequent 9p and 19q loss (in anaplastic astrocytoma) Rare: • *TERT* mutation (26%) • *EGFR* amplification (4%)	• *TERT* mutation (80%) • 10q loss (70%) • *CDKN2A/2B* loss (60%) • *EGFR* alterations (55%) • *PTEN* alterations (40%) • MGMT*p* methylation (40%) Rare or absent: • *TP53* mutation (25%) • *ATRX* loss (0%)	• *H3K27M* change in *H3F3A* (75%), or *HIST1H3B/C* (25%) • *TP53* mutation (50%) • *PDGFRA* amp. (50%) Rare or absent: • *TERT* mutation (~20%) • *ATRX* loss (15%) • MGMT*p* methylation (<10%) • *IDH* mutation (0%)	Anaplastic pleomorphic xanthoastrocytoma: • *BRAF* V600E mutation (~50%) Anaplastic ganglioglioma: • *BRAF* V600E (~50%) • Absent: *IDH*, 1p/19q, *TP53*, *PTEN*, or *EGFR* alteration Anaplastic ependymoma: • RELA-fusion

AA, Anaplastic astrocytoma; *GB*, glioblastoma; *IDH*, isocitrate dehydrogenase.

gliomas have a distinct molecular profile often characterized by *TERT* promoter mutation. Also common are *CDKN2A/B* and/or *EGFR* alterations, whereas *TP53* mutations are rare (Table 12.1). A small fraction of *IDH* wild-type astrocytomas are diagnosed as grade II and III. These are thought to represent an early transient phase of the same disease spectrum. Their clinical course therefore closely resembles primary glioblastoma and differs substantially from *IDH* mutant astrocytomas of the same grade. A unique subgroup of *IDH* wild-type astrocytomas harbor a mutation at locus K27 in the *histone 3 (H3)* gene. Based on their predilection to the thalamus, pons, and spinal cord, these tumors are referred to as diffuse midline gliomas. Given their aggressive behavior noted in the pediatric population, these tumors are automatically classified grade IV even though ~15% of them lack necrosis or neovascularization.

Methylation of the O6–methylguanine–DNA methyltransferase gene promoter (MGMT*p*) is the most important predictor of response to alkylating chemotherapy in *IDH* wild-type astrocytomas, whereas it is much less significant in the presence of an *IDH* mutation. Additional mutations that exhibited survival benefit when targeted with second-line therapies include *BRAF*-V600E and *NTRK1* gene fusion, yet these are seen in ~1% of adult gliomas.[3,4]

Clinical cases

CASE 12.1 NEW CONTRAST ENHANCEMENT IN A LOW-GRADE OLIGODENDROGLIOMA: APPROACH TO ANAPLASTIC OLIGODENDROGLIOMA

Case. A 54-year-old female has a history of right frontal grade II oligodendroglioma, *IDH1*-mutated, 1p19q co-deleted that was treated 11 years ago with radiation with procarbazine, CCNU (lomustine), and vincristine (PCV) chemotherapy. After a long history of well-controlled seizures, she presented with refractory breakthrough focal seizures despite escalating levetiracetam to 2000 mg twice daily and lacosamide to 300 mg twice daily. A contrast-enhanced brain MRI revealed an enlarging T2/fluid attenuated inversion recovery (FLAIR) hyperintense in the right frontal lobe with a new faint region of gadolinium enhancement in the lateral right frontal lobe that had not previously been visible and was concerning for progression to higher grade. The patient was taken to the operating room where maximal safe subtotal resection was performed. Pathology revealed an infiltrative glial neoplasm with round nuclei, perinuclear halos, rare microcalcifications, and an elevated Ki-67 labeling index up to 10%. A final diagnosis of anaplastic oligodendroglioma (WHO grade III) was made. The patient was treated with repeat radiation with concurrent and adjuvant temozolomide chemotherapy with clinical response to treatment and was able to taper antiepileptic regimen to levetiracetam monotherapy at 1500 mg twice daily.

Teaching Points: Approach to Anaplastic Oligodendrogliomas. Anaplastic oligodendrogliomas (AOs) are rare high-grade diffuse gliomas. They are responsible for less than 1% of all primary intracranial neoplasms. Although the annual incidence of AO is 1–2 in a million,[5] they are not uncommon in neuro-oncology subspecialty clinics due to their 10-fold longer survival than those with glioblastoma. Patients' median age of 50 years at diagnosis places AOs on the older end of the spectrum of *IDH* mutant tumors. However, they are much younger than those with glioblastomas. AOs are thought to be tumors that develop slowly, and are usually diagnosed *de novo*. They less commonly progress from a grade II oligodendroglioma after an approximate 6–7-year lead time.[6,7]

Pathology. Anaplastic oligodendrogliomas are characterized by infiltrative cells with round nuclei and perinuclear halo producing a "fried egg" appearance. They have delicate networks of branching capillaries resembling "chicken wire" and variable amounts of microcalcification (Fig. 12.2). Unlike the three-tiered grading system of astrocytomas, oligodendrogliomas are either classified as WHO grade II or III, where the presence of brisk mitotic activity, microvascular proliferation, and necrosis denote the anaplastic (grade III) group. Molecularly, AOs are *IDH* mutant and 1p/19q co-deleted similarly to their low-grade counterparts; polyploidy is a feature that is more commonly seen in high-grade oligodendrogliomas.

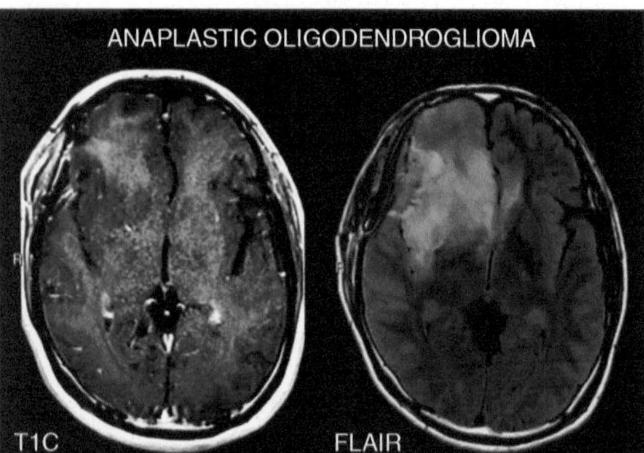

Fig. 12.2 Conventional MRI of an anaplastic oligodendroglioma. This patient was initially diagnosed with a grade II oligodendroglioma with an extensive T2/FLAIR hyperintense volume. Over time, faint gadolinium enhancement developed on the T1-weighted images (see in the right frontal lobe), which was confirmed to be grade III oligodendroglioma on subsequent resection. *FLAIR*, Fluid attenuated inversion recovery.

Location and presentation. AOs are almost exclusively supratentorial with a strong predilection to the frontal lobe. They seldom affect infratentorial structures or the spine through leptomeningeal spread. There are a few case reports describing spread beyond the confines of the central nervous system (CNS); however, this is exceedingly rare.[8] As expected, the presenting symptoms depend on the location of the tumor. Partial seizures with or without secondary generalization are by far the most common presenting symptoms of AOs. Seizures affect about 60% AOs, which is only slightly less common than in their low-grade counterparts.[9] The high seizure frequency in these tumors may be explained by the combination of frequent cortical infiltration and 2HG production (see *Management of tumor-induced seizures*, below). Only 20% of patients present with focal neurologic deficits, which are typically less pronounced than one would expect based on the tumor's localization and extent. This is most likely due to the slow growth allowing concurrent functional brain reorganization and thus compensation for potential neurologic deficits.[10]

Imaging. AOs present with heterogeneous signal intensity on T2/FLAIR. They often infiltrate the cerebral cortex with variable amount of mass effect on adjacent brain parenchyma (Fig. 12.2). Their margins are relatively indistinct, although they tend to be better demarcated on MRI than glioblastomas. More than 70% of AOs enhance gadolinium-contrast with a typically diffuse and often dotty configuration. This is thought to be the radiographic manifestation of the histologic "chicken wire" vascular pattern and is shared with many grade II oligodendrogliomas. Consequently, contrast-enhanced MRI has a very limited ability to distinguish high- and low-grade oligodendrogliomas.[11] Intratumoral microhemorrhages are common in AOs and can often present with T1-hyperintensities. Oligodendrogliomas in general are the most commonly calcified brain tumors.[12] However, calcification can be observed with other neoplasms such as in pilocytic astrocytomas, ependymal, and glioneuronal tumors and is therefore not pathognomonic.

MR spectroscopy can detect a signal derived from 2HG *in vivo*. This method may be used to identify and monitor the *IDH* mutant tumor volume. However, these images are technically difficult to acquire and therefore have not yet made into day-to-day clinical practice.[13,14] AOs seem to have the highest apparent diffusion coefficients (ADCs) among high-grade gliomas. Interestingly, oligodendrogliomas generally have elevated relative cerebral blood volume (rCBV) regardless of grade and prognosis. This is again thought to be a correlate of the underlying tortuous microvascular system. Consequently, perfusion-weighted imaging has limited role in the diagnosis or surveillance of these tumors.[15,16] A similar phenomenon had been described with PET using amino acid tracers, where both low- and high-grade oligodendrogliomas exhibit high uptake compared with astrocytomas.[17,18]

Surgical approach. The diagnosis of high-grade glioma requires histopathologic confirmation unless such cannot be achieved without significant morbidity. Even with a prior history of histologically proven low-grade oligodendroglioma, surgical confirmation of grade may be helpful, as these tumors often exhibit contrast enhancement without underlying malignant transformation. Furthermore, adequate surgical samples are essential as genetic profiling may have immediate clinical implications. Although resection in anaplastic oligodendroglial tumors has been consistently associated with favorable outcomes, data is lacking from a purely 1p/19q co-deleted AO population.[19,20] Hence, the current recommendation of maximal safe resection of the T2/FLAIR hyperintense and/or contrast enhancing volume is extrapolated from low-grade oligodendroglial and mixed high-grade glioma cohorts.[21–23] Of note, reorganization of functional brain networks is often observed in slower growing tumors, such as AOs progressing from a low-grade intermediary. Consequently, extensive resections are often achievable in tumors situated in conventionally "eloquent" regions. Surgical removal of epileptogenic foci may also improve seizure control in AOs. Nonetheless, surgery is virtually never curative in AOs, and additional treatment covering the infiltrative part of the tumor is fundamental for prolonging survival. *Radiation and chemotherapy.* Anaplastic oligodendrogliomas are relatively radiosensitive. Monotherapy via standard fractionated external beam radiation has been associated with a median overall survival of approximately 8 years (Table 12.2). Addition of a chemotherapy regimen combining procarbazine, CCNU (lomustine), and vincristine (PCV) administered in 6-week cycles has nearly doubled survival in these patients, as evidenced by two independent randomized controlled phase III trials.[19,24] One of these studies reported an almost 15-year overall survival with this regimen. Thus, radiotherapy preceded or followed by PCV has become the standard approach for anaplastic oligodendrogliomas (Fig. 12.3A). Although PCV was proven effective, it was also proven relatively toxic, as only

Table 12.2 Prognosis of high-grade gliomas

Diagnosis	WHO Grade	Prognosis (overall survival, unless indicated)
Glioblastoma, *IDH* wild-type, NOS	IV	Resection only: 4 mo. XRT only: 12.1 mo. XRT/TMZ + adjuvant TMZ: 14.6 mo. XRT/TMZ + adjuvant TMZ/TTF: 20.9 mo.
Glioblastoma, *IDH* wild-type, MGMT*p* methylated	IV	XRT only: 15.3 mo. XRT/TMZ + adjuvant TMZ: 23.4 mo.
Glioblastoma, *IDH* wild-type MGMT*p* unmethylated	IV	XRT only: 11.8 mo. XRT/TMZ + adjuvant TMZ: 12.6 mo.
Diffuse midline glioma, H3K27M mutant	IV	Median OS: 17–31 mo (may be better than in children)
Glioblastoma, *IDH* mutant	IV	Surgery + XRT: 24 mo. Surgery, XRT/TMZ + adjuvant TMZ: 31 mo. (similar to *IDH* wild-type AA)
Anaplastic Astrocytoma, *IDH* wild-type	III	Median OS: 19.2 months
Anaplastic Astrocytoma, *IDH* mutant	III	Median OS: 9.8 years, likely benefit from combined XRT/TMZ + adjuvant TMZ
Anaplastic Oligodendroglioma, *IDH* mutant, 1p/19q co-deleted	III	XRT only: 7.3–9.3 years XRT and PCV: 14.7 years
Anaplastic pleomorphic xanthoastrocytoma	III	5-year OS: 76%
Anaplastic ganglioglioma	III	Median OS: 24.7 mo.
Anaplastic ependymoma	III	Progression-free survival: 27.6 months

AA, Anaplastic astrocytoma; *NOS*, not otherwise specified; *OS*, overall survival; *TMZ*, Temozolomide; *TTF*, tumor treating fields (Optune); *XRT*, fractionated external beam radiotherapy; *XRT/TMZ*, XRT with concurrent TMZ.

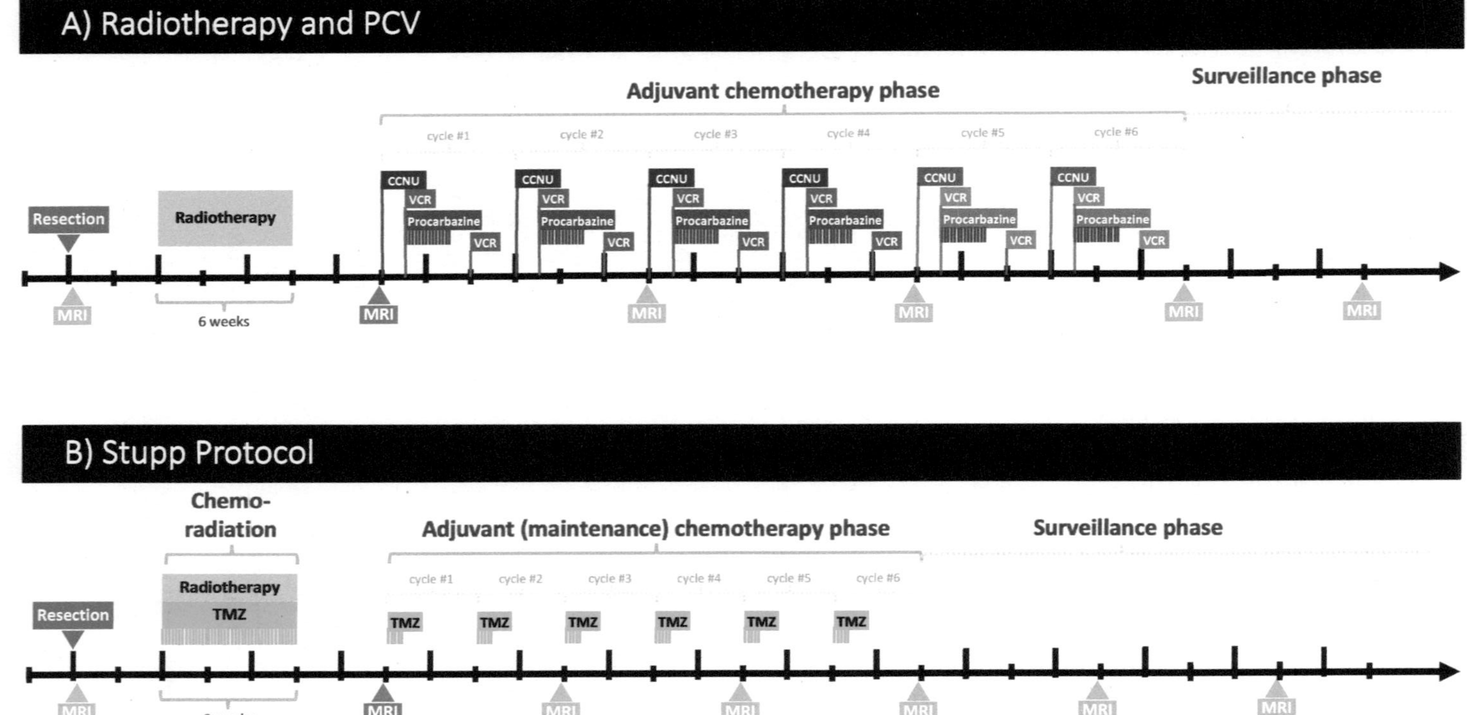

Fig. 12.3 (A) illustrates the timeline of the PCV protocol with radiotherapy followed by 6-week cycles of CCNU on day 1, vincristine (VCR) on day 8 and 29, and daily procarbazine from day 8 through day 21. (B) illustrates the Stupp protocol with 6 weeks of combined radiotherapy and low-dose temozolomide (TMZ) followed by 4-week cycles of standard dose temozolomide given day 1 through day 5.

half of the patients tolerated four or more cycles. Dose reductions and treatment delays were frequent. Grade III hematologic toxicities were noted in more than 50% of patients enrolled in these trials with neutropenia and thrombocytopenia being the most common.[20,25] Myelosuppression is mainly attributed to CCNU and procarbazine, and typically occurs 2–8 weeks after the start of treatment, with a recovery taking 4–6 weeks or longer. CCNU is often associated with a cumulative and even more prolonged cytopenias that may persist years after completion of the treatment. Nausea and emesis affect up to 90% of patients taking this regimen and can be controlled with antiemetics in most cases. Procarbazine also has a weak monoamine oxidase inhibitor effect and thus interacts with enzyme-inducing antiepileptic drugs (AEDs) and selective serotonin reuptake inhibitors and necessitates a low-tyramine diet. Additionally, vincristine's penetration into brain tumors has been called into question,[26] yet it is a common culprit of peripheral neurotoxicity. This typically manifests as a dose-dependent distal symmetrical sensorimotor axonal neuropathy first presenting with loss of the ankle jerk reflex, followed by often painful paresthesia, and loss of distal vibratory sensation.[27] Vincristine may also contribute to significant constipation due to autonomic neuropathy.

Considering all the above, a practical approach to this regimen is to first administer radiotherapy, which is generally well tolerated and "secures" the tumor, then proceed with PCV about 4 weeks after completion of radiation. Although the goal is to administer up to six cycles of PCV, dose reductions are almost always necessary, and maintaining CCNU dosing should be prioritized over procarbazine, whereas discontinuation of vincristine should be considered if any sign of neuropathy emerges (Fig. 12.3A).

There is a great desire to adopt a less toxic regimen than PCV, yet it is the regimen with the most evidence of long-term efficacy at the present time. In a trial of anaplastic gliomas comparing monotherapy of radiation, or chemotherapy with either temozolomide or PCV, neither treatment modalities provided superior overall survival to one another.[28] In a retrospective analysis of 1p/19q co-deleted AOs, PCV monotherapy was associated with longer progression-free survival compared with temozolomide alone; those who received radiotherapy combined with either chemotherapy regimen did better than those receiving monotherapy.[29] The results suggest that radiotherapy with concurrent temozolomide, followed by adjuvant temozolomide (i.e., Stupp protocol, Fig. 12.3B), could serve as an alternative to PCV. This question is currently assessed in the phase III CODEL trial (NCT00887146) comparing the two regimens. Using temozolomide as initial treatment of AOs outside the above trial is generally discouraged unless there are well-justified concerns about PCV not being tolerated or inaccessible.

Clinical Pearls

1. Oligodendrogliomas are defined by co-deletion of chromosomes 1p/19q and respond well to radiation and PCV chemotherapy.
2. Maximum safe resection may prolong survival but is never curative and may not be feasible in deeply infiltrative lesions that cross the midline or are adjacent to eloquent structures.
3. New or worsening seizures are an indicator of tumor progression in high-grade gliomas and should be evaluated with contrast-enhanced MRI and, if necessary, biopsy or resection.
4. Besides antiepileptic drugs (AEDs), antineoplastic therapy may help improve seizure control.

CASE 12.2 PATCHY CONTRAST ENHANCEMENT IN A HIGH-GRADE BRAIN LESION: APPROACH TO ANAPLASTIC ASTROCYTOMA

Case. A 24-year-old woman presents with a 2-month history of progressive worsening left leg weakness, falls, and tripping. She is an extremely active triathlete who was seen by her primary physician for difficulty in competition and underwent contrast-enhanced MRI brain revealing an infiltrating T2/FLAIR hyperintense lesion in the right posterior frontal lobe with a small focus of contrast enhancement in the anterior portion of the lesion (Fig. 12.4). She underwent awake craniotomy with near complete resection of the lesion and transiently worsening left-sided weakness, which improved postoperatively. Pathology revealed abundant astrocytic cells with nuclear atypia, mitotic activity, and elevated Ki-67 labeling index up to 8% and regions of increased vascular endothelial proliferation. On immunohistochemistry, there was strong nuclear staining for mutant *IDH1* R132H and p53 with loss of ATRX staining. A final diagnosis of anaplastic astrocytoma (WHO grade III), *IDH* mutant was made. Standard radiation with concurrent temozolomide was initiated 4 weeks postoperatively, which was tolerated well except for thrombocytopenia (nadir 65,000/μL), prompting discontinuation of temozolomide 1 week early. One month after completion of the concurrent therapy she had a Karnofsky performance scale score of 80%, a stable neurologic examination, and blood counts that revealed normal platelet counts but substantial lymphopenia (TLC 400). Adjuvant temozolomide was pursued, and she completed six cycles of treatment with stable imaging findings.

Teaching Points: Approach to Anaplastic Astrocytomas. Anaplastic astrocytomas (AAs) are responsible for approximately 10% of all gliomas. They are typically found *de novo* but can progress from a low-grade intermediary. About 50% of low-grade astrocytomas progress into anaplastic glioma within 5 years of diagnosis. AAs consist of two sharply distinct groups based on *IDH* status. *IDH* mutants represent 70–80% of AAs and are the youngest population of high-grade gliomas with a typical presentation in the late 30s and a prognosis closer to AOs. *IDH* wild-type AAs are much less

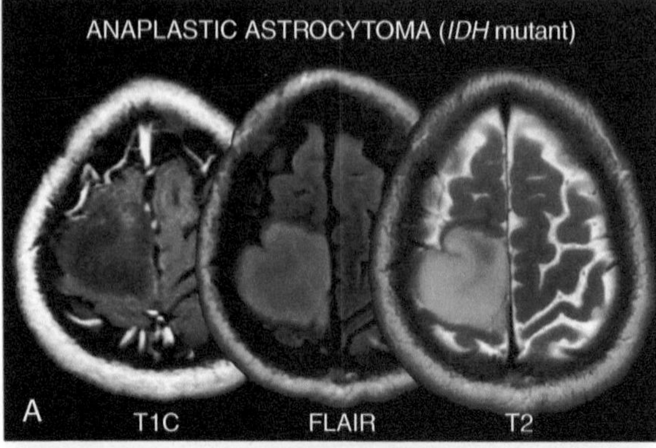

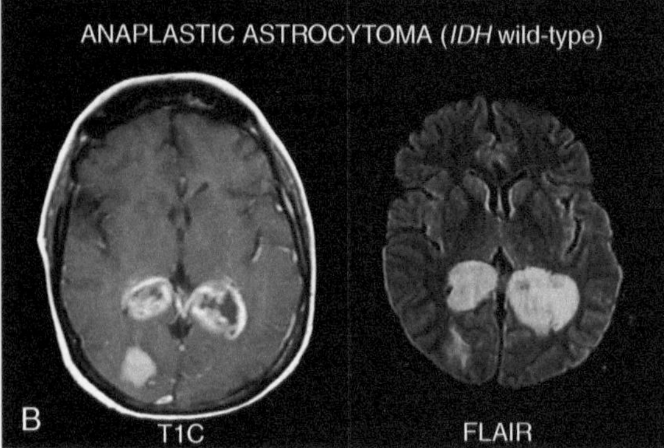

Fig. 12.4 (A) Anaplastic astrocytoma with the characteristic T2/FLAIR mismatch sign for *IDH* mutant tumors. Note the mostly homogeneous T2 signal with the relatively hypointense FLAIR abnormality with a hyperintense halo. (B) This patient has a multifocal high-grade astrocytoma. Although the biopsy of the right occipital lesion suggested anaplastic astrocytoma, the presence of necrosis in the trigonum bilaterally is suggestive of glioblastoma. The histopathologic diagnosis is likely a result of sampling error. *FLAIR*, Fluid attenuated inversion recovery.

common. They typically present at older ages, between 45 and 55, and have a prognosis similar to glioblastoma. Although the current diagnostic and treatment approach is essentially the same for all astrocytic high-grade gliomas, this chapter will focus on some of the unique features and nuances that distinguish AAs from other high-grade gliomas with emphasis on those with *IDH* mutation.

Pathology and predictive markers. As mentioned in the general histopathology section, AAs are characterized by astrocytic cells showing nuclear atypia, increased cellularity, and mitotic activity (Ki-67 5–10%), while they lack necrosis or vascular proliferation. Oligodendroglioma-like components are often present, but lack of 1p/19q co-deletion rules out oligodendroglioma. If *IDH* mutation is present, most patients have the canonical R132H alteration, whereas *IDH2* mutations such as R172K are very rare. On immunohistochemistry, *IDH* mutant AAs typically exhibit strong nuclear staining for p53 because of mutation in gene TP53 (Table 12.1). Mutation of the ATRX gene manifests as loss of ATRX staining. Although ATRX may be preserved in low-grade *IDH* mutant astrocytomas, this mutation is ubiquitous for *IDH* mutant AAs. In contrast, *IDH* wild-type AAs often have a *TERT* mutation, *EGFR* gene amplification, or whole chromosome 7 gain or 10 loss. The presence of any of these alterations confer the diagnosis of "molecular glioblastoma" based on the similarly poor prognosis.[2]

IDH mutation is a decisive factor in the cascade of hypermethylation in diffuse gliomas. As a result, those hypermethylated (often referred to as G-CIMP positive) have higher sensitivity to both radiation and chemotherapy. MGMT*p* methylation is mostly the result of the hypermethylated state as reflected by its similar incidence to *IDH* mutations, and has limited predictive value in the *IDH* mutant population. In contrast, MGMT*p* methylation is indeed predictive of higher chemotherapy sensitivity in *IDH* wild-type AAs.[30]

Location and presentation. Similar to other high-grade gliomas, AAs are supratentorial tumors. They have a predilection to the frontal lobe, but often present in a gliomatosis cerebri pattern, involving three or more lobes in the brain. Consequently, their presenting symptoms develop and progress slowly over months. These most commonly include cognitive impairment and hemiparesis aphasia, whereas signs and symptoms related to ICP elevation are rare. Inaugural seizures may happen in all AAs, but are more common in those with *IDH* mutation as attributed to the production of 2HG.

Imaging. AAs are T2/FLAIR hyperintense on MRI with blurry margins and no intralesional calcification. Most of them enhance contrast in a nodular, patchy, or less commonly ring pattern. According to a 1p/19q agnostic analysis, 32% of *IDH1* mutant anaplastic gliomas lack enhancement, compared with 12% of non-enhancing *IDH* wild-type tumors.[31] More recently, a constellation of hyperintense T2 and relatively hypointense FLAIR signal with a hyperintense peripheral rim has been described *IDH* mutant astrocytomas. Although this "T2-FLAIR mismatch" sign was found to be 100% specific yet only 51% sensitive for *IDH* mutants in independent cohorts, caution should be exercised when interpreting these findings (Fig. 12.4).[32–34]

Advanced MRI may be useful in the initial evaluation of these tumors. Elevated rCBV is highly sensitive in the distinction of high- and low-grade gliomas, but this feature lacks specificity.[35] MR spectroscopic detection of 2HG peak may also be helpful in identifying *IDH* mutant AAs, yet again this technique is not yet widely adopted. Additionally, 2HG production may be a less important factor in these tumors as they had already undergone malignant transformation. *IDH* wild-type AAs have distinctly low ADCs only comparable with *IDH* wild-type glioblastomas. In comparison, oligodendrogliomas have the highest ADC of all high-grade gliomas, and *IDH* mutant AAs are in between.[16] Of course, none of these techniques replace histopathologic confirmation.

Initial treatment approach. The *IDH* mutation is being evaluated as a direct or indirect therapeutic target. However, at present, the standard initial treatment approach of high-grade astrocytomas is *IDH* agnostic. It includes maximal safe resection followed by chemoradiation and adjuvant temozolomide. The exact benefit of concurrent and/or adjuvant temozolomide was evaluated by the CATNON trial (NCT00626990).[36] Preliminary data from this study suggest that *IDH* mutant AAs may benefit from temozolomide and radiotherapy. In this cohort, patients with *IDH* mutant AAs had an overall survival of 9.7 years versus the 1.6 years in the *IDH* wild-type group.[37]

Clinical Pearls

1. High-grade astrocytomas are treated with radiotherapy with concurrent and adjuvant temozolomide chemotherapy.
2. *IDH* mutant astrocytomas have a more favorable prognosis and response to treatment than those with wild-type *IDH*.

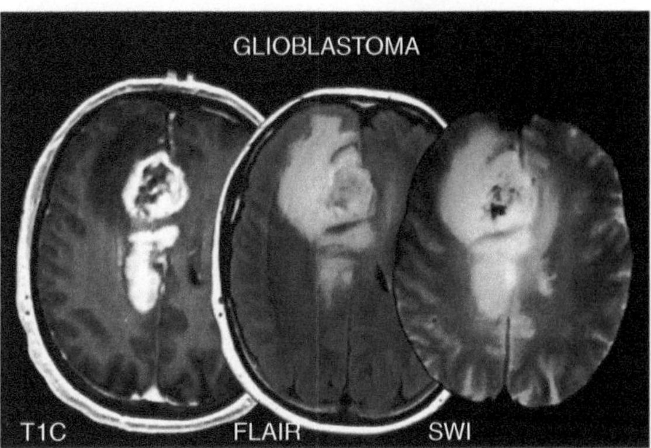

Fig. 12.5 Glioblastoma with classic centrally necrotic ring enhancing anterior portion with extensive surrounding edema and contralateral expansion through the corpus callosum and a homogeneously enhancing posterior portion, which became necrotic on subsequent follow-up. T1C, T1-weighted contrast-enhanced; FLAIR, fluid attenuated inversion recovery; SWI, susceptibility weighted image.

CASE 12.3A ACUTE-ONSET NEUROLOGICAL DEFICIT FROM A HIGH-GRADE BRAIN LESION: APPROACH TO GLIOBLASTOMA

Case. A 61-year-old male with a history of hypertension was evaluated in the Emergency Department (ED) after he sustained a fall at work. In retrospect, he started tripping over thresholds and rugs with his left foot about 10 days prior to presentation. His neurologic examination revealed a subtle left pronator drift with moderate, flexor predominant weakness in the left lower extremity with hyperreflexia. A contrast-enhanced brain MRI confirmed the presence of a T2/FLAIR hyperintense lesion spanning across the medial part of right frontal and parietal convexity with an irregular ring enhancing focus centrally (Fig. 12.5). He was started on dexamethasone 4 mg every 6 hours and levetiracetam 500 mg twice daily and was taken to the operating room for a subtotal resection of the enhancing mass 2 days later. The pathology revealed a glioblastoma with bizarre glial cells with foci resembling astrocytic morphology, and palisading necrosis accompanied by vascular proliferation and an elevated Ki-67 labeling index up to 25%. Immunohistochemistry was negative for mutant *IDH* or H3K27M proteins and showed preserved staining for ATRX. Subsequent next-generation sequencing revealed a mutation in the *TERT* promoter and concurrent *EGFR* gene mutation and amplification. Additional testing revealed MGMT promoter methylation. Standard radiation with concurrent temozolomide was initiated 5 weeks postoperatively, which was tolerated well.

Teaching Points: Approach to Glioblastomas. Glioblastomas are the most aggressive and by far the most common primary brain tumors. With their annual incidence of 3.2 per 100.000, they represent more than half of all gliomas, and about 15% of all intracranial neoplasms.[5] More than 90% of glioblastomas are *IDH* wild-type and present *de novo*. Hence these are also referred to as "primary glioblastoma". The remainder have an *IDH* mutation and mostly develop from a lower-grade intermediary ("secondary glioblastomas"). Because of relative homogeneity, reports on primary glioblastoma from before the molecular era are much less likely to have been skewed by the *IDH* mutants. Thus, this section will generally refer to *IDH* wild-type glioblastoma, whereas specific differences in those with *IDH* mutation will be pointed out. Such is the case with the age distribution where the incidence peaks in the seventh decade of life in those with *IDH* wild-type tumors, whereas the *IDH* mutant subgroup presents in the late 40s.

Pathology. As discussed above, anaplastic features and elevated proliferative activity (Ki-67 >10%) are coupled with microvascular proliferation and/or palisading necrosis in glioblastomas (Fig. 12.2C). They are among the most morphologically heterogeneous tumors (hence the now-abandoned adjective *multiforme*), with a microscopic appearance ranging from small to multinucleated giant cells, and granular, lipidized, oligodendroglia-like, gemistocytic, primitive neuronal, or even metaplastic/sarcomatous components. Molecularly, *IDH* wild-type glioblastomas are characterized by TERT*p* mutation, 10q loss, CDKN2A/B, and EGFR mutations, whereas TP53 and ATRX loss are only typical for *IDH* mutants. These mutational signatures can also be divided into proneural, neural, classic, and mesenchymal types; however, these may vary regionally within the same tumor and change over time.

The 2016 WHO classification specifies three subtypes of *IDH* wild-type glioblastoma including epithelioid, giant cell, and gliosarcoma variants, each with some unique features. For example, 50% of epithelioid glioblastomas harbor a BRAF-V600E mutation and may progress from a low-grade intermediary and may be related to pleomorphic xanthoastrocytoma. They also have a higher tendency for leptomeningeal spread.[38]

Giant cell glioblastomas have bizarre-appearing multinucleated cells that accumulate around vessels and tend to lack microvascular proliferation. Their molecular profile resembles *IDH* mutant astrocytomas with common TP53 and rare EGFR mutations and have slightly better (though still short) survival. Lastly, gliosarcomas have sarcomatous components and may pose a challenge distinguishing them from metastatic disease. Irrespective of the above-mentioned differences, glioblastoma subtypes are treated similarly in clinical practice.

Location and presentation. Similar to other high-grade gliomas, glioblastomas are typically supratentorial and present with neurologic symptoms that develop over weeks to a few months. These include focal neurologic deficits attributable to the area of involvement or mass effect. About 30–50% of patients present with seizures that are more common in the presence of *IDH* mutation. Intracranial hemorrhage is a less common culprit of hyperacute deficits and is seen in about 2% of patients.

Imaging and radiographic mimics. Most patients present to the ED and undergo non-contrast CT of the head, which visualizes extensive edema, mass effect, and, occasionally, hemorrhage; however, contrast-enhanced brain MRI is necessary to identify the most characteristic radiographic features of glioblastoma (Fig. 12.5). These include heterogeneous rim enhancement with often multilobulated cystic central clearing (T1-hypointensity) surrounded by extensive T2/FLAIR hyperintensity. The enhancing nodular part can be considered as the solid portion of the tumor with the highest concentration of neoplastic cells with highly permeable immature capillaries contributing to the gadolinium contrast leakage. The T2/FLAIR hyperintensity represents the infiltrating part of the tumor that extends into the normal-appearing MRI regions with a gradually decreasing tumor cell concentration.[39] Some of these tumors present with multiple foci of contrast enhancement, which, if connected by contiguous T2/FLAIR hyperintensity, are referred to as multifocal. Less commonly, radiographically isolated enhancing foci are observed and these tumors are referred to as multicentric and are most commonly clonally-related to the dominant lesion.

Differential diagnosis. Although the radiographic features tend to be quite suggestive, they overlap with other tumors such as primary CNS lymphoma or brain metastases, whereas non-neoplastic differential diagnoses include Baló's concentric sclerosis and other tumefactive demyelinating lesions. Rarely, infectious processes such as abscesses or ischemia may also mimic the appearance of glioblastoma. The presence of incomplete ("C"-shaped) ring enhancement suggests against gliomas and is typical for autoimmune diseases and may also be seen in lymphoma. Advanced MRI techniques can narrow the differential diagnoses; for example, glioblastomas have low ADC in general, especially compared with subacute demyelination. The extent of diffusion restriction can occasionally mimic ischemia, though it is mostly attributed to hypercellularity or recent seizures in the context of glioblastoma. Decreased *N*-acetyl-aspartate (NAA)/Choline ratio on MR spectroscopy and elevated rCBV on perfusion-weighted imaging are also suggestive of glioblastoma. Amino acid tracers, such as FET and FDOPA, may also have a role clarifying the diagnosis, as glioblastomas have much higher tracer uptake and different uptake dynamics compared with non-neoplastic or even metastatic lesions.[40] Lastly, some glioblastomas present with spontaneous intracerebral hemorrhage (ICH), which may obscure the underlying tumor in the acute setting. Thus, in ICH cases where there is no clear etiology identified, follow-up imaging after the resorption of the hematoma may reveal the underlying tumor.

Irrespective of the current advances in imaging, the diagnosis of glioblastoma requires histopathologic confirmation. In extremely rare cases, where the suspicious lesion is confined to a location with high-risk of biopsy-associated morbidity or even mortality (e.g., medullary lesions), multidisciplinary tumor board discussion involving neurosurgeons, medical neuro-oncologists, radiation oncologists, and neuroradiologists may help the decision-making process and treatment planning.

Surgical approach. Due to their infiltrative nature, glioblastomas are surgically incurable, as evidenced by failed attempts of hemispherectomies for glioma patients in the early 20th century[41] and the historical median overall survival of 4 months in those treated with surgery only.[42] Nonetheless, surgery plays an integral role in the management of these patients, from obtaining adequate samples for both histopathologic and molecular analysis to cytoreduction. The extent of resection has been consistently found predictive of survival in glioblastomas, and traditionally, 80% or more removal of the contrast-enhancing volume has been associated with improved outcomes.[43] However, in a hypothetical comparison, the residual enhancing volume will still be higher after 90% resection of a 60 cc tumor than after resecting 60% of a 10 cc tumor. The issue of assessing totality of resection is even further complicated when the T2/FLAIR hyperintense area is also factored into the tumor volume. The importance of the residual contrast-enhancing and T2/FLAIR-defined tumor volume was subsequently confirmed to be a more robust independent predictor of survival.[44] These data tailored the current standard approach of maximal safe resection attempting to remove as much of the radiographic tumor volume as possible without introducing new neurologic deficits. Worsened postoperative performance status cancels out the benefits of surgery both from a quality-of-life and survival stand point. Recent publications have also proposed the use of amino acid PET as a potentially valuable imaging adjunct for better delineation of a metabolically active tumor; however, these techniques are not readily available in the United States at present.[40,45]

The timing of surgery in patients with suspected glioblastoma is guided by indirect evidence and pragmatic considerations. First, emergency resection is not indicated in most cases. However, inferring from the above data indicating better survival with higher performance status and smaller tumors, a resection may be more successful before further radiographic or clinical progression of the disease. Additionally, the potential risk of losing patients to follow-up also needs to be taken into consideration. In practice, this equation usually translates into surgery performed within days of initial presentation.

Radiation and chemotherapy. Prior to 2005, the standard of care for glioblastoma was fractionated external beam radiotherapy with a total dose of 60 Gy administered over 6 weeks. Monotherapy with radiation offers a median overall survival of 12 months, as compared with the 4 months in historical controls treated with surgery only. Stupp et al., in their landmark study, were the first to prove survival benefit using chemotherapy in glioblastomas.[46] They added low-dose daily oral temozolomide (75 mg/m^2) administered concurrently with radiotherapy followed by adjuvant standard dose temozolomide (150–200 mg/m^2), given for 5 days for 6–12 four-week cycles (Fig. 12.3B). The pooled survival was 14.6 months in those treated with this regimen, 2.5 months longer than in those treated with radiation only. Subsequent analyses showed that most survival benefit was seen in those with MGMT*p* methylated tumors, reaching a median overall survival of 23.4 months in this cohort.[47,48] The benefit of the Stupp protocol is a matter of debate in those with unmethylated MGMT*p*. However, the long-term analysis of this study showed 0% survival in those patients who received radiation as monotherapy, versus 11% in those who also received chemotherapy. Whether the long-term survivors in this group had other genetic determinants of superior chemotherapy response, such as *IDH* mutations, remains a question. Thus, at present, all patients with glioblastoma are treated with chemoradiation followed by adjuvant temozolomide.

Temozolomide is a generally well-tolerated chemotherapy agent. Its most common severe complications warranting dose adjustments include thrombocytopenia (~11%) and neutropenia (~7%).[46] On the other hand, the lymphopenia related to chemoradiation tends to be underreported and increase risk for *Pneumocystis jirovecii* pneumonia (PJP) warranting prophylactic antibiotic treatment. Severe non-hematologic complications of temozolomide are rare and include fatigue, nausea, and hair thinning, which are seen in 50% or more of patients (although patients usually do not develop alopecia). Rash is described in less than 20% of patients and can often be attributed to drugs used for PJP prophylaxis.

Unfortunately, there has been no prospective study aiming to identify whether the concurrent or the adjuvant use of temozolomide is more valuable to prolong survival. The identification of survival benefit for those with lower MGMT expression suggested that MGMT depletion could be a viable strategy to improve survival. However, alternative or prolonged schedules attempting to achieve this, such as using "dose-dense" temozolomide (75–100mg/m^2 per day for 21 days a month), or extending standard adjuvant temozolomide beyond six cycles, increased hematologic toxicity without added survival benefit.[49–51]

Tumor treating fields. A novel treatment approach called tumor treating fields (TTF) has been developed to generate low-intensity alternating electric fields within the cranium, which proposedly disrupts mitotic spindle formation as an antineoplastic measure. The signal is delivered via an array of transducers placed over the shaven scalp. The leads are attached to a battery pack that is fitted into a small shoulder bag, and the device is worn at least 18 hours a day. In 2017, the open-label randomized phase III clinical trial adding TTF to the standard adjuvant temozolomide had shown prolonged survival for those with glioblastoma.[52] Unfortunately, limitations in the study design, such as lack of blinding and no sham control, makes it difficult to interpret the exact survival benefit of this regimen.

Special populations. Lastly, patients with many comorbidities, poor performance status, and shorter radiotherapy courses ranging from 2–4 weeks with or without concurrent chemotherapy had been shown to have comparable outcomes to their counterparts receiving standard therapy. Therefore, these modified regimens can be considered for frail patients.

Clinical Pearls

In this case, the initial histology was consistent with glioblastoma. Subsequent molecular analysis did not reveal *IDH* gene mutation. This supports a final integrated diagnosis of *IDH* wild-type glioblastoma, WHO grade IV. In this case, MGMT promoter was found to be methylated, which is seen in approximately 40% of *IDH* wild-type glioblastomas and associated with a more favorable response to chemotherapy with temozolomide.

1. High-grade diffuse gliomas include glioblastomas, anaplastic astrocytomas, and oligodendrogliomas.
2. Diagnosis of a high-grade glioma begins with histologic assessment and integrates molecular alterations to identify high-grade glioma subgroups that have distinct prognoses and therapy responses.
3. MGMT promoter methylation predicts favorable response to temozolomide in *IDH* wild-type astrocytomas.

CASE 12.3B SEIZURES, EDEMA, AND POST-TREATMENT NEUROLOGICAL COMPLICATIONS IN HIGH-GRADE GLIOMA

Case. The 61-year-old male in Case 12.3a with a right frontoparietal glioblastoma, *IDH* wild-type, and MGMT promoter methylated completed concurrent chemoradiation. One month after completing radiation, his brain MRI revealed a thickened enhancement in the margin of the surgical bed with a 1 cm nodular focus anteriorly, increased edema throughout the right hemisphere, and a 3-mm midline shift. He was admitted with a generalized tonic-clonic seizure. His dexamethasone dose was increased to 8 mg twice daily. He was restarted on levetiracetam, which had been discontinued after his initial surgery as he had not had seizures at the time of presentation. He had no further breakthrough seizures. Imaging findings were felt to be consistent with pseudoprogression in an MGMT*p* methylated glioblastoma; however, early tumor progression could not be excluded. After discharge from the hospital in stable condition, the first adjuvant cycle of temozolomide was able to be initiated at 150 mg/m^2 per day on a 5/28-day cycle. Repeat imaging after cycle one of adjuvant therapy revealed reduced contrast enhancement, improved perilesional edema, and midline shift decreasing to 1 mm consistent with pseudoprogression.

Teaching Points: Diagnosis and Treatment of Common Neurological Complications in High-Grade Glioma Patients. This case highlights the neurological complications that may occur in glioma patients, including but not limited to tumor-associated seizures, cerebral edema, and intracranial hemorrhage.

Management of tumor-induced seizures. Other than focal deficits, the most notable neurologic complications of high-grade gliomas include seizures, brain edema with or without herniation, and intracranial hemorrhages. Seizures affect about half of glioblastoma patients and up to 70% of those with anaplastic gliomas, yet are much less common than in low-grade gliomas.[53] The differences in seizure prevalence seem to correspond to the distribution of *IDH* mutants among these groups. Mutant *IDH* is directly implicated in glioma related epileptogenesis via its product, 2HG, which elicits its effect in a direct glutamatergic fashion.[54] This observation also explains why molecularly agnostic analyses found epilepsy prognostically favorable in high-grade glioma but neutral in low-grade.

Despite what the high seizure incidence might suggest, there is no evidence to support the use of prophylactic AEDs in gliomas.[55] Most of the data come from the study of enzyme-inducing AEDs in the perioperative setting, whereas the question remains debated using newer generation AEDs.[56–58] Regardless, levetiracetam is frequently used by neurosurgeons for perioperative seizure prophylaxis and is typically to be stopped a week after surgery. However, in practice, the decision whether to discontinue prophylactically initiated AEDs is often left at the discretion of the neuro-oncologist. In contrast, the initiation and prolonged use of AEDs is warranted in patients who had one or more seizures, as, similarly to other lesional epilepsies, they are more likely to have recurrent events.

Similar to other epilepsies, the choice of AED should be guided by the drug's side-effect profile and efficacy. In general, enzyme-inducing and myelotoxic AEDs should be avoided. When applied concurrently, these may reduce the levels of dexamethasone and anticancer agents (temozolomide is typically an exception). They can also promote production of toxic metabolites, and increase the severity of bone marrow impairment such as thrombocytopenia. Levetiracetam has proven efficacy in glioma-related epilepsy,[59] and is the most commonly used agent in this setting. Lacosamide is a potent and generally well-tolerated, but expensive, alternative or adjunct to levetiracetam. Lamotrigine is also a good alternative for select patients who cannot tolerate other AEDs due to fatigue, cognitive, or behavior issues. Given the lack of IV formulation and slow titration, lamotrigine is most appropriate for those who have finished chemotherapy and have stable disease. Topiramate and zonisamide are also effective, and, in certain cases, the use of valproate and oxcarbazepine may be justified.

Unlike low-grade gliomas, about 70% of new or breakthrough seizures are closely associated with progressive disease in high-grade gliomas.[60] Therefore, these events warrant clinical and radiographic evaluation besides the adjustment of AEDs. EEG may be helpful if the semiology localizes outside a radiographically abnormal area or when there is persistently altered mental status. Distal spread, leptomeningeal disease, or remote epileptogenesis from inhibitory deafferentation may be alternative etiologies to local progression. Assessing for inadequate compliance, and, in some cases, measurement of drug levels may be helpful in adjusting AED dosage. Combination therapy with one of the above-mentioned agents may improve seizure control. Additionally, in the presence of MRI changes, reducing edema using dexamethasone may also complement the AED regimen. In select patients, surgical debulking, radiotherapy, and even chemotherapy were associated with improved seizure control as well.

Withdrawing AEDs is a peculiar issue for patients with high-grade gliomas who had a seizure in the past. Although hypothetical factors to predict successful AED withdrawal follow similar lines to the general epilepsy population, such as prolonged seizure freedom (measured in years), or normal neurologic status and cognition, tumor specific factors such as distance from cerebral cortex and extratemporal tumor location and, of course, overall good prognosis may be favorable predictors. However, many of these favorable characteristics are associated with *IDH* mutant tumors that have a higher prevalence of seizures as well.

Management of cerebral edema. Cerebral edema is a common complication of high-grade gliomas. It develops because of blood-brain barrier (BBB) breakdown and can present with isolated headaches due to stretching of the cerebral vasculature, focal neurologic deficits, and, rarely, seizures. Altered mental status may be the result of focal compression of structures responsible for attention and wakefulness, or secondary to global elevation of intracranial pressure. Cerebral edema most commonly occurs during the second half of, or within weeks after the completion of radiation therapy, but it can occur in any phase of the disease. Exogenous corticosteroids are the mainstay of symptomatic treatment. Of these, dexamethasone is preferred in neuro-oncology given its good BBB penetration and minimal mineralocorticoid effect. It acts through reducing BBB permeability at the capillary level, thus improving BBB integrity. Whereas its pharmacologic half-life is 4–6 hours, its biologic half-life is 36–52 hours.[61] The every 6-hour dosing of dexamethasone is derived from the 1960s when its efficacy to reduce neurosurgical complication was described.[61] However, the effect on capillaries lasts at least 12 hours. The use of corticosteroids poses additional risk for those with insomnia, psychosis, weight gain, loss of muscle mass and idiosyncratic myopathy, immunosuppression, peptic ulcers, adrenal insufficiency, and even venous thromboembolisms (VTEs).[62,63] Therefore, in a non-emergency setting, dexamethasone should be used at the lowest effective dose for symptom control, for the shortest duration necessary. It should be administered in one or two doses a day, with the second dose no later than the afternoon to avoid insomnia. Tapering in 5–7-day intervals allows assessment whether the lower dose is tolerated. For patients with significant intracranial swelling, and failure to wean steroids, the use of bevacizumab can be considered. Bevacizumab is a monoclonal antibody that sequestrates VEGF and helps reduce cerebral edema via restoration of BBB integrity. Unfortunately, bevacizumab also has a set of side effects that are thought to be due to endothelial dysfunction and include renal impairment, uncontrolled hypertension, increased risk for major hemorrhage, VTEs, and ischemic events including stroke. It also impairs wound healing and thus surgeries are contraindicated for 4–6 weeks after the last bevacizumab infusion.

Altered mental status in the setting of impending herniation is a neurologic emergency. Its management includes intravenous use of high-dose corticosteroids in addition to standard methods of brain resuscitation, including elevation of the head to improve venous outflow, hyperventilation to induce vasoconstriction and reduce intracranial volume, with or without concurrent use of hypertonic saline, or mannitol for further intracranial volume reduction. In certain cases, surgery can also be attempted to reduce tumor volume that contributes to tissue shift and intracranial pressure elevation.

Approach to intracranial hemorrhage. Approximately 2% of patients with glioblastoma develop an ICH, whereas these events are exceedingly rare in other gliomas.[64–66] Microhemorrhages are commonly seen in treatment naïve oligodendrogliomas and in all gliomas following radiotherapy. Asymptomatic lesional hemorrhages should be interpreted within the context. Most small bleeds tend to remain asymptomatic, and the main management strategy of these should be to control potential risk factors that could lead to hematoma expansion. In other cases, even small bleeds may trigger seizures, which require adjustment of AEDs. Major bleeds most commonly occur within the contrast-enhancing tumor volume, in the setting of anticoagulation, whereas those without enhancement are unlikely to develop ICH. In contrast to the general population, hypertension does not have a strong association with glioma-related major ICH.[66] Additional risk factors include thrombocytopenia and treatment with bevacizumab with or without concurrent anticoagulation. ICH affects about 3% of those on bevacizumab, 6% of those anticoagulated, and 11% of those on the combination of the two, whereas only 3% of those on the combination regimen develop life-threatening hemorrhages.[66,67] Furthermore, as anticoagulation does not seem to have a detrimental effect on survival, the benefits of anticoagulation often outweigh the risk of ICH. If major ICH occurs, the treatment requires ICU level of care in most patients, and following similar strategies as with bleeds of other etiologies.

Clinical Pearls

1. Multidisciplinary symptom-oriented care may provide improved quality-of-care in complex cases.
2. Corticosteroids are used to manage symptoms caused by tumor-induced edema.
3. Corticosteroids can be effectively administered in one or two doses a day and evening doses should be avoided to minimize steroid-related insomnia.
4. Bevacizumab can be utilized as a steroid-sparing agent in select cases.

CASE 12.3C VENOUS THROMBOSIS, *PNEUMOCYSTIS*, STEROID MYOPATHY, AND NON-NEUROLOGICAL COMPLICATIONS OF HIGH-GRADE GLIOMA

Case. The 61-year-old male in Case 12.3a with an *IDH* wild-type, MGMT promoter methylated glioblastoma presented clinically stable after cycle 1 of adjuvant temozolomide with improving MRI scan consistent with early pseudoprogression. The decision was made to escalate temozolomide to 200 mg/m^2 per day according to the standard protocol. His subsequent 6 months of adjuvant treatment were complicated by: (1) inability to reduce steroids without increasing headaches, (2) deep venous thrombosis (DVT) of the left lower extremity that was treated with anticoagulation, (3) acute onset dyspnea and low-grade fever with a CT angiogram of the chest that was negative for a pulmonary embolus, but revealed ground glass opacities scattered throughout the lungs bilaterally. Bronchoscopy confirmed the diagnosis of *Pneumocystis jirovecii* pneumonia (PJP) and intravenous trimethoprim-sulfamethoxazole. After completing the intended six cycles of adjuvant temozolomide, he reported chronic fatigue and difficulty climbing stairs. His brain MRI remained stable. In an effort to mitigate the fatigue and the steroid-induced myopathy, levetiracetam and dexamethasone were tapered and discontinued.

Teaching Points: Common Non-Neurological Complications in Patients With High-Grade Glioma. In addition to neurological symptoms, non-neurological complications are common in patients with high-grade glioma. This case highlights several of the more common complications including treatment-induced lymphopenia, venous thromboembolism, *Pneumocystis* pneumonia, and corticosteroid induced myopathy.

Iatrogenic lymphopenia. Blood counts are routinely followed in patients with high-grade gliomas receiving radiation and temozolomide. Temozolomide is routinely held for significant neutropenia and thrombocytopenia. However, the most frequent change in blood counts is usually in the total lymphocyte counts. In general, lymphocyte and CD4 counts are within the normal range at the beginning of radiation but fall by about 70% immediately after the completion of radiation with concurrent temozolomide and may not fully recover for over 1 year.[68] Forty percent of these patients develop CD4 counts below 200 cells/mm^2, which is the level used to begin prophylactic antibiotics in patients with HIV. *Pneumocystis* pneumonia is a highly lethal complication of severe lymphopenia, especially when patients are also receiving glucocorticoids, which has been repeatedly reported in this patient population. As a result, prophylactic sulfamethoxazole-trimethoprim is routinely provided to patients until their lymphopenia resolves. In addition, early tumor progression and death in patients with high-grade gliomas has been independently associated severe treatment-related lymphopenia.[68]

Recent studies strongly suggest that this iatrogenic lymphopenia is related to the inadvertent radiation of circulating lymphocytes as they pass through the radiation field rather than to steroids or the temozolomide.[69–72] Severe radiation-related lymphopenia associated with early death from tumor progression has also been reported in patients with a variety of other solid tumors including head and neck cancer, lung, pancreatic, and cervical cancers.[73] It is likely that the number of radiation fractions, the volume of the radiation field, the radiation dose rates, and the inclusion of lymphoid storage sites (i.e., bone marrow and lymphoid organs) play a significant role in determining the extent of this lymphopenia. Studies are underway to modify radiation fields and fractions and to stimulate the production of lymphocytes using IL-7 in an effort to prevent or repair this recently described radiation injury. This becomes increasingly important as recent reports suggest that lymphopenia compromises responses to immunologic interventions such as vaccines or checkpoint inhibitors.[74] Currently, there are no specific clinical interventions or modifications suggested for lymphopenic patients other than the rapid assessment of shortness of breath and hypoxia for those at high risk for PJP infections.

Venous thromboembolism. VTE is a common complication of cancer and its treatment. Overall it has been estimated that patients with cancer have a 4–20-fold increased risk of VTE that is further accentuated by the administration of chemotherapy.[75]

Furthermore, VTE has been identified as prominent cause of death in cancer patients undergoing chemotherapy.[76] Patients with high-grade gliomas are at particularly high risk for VTE.[77,78] The cumulative incidence of symptomatic VTE among glioma patients has been estimated to be as high as 36% during their illness. The risk of VTE is highest in the postoperative period but remains increased through the entire course of the disease.[77]

Factors associated with an increased risk of VTE in patients with primary malignant brain tumors can be divided into three distinct categories. The patient-related factors include older age, obesity, tumor size, immobility, and leg paresis. Treatment-related factors include recent surgery especially with long operative times (>4 hours), chemotherapy, and antiangiogenic therapy (bevacizumab). Tumor-related risk factors also play a significant role in the incidence of VTE. VTE are more common in high-grade gliomas, in patients with intracranial hemorrhages related to their tumors, and in patients with elevated factor VIII activity. Recently, a striking association has been noted between the tumor's *IDH* mutational status and VTE.[79] Patients with mutant *IDH1*, which is much more common in grade II and III gliomas, appear to be at strikingly lower risk for VTE than those with wild-type *IDH* status, which is more common in older patients with glioblastoma. Similarly, tumors that express the glycoprotein podoplanin appear to be associated with both intratumoral thrombi and a high risk of VTE. This glycoprotein expression is most common in high-grade *IDH* wild-type gliomas.[80]

Prevention of VTE is important, as thrombosis and its treatment are associated with significant morbidity, mortality, and reduced quality of life. In general, thromboprophylaxis is recommended in hospitalized cancer patients and especially in the perioperative setting.[81] These recommendations also apply to patients with brain tumors, and as a result, low molecular weight heparin (LMWH) is generally recommended for 7–10 days after craniotomy. As the risk of VTE in patients with high-grade gliomas remains high throughout this illness, a randomized placebo-controlled study (PRODIGE) was initiated to evaluate the safety and efficacy of prophylactic LMWH (dalteparin) for up to 12 months in patients with high-grade gliomas.[82] Although this study was terminated prematurely due to poor accrual, 99 patients were randomized to LMWH and 87 to placebo. The results suggest a somewhat lower VTE rate and a trend toward increased major intracranial bleeding in patients on LMWH. A phase 1 study of tinzaparin reported similar results,[83] whereas Robins et al. did not note any VTE or bleeding events among 42 patients receiving dalteparin.[84] Given the currently available data, primary pharmacologic prophylaxis is not recommended for patients with malignant glioma after the postoperative period.[85] Instead, the emphasis is on early diagnosis and treatment of VTE.

VTEs in patients with brain tumors commonly present with unilateral lower extremity swelling with or without calf pain. These findings may be accompanied by dyspnea on exertion, hypoxia, pleuritic chest pain and/or hemoptysis if a lower extremity clot dislodges and travels to the lung. As a rule, any patient with lower extremity or pulmonary signs or symptoms deserves a formal evaluation to rule out a DVT (ultrasound of the lower extremity) or pulmonary embolism (PE; CT angiogram). These studies are frequently positive as about 30% of patients with high-grade gliomas will develop DVT or PE during their illness.

Treatment of VTE. Treatment of established VTE is very similar to that in other cancer settings. Current guidelines recommend LMWH over a vitamin-K antagonist. This recommendation is largely based on the results of the CLOT trial, which revealed better efficacy and safety in cancer patients.[86] However, this study included fewer than 30 patients with brain tumors and did not provide results from this small subpopulation. In 2018, LMWH was directly compared with a direct oral anticoagulant (DOAC) in cancer patients with a documented VTE.[87] Edoxaban was noted to be non-inferior to LMWH but was associated with higher rates of major bleeding. In the 74 patients accrued to this study with either primary brain tumors or brain metastases, efficacy and complications were similar but intracranial bleeding rates were not specifically reported. Another similar study of LMWH and a DOAC again revealed a higher risk of clinically relevant bleeding but included only three patients with brain tumors.[88] Based on the available data and the relatively low risk of fatal ICH, at this time the recommended first-line therapy for documented VTE in this unique patient population is systemic anticoagulation with LMWH.

Anticoagulation for VTE. Given the potential risk of intracranial hemorrhage with anticoagulation in patients with primary brain tumors, clinicians are generally cautious in initiating anticoagulation. A brain CT scan without contrast before starting anticoagulation provides an important baseline evaluation. Patients are then evaluated for relative contraindications to anticoagulation. These would include fresh blood on the pre-treatment brain CT, significant thrombocytopenia or an underlying coagulation disorder, or evident sources of active bleeding. If no contraindications exist, patients are often started on a heparin drip (which is reversible and can be given without a bolus dose in a stable patient) for 12–24 hours, and a brain CT scan without contrast is repeated to ensure that this has not precipitated a CNS bleed. If the patient's clinical and radiographic evaluations are stable, LMWH is initiated. Although anticoagulation for VTE is frequently discontinued months later, many patients with high-grade gliomas develop a recurrent VTE with discontinuation of LMWH. As a result, it is frequently continued indefinitely. For patients where systemic anticoagulation is contra indicated, treatment options include placing an inferior vena cava (IVC) filter until clinical conditions improve and then adding LMWH, relying on the filter alone, which is associated with a failure rate of about 30%, or using he IVC filter with low doses of LMWH.

Clinical Pearls

1. Thirty percent of patients with *IDH* wild-type gliomas develop VTEs.
2. Anticoagulation is safe in most glioma patients with VTE.
3. Lymphopenia is a common complication of chemoradiation and is associated with shorter survival and increased risk for infection.
4. PJP prophylaxis is recommended in lymphopenic patients.

CASE 12.3D RECURRENT DISEASE AND END-OF-LIFE CARE IN HIGH-GRADE GLIOMA

Case. The 61-year-old male in Case 12.3a with an *IDH* wild-type, MGMT promoter methylated glioblastoma completed treatment with concurrent and adjuvant temozolomide and was clinically and radiographically stable until approximately 6 months after finishing adjuvant temozolomide. He then reported worsening left-sided upper and lower extremity weakness with headaches. MRI showed nodular enhancement extending toward the right frontal convexity and increased T2/FLAIR hyperintensity spreading to the left hemisphere through the corpus callosum and there was also a 5-mm midline shift. Perfusion-weighted images revealed elevated blood volume in the enhancing area, as well as in additional non-enhancing foci. The findings were consistent with tumor pseudoprogression. The patient was monitored closely for the subsequent months and remained stable until his clinical deterioration 14 months later. Due to his poor functional status, he elected not to undergo further anticancer treatment and enrolled in hospice. He died 3 months later.

Teaching Points: Imaging Surveillance, Detection of Recurrent Disease, and End-of-Life Care. This case highlights several important aspects of clinical care in high-grade glioma. First, post-treatment pseudoprogression may not only occur early after chemoradiation but can also occur late and is more common in patients with MGMT*p* methylated gliomas. Perfusion-weighted and diffusion-weighted imaging can be helpful but is not diagnostic, and serial imaging is often needed, at times with biopsy or repeat resection. Ultimately, all patients will suffer from recurrent disease for which treatment options quickly become limited, and early consideration for concurrently managing end-of-life care is important.

Treatment monitoring and surveillance. Standard time points to perform imaging evaluations include the pre- and postoperative period, 4 weeks after radiation, and approximately every other chemotherapy cycle (i.e., every 2 to 3 months depending on the regimen).[89] The goal of the postoperative MRI is to assess the extent of the surgical intervention and is best acquired after 24–48 hours to minimize confounding postoperative changes.[89,90] The purpose of the post-radiation MRI is to establish a new radiographic baseline for patients and is to be used for comparison and response assessment on subsequent scans. As conventional MRI alone cannot differentiate tumor progression from treatment-related changes at this time point, these post-radiations scans often show worsening enhancement and edema, especially those of MGMT*p* methylated glioblastomas. This underlines the importance of concurrent clinical evaluation of patients with an attentive neurological examination, which may be discrepant from what is expected based on merely imaging.[90] Lastly, the imaging during the chemotherapy-only phase is to allow early identification of therapy failure and enable timely decision making about second-line or experimental treatments. Although the current National Comprehensive Cancer Network guidelines recommend every 2–4-month imaging for the first 3 years of post-treatment surveillance phase,[89] in practice, these intervals can be individualized based on tumor and patient characteristics.

Recurrent disease. Virtually all high-grade gliomas recur, and thus the decision making in this setting must factor in the extent of recurrence, prior treatment history, the type, and molecular profile of the tumor, as well as the performance status and the wishes and values of the patient. Thus, localized recurrence can be treated with localized therapy including surgery and radiation, whereas more extensive, multifocal, or leptomeningeal recurrence warrant systemic therapy or hospice enrollment.

Repeat surgery has many potential benefits including confirmation of recurrence versus treatment-related changes, cytoreduction, and, in select cases, may allow local chemotherapy. The former is often mandatory for those with anaplastic astrocytomas, as many trials require confirmation of glioblastoma on histology. Furthermore, surgery may allow placement of BCNU (carmustine) wafers for those who are not suitable candidates to receive systemic therapy. The use of BCNU wafers showed a 2-month survival benefit compared with placebo in patients diagnosed with recurrent high-grade gliomas, and fully resorb within weeks of placement.[91]

Repeat radiation treatment follows a similar approach to repeat surgery. Those with prolonged stability after radiation, especially in tumors that are more radiosensitive, such as those with *IDH* mutations, seem to be the best candidates, whereas brainstem and spinal cord locations are highly limiting due to the inherently lower radio-tolerance of these structures.

The use of systemic chemotherapy with or without radiation should be determined along the same principles. Of note, there is no currently known second-line systemic therapy that prolongs overall survival for glioblastoma; this includes trials using a great variety of agents such as bevacizumab, lomustine, irinotecan, sunitinib, rindopepimut, or even TTF, among many others.[92–96] Targeted therapies have limited evidence, but may be attempted based on the molecular profile of the tumor in question. Of these, the use of BRAF inhibitors to treat *BRAF*-V600E mutant tumors and targeting *NTRK* fusion has shown some signal of efficacy.[3,4]

Lastly, those with suitable functional status should be considered for clinical trials that may include all the above-mentioned treatment modalities. Selection of patients based on molecular characteristics has been an increasing trend in clinical trial design, and among many targets, include *IDH* mutants either direct targeting using vaccines, enzymatic inhibitors, or inhibitors of downstream products of the enzyme. Regardless of data-driven drug design and promising preclinical data, a successful trial requires the drug to pass the BBB not only in the contrast-enhancing tumor but in radiographically normal brain as well, in sufficiently high concentrations and for an adequate duration without intolerable toxicity. The recognition of this has led to a trend of adding surgery to assess pharmacokinetic and pharmacodynamic properties of the drug in question; however, a paradigm shift in drug and trial design is needed to improve the efficacy of studies.

End-of-life care. Sadly, virtually all high-grade glioma patients succumb to their illness. When the timing is appropriate, conversations about advance directives and end-of-life care should take place, preferably early in the course of the disease. Neuro-oncologists are well equipped to manage numerous symptoms that may limit quality of life, such as headaches due to brain edema, seizures, impaired sleep, etc.[97] However, patients with complex issues may benefit from a multidisciplinary, symptom-focused approach with the help of palliative care and hospice providers. Pain is a less prominent symptom at the end-stages of primary brain tumors, and these patients tend to be different from the general cancer population in many other respects as well. Therefore, neuro-oncologists need to be familiar with resources available in a hospice setting (e.g., staffing, AEDs, and parenteral dosing alternatives, etc.) and should form a close collaboration with the hospice team to help manage symptoms near the end of life.

Clinical Pearls

1. Guidelines recommend surveillance imaging of a high-grade glioma every 2–4 month for the first 3 years and these recommendations are often individualized based on prognostic factors and risk of early recurrence.
2. Virtually all high-grade gliomas will recur, at which time repeat surgery, radiation, salvage chemotherapy, or clinical trials are considered.
3. There is no currently known second-line systemic therapy that prolongs overall survival for glioblastoma.
4. Palliative care is optimally integrated into the management of high-grade gliomas early and contemporaneously with aggressive tumor-directed therapy, particularly once these tumors recur.

Approach to H3K27M mutant diffuse midline gliomas

Gliomas that preferentially affect the pons, the spinal cord, and the thalamus are referred to as diffuse midline gliomas and are relatively common in the pediatric population. The shift toward tissue sampling and molecular profiling of these tumors led to the identification of the canonical K27M mutation in the histone-3 gene. As these H3K27M mutant tumors were consistently identified to be a predictor of poorer survival in children, the 2016 WHO classification declared them as a new category. They are considered grade IV, although 15% of them have histopathologic features more consistent with grade II or III tumors. They are almost invariably *IDH* wild-type, and are hypomethylated. According to preliminary data, MGMT*p* methylation may be present in less than 10% of them and they are therefore considered chemoresistant (Table 12.1). Data is currently being accumulated in the adult population. According to preliminary studies, these mutations seem to be present in about 15% of adult midline gliomas and appear to have a favorable overall survival of 17–31 months, compared with their *IDH* wild-type counterparts without H3K27 mutations.[98,99]

References

1. Louis DN, World Health Organisation. *WHO Classification of Tumours of the Central Nervous System*. 4th ed. Lyon, France: International Agency for Research on Cancer; 2016.
2. Louis DN, Ellison DW, Brat DJ, et al. cIMPACT-NOW: a practical summary of diagnostic points from Round 1 updates. *Brain Pathol*. 2019;29:469–472.
3. Schreck KC, Guajardo A, Lin DDM, Eberhart CG, Grossman SA. Concurrent BRAF/MEK inhibitors in BRAF V600-mutant high-grade primary brain tumors. *J Natl Compr Canc Netw*. 2018;16:343–347.
4. Ziegler DS, Wong M, Mayoh C, et al. Brief report: potent clinical and radiological response to larotrectinib in TRK fusion-driven high-grade glioma. *Br J Cancer*. 2018;119:693–696.
5. Ostrom QT, Gittleman H, Truitt G, Boscia A, Kruchko C, Barnholtz-Sloan JS. CBTRUS Statistical Report: primary brain and other central nervous system tumors diagnosed in the United States in 2011–2015. *Neuro Oncol*. 2018;20:iv1–iv86.
6. Lebrun C, Fontaine D, Ramaioli A, et al. Long-term outcome of oligodendrogliomas. *Neurology*. 2004;62:1783–1787.
7. Ohgaki H, Kleihues P. Population-based studies on incidence, survival rates, and genetic alterations in astrocytic and oligodendroglial gliomas. *J Neuropathol Exp Neurol*. 2005;64:479–489.
8. Demeulenaere M, Duerinck J, DU Four S, Fostier K, Michotte A, Neyns B. Bone marrow metastases from a 1p/19q Co-deleted oligodendroglioma—a case report. *Anticancer Res*. 2016;36:4145–4149.
9. Lebrun C, Fontaine D, Ramaioli A, et al. Long-term outcome of oligodendrogliomas. *Neurology*. 2004;62:1783–1787.
10. Wunderlich G, Knorr U, Herzog H, Kiwit JC, Freund HJ, Seitz RJ. Precentral glioma location determines the displacement of cortical hand representation. *Neurosurgery*. 1998;42:18–26; discussion 26–27.
11. White ML, Zhang Y, Kirby P, Ryken TC. Can tumor contrast enhancement be used as a criterion for differentiating tumor grades of oligodendrogliomas? *AJNR Am J Neuroradiol*. 2005;26:784–790.
12. Smits M. Imaging of oligodendroglioma. *Br J Radiol*. 2016;89:20150857.
13. Choi C, Ganji SK, DeBerardinis RJ, et al. 2-hydroxyglutarate detection by magnetic resonance spectroscopy in IDH-mutated patients with gliomas. *Nat Med*. 2012;18:624–629.
14. Verma G, Mohan S, Nasrallah MP, et al. Non-invasive detection of 2-hydroxyglutarate in IDH-mutated gliomas using two-dimensional localized correlation spectroscopy (2D L-COSY) at 7 Tesla. *J Transl Med*. 2016;14:274.
15. Jenkinson MD, Smith TS, Joyce KA, et al. Cerebral blood volume, genotype and chemosensitivity in oligodendroglial tumours. *Neuroradiology*. 2006;48:703–713.
16. Leu K, Ott GA, Lai A, et al. Perfusion and diffusion MRI signatures in histologic and genetic subtypes of WHO grade II-III diffuse gliomas. *J Neurooncol*. 2017;134:177–188.
17. Jansen NL, Schwartz C, Graute V, et al. Prediction of oligodendroglial histology and LOH 1p/19q using dynamic [18F] FET-PET imaging in intracranial WHO grade II and III gliomas. *Neuro Oncol*. 2012;14:1473–1480.
18. Saito T, Maruyama T, Muragaki Y, et al. 11C-methionine uptake correlates with combined 1p and 19q loss of heterozygosity in oligodendroglial tumors. *AJNR Am J Neuroradiol*. 2013;34:85–91.
19. Cairncross G, Wang M, Shaw E, et al. Phase III trial of chemoradiotherapy for anaplastic oligodendroglioma: long-term results of RTOG 9402. *J Clin Oncol*. 2013;31:337–343.
20. van den Bent MJ, Carpentier AF, Brandes AA, et al. Adjuvant procarbazine, lomustine, and vincristine improves progression-free survival but not overall survival in newly diagnosed anaplastic oligodendrogliomas and oligoastrocytomas: a randomized european organisation for research and treatment of cancer phase III trial. *J Clin Oncol*. 2006;24:2715–2722.
21. Smith JS, Chang EF, Lamborn KR, et al. Role of extent of resection in the long-term outcome of low-grade hemispheric gliomas. *J Clin Oncol*. 2008;26:1338–1345.
22. Snyder LA, Wolf AB, Oppenlander ME, et al. The impact of extent of resection on malignant transformation of pure oligodendrogliomas: clinical article. *J Neurosurg*. 2014;120:309–314.
23. Hervey-Jumper SL, Berger MS. Evidence for improving outcome through extent of resection. *Neurosurg Clin N Am*. 2019;30:85–93.
24. van den Bent MJ, Brandes AA, Taphoorn MJ, et al. Adjuvant procarbazine, lomustine, and vincristine chemotherapy in newly diagnosed anaplastic oligodendroglioma: long-term follow-up of EORTC brain tumor group study 26951. *J Clin Oncol*. 2013;31:344–350.
25. Cairncross G, Berkey B, Shaw E, et al. Phase III trial of chemotherapy plus radiotherapy compared with radiotherapy alone for pure and mixed anaplastic oligodendroglioma: Intergroup Radiation Therapy Oncology Group Trial 9402. *J Clin Oncol*. 2006;24:2707–2714.
26. Boyle FM, Eller SL, Grossman SA. Penetration of intra-arterially administered vincristine in experimental brain tumor. *Neuro Oncol*. 2004;6:300–306.
27. Pal PK. Clinical and electrophysiological studies in vincristine induced neuropathy. *Electromyogr Clin Neurophysiol*. 1999;39:323–330.
28. Wick W, Roth P, Hartmann C, et al. Long-term analysis of the NOA-04 randomized phase III trial of sequential radiochemotherapy of anaplastic glioma with PCV or temozolomide. *Neuro Oncol*. 2016;18:1529–1537.
29. Lassman AB, Iwamoto FM, Cloughesy TF, et al. International retrospective study of over 1000 adults with anaplastic oligodendroglial tumors. *Neuro Oncol*. 2011;13:649–659.
30. Wick W, Meisner C, Hentschel B, et al. Prognostic or predictive value of MGMT promoter methylation in gliomas depends on IDH1 mutation. *Neurology*. 2013;81:1515–1522.
31. Wang YY, Wang K, Li SW, et al. Patterns of tumor contrast enhancement predict the prognosis of anaplastic gliomas with IDH1 mutation. *AJNR Am J Neuroradiol*. 2015;36:2023–2029.
32. Patel SH, Poisson LM, Brat DJ, et al. T2–FLAIR mismatch, an imaging biomarker for IDH and 1p/19q status in lower-grade gliomas: a TCGA/TCIA project. *Clin Cancer Res*. 2017;23:6078–6085.
33. Broen MPG, Smits M, Wijnenga MMJ, et al. The T2-FLAIR mismatch sign as an imaging marker for non-enhancing IDH-mutant, 1p/19q-intact lower-grade glioma: a validation study. *Neuro Oncol*. 2018;20:1393–1399.
34. Johnson DR, Kaufmann TJ, Patel SH, Chi AS, Snuderl M, Jain R. There is an exception to every rule—T2-FLAIR mismatch sign in gliomas. *Neuroradiology*. 2019;61:225–227.

35. Abrigo JM, Fountain DM, Provenzale JM, et al. Magnetic resonance perfusion for differentiating low–grade from high–grade gliomas at first presentation. *Cochrane Database Syst Rev*. 2018;1:CD011551.
36. U. S. National Library of Medicine. Phase III trial of anaplastic glioma without 1p/19q LOH. *ClinicalTrials.gov*. Available at: https://clinicaltrials.gov/ct2/show/NCT00626990. Accessed October 9, 2019.
37. Van Den Bent MJ, et al. Second interim and first molecular analysis of the EORTC randomized phase III intergroup CATNON trial on concurrent and adjuvant temozolomide in anaplastic glioma without 1p/19q codeletion. *J Clin Oncol*. 2019;37:2000.
38. Alexandrescu S, Korshunov A, Lai SH, et al. Epithelioid glioblastomas and anaplastic epithelioid pleomorphic xanthoastrocytomas-same entity or first cousins? Epithelioid GBM and Anaplastic Epithelioid PXA. *Brain Pathol*. 2016;26:215–223.
39. Kamson DO, Juhász C, Buth A, et al. Tryptophan PET in pretreatment delineation of newly-diagnosed gliomas: MRI and histopathologic correlates. *J Neurooncol*. 2013;112:121–132.
40. Juhász C, Dwivedi S, Kamson DO, Michelhaugh SK, Mittal S. Comparison of amino acid positron emission tomographic radiotracers for molecular imaging of primary and metastatic brain tumors. *Mol Imaging*. 2014;13. https://doi.org/10.2310/7290.2014.00015.
41. Dandy WE. Physiological studies following extirpation of the right cerebral hemisphere in man. *Bull Johns Hopkins Hosp*. 1933;53:31–35.
42. Salcman M. Survival in glioblastoma: historical perspective. *Neurosurgery*. 1980;7:435–439.
43. Sanai N, Polley MY, McDermott MW, Parsa AT, Berger MS. An extent of resection threshold for newly diagnosed glioblastomas. *J Neurosurg*. 2011;115:3–8.
44. Grabowski MM, Recinos PF, Nowacki AS, et al. Residual tumor volume versus extent of resection: predictors of survival after surgery for glioblastoma. *J Neurosurg*. 2014;121:1115–1123.
45. Albert NL, Weller M, Suchorska B, et al. Response assessment in neuro-oncology working group and European Association for neuro-oncology recommendations for the clinical use of PET imaging in gliomas. *Neuro Oncol*. 2016;18:1199–1208.
46. Stupp R, Mason WP, van den Bent MJ, et al. Radiotherapy plus concomitant and adjuvant temozolomide for glioblastoma. *N Engl J Med*. 2005;352:987–996.
47. Hegi ME, Diserens AC, Gorlia T, et al. MGMT gene silencing and benefit from temozolomide in glioblastoma. *N Engl J Med*. 2005;352:997–1003.
48. Stupp R, Hegi ME, Mason WP, et al. Effects of radiotherapy with concomitant and adjuvant temozolomide versus radiotherapy alone on survival in glioblastoma in a randomised phase III study: 5-year analysis of the EORTC-NCIC trial. *Lancet Oncol*. 2009;10:459–466.
49. Gilbert MR, Wang M, Aldape KD, et al. RTOG 0525: a randomized phase III trial comparing standard adjuvant temozolomide (TMZ) with a dose-dense (dd) schedule in newly diagnosed glioblastoma (GBM). *J Clin Oncol*. 2011;29. 2006–2006.
50. Blumenthal DT, Gorlia T, Gilbert MR, et al. Is more better? The impact of extended adjuvant temozolomide in newly diagnosed glioblastoma: a secondary analysis of EORTC and NRG Oncology/RTOG. *Neuro Oncol*. 2017;19:1119–1126.
51. Gramatzki D, Kickingereder P, Hentschel B, et al. Limited role for extended maintenance temozolomide for newly diagnosed glioblastoma. *Neurology*. 2017;88:1422–1430.
52. Stupp R, Taillibert S, Kanner A, et al. Effect of tumor-treating fields plus maintenance temozolomide vs maintenance temozolomide alone on survival in patients with glioblastoma: a randomized clinical trial. *JAMA*. 2017;318:2306–2316.
53. Lote K, Stenwig AE, Skullerud K, Hirschberg H. Prevalence and prognostic significance of epilepsy in patients with gliomas. *Eur J Cancer*. 1998;34:98–102.
54. Chen H, Judkins J, Thomas C, et al. Mutant IDH1 and seizures in patients with glioma. *Neurology*. 2017;88:1805.
55. Wali AR, Rennert RC, Wang SG, Chen CC. Prophylactic anticonvulsants in patients with primary glioblastoma. *J Neurooncol*. 2017;135:229–235.
56. Glantz MJ, Cole BF, Forsyth PA, et al. Practice parameter: anticonvulsant prophylaxis in patients with newly diagnosed brain tumors. *Neurology*. 2000;54:1886.
57. Perucca E. Optimizing antiepileptic drug treatment in tumoral epilepsy. *Epilepsia*. 2013;54:97–104.
58. Iuchi T, Kuwabara K, Matsumoto M, Kawasaki K, Hasegawa Y, Sakaida T. Levetiracetam versus phenytoin for seizure prophylaxis during and early after craniotomy for brain tumours: a phase II prospective, randomised study. *J Neurol Neurosurg Psychiatry*. 2015;86:1158–1162.
59. Rosati A, Buttolo L, Stefini R, Todeschini A, Cenzato M, Padovani A. Efficacy and safety of levetiracetam in patients with glioma: a clinical prospective study. *Arch Neurol*. 2010;67:343–346.
60. Kim YH, Park CK, Kim TM, et al. Seizures during the management of high-grade gliomas: clinical relevance to disease progression. *J Neurooncol*. 2013;113:101–109.
61. Galicich JH, French LA, Melby JC. Use of dexamethasone in treatment of cerebral edema associated with brain tumors. *J Lancet*. 1961;81:46–53.
62. Johannesdottir SA, Horváth-Puhó E, Dekkers OM, et al. Use of glucocorticoids and risk of venous thromboembolism: a nationwide population-based case-control study. *JAMA Intern Med*. 2013;173:743–752.
63. Stuijver DJ, Majoor CJ, van Zaane B, et al. Use of oral glucocorticoids and the risk of pulmonary embolism: a population-based case-control study. *Chest*. 2013;143:1337–1342.
64. Stark AM, Nabavi A, Mehdorn HM, Blömer U. Glioblastoma multiforme—report of 267 cases treated at a single institution. *Surg Neurol*. 2005;63:162–169.
65. Joseph DM, O'Neill AH, Chandra RV, Lai LT. Glioblastoma presenting as spontaneous intracranial haemorrhage: case report and review of the literature. *J Clin Neurosci*. 2017;40:1–5.
66. Khoury MN, Missios S1, Edwin N, et al. Intracranial hemorrhage in setting of glioblastoma with venous thromboembolism. *Neurooncol Pract*. 2016;3:87–96.
67. Norden AD, Bartolomeo J, Tanaka S, et al. Safety of concurrent bevacizumab therapy and anticoagulation in glioma patients. *J Neurooncol*. 2012;106:121–125.
68. Grossman SA, Ye X, Lesser G, et al. Immunosuppression in patients with high-grade gliomas treated with radiation and temozolomide. *Clin Cancer Res*. 2011;17:5473–5480.
69. Yovino S, Grossman SA. Severity, etiology and possible consequences of treatment-related lymphopenia in patients with newly diagnosed high-grade gliomas. *CNS Oncol*. 2012;1:149–154.
70. Yovino S, Kleinberg L, Grossman SA, Narayanan M, Ford E. The etiology of treatment-related lymphopenia in patients with malignant gliomas: modeling radiation dose to circulating lymphocytes explains clinical observations and suggests methods of modifying the impact of radiation on immune cells. *Cancer Invest*. 2013;31:140–144.

71. Ellsworth S, Balmanoukian A, Kos F, et al. Sustained CD4+ T cell-driven lymphopenia without a compensatory IL-7/IL-15 response among high-grade glioma patients treated with radiation and temozolomide. *Oncoimmunology*. 2014;3:e27357.
72. Piotrowski AF, Nirschi TR, Velarde E, et al. Systemic depletion of lymphocytes following focal radiation to the brain in a murine model. *Oncoimmunology*. 2018;7:e1445951.
73. Grossman SA, Ellsworth S, Campian J, et al. Survival in patients with severe lymphopenia following treatment with radiation and chemotherapy for newly diagnosed solid tumors. *J Natl Compr Canc Netw*. 2015;13:1225–1231.
74. Diehl A, Yarchoan M, Hopkins A, Jaffee E, Grossman SA. Relationships between lymphocyte counts and treatment-related toxicities and clinical responses in patients with solid tumors treated with PD-1 checkpoint inhibitors. *Oncotarget*. 2017;8:114268–114280.
75. Streiff MB, Ye X, Kickler TS, et al. A prospective multicenter study of venous thromboembolism in patients with newly-diagnosed high-grade glioma: hazard rate and risk factors. *J Neurooncol*. 2015;124:299–305.
76. Khorana AA, Francis CW, Culakova E, Kuderer NM, Lyman GH. Thromboembolism is a leading cause of death in cancer patients receiving outpatient chemotherapy. *J Thromb Haemost*. 2007;5:632–634.
77. Marras LC, Geerts WH, Perry JR. The risk of venous thromboembolism is increased throughout the course of malignant glioma. *Cancer*. 2000;89:640–646.
78. Edwin NC, Khoury MN, Sohal D, McCrae KR, Ahluwalia MS, Khorana AA. Recurrent venous thromboembolism in glioblastoma. *Thromb Res*. 2016;137:184–188.
79. Unruh D, Schwarze SR, Khoury L, et al. Mutant IDH1 and thrombosis in gliomas. *Acta Neuropathol*. 2016;132:917–930.
80. Riedl J, Ay C. Venous thromboembolism in brain tumors: risk factors, molecular mechanisms, and clinical challenges. *Semin Thromb Hemost*. 2019;45:334–341.
81. Lyman GH, Bohlke K, Khorana AA, et al. Venous thromboembolism prophylaxis and treatment in patients with cancer: American Society of Clinical Oncology Clinical Practice Guideline Update 2014. *J Clin Oncol*. 2015;33:654–656.
82. Perry JR, Julian JA, Laperriere NJ, et al. PRODIGE: a randomized placebo-controlled trial of dalteparin low-molecular-weight heparin thromboprophylaxis in patients with newly diagnosed malignant glioma. *J Thromb Haemost*. 2010;8:1959–1965.
83. Perry SL, Bohlin C, Reardon DA, et al. Tinzaparin prophylaxis against venous thromboembolic complications in brain tumor patients. *J Neurooncol*. 2009;95:129–134.
84. Robins HI, O'Neill A, Gilbert M, et al. Effect of dalteparin and radiation on survival and thromboembolic events in glioblastoma multiforme: a phase II ECOG trial. *Cancer Chemother Pharmacol*. 2008;62:227–233.
85. Jo JT, Schiff D, Perry JR. Thrombosis in brain tumors. *Semin Thromb Hemost*. 2014;40:325–331.
86. Lee AY, Levine MN, Baker RI, et al. Low-molecular-weight heparin versus a coumarin for the prevention of recurrent venous thromboembolism in patients with cancer. *N Engl J Med*. 2003;349:146–153.
87. Raskob GE, van Es N, Verhamme P, et al. Edoxaban for the treatment of cancer-associated venous thromboembolism. *N Engl J Med*. 2018;378:615–624.
88. Young AM, Marshall A, Thirlwall J, et al. Comparison of an oral factor Xa inhibitor with low molecular weight heparin in patients with cancer with venous thromboembolism: results of a randomized trial (SELECT-D). *J Clin Oncol*. 2018;36:2017–2023.
89. Nabors LB, Portnow J, Ahluwalia M, et al. NCCN Clinical Practice Guidelines in Oncology - Central Nervous System Cancers, Version 1.2019. Available at: https://www.nccn.org/professionals/physician_gls/pdf/cns.pdf. Accessed March 3, 2020.
90. Wen PY, Macdonald DR, Reardon DA, et al. Updated response assessment criteria for high-grade gliomas: response assessment in neuro-oncology working group. *J Clin Oncol*. 2010;28:1963–1972.
91. Brem H, Piantadosi S, Burger PC, et al. Placebo-controlled trial of safety and efficacy of intraoperative controlled delivery by biodegradable polymers of chemotherapy for recurrent gliomas. *Lancet*. 1995;345:1008–1012.
92. Weller M, Butowski N, Tran DD, et al. Rindopepimut with temozolomide for patients with newly diagnosed, EGFRvIII-expressing glioblastoma (ACT IV): a randomised, double-blind, international phase 3 trial. *Lancet Oncol*. 2017;18:1373–1385.
93. Wick W, Gorlia T, Bendszus M, et al. Lomustine and bevacizumab in progressive glioblastoma. *N Engl J Med*. 2017;377:1954–1963.
94. Grisanti S, Ferrari VD, Buglione M, et al. Second line treatment of recurrent glioblastoma with sunitinib: results of a phase II study and systematic review of literature. *J Neurosurg Sci*. 2019;63:458–467.
95. Gerstner ER. ACT IV: the final act for rindopepimut? *Lancet Oncol*. 2017;18:1294–1296.
96. Stupp R, Wong ET, Kanner AA, et al. NovoTTF-100A versus physician's choice chemotherapy in recurrent glioblastoma: a randomised phase III trial of a novel treatment modality. *Eur J Cancer*. 2012;48:2192–2202.
97. Walbert T. Palliative care, end-of-life care, and advance care planning in neuro-oncology. *Continuum (Minneap Minn)*. 2017;23:1709–1726.
98. Buerki R, Lapointe S, Solomon D, et al. Clinical and pathological characteristics of 52 adults with H3 K27M-mutant diffuse midline gliomas at UCSF (S14.004). *Neurology*. 2019;92:S14.
99. Schreck KC, Ranjan S, Skorupan N, et al. Incidence and clinicopathologic features of H3 K27M mutations in adults with radiographically-determined midline gliomas. *J Neurooncol*. 2019;143:87–93.

Chapter 13

Approach to the patient with CNS lymphoma

Ahmad N. Kassem and David M. Peereboom

CHAPTER OUTLINE

Introduction

Primary central nervous system lymphoma (PCNSL) is defined as lymphoma confined to the central nervous system (CNS) at presentation. By contrast, secondary CNS lymphoma represents a systemic lymphoma (i.e., outside the CNS) that has metastasized to the CNS (e.g., secondary site) either as part of the initial presentation or at relapse. Secondary CNS lymphoma can also manifest as isolated CNS relapse despite systemic remission. Although this chapter focuses on PCNSL, secondary CNS lymphoma shares many similarities in the approach and management.

PCNSL is a rare, aggressive extranodal non-Hodgkin lymphoma (NHL) that is confined to the CNS with no evidence of prior or current systemic disease. It may involve the brain, eyes, leptomeninges, or the spinal cord. Of note, eye involvement in this context refers to involvement of the vitreous and retina—i.e., *ocular* lymphoma. In contrast, *orbital* lymphoma refers to a non-CNS site of extranodal lymphoma; as such, it is not germane to the discussion of CNS lymphoma. PCNSL accounts for 2 to 3% of all primary CNS tumors.[1] The median age of patients with PCNSL is approximately 60 years. Over 90% of cases of PCNSL are classified histologically as diffuse large B-cell lymphoma (DLBCL).[2]

Patients present with progressive and relatively rapid progression of focal neurological symptoms. Over two-thirds of patients present with a focal neurological deficit and over 40% have neuropsychiatric symptoms. Other presenting symptoms include increased intracranial pressure, seizures, and visual disturbances.[3]

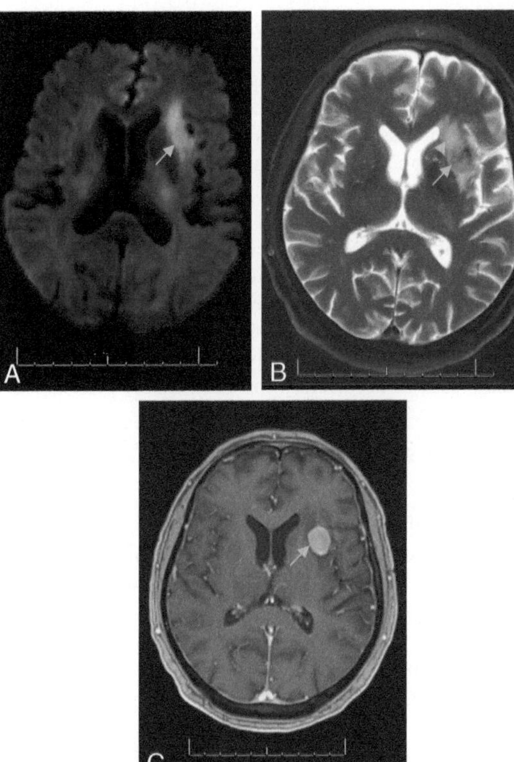

Fig. 13.1 MRI of the brain including (A) axial diffusion-weighted imaging showing an area of restricted diffusion in the left insular cortex (arrow), (B) axial T2-weighted imaging showing a central round mass lesion (arrow) with surrounding cerebral edema (arrowhead), and (C) axial T1-weighted homogeneously gadolinium-enhanced lesion (arrow) measuring 1.4 × 1.8 cm^2.

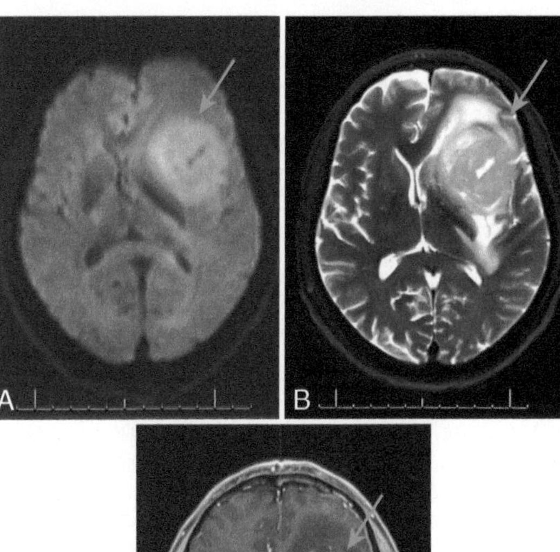

Fig. 13.2 MRI of the brain including (A) axial diffusion-weighted imaging showing a large area of restricted diffusion in the insular cortex (arrow), (B) axial T2-weighted imaging showing an enlarged lesion (arrow) with surrounding mass effect, expansion into the region of the Sylvian fissure and surrounding cerebral edema with left to right midline shift, and (C) axial T1-weighted imaging showing a large homogeneous enhancing 3.6 × 4.6 cm^2 lesion (arrow).

Clinical case

CASE 13.1 PRIMARY CNS LYMPHOMA

Case. A 61-year-old female presented in 2009 to an outside hospital with confusion, word-finding difficulties, and absence episodes. MRI of the brain demonstrated a 1.8 cm × 1.4 cm diffusely enhancing mass in the left frontal lobe (Fig. 13.1A–C). The patient received corticosteroids. A lumbar puncture (LP) yielded cerebrospinal fluid (CSF) that was abnormal but nondiagnostic by cytology and flow cytometry. A brain biopsy was performed and the specimen was read as suspicious but nondiagnostic for lymphoma. The mass gradually shrunk, the corticosteroids were tapered off, and the patient felt well for 2 years. In 2011, the patient developed floaters; a vitrectomy showed scattered atypical cells but was nondiagnostic. Six months later, a brain mass appeared. A second brain biopsy demonstrated chronic inflammatory cells. The patient came off corticosteroids and was monitored until 2014, when the lesion grew (Fig. 13.2A–C). A brain biopsy demonstrated DLBCL. Systemic staging including CT chest, abdomen, and pelvis was negative for systemic involvement. Ocular examination did not reveal involvement of the vitreous. A diagnosis of primary CNS DLBCL was made and the patient enrolled in a clinical trial of high-dose methotrexate (HD-MTX)–based combination chemotherapy. She completed the 6-month regimen and achieved a complete response (CR) that lasted for 3 years. In 2017, the patient had a relapse. She was re-challenged with HD-MTX and again achieved a CR. In 2018, she developed an isolated ocular recurrence and received intravitreal chemotherapy. She continues with stable ocular disease on intravitreal therapy without relapse in the brain or CSF.

Teaching Points: Approach to Evaluation and Management of PCNSL. This patient's case illustrates several important aspects of the evaluation and management of PCNSL. At presentation, she received corticosteroids, which likely contributed to the initial nondiagnostic pathological specimens. Because of this nondiagnostic pathology, she underwent an LP, vitrectomy, and three brain biopsies before her PCNSL was able to be diagnosed, 5 years after her initial symptoms. Thus, corticosteroids should be withheld in any patient for whom PCNSL (or any lymphoma) is suspected but not yet diagnosed.

In terms of management, she was enrolled in a clinical trial at diagnosis. Although she eventually relapsed, participation in a well-designed clinical trial is the treatment of choice for aggressive primary CNS malignancies including CNS lymphoma. She had a good initial response to HD-MTX–based chemotherapy and when her disease recurred 3 years later, she was able to be re-challenged with methotrexate with good response. Thus, for a patient with a durable response to chemotherapy, re-challenge with the same regimen is a reasonable option.

Her isolated ocular relapse was treated with isolated ocular therapy while her brain and CSF remained disease free. For a patient with isolated ocular disease, local therapy to the eyes is a reasonable option.

This case raises several important clinical questions for consultants evaluating and managing these patients. The remainder of the chapter will address each of these clinical questions:

1. Is lymphoma in the differential diagnosis for this new brain lesion?
2. In biopsied-confirmed CNS lymphoma, is this primary or secondary CNS lymphoma?
3. Is the patient immune competent or immunocompromised?
4. What is the approach to management of immunocompetent PCNSL?
5. What is the approach to management of immunocompromised PCNSL?
6. What is the approach to management of relapsed or refractory PCNSL?

Approach to the initial diagnosis of CNS lymphoma

About two-thirds of immunocompetent patients with PCNSL initially present with a solitary brain mass. Involvement of the brain hemispheres is the most common localization (38%), followed by thalamus and basal ganglia (16%), corpus callosum and related structures (14%), periventricular loci (12%), and the cerebellum (9%).[4] MRI of the brain typically demonstrates periventricular homogenous contrast enhancement with well-defined borders, low signal on T2-weighted imaging, and restricted diffusion on diffusion-weighted imaging.[5] Less typical presentations such as an intraventricular mass, cranial or radicular nerve enhancement, or isolated meningeal enhancement have been described. In patients who are immunocompromised, imaging findings may be atypical with multiple, ring-enhancing, or patchy enhancing lesions being observed.

Suggestive imaging must be followed by histopathologic confirmation. Tissue diagnosis is essential as the differential diagnosis on MRI of the brain includes multiple sclerosis, sarcoidosis, and occasionally gliomas. Like lymphoma, these entities may demonstrate a transient response to corticosteroids.[5] Therefore, unless the patient is deteriorating, one must avoid corticosteroid administration prior to the proper evaluation of the patient with suspected PCNSL. The potent lympholytic property of corticosteroids will commonly lead to necrosis of lymphoma, rendering tissue nondiagnostic as occurred in the patient described above.

Clinical pearls

1. Immunosuppression and older age are the major risk factors for the development of PCNSL.
2. The typical clinical presentation of PCNSL involves progressive and relatively rapid focal neurological symptoms associated with the neuroanatomic localization of the tumor.
3. Treatment with corticosteroids should be deferred until pathologic confirmation.

Differentiating primary and secondary CNS lymphoma

For a patient presenting with a possible CNS lymphoma on imaging, the initial decision on the site of tissue diagnosis will also depend on imaging of the chest, abdomen, and pelvis, typically with CT. Some centers use positron emission tomography (PET) CT scan with fluorodeoxyglucose (FDG) (PET-CT). Imaging of these sites accomplishes two purposes: (1) It distinguishes primary from secondary CNS lymphoma and, (2) if suggestive of systemic lymphoma, it determines a site for biopsy. If systemic lymphadenopathy is present, a lymph node biopsy is the biopsy site of choice, as it will reveal the lymph node architecture that informs the subtype of lymphoma and allows comprehensive molecular analysis, which in turn oftentimes will guide therapy. Men with negative systemic imaging should have a testicular ultrasound (US) to rule out primary testicular lymphoma, which, though uncommon as a primary site, has a significant risk of CNS metastasis.[6] Bone marrow aspirate and biopsy have been recommended in some guidelines as part of the evaluation for systemic lymphoma. If the described staging is negative, however, the likelihood of finding isolated bone marrow lymphoma as a source of CNS involvement is 2.5%, calling into question the utility of this procedure.[7]

Once the CT of chest, abdomen, and pelvis and, in men, testicular US are confirmed negative, three options exist for tissue diagnosis and should be pursued in order from least to most invasive.

1. *Lumbar puncture.* If not contraindicated by elevated intracranial pressure, the least invasive method to diagnose PCNSL is an LP. Importantly, the CSF analysis should be of high volume (>10 mL) and must include flow cytometry and ideally reviewed by a hematopathologist, in addition to routine analysis and cytology. CSF cultures are not necessary in the absence of symptoms or signs of infection and allows for prioritizing CSF to more relevant tests. MRI should be performed prior to the LP to avoid nonspecific meningeal enhancement caused by the procedure. This enhancement can mimic leptomeningeal disease. For patients with immunocompromised PCNSL, the presence of positive CSF Epstein-Barr virus (EBV)-polymerase chain reaction (PCR) in the setting of typical imaging of CNS lymphoma is diagnostic and can mitigate the need for brain biopsy.
2. *Slit lamp examination (SLE).* SLE should be performed to detect cells in the vitreous and/or retinal infiltrates. A suspicious finding on SLE would be followed by a vitrectomy or, in some cases, by a retinal biopsy.
3. *Brain biopsy.* If both the LP and SLE are negative, the patient should have a brain biopsy. Although a positive LP or vitrectomy will spare the patient a brain biopsy, the patient who has been diagnosed by brain biopsy first should still undergo an LP and SLE to establish the presence or absence of disease in the CSF and/or ocular compartment, respectively. The latter patient with suspicious findings on SLE would not require a vitrectomy to establish ocular involvement. As mentioned earlier, corticosteroid administration increases the risk of a nondiagnostic biopsy usually characterized by necrosis. In case of a nondiagnostic biopsy after corticosteroid administration, serial imaging after withdrawal of corticosteroid therapy may be performed with repeat biopsy after radiologic evidence of tumor regrowth.[8]

Whereas the vast majority of PCNSL are DLBCL, the finding of Burkitt, low-grade, or T-cell lymphoma will alter the management.[9] Clinically, the most important tumor cell marker is the lymphocyte surface CD20, which predicts therapeutic response to anti-CD20 antibodies such as rituximab.

The pathologic evaluation of CSF should include cell counts, protein, glucose, histology, cytology, and flow cytometry. The latter three tests should also be performed on vitreous fluid. The sensitivity of CSF cytology in diagnosis of PCNSL is only 15%.[10] Flow cytometry is more sensitive.[11] If the initial CSF analysis suggests but does not confirm (e.g., elevated protein concentration or presence of lymphocytes read as "atypical" or "suspicious") lymphoma, a repeat LP may be diagnostic. If the initial CSF is normal, however, a repeat sample will have a low diagnostic yield. Finally, PCR detection of immunoglobulin (IgH) gene rearrangements in CSF may also be helpful, as it does not require intact cells.[10]

Clinical pearls

1. Ninety to ninety-five percent of cases of PCNSL are classified histologically as DLBCL.
2. MRI with contrast is the most sensitive imaging modality for the detection of PCNSL.
3. Diagnosis and staging require a HIV serology, full-body CT or PET-CT, detailed ophthalmologic examination, LP, and in older males, a testicular US.

Approach to the immunocompetent patient with PCNSL

Once a diagnosis of PCNSL is established, the immune function of the host is a critical first step in determining the optimal approach to managing the patient. Although immunodeficiency and immunosuppression are the main risk factors for the development of PCNSL, most cases occur in immunocompetent individuals.[3]

PCNSL should be approached as a "whole brain disease."[12] Pretreatment clinical evaluation should include a detailed history and physical examination with careful assessment of neurologic deficits and lymphadenopathy that may suggest systemic disease. Cognitive function testing with neuropsychologic batteries should be performed at baseline and during follow-up visits to watch for potential treatment toxicities.[13] Often, patients at diagnosis are floridly ill and cannot participate in such testing. Laboratory testing should include HIV and hepatitis serologies, lactate dehydrogenase, and hepatic and renal function tests. Although some guidelines recommend a bone marrow aspirate and biopsy, this procedure has a yield of only 2.5% in detecting isolated bone marrow lymphoma as a source of secondary CNS lymphoma.[14] Therefore, many centers do not perform this procedure as part of the evaluation for CNS lymphoma.

Prognosis. The prognostic significance of the classic Ann Arbor staging system does not apply to PCNSL. Several prognostic scoring systems are used for PCNSL.[15,16] The simplest prognostic score distinguishes three groups on the basis of age and Karnofsky performance status (KPS)—age <50 years, age >50 years plus KPS >70, or age >50 years plus KPS less than 70—which correlate with median overall survivals of 8.5, 3.2, and 1.1 years, respectively.[15] In daily practice, this system is simple to use and offers at least a rough estimate of prognosis.

Treatment of immunocompetent PCNSL

As with any serious illness, the optimal patient management is entry onto a clinical trial, as was the case in the patient described previously. Unlike most CNS malignancies, the goal of therapy for PCNSL is long-term disease control. Because PCNSL generally responds very well to therapy, most patients, even if severely ill, should be considered for aggressive treatment.

Surgery. Traditionally, surgery has had no role in the management of PCNSL with the exception of placement of an Ommaya reservoir for the administration of intrathecal therapy. The rapid response to corticosteroids, chemotherapy, and radiation therapy obviate a role for surgical resection. The occasional patient whose brain mass has a radiographic appearance of a glioma may undergo a resection with the unexpected pathologic finding of lymphoma.

Phases of treatment. Therapy for newly diagnosed hematologic malignancies including PCNSL is often divided into three phases: induction, consolidation, and maintenance. Induction refers to the initial therapy, generally with multiagent chemotherapy, with the goal of cure or at least a CR (i.e., no evidence of active cancer detectable on physical examination, CNS imaging, repeat SLE, and, if positive at diagnosis, a repeat LP). Successful induction is then followed by consolidation, which may involve chemotherapy and/or radiation therapy with the goal of consolidating the CR. Thereafter, maintenance therapy may be given with the goal of preventing or delaying disease recurrence, although the efficacy of maintenance therapy in PCNSL is unproven.

Induction therapy

Before the advent of effective chemotherapy for PCNSL, whole-brain radiation therapy (WBRT) was the only treatment offered to PCNSL patients. WBRT resulted in short-lived responses with overall survival (OS) between 10 and 18 months with a 5-year survival of <20%.[17,18] Furthermore, the neurocognitive decline seen in PCNSL survivors can be severe, although lower radiation dose regimens (23.4 Gy instead of 45 Gy) likely have a better toxicity profile and have recently been tested in a randomized clinical trial.[19] Off study, however, most centers defer WBRT until failure of effective chemotherapy regimens.[20] CHOP chemotherapy regimen (cyclophosphamide, doxorubicin, vincristine, and prednisone), typically used in aggressive systemic lymphomas, failed to show adequate disease control due to the poor blood-brain barrier (BBB) penetration of these agents.

High-dose methotrexate. HD-MTX emerged in the 1970s as an effective treatment for PCNSL. It is still regarded as the most important and beneficial single drug. Penetration of methotrexate into the CNS depends on the total dose and the rate of infusion. Although doses of at least 3.5 grams (G)/m^2 can cross the BBB and reach tumoricidal concentrations in the brain parenchyma, tumoricidal concentrations in the CSF require doses of 3 G/m^2 by rapid infusion—over 3 hours maximum.[21] Doses of 8 G/m^2 can achieve cytotoxic concentrations in the vitreous and is often used for patients with ocular involvement.[22] HD-MTX intravenously provides sufficient cytotoxic levels in the CNS with no added benefit from intrathecal MTX.[23,24] Therefore, intrathecal MTX is generally not part of the therapy for newly diagnosed patients. Infusions of HD-MTX require pretreatment and posttreatment hyperhydration, urine alkalinization, leucovorin rescue, and monitoring of MTX concentration. Multiagent chemotherapy with a HD-MTX backbone is essential, yet the choice of agents to be used with MTX is still a matter of discussion.[25,26]

Rituximab. Rituximab, an anti-CD20 monoclonal antibody that has been the mainstay of treatment of systemic NHLs, has poor CNS penetration due to the large size of the molecule.[26,27] The highest concentration and resultant efficacy of rituximab occurs during the early treatment phase when the integrity of the BBB is reduced at the location of the contrast-enhancing tumors.[28] Addition of rituximab to MTX-based regimens has shown significant improvement in complete remission rates and OS. Although one randomized trial did not show benefit with the addition of rituximab, the backbone of that regimen was atypical.[29] As a result, rituximab remains part of all induction protocols for PCNSL.

Methotrexate-based regimens. Multiple methotrexate-based chemotherapy regimens including rituximab have been investigated. Rituximab, methotrexate, vincristine, and procarbazine (R-MVP); rituximab, methotrexate, and temozolomide (MR-T); rituximab, methotrexate, etoposide, carmustine, and prednisone (RMBVP); and rituximab, methotrexate, cytarabine, and thiotepa (MATRix) were all tried with different consolidation therapies. A prospective randomized comparison trial has been performed in the general population, demonstrating the superiority of MATRix over a two- or three-drug combination of the same agents.[30] The only comparison study compared HD-MTX and temozolomide with HD-MTX, vincristine, and procarbazine (MVP) in an elderly population (age >59 years) in a multicenter phase II trial. Toxicity profiles were similar between the groups. The objective response rate was 82% in the MVP group and 71% in the HD-MTX and temozolomide group, and median OS was 31 and 14 months, respectively. Although these trends were not statistically significant, the results favor the MVP regimen.[31] No single regimen appears to be clearly superior. The choice of induction regimen is largely determined by geographic tendencies and physician preferences. Prospective trials are needed to compare these regimens.

Blood-brain barrier disruption therapy. BBB disruption (BBBD) with hyperosmotic mannitol increases CNS drug concentrations.[32] When followed by intraarterial methotrexate, patients who had the procedure achieved similar outcomes to patients treated with HD-MTX based chemotherapy.[33] Durable responses can be achieved, but the procedure is quite complex and requires general anesthesia. Because few centers perform the procedure, randomized trials that compare this strategy with conventional HD-MTX–based chemotherapy are not feasible. As a result, BBBD with intraarterial chemotherapy has not been widely implemented.

Assessment of response. OS is the most important measure of efficacy of treatment for PCNSL. Radiographic response is assessed after induction and then after consolidation and with regular assessments after the completion of therapy. Radiographic responses are scored as complete response (CR), partial response, stable disease, and progressive disease (PD). The most important of these is the CR, which requires (1) complete disappearance of all enhancing abnormalities on contrast-enhanced MRI; (2) absence of malignant cells in the vitreous and resolution of any previously documented retinal or optic nerve infiltrates if present at initial staging; and (3) negative CSF cytology if previously positive.[33]

Consolidation therapy

Patients who achieve complete remission after induction therapy are offered consolidation therapy to achieve a durable response. Current consolidation therapy options include radiation, chemotherapy, or myeloablative chemotherapy with autologous stem cell rescue.

Radiation. The role of WBRT as a consolidation therapy after inducing remission is a matter of controversy in PCNSL. The only phase III randomized study conducted in PCNSL examined whether the omission of WBRT affected survival. All patients received HD-MTX with or without ifosfamide, and those who achieved a CR were randomly assigned to receive 45 Gy WBRT or observation; those patients with less than a CR were randomly assigned to receive 45 Gy WBRT or high-dose cytarabine. WBRT prolonged progression-free survival (PFS) but not OS.[34,35] Whereas some experts have retained WBRT as part of standard consolidation based on improved PFS, most have omitted WBRT based on the lack of OS advantage and the high rate of neurotoxicity with WBRT.[35,36] There is growing evidence that reduced-dose WBRT consolidation after MTX-based induction therapy provides satisfying OS and PFS with superior patient neurocognitive profiles on follow-up compared with 45 Gy WBRT.[37]

High-dose chemotherapy with autologous stem-cell rescue. Consolidation therapy with high-dose chemotherapy and ASCR (HDC-ASCR) should be considered for younger patients with good organ function who achieve CR or near CR after induction therapy. Two trials suggested that HDC-ASCR after remission with methotrexate-based induction therapy is as effective as WBRT without neurocognitive toxicity seen with WBRT.[38–40] Patients should be carefully selected before undergoing such an aggressive treatment approach; however, the population eligible for HDC-ASCR is becoming more and more inclusive.

Consolidation chemotherapy. Non-myeloablative consolidative chemotherapy is developing as an option for PCNSL patients in remission. The Cancer and Leukemia Group B (CALGB) 50202 multicenter phase 2 trial reported promising results using high doses of cytarabine and etoposide as non-myeloablative consolidation, without WBRT, after induction therapy with MTX, temozolomide, and rituximab.[41] Non-myeloablative consolidation may be an attractive option to a wide population of patient who may not be eligible for ASCR.

Maintenance treatment

The progress achieved in inducing remission in PCNSL opened the door for discussion about maintenance treatment. Maintenance therapy is of significant value for patients who are not candidates for aggressive consolidative therapies or when WBRT is avoided. The continuation of methotrexate at longer intervals has been considered as a form of maintenance therapy.[42,43] Oral alkylating agents such as procarbazine and temozolomide have been explored as potential agents used for maintenance with no clear evidence of benefit, especially with the studies being non-comparative.[44] The oral immunomodulator lenalidomide has also been studied as a single-agent maintenance with promising results.[45] Prospective studies are needed to confirm the benefit of maintenance therapy and to define the optimal agent.

Follow-up

There is currently no consensus regarding a standardized follow-up for PCNSL patients. The benefit of routine imaging has not been established. A 10-year retrospective multicenter study in Denmark, including 86 patients, showed no role for routine radiologic follow up, with 97% of relapses being suspected based on symptoms and only one case detected on routine imaging.[46] On the other hand, asymptomatic patients who tend to have higher performance scores at relapse may be offered more aggressive and effective therapy with a higher chance of achieving remission; an argument in favor of routine surveillance imaging. The vast majority of centers perform routine surveillance with history, physical examination including a Mini-Mental State Examination (MMSE), and gadolinium-enhanced MRI scan of the brain. Patients with initial involvement of the eyes or spinal fluid should undergo repeat ophthalmologic examinations and LPs, respectively.[13] Patients should be reassessed after completion of therapy, at a minimum of every 3 months for 2 years, then every 6 months for 3 years, and annually for at least 5 years, for a total of 10 years of follow-up. Minimum testing at follow-up should include history, physical examination including an MMSE, and gadolinium enhanced MRI scan of the brain.

Special populations

PCNSL in the elderly. The incidence of PCNSL is increasing among the elderly, who comprise at least half of the individuals with the disease. Many PCNSL clinical trials exclude the elderly.[47] Elderly patients are at a higher risk of treatment toxicity due to declining organ function, decreased drug metabolism and elimination, comorbidities, and polypharmacy. The choice of induction therapy is particularly important in the elderly as they are often poor candidates for consolidation treatments. HD-MTX, however, is the treatment of choice for induction and is well tolerated by elderly patients with adequate supportive measures and frequent checks of renal function.[48] Methotrexate and temozolomide; or methotrexate, vincristine, procarbazine, and cytarabine are potential induction regimens for elderly patients with PCNSL, with some studies slightly favoring the latter.[32]

Intraocular lymphoma. Approximately 25% of PCNSL patients have intraocular involvement at the time of diagnosis.[49] Conversely 60–90% of patients with primary vitreoretinal lymphoma will develop PD in other sites of the CNS.[50] The prognostic significance of intraocular involvement is not clear, although it may suggest a worse prognosis on the basis of a more aggressive histology and a heavier burden of disease. More than one-third of patients with intraocular lymphoma have no visual symptoms, highlighting the importance of a dedicated ophthalmic examination for staging PCNSL at the time of diagnosis. Failure to diagnose intraocular lymphoma (IOL) may lead to the persistence of a malignant reservoir that increases the risk of recurrence. Furthermore, a vitrectomy or retinal biopsy may save the patient the risks of a brain biopsy.[51] Treatment for IOL includes local and systemic therapeutic interventions. Local therapy includes external beam radiotherapy to the eyes or intravitreal MTX and rituximab.[51] Treatment-related complications of intravitreal MTX include vitreous hemorrhage, endophthalmitis, retinal detachment, and hypotony.[52] Ocular radiotherapy or intraocular chemotherapy is associated with prolonged ocular disease control but without impact on OS.[52]

Clinical pearls

1. HD-MTX is the single most important treatment agent for PCNSL. Current therapy consists of a methotrexate-based combination chemotherapy with rituximab for B-cell lymphomas. Intrathecal therapy may be considered in patients with evidence of leptomeningeal involvement.
2. In patients who achieve a CR to induction therapy, high-dose chemotherapy with autologous stem cell rescue should be offered as consolidation to fit patients.
3. In patients who achieve a CR to induction therapy and are not candidates for autologous stem cell rescue, consolidation chemotherapy is considered or, in some cases, clinicians may consider WBRT.

Approach to the immunosuppressed patient with PCNSL

Immune suppression either by HIV or immunosuppressive agents allows growth of EBV. Because EBV drives lymphomagenesis, immune suppression increases the risk of NHL and consequently PCNSL. The general strategy for management of these patients involves immune reconstitution with or without cytotoxic therapy.

HIV-associated PCNSL

Before 1996, 40% of AIDS patients presented with malignancy (60% with an opportunistic infection).[53] Because the management of AIDS-related PCNSL (AR-PCNSL) differs substantially from that of immunocompetent patients, all patients with suspected PCNSL and an unknown HIV status require HIV testing. PCNSL accounts for 15% of NHL in HIV patients versus less than 1% of NHL in the general population.[54] AIDS patients have an absolute risk of 2–6% of developing PCNSL, a risk 1000 higher than the general population.[55] AR-PCNSL typically occurs in patients with CD4 counts below 50 cells/μL blood.[55,56] PCNSL constitutes up to 30% of CNS lesions in patients with AIDS.[57]

The frequency of HIV-associated PCNSL has diminished with the development of highly active antiretroviral therapy (HAART).[58] Despite HAART, PCNSL has the worst prognosis of any HIV-associated malignancy, with an estimated 2-year mortality as high as 90%.[59]

Patients with AR-PCNSL often present with florid acute organic brain syndrome, unlike the more insidious neurological decline seen in immunocompetent individuals.[54] The diagnostic approach is similar to that in immunocompetent patients with a few differences. CSF should be assayed for toxoplasma gondii and EBV. Detection of EBV activity in the CSF is suggestive of PCNSL. If CSF evaluation and ocular examination are negative and a brain biopsy cannot be performed, an elevated CSF EBV load in the setting of an FDG-avid CNS lesion on PET is highly specific and may justify treatment initiation.[60]

In HIV/AIDS patients, cerebral toxoplasmosis is on the differential diagnosis as it presents similarly with ring-enhancing lesions. Prior to the HAART era, a trial of empirical treatment for toxoplasmosis was common; resolution of the mass would rule out lymphoma. This approach is no longer recommended, as timely diagnosis and treatment of PCNSL can minimize the risk of neurological deterioration.[61]

Because AR-PCNSL is typically an end-stage manifestation of AIDS, these patients need urgent immune reconstitution, to control both opportunistic infections as well as lymphoma. A challenge in AR-PCNSL is to effectively target the malignancy while allowing immune reconstitution. Unfortunately, HIV seropositive individuals have been excluded from key studies in PCNSL treatment.

Upfront WBRT with HAART had been considered the standard of care of AR-PCNSL but has largely been replaced by chemotherapy. HAART and HD-MTX should be considered as the first-line for AR-PCNSL. Rituximab is safe in HIV-infected individuals and may be introduced when CD counts exceed 50 cells/μL.[62,63] Alkylating agents, vincristine and cytarabine, however, may be associated with an increased rate of neutropenic complications and a potentially more attenuated rate of CD4 recovery with HAART in HIV patients.[55] Intensive chemotherapy with ASCR has not been traditionally offered to patient with AR-PCNSL, although several series have described the use of chemotherapy with ASCR.[64,65]

Clinical pearls

1. Patients with AIDS-related PCNSL require HAART therapy and chemotherapy.
2. An elevated CSF EBV PCR in the setting of a typical brain lesion on MRI or FDG-avid CNS lesion on PET is highly specific for primary CNS lymphoma and may justify treatment initiation.

Iatrogenic immunosuppression-related PCNSL

The population of immunosuppressed individuals is steadily increasing with the wide use of immunosuppressive therapies and the advancements in the field of solid organ or allogeneic hematopoietic stem cell transplantation. Posttransplant lymphoproliferative disorder (PTLD) is a well-known complication of organ transplantation. Although brain involvement occurs in 7–15% of PTLD, isolated CNS disease is rare.[66,67] For patients with PTLD, reduction of immunosuppressive drugs carries the risk of graft failure, which contributes to the high mortality.[68] As a single strategy, reduction of immunosuppression is not adequate and must be accompanied by chemotherapy.[66] The management of these patients requires close collaboration with the transplant providers in order to decide on how much to reduce the transplant antirejection regimen. The chemotherapy treatment regimens are similar to those used for immunocompetent patients.

Clinical pearls

1. Patients with PTLD and PCNSL require reduction in immunosuppression and chemotherapy.

Approach to recurrent PCNSL

Despite the significant improvement in the management of PCNSL in the past years, up to 60% of patients experience relapse and one-third of patients have refractory disease (no response to initial therapy).[69,70] Treatment for PD depends on performance status, site of relapse, prior treatment, and duration of response.[35] In patients with long-lasting remission after initial treatment, re-challenge with a HD-MTX–containing chemotherapy should be considered.[6,8] If HDC-ASCR was not attempted as a consolidation therapy, it may be offered upon relapse.

Several newer strategies have emerged in recent years. Immunotherapy using single agent PD1 inhibitors or combination immunotherapy using a CD20 inhibitor (e.g., rituximab) and a PD1 inhibitor (e.g., nivolumab, pembrolizumab) is an approach under investigation.[71,72] The immunomodulatory agents lenalidomide and pomalidomide have activity against progressive PCNSL.[45,73] Ibrutinib, a Bruton tyrosine kinase inhibitor, also has activity against progressive PCNSL.[74,75] Other single agents or combinations with modest efficacy include temozolomide (with or without rituximab), topotecan, pemetrexed, bendamustine, ifosfamide/etoposide, cisplatin/cytarabine, buparlisib, and intraarterial carboplatin. Although rituximab has limited penetration across the BBB, intrathecal administration somewhat surprisingly can yield parenchymal responses.[76] Chimeric antigen receptor (CAR) T-cells penetrate the CNS, and responses have been observed in secondary CNS lymphoma patients (see Chapter 30 for discussion of

CAR T cells).[77] Trials of this strategy for progressive PCNSL are expected in the near future. Because the efficacy of WBRT at relapse is comparable with that when employed as initial therapy, most experts reserve WBRT for patients in whom medical salvage treatment fails.[78]

Clinical pearls

1. More than half of PCNSL patients who respond to treatment suffer from relapse. PCNSL relapse is treated with chemotherapy, immunotherapy, or WBRT.

Approach to PCNSL with leptomeningeal involvement

Leptomeningeal dissemination occurs in 11–42% of patients with PCNSL.[79,80] Patients with leptomeningeal PCNSL may present with multifocal symptoms, headaches, cranial nerve palsies, and spinal radiculopathies but often present without localizing symptoms.[4,81] Primary leptomeningeal lymphoma (PLML) without synchronous parenchymal brain/spine or systemic disease is rare and constitutes about 7% of PCNSL cases.[82]

Contrast-enhanced MRI of the entire neuraxis to define total tumor burden should be performed before initiating treatment. If a patient has already been diagnosed with PCNSL and imaging reveals classic leptomeningeal enhancement, the diagnosis of leptomeningeal lymphoma can be made and CSF sampling can be deferred. Otherwise, histologic confirmation by CSF sampling is essential. CSF should be sent for cytology, flow cytometry, and ideally review of an unfixed, stained sample by a hematopathologist. Repeat sampling with the addition of gene rearrangement studies can be performed if the initial sample is suspicious but nonconfirmatory.

In PLML, the CSF profile is always abnormal, and findings may include leukocytosis, elevated protein concentration, and hypoglycorrhachia. Definitive diagnosis may be established by detection of malignant lymphocytes on cytology, or a monoclonal population by flow cytometry or gene rearrangement studies, which may be more sensitive.[81] Despite the afore mentioned workup, the confirmation of the diagnosis by CSF sampling is sometimes not possible. If the suspicion remains high, diagnosis is sometimes possible with a meningeal biopsy from an enhancing area on MRI.[83]

A high rate of false-positive and false-negative results has been reported in CSF studies in PCNSL with leptomeningeal involvement.[84,85] False-negative results can be avoided by collection of high volumes (e.g., at least 10 mL), withholding of corticosteroids before the procedure, and prompt transfer of samples to the laboratory for analysis to preserve integrity of the sample.[86,87] Demonstration of T-cell receptor gene rearrangement may help differentiate true T-cell lymphoma from reactive T lymphocytes, which may accompany a B-cell malignancy.[88,89]

The impact of leptomeningeal involvement on prognosis has been reported inconsistently in the literature, with some studies associating it with a worse outcomes and other analyses showing no significant differences in prognosis between PCNSL patients who present with or without leptomeningeal dissemination.[79,80]

Current guidelines of the National Comprehensive Cancer Network (NCCN) recommends treatment with intrathecal MTX, cytarabine, or rituximab in cases of positive CSF studies or meningeal enhancement on MRI. In patients with obvious meningeal enhancement, intrathecal chemotherapy may have limited efficacy due to its very shallow penetration into the meninges. A significant toxicity of intrathecal chemotherapy is leukoencephalopathy (see Chapter 27, Case 27.5 for further discussion of approach to treatment-induced leukoencephalopathy). Radiation therapy could be considered for the unusual patient in whom deficits and sites of disease are focal and chemotherapy by any route is not an option.

Bing-Neel syndrome

Bing-Neel syndrome (BNS) is a CNS complication of Waldenström macroglobulinemia (WM), a B-cell lymphoproliferative disorder characterized by the presence of a serum IgM paraprotein associated with bone marrow infiltration by lymphoplasmacytic lymphoma.[90] Extranodal involvement of WM is exceedingly uncommon, and in BNS, malignant lymphoplasmacytic cells invade the CNS.[91] In the most common form, lymphocytes invade the leptomeningeal sheaths and perivascular spaces; it thus appears as enhancement and/or thickening of the meninges. A less common tumoral form presents as an intraparenchymal mass.

The clinical symptoms of BNS are diverse and may include headaches, cognitive deficit, cranial nerve palsies, and gait disorders.[92] The diagnosis of BNS is usually made within months after confirming the diagnosis of WM, yet it may be found in patients in whom a diagnosis of WM has not been made on presentation in up to one-third of cases.[93,94] BNS should be suspected in any WM patient with neurological manifestations. These symptoms and signs, however, could also result from neurological complications of WM caused by IgM deposition centrally leading to hyperviscosity syndrome, or deposition peripherally causing a demyelinating peripheral neuropathy.[94] Some references divide BNS into type A, where the symptoms are caused by lymphoplasmacytic infiltration into the CNS, and type B, where the symptoms are explained by IgM deposition.[95] Patients with either presentation should undergo contrast-enhanced MRI of the brain and spinal cord where BNS typically presents as thickening and enhancement of cranial nerves or the cauda equina. Less commonly, a tumoral form occurs and is most commonly seen in the deep subcortical parenchyma.[96]

Treatment should be offered to symptomatic patients with BNS. Because BNS is an indolent disease, asymptomatic patients may be monitored every 2–3 months off treatment. The goal of therapy is to treat the neurological symptoms. Treatment is guided by the clearance of neurological symptoms even if the disease is detectable by CSF analysis or radiological evidence.[93]

Like other lymphomas, BNS responds to corticosteroids, yet the effect is short-lasting. Corticosteroids should be reserved for rapid relief of symptoms after histopathologic confirmation of the diagnosis if possible. Overall response to first-line therapy is about 70% according to retrospective data, with no significant difference between different systemic therapeutic agents.[94,97] Treatment options for BNS are mostly adapted from PCNSL treatment. Patients with isolated meningeal involvement may be treated with intrathecal treatment alone. Other options include HD-MTX, high-dose cytarabine fludarabine, cladribine, bendamustine, or ibrutinib. Rituximab is often added to treatment regimens, with no clear evidence supporting its benefit.[94] Although BNS is radiosensitive, radiation therapy is not recommended as first-line regimen; it may be offered to patients for whom other treatments have failed, or patients with localized symptomatic spinal disease. In case of relapse, challenging with the same therapeutic agent may be considered if the initial response was complete and long standing.[97]

Clinical pearls

1. Bing-Neel syndrome is a rare and slowly progressing complication of Waldenström macroglobulinemia whereby malignant lymphoplasmacytic cells invade the CNS.
2. Treatment of Bing-Neel syndrome aims at treating neurological symptoms of the disease.

Primary T-cell CNS lymphoma

T-cell primary CNS lymphoma (TPCNSL) is a rare form of PCNSL and comprises 2 to 8.5% of cases, with higher incidences reported in eastern countries such as Japan and Korea.[3,98–100]

Of note, B-cell lymphomas are often infiltrated by T-cells, which may complicate the interpretation of immunophenotyping. Therefore, reactive T-cells in a B-cell tumor must be distinguished from a true T-cell lymphoma. This is especially true if a biopsy is collected after corticosteroid treatment, which would cause lysis of B-cells and the collection of reactive T-cells.[101] This distinction can be made with immunohistochemical staining and PCR for TCR gene rearrangement.[102,103] The clinical picture and treatment modalities for T-cell PCNSL is similar to DLBCL with similar agents used in treatment, with the exception of rituximab, which is used only for B-cell malignancies that express CD20.

Clinical pearls

1. T-cell primary CNS lymphoma (TPCNSL) is a rare form of PCNSL. The clinical picture and treatment modalities for TPCNSL are similar to DLBCL with similar agents used in treatment.

Diagnosis and management of neurological complications of treatment for PCNSL

With the improvement in survival of patients with PCNSL, complications of treatment are more commonly observed and require significant attention. Treatment-related neurotoxicity is defined as progressive neurological or cognitive impairment noted on serial examinations in the absence of lymphoma recurrence.[104] Although it is classically considered a late complication of PCNSL treatment, some studies suggest that leukoencephalopathy may begin within weeks after treatment completion.

Whole-brain radiation therapy (also see Chapter 25 for discussion of radiation-induced neurocognitive dysfunction). WBRT alone or with systemic chemotherapy is a significant risk factor for the development of late neurotoxicity, with patients over 60 years of age being at higher risk. Common symptoms and signs include deficits in attention, memory, executive function, gait ataxia, and incontinence. The MMSE is commonly used on follow-up to screen for neurotoxicity but has a low sensitivity for the detection of all of the symptoms of neurotoxicity. The actual incidence of neurotoxicity may thus be underestimated. A more detailed assessment such as a neuropsychologic evaluation usually reveals a more significant reduction in cognitive and psychomotor function in addition to a reduction in overall quality of life after early WBRT.[105] Periventricular white matter changes, ventricular enlargement, and cortical atrophy are common radiologic findings. In addition to demyelination and neuronal loss, pathologic studies suggest a possible vascular component.[106] Although reduced-dose WBRT is associated with milder cognitive dysfunction among PCNSL survivors compared with standard-dose WBRT, reduced dose WBRT as consolidation is still associated with impairments of verbal memory and motor speed.[50,107]

High-dose methotrexate (also see Chapter 27 for discussion of complications of systemic chemotherapy). Neurologic toxicity of HD-MTX can consist of stroke-like symptoms, an acute or subacute encephalopathy, and in the long term, a delayed multifocal leukoencephalopathy.[108] PCNSL patients treated with HD-MTX–based therapies without consolidative WBRT do not appear to exhibit severe cognitive dysfunction as determined by posttreatment neuropsychologic testing but nevertheless score lower than normative control subjects in several cognitive domains.[109]

Other chemotherapeutics (also see Chapter 27). Other chemotherapeutic agents can cause neurotoxicity. Rituximab uncommonly causes reactivation of John Cunningham (JC) virus leading to progressive multifocal leukoencephalopathy.[110] Vincristine neurotoxicity most commonly presents as a peripheral neuropathy, which can be severe, necessitating discontinuation of the drug. Vincristine should be stopped at the first manifestation of neuropathy, as this toxicity is cumulative and often permanent. Less common neurological toxicities include autonomic neuropathy, cranial nerve palsies, gait disorders, and encephalopathy. Cytarabine can cause an acute cerebellar ataxia. Unfortunately, there are no known protective measures or treatments for the effects of iatrogenic neurotoxicity in PCNSL, although patients who receive WBRT for brain metastases benefit from the addition of memantine.[111] Memantine could be considered for patients who require WBRT.

Clinical pearls

1. Treatment-related neurotoxicity including neurocognitive dysfunction after WBRT, delayed-onset leukoencephalopathy after methotrexate, or progressive multifocal leukoencephalopathy are major complications of PCNSL treatment and require frequent follow up after treatment.

References

1. Ostrom QT, Gittleman H, Liao P, et al. CBTRUS statistical report: primary brain and central nervous system tumors diagnosed in the United States in 2007–2011. *Neuro Oncol.* 2014;16(suppl 4):iv1–63.
2. Phillips EH, Fox CP, Cwynarski K. Primary CNS lymphoma. *Curr Hematol Malig Rep.* 2014;9:243–253.
3. Bataille B, Delwail V, Menet E, et al. Primary intracerebral malignant lymphoma: report of 248 cases. *J Neurosurg.* 2000;92:261–266.
4. Fine HA, Mayer RJ. Primary central nervous system lymphoma. *Ann Intern Med.* 1993;119:1093–1104.
5. Küker W, Nägele T, Korfel A, et al. Primary central nervous system lymphomas (PCNSL): MRI features at presentation in 100 patients. *J Neuro Oncol.* 2005;72:169–177.
6. Abrey LE, Batchelor TT, Ferreri AJ, et al. Report of an international workshop to standardize baseline evaluation and response criteria for primary CNS lymphoma. *J Clin Oncol.* 2005;23:5034–5043.
7. Hall KH, Panjic EH, Valla K, Flowers CR, Cohen JB. How to decide which DLBCL patients should receive CNS prophylaxis. *Oncology (Williston Park).* 2018;32:303–309.
8. Porter AB, Giannini C, Kaufmann T, et al. Primary central nervous system lymphoma can be histologically diagnosed after previous corticosteroid use: a pilot study to determine whether corticosteroids prevent the diagnosis of primary central nervous system lymphoma. *Ann Neurol.* 2008;63:662–667.
9. Camilleri-Broët S, Martin A, Moreau A, et al. Primary central nervous system lymphomas in 72 immunocompetent patients: pathologic findings and clinical correlations. *Am J Clin Pathol.* 1998;110:607–612.
10. Ekstein D, Ben-Yehuda D, Slyusarevsky E, Lossos A, Linetsky E, Siegal T. CSF analysis of IgH gene rearrangement in CNS lymphoma: relationship to the disease course. *J Neurol Sci.* 2006;247:39–46.
11. Quijano S, López A, Manuel Sancho J, et al. Identification of leptomeningeal disease in aggressive B-cell non-Hodgkin's lymphoma: improved sensitivity of flow cytometry. *J Clin Oncol.* 2009;27:1462–1469.
12. Kerbauy MN, Moraes FY, Lok BH, et al. Challenges and opportunities in primary CNS lymphoma: a systematic review. *Radiother Oncol.* 2017;122:352–361.
13. Grommes C, DeAngelis LM. Primary CNS lymphoma. *J Clin Oncol.* 2017;35:2410–2418.
14. Hall KH, Panjic EH, Valla K, Flowers CR, Cohen JB. How to decide which DLBCL patients should receive CNS prophylaxis. *Oncology (Williston Park).* 2018;32:303–309.
15. Abrey LE, Ben-Porat L, Panageas KS, et al. Primary central nervous system lymphoma: the Memorial Sloan-Kettering Cancer Center prognostic model. *J Clin Oncol.* 2006;24:5711–5715.
16. Ferreri AJM, Blay JY, Reni M, et al. Prognostic scoring system for primary CNS lymphomas: the international extranodal lymphoma study group experience. *J Clin Oncol.* 2003;21:266–272.
17. Shibamoto Y, Ogino H, Hasegawa M, et al. Results of radiation monotherapy for primary central nervous system lymphoma in the 1990s. *Int J Radiat Oncol Biol Phys.* 2005;62:809–813.
18. Nelson DF, Martz KL, Bonner H, et al. Non-Hodgkin's lymphoma of the brain: can high dose, large volume radiation

therapy improve survival? Report on a prospective trial by the Radiation Therapy Oncology Group (RTOG): RTOG 8315. *Int J Radiat Oncol Biol Phys*. 1992;23:9–17.
19. Morris PG, Correa DD, Yahalom J, et al. Rituximab, methotrexate, procarbazine, and vincristine followed by consolidation reduced-dose whole-brain radiotherapy and cytarabine in newly diagnosed primary CNS lymphoma: final results and long-term outcome. *J Clin Oncol*. 2013;31:3971–3979.
20. Citterio G, Ferreri AJ, Reni M. Current uses of radiation therapy in patients with primary CNS lymphoma. *Expert Rev Anticancer Ther*. 2013;13:1327–1337.
21. Lippens RJ, Winograd B. Methotrexate concentration levels in the cerebrospinal fluid during high-dose methotrexate infusions: an unreliable prediction. *Pediatr Hematol Oncol*. 1988;5:115–124.
22. Batchelor T, Carson K, O'Neill A, et al. Treatment of primary CNS lymphoma with methotrexate and deferred radiotherapy: a report of NABTT 96-07. *J Clin Oncol*. 2003;21:1044–1049.
23. Glantz MJ, Cole BF, Recht L, et al. High-dose intravenous methotrexate for patients with nonleukemic leptomeningeal cancer: is intrathecal chemotherapy necessary? *J Clin Oncol*. 1998;16:1561–1567.
24. Khan RB, Shi W, Thaler HT, DeAngelis LM, Abrey LE. Is intrathecal methotrexate necessary in the treatment of primary CNS lymphoma? *J Neuro Oncol*. 2002;58:175–178.
25. Graham MS, DeAngelis LM. Improving outcomes in primary CNS lymphoma. *Best Pract Res Clin Haematol*. 2018;31:262–269.
26. Ferreri AJ, Reni M, Foppolo M, et al. High-dose cytarabine plus high-dose methotrexate versus high-dose methotrexate alone in patients with primary CNS lymphoma: a randomised phase 2 trial. *Lancet*. 2009;374:1512–1520.
27. Shah GD, Yahalom J, Correa DD, et al. Combined immunochemotherapy with reduced whole-brain radiotherapy for newly diagnosed primary CNS lymphoma. *J Clin Oncol*. 2007;25:4730–4735.
28. Rubenstein JL, Combs D, Rosenberg J, et al. Rituximab therapy for CNS lymphomas: targeting the leptomeningeal compartment. *Blood*. 2003;101:466–468.
29. Bromberg JEC, Issa S, Bakunina K, et al. Rituximab in patients with primary CNS lymphoma (HOVON 105/ALLG NHL 24): a randomised, open-label, phase 3 intergroup study. *Lancet Oncol*. 2019;20:216–228.
30. Ferreri AJM, Cwynarski K, Pulczynski E, et al. Chemoimmunotherapy with methotrexate, cytarabine, thiotepa, and rituximab (MATRix regimen) in patients with primary CNS lymphoma: results of the first randomisation of the International Extranodal Lymphoma Study Group-32 (IELSG32) phase 2 trial. *Lancet Haematol*. 2016;3:e217–e227.
31. Omuro A, Chinot O, Taillandier L, et al. Methotrexate and temozolomide versus methotrexate, procarbazine, vincristine, and cytarabine for primary CNS lymphoma in an elderly population: an intergroup ANOCEF-GOELAMS randomised phase 2 trial. *Lancet Haematol*. 2015;2:e251–e259.
32. Neuwelt EA, Goldman DL, Dahlborg SA, et al. Primary CNS lymphoma treated with osmotic blood-brain barrier disruption: prolonged survival and preservation of cognitive function. *J Clin Oncol*. 1991;9:1580–1590.
33. Angelov L, Doolittle ND, Kraemer DF, et al. Blood-brain barrier disruption and intra-arterial methotrexate-based therapy for newly diagnosed primary CNS lymphoma: a multi-institutional experience. *J Clin Oncol*. 2009;27:3503–3509.
34. Thiel E, Korfel A, Martus P, et al. High-dose methotrexate with or without whole brain radiotherapy for primary CNS lymphoma (G-PCNSL-SG-1): a phase 3, randomised, non-inferiority trial. *Lancet Oncol*. 2010;11:1036–1047.
35. Korfel A, Thiel E, Martus P, et al. Randomized phase III study of whole-brain radiotherapy for primary CNS lymphoma. *Neurology*. 2015;84:1242–1248.
36. Citterio G, Reni M, Gatta G, Ferreri AJM. Primary central nervous system lymphoma. *Crit Rev Oncol Hematol*. 2017;113:97–110.
37. Morris PG, Correa DD, Yahalom J, et al. Rituximab, methotrexate, procarbazine, and vincristine followed by consolidation reduced-dose whole-brain radiotherapy and cytarabine in newly diagnosed primary CNS lymphoma: final results and long-term outcome. *J Clin Oncol*. 2013;31:3971–3979.
38. Ferreri AJM, Cwynarski K, Pulczynski E, et al. Whole-brain radiotherapy or autologous stem-cell transplantation as consolidation strategies after high-dose methotrexate-based chemoimmunotherapy in patients with primary CNS lymphoma: results of the second randomisation of the International Extranodal Lymphoma Study Group-32 phase 2 trial. *Lancet Haematol*. 2017;4:e510–e523.
39. Houillier C, Taillandier L, Lamy T, et al. Whole brain radiotherapy (WBRT) versus intensive chemotherapy with haematopoietic stem cell rescue (IC + HCR) for primary central nervous system lymphoma (PCNSL) in young patients: an intergroup Anocef-Goelams randomized phase II trial (PRECIS). *Blood*. 2016;128:782.
40. Correa D, Anderson ND, Glass A, Mason WP, DeAngelis LM, Abrey LE. Cognitive functions in primary central nervous system lymphoma patients treated with chemotherapy and stem cell transplantation: preliminary findings. *Clin Adv Hematol Oncol*. 2003;1:490.
41. Rubenstein JL, His ED, Johnson JL, et al. Intensive chemotherapy and immunotherapy in patients with newly diagnosed primary CNS lymphoma: CALGB 50202 (Alliance 50202). *J Clin Oncol*. 2013;31:3061–3068.
42. Cher L, Glass J, Harsh GR, Hochberg FH. Therapy of primary CNS lymphoma with methotrexate-based chemotherapy and deferred radiotherapy: preliminary results. *Neurology*. 1996;46:1757–1759.
43. Chamberlain MC, Johnston SK. High-dose methotrexate and rituximab with deferred radiotherapy for newly diagnosed primary B-cell CNS lymphoma. *Neuro Oncol*. 2010;12:736–744.
44. Pulczynski EJ, Kuittinen O, Erlanson M, et al. Successful change of treatment strategy in elderly patients with primary central nervous system lymphoma by de-escalating induction and introducing temozolomide maintenance: results from a phase II study by the Nordic Lymphoma Group. *Haematologica*. 2015;100:534–540.
45. Rubenstein JL, Geng H, Fraser EJ, et al. Phase 1 investigation of lenalidomide/rituximab plus outcomes of lenalidomide maintenance in relapsed CNS lymphoma. *Blood Adv*. 2018;2:1595–1607.
46. Mylam KJ, Michaelsen TY, Hutchings M, et al. Little value of surveillance magnetic resonance imaging for primary CNS lymphomas in first remission: results from a Danish multicentre study. *Br J Haematol*. 2017;176:671–673.
47. Graham MS, DeAngelis LM. Improving outcomes in primary CNS lymphoma. *Best Pract Res Clin Haematol*. 2018;31:262–269.

48. Bessell EM, Dickinson P, Dickinson S, Salmon J. Increasing age at diagnosis and worsening renal function in patients with primary central nervous system lymphoma. *J Neuro Oncol*. 2011;104:191–193.
49. Chan CC, Wallace DJ. Intraocular lymphoma: update on diagnosis and management. *Cancer Control*. 2004;11:285–295.
50. Wang CC, Carnevale J, Rubenstein JL. Progress in central nervous system lymphomas. *Br J Haematol*. 2014;166:311–325.
51. Grimm SA, McCannel CA, Omuro AM, et al. Primary CNS lymphoma with intraocular involvement: international PCNSL collaborative group report. *Neurology*. 2008;71:1355–1360.
52. Chan CC, Rubenstein JL, Coupland SE, et al. Primary vitreoretinal lymphoma: a report from an international primary central nervous system lymphoma collaborative group symposium. *Oncol*. 2011;16:1589–1599.
53. Sepkowitz KA. Aids — the first 20 years. *N Engl J Med*. 2001;344:1764–1772.
54. Rios A. HIV-related hematological malignancies: a concise review. *Clin Lymphoma Myeloma Leuk*. 2014;14:S96–S103.
55. Gupta NK, Nolan A, Omuro A, et al. Long-term survival in AIDS-related primary central nervous system lymphoma. *Neuro Oncol*. 2017;19:99–108.
56. Skolasky RL, Dal Pan GJ, Olivi A, Lenz FA, Abrams RA, McArthur JC. HIV-associated primary CNS lymorbidity and utility of brain biopsy. *J Neurol Sci*. 1999;163:32–38.
57. Forsyth PA, DeAngelis LM. Biology and management of AIDS-associated primary CNS lymphomas. *Hematol Oncol Clin North Am*. 1996;10:1125–1134.
58. Shiels MS, Pfeiffer RM, Hall HI, et al. Proportions of Kaposi sarcoma, selected non-Hodgkin lymphomas, and cervical cancer in the United States occurring in persons with AIDS, 1980–2007. *J Am Med Assoc*. 2011;305:1450.
59. Achenbach CJ, Cole SR, Kitahata MM, et al. Mortality after cancer diagnosis in HIV-infected individuals treated with antiretroviral therapy. *AIDS*. 2011;25:691–700.
60. Antinori A, De Rossi G, Ammassari A, et al. Value of combined approach with thallium-201 single-photon emission computed tomography and Epstein-Barr virus DNA polymerase chain reaction in CSF for the diagnosis of AIDS-related primary CNS lymphoma. *J Clin Oncol*. 1999;17. 554–554.
61. Yarchoan R, Uldrick TS. HIV-associated cancers and related diseases. *N Engl J Med*. 2018;378:1029–1041.
62. Sparano JA, Lee JY, Kaplan LD, et al. Rituximab plus concurrent infusional EPOCH chemotherapy is highly effective in HIV-associated B-cell non-Hodgkin lymphoma. *Blood*. 2010;115:3008–3016.
63. Noy A, Lee JY, Cesarman E, et al. Amc 048: modified CODOX-M/IVAC-rituximab is safe and effective for HIV-associated Burkitt lymphoma. *Blood*. 2015;126:160–166.
64. Wolf T, Kiderlen T, Atta J, et al. Successful treatment of AIDS-associated, primary CNS lymphoma with rituximab-and methotrexate-based chemotherapy and autologous stem cell transplantation. *Infection*. 2014;42:445–447.
65. O'Neill A, Mikesch K, Fritsch K, et al. Outcomes for HIV-positive patients with primary central nervous system lymphoma after high-dose chemotherapy and auto-SCT. *Bone Marrow Transplant*. 2015;50:999–1000.
66. Evens AM, Choquet S, Kroll-Desrosiers AR, et al. Primary CNS posttransplant lymphoproliferative disease (PTLD): an international report of 84 cases in the modern era. *Am J Transplant*. 2013;13:1512–1522.
67. Morgans AK, Reshef R, Tsai DE. Posttransplant lymphoproliferative disorder following kidney transplant. *Am J Kidney Dis*. 2010;55:168–180.
68. Mahale P, Shiels MS, Lynch CF, Engels EA. Incidence and outcomes of primary central nervous system lymphoma in solid organ transplant recipients. *Am J Transplant*. 2018;18:453–461.
69. Jahnke K, Thiel E, Martus P, et al. Relapse of primary central nervous system lymphoma: clinical features, outcome and prognostic factors. *J Neuro Oncol*. 2006;80:159–165.
70. Langner-Lemercier S, Houillier C, Soussain C, et al. Primary CNS lymphoma at first relapse/progression: characteristics, management, and outcome of 256 patients from the French LOC network. *Neuro Oncol*. 2016;18:1297–1303.
71. Nayak L, Iwamoto FM, LaCasce A, et al. PD-1 blockade with nivolumab in relapsed/refractory primary central nervous system and testicular lymphoma. *Blood*. 2017;129:3071–3073.
72. Ambady P, Szidonya L, Firkins J, et al. Combination immunotherapy as a non-chemotherapy alternative for refractory or recurrent CNS lymphoma. *Leuk Lymphoma*. 2019;60:515–518.
73. Tun HW, Johnston PB, DeAngelis LM, et al. Phase 1 study of pomalidomide and dexamethasone for relapsed/refractory primary CNS or vitreoretinal lymphoma. *Blood*. 2018;132:2240–2248.
74. Grommes C, Pastore A, Palaskas N, et al. Ibrutinib unmasks critical role of Bruton tyrosine kinase in primary CNS lymphoma. *Cancer Discov*. 2017;7:1018–1029.
75. Soussain C, Choquet S, Blonski M, et al. Ibrutinib monotherapy for relapse or refractory primary CNS lymphoma and primary vitreoretinal lymphoma: final analysis of the phase II 'proof-of-concept' iLOC study by the lymphoma study association (LYSA) and the French oculo-cerebral lymphoma (LOC) network. *Eur J Cancer*. 2019;117:121–130.
76. Rubenstein JL, Fridlyand J, Abrey L, et al. Phase I study of intraventricular administration of rituximab in patients with recurrent CNS and intraocular lymphoma. *J Clin Oncol*. 2007;25:1350–1356.
77. Abramson JS, McGree B, Noyes S, et al. Anti-CD19 CAR T cells in CNS diffuse large-B-cell lymphoma. *N Engl J Med*. 2017;377:783–784.
78. Löw S, Han CH, Batchelor TT. Primary central nervous system lymphoma. *Ther Adv Neurol Disord*. 2018;11: 1756286418793562.
79. Balmaceda C, Gaynor JJ, Sun M, Gluck JT, DeAngelis LM. Leptomeningeal tumor in primarchy central nervous system lymphoma: recognition, significance, and implications. *Ann Neurol*. 1995;38:202–209.
80. Korfel A, Weller M, Martus P, et al. Prognostic impact of meningeal dissemination in primary CNS lymphoma (PCNSL): experience from the G-PCNSL-SG1 trial. *Ann Oncol*. 2012;23:2374–2380.
81. Taylor JW, Flanagan EP, O'Neill BP, et al. Primary leptomeningeal lymphoma: international primary CNS lymphoma Collaborative Group report. *Neurology*. 2013;81:1690–1696.
82. Lachance DH, O'Neill BP, Macdonald DR, et al. Primary leptomeningeal lymphoma: report of 9 cases, diagnosis with immunocytochemical analysis, and review of the literature. *Neurology*. 1991;41:95–100.
83. Cheng TM, O'Neill BP, Scheithauer BW, Piepgras DG. Chronic meningitis. *Neurosurgery*. 1994;34:590–596.
84. Freilich RJ, Krol G, DeAngelis LM. Neuroimaging and cerebrospinal fluid cytology in the diagnosis of leptomeningeal metastasis. *Ann Neurol*. 1995;38:51–57.

85. Glass JP, Melamed M, Chernik NL, Posner JB. Malignant cells in cerebrospinal fluid (CSF): the meaning of a positive CSF cytology. *Neurology*. 1979;29:1369–1375.
86. Bromberg JEC, Breems DA, Kraan J, et al. CSF flow cytometry greatly improves diagnostic accuracy in CNS hematologic malignancies. *Neurology*. 2007;68:1674–1679.
87. Glantz MJ, Cole BF, Glantz LK, et al. Cerebrospinal fluid cytology in patients with cancer: minimizing false-negative results. *Cancer*. 1998;82:733–739.
88. Dulai MS, Park CY, Howell WD, et al. CNS T-cell lymphoma: an under-recognized entity? *Acta Neuropathol*. 2008;115:345–356.
89. Hegde U, Filie A, Little RF, et al. High incidence of occult leptomeningeal disease detected by flow cytometry in newly diagnosed aggressive B-cell lymphomas at risk for central nervous system involvement: the role of flow cytometry versus cytology. *Blood*. 2005;105:496–502.
90. Owen RG, Treon SP, Al-Katib A, et al. Clinicopathological definition of Waldenstrom's macroglobulinemia: consensus panel recommendations from the second international workshop on Waldenstrom's macroglobulinemia. *Semin Oncol*. 2003;30:110–115.
91. Treon SP. How I treat Waldenström macroglobulinemia. *Blood*. 2015;126:721–732.
92. Malkani RG, Tallman M, Gottardi-Littell N, et al. Bing–Neel syndrome: an illustrative case and a comprehensive review of the published literature. *J Neuro Oncol*. 2010;96:301–312.
93. Minnema MC, Kimby E, D'Sa S, et al. Guideline for the diagnosis, treatment and response criteria for Bing-Neel syndrome. *Haematologica*. 2017;102:43–51.
94. Simon L, Fitsiori A, Lemal R, et al. Bing-Neel syndrome, a rare complication of Waldenström macroglobulinemia: analysis of 44 cases and review of the literature. A study on behalf of the French Innovative Leukemia Organization (FILO). *Haematologica*. 2015;100:1587–1594.
95. Fintelmann F, Forghani R, Schaefer PW, Hochberg EP, Hochberg FH. Bing-Neel syndrome revisited. *Clin Lymphoma Myeloma*. 2009;9:104–106.
96. Kim HJ, Suh SI, Kim JH, Kim BJ. Brain magnetic resolution imaging to diagnose Bing-Neel syndrome. *J Korean Neurosurg Soc*. 2009;46:588–591.
97. Castillo JJ, D'Sa S, Lunn MP, et al. Central nervous system involvement by Waldenström macroglobulinaemia (Bing-Neel syndrome): a multi-institutional retrospective study. *Br J Haematol*. 2016;172:709–715.
98. Shenkier TN, Blay JY, O'Neill BP, et al. Primary CNS lymphoma of T-cell origin: a descriptive analysis from the international primary CNS lymphoma collaborative group. *J Clin Oncol*. 2005;23:2233–2239.
99. Hayabuchi N, Shibamoto Y, Onizuka Y. Primary central nervous system lymphoma in Japan: a nationwide survey. *Int J Radiat Oncol Biol Phys*. 1999;44:265–272.
100. Choi JS, Nam DH, Ko YH, et al. Primary central nervous system lymphoma in Korea: comparison of B- and T-cell lymphomas. *Am J Surg Pathol*. 2003;27:919–928.
101. Gijtenbeek JM, Rosenblum MK, DeAngelis LM. Primary central nervous system T-cell lymphoma. *Neurology*. 2001;57:716–718.
102. Schniederjan MJ, Brat DJ. *Biopsy Interpretation of the Central Nervous System*. Philadelphia: Wolters Kluwer/Lippincott Williams & Wilkins Health; 2011.
103. van Krieken JH, Elwood L, Andrade RE, Jaffe ES, Cossman J, Medeiros LJ. Rearrangement of the T-cell receptor delta chain gene in T-cell lymphomas with a mature phenotype. *Am J Pathol*. 1991;139:161–168.
104. Ferreri AJ, DeAngelis L, Illerhaus G, et al. Whole-brain radiotherapy in primary CNS lymphoma. *Lancet Oncol*. 2011;12:119–120.
105. Herrlinger U, Schäfer N, Fimmers R, et al. Early whole brain radiotherapy in primary CNS lymphoma: negative impact on quality of life in the randomized G-PCNSL-SG1 trial. *J Cancer Res Clin Oncol*. 2017;143:1815–1821.
106. Lai R, Abrey LE, Rosenblum MK, DeAngelis LM. Treatment-induced leukoencephalopathy in primary CNS lymphoma: a clinical and autopsy study. *Neurology*. 2004;62:451–456.
107. Correa DD, Rocco-Donovan M, DeAngelis LM, et al. Prospective cognitive follow-up in primary CNS lymphoma patients treated with chemotherapy and reduced-dose radiotherapy. *J Neuro Oncol*. 2009;91:315–321.
108. Schaff LR, Grommes C. Updates on primary central nervous system lymphoma. *Curr Oncol Rep*. 2018;20:11.
109. Correa DD, Shi W, Abrey LE, et al. Cognitive functions in primary CNS lymphoma after single or combined modality regimens. *Neuro Oncol*. 2012;14:101–108.
110. Carson KR, Evens AM, Richey EA, et al. Progressive multifocal leukoencephalopathy after rituximab therapy in HIV-negative patients: a report of 57 cases from the Research on Adverse Drug Events and Reports project. *Blood*. 2009;113:4834–4840.
111. Brown PD, Pugh S, Laack NN, et al. Memantine for the prevention of cognitive dysfunction in patients receiving whole-brain radiotherapy: a randomized, double-blind, placebo-controlled trial. *Neuro Oncol*. 2013;15:1429–1437.

Chapter | 14 |

Approach to a patient with brain metastasis

Michael H. Soike and Michael D. Chan

CHAPTER OUTLINE

Introduction

Brain metastases are a frequent occurrence in patients with solid malignancies. Up to 40% of patients with solid tumors will develop brain metastases at some point in their disease course, and 170,000 patients are diagnosed with brain metastases each year.[1] The most common solid tumors that metastasize to the brain are lung, breast, melanoma, renal cell carcinoma, and gastrointestinal (GI) malignancies. The incidence of brain metastases appears to be rising, as better diagnostic methods have evolved (i.e., MRI) and, perhaps more important, systemic therapy has improved. These therapies have improved control of malignant disease outside of the central nervous system (CNS), and patients with metastatic disease are living longer. Because of longer life spans in patients with metastatic cancer, the length of time for patients to develop brain metastases is extended. Although many chemotherapeutic agents work well outside the CNS, they often fail to cross the blood-brain barrier, and many are unable to prevent tumor cells from seeding the brain parenchyma.

The life expectancy of patients with brain metastases is highly variable. The median survival is about 7.2 months, but ranges from 2.8 to 25 months.[2] When considering appropriate management for brain metastasis, clinicians commonly consider histology, age, performance status, and extent of systemic disease (i.e., few sites of metastatic disease vs numerous sites of disease). Clinicians often use a tool called the Diagnosis-Specific Graded Prognostic Assessment (DS-GPA) to aid prognostication.[2] The tool helps predict overall survival in patients with brain metastases. For instance, the estimated survival for a patient with melanoma, poor performance status, and four brain metastases is 3.5 months, whereas for a patient with breast cancer with two brain metastases and a favorable phenotype (estrogen and progesterone positive, HER2 negative), the median survival is 25 months.

MRI is the recommended imaging modality for routine staging particularly with cancers that have a high frequency of brain metastasis (Table 14.1). In lung cancer, due to the high frequency of brain metastases, an MRI is accepted as a standard component of screening for all stages of disease. Additionally, an MRI is reasonable to obtain in an aggressive locally advanced melanoma with nodal disease. In patients with neurologic symptoms such as headaches, seizures, ataxia, or focal neurologic deficits, an MRI is indicated for patients with breast cancer, renal cell carcinoma, or GI malignancies. It is also useful to know that squamous cell carcinoma of the head and neck, such as HPV-related oropharyngeal cancer, nasopharyngeal cancer, laryngeal cancer, or tongue cancer, rarely metastasize to the brain. Direct perineural invasion via cranial nerve foramen may be seen in these patients and result in intracranial spread of malignancy as opposed to parenchymal brain metastasis.[3] Prostate and pancreatic cancer rarely metastasize to the brain.

Table 14.1 Indications for MRI in patients with cancer to detect brain metastases

MRI recommended as staging for initial diagnosis without symptoms	MRI recommended for patients with focal neurologic symptoms	Rarely metastasize to brain
Small-cell lung cancer	Breast cancer	Squamous cell carcinoma of the head and neck
Non–small-cell lung cancer	Renal cell carcinoma	Pancreatic cancer
Advanced melanoma (Stage IIIC or higher)	Colon, rectal, and esophageal cancer	Prostate cancer

In the following cases, we will describe common clinical scenarios and available treatment options for patients with brain metastasis.

CASE 14.1 LARGE, SYMPTOMATIC BRAIN METASTASIS WITHOUT KNOWN CANCER DIAGNOSIS

Case. A 56-year-old male with a 20 pack-year history of smoking presents to the emergency room with 3 weeks of headache and confusion (Fig. 14.1). There is no history of seizures and no known cancer diagnosis. The patient's vital signs are stable and an MRI demonstrates a large, 2.3 × 2.5 cm^2 enhancing lesion in the left cerebellum, as well as lesions in the right cerebellum and right frontal lobe concerning for metastases (Fig. 14.2). Neurologic examination is significant for dysdiadochokinesia and a wide-based gait. Upon admission, a CT scan of the chest abdomen pelvis reveals a 1.5-cm nodule in the right upper lobe of the lung and a 3-cm enhancing mass in the right lobe of the liver.

Craniotomy is performed and final pathology reveals adenocarcinoma of the colon. The patient is discharged and returns 3 weeks later for adjuvant radiation therapy to the cavity as an outpatient. An MRI, obtained for treatment-planning purposes, shows a resected tumor cavity as well as slight interval enlargement of the two previously identified frontal lobe metastases.

The patient is treated with stereotactic radiosurgery (SRS) to the cavity, as well as to the two small brain metastases in one session lasting about an hour and a half. The following week, he begins chemotherapy for colon cancer.

Teaching Points: Role of Craniotomy in Management of Brain Metastases. This case highlights the role of surgical resection and postoperative cavity-directed radiotherapy in brain metastasis patients.

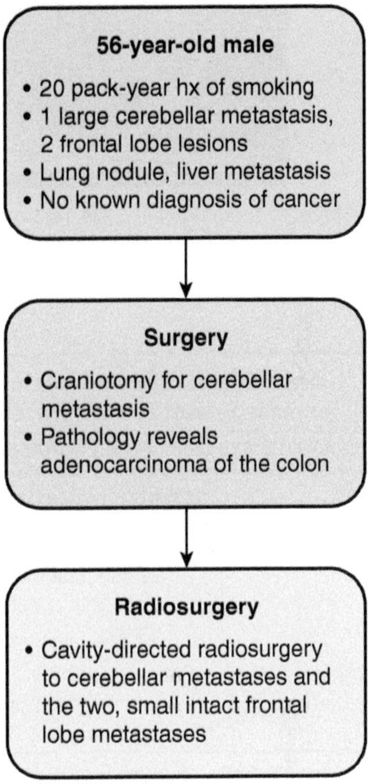

The role of craniotomy

Surgical resection is utilized in several clinical scenarios including metastases that are: (1) large size (≥3 cm), (2) in patients without a known cancer diagnosis, or (3) for selected cases of local recurrence of brain metastasis at a site of prior radiation therapy (Table 14.2). In the case of this patient, he presented with no known history of malignancy and several indeterminate findings on CT scan. The primary etiology of the lesion was not easily identifiable on imaging, and tissue diagnosis was needed before appropriate chemotherapy could be selected. If the patient is symptomatic, it is reasonable to start steroids (4 mg dexamethasone every 6 or 12 hours) prior to resection to help reduce mass effect and clinically significant vasogenic edema. Histologic diagnosis obtained from tumor tissue can be particularly useful to identify unsuspected or unknown primary tumors. In a seminal series by Patchell et al., 11% of the craniotomies performed for *presumed* brain metastases actually revealed primary brain tumors or abscesses.[4] Thus, pathologic confirmation of malignancy is critical in patients without a known cancer diagnosis.

56-year-old male
- 20 pack-year hx of smoking
- 1 large cerebellar metastasis, 2 frontal lobe lesions
- Lung nodule, liver metastasis
- No known diagnosis of cancer

↓

Surgery
- Craniotomy for cerebellar metastasis
- Pathology reveals adenocarcinoma of the colon

↓

Radiosurgery
- Cavity-directed radiosurgery to cerebellar metastases and the two, small intact frontal lobe metastases

Fig. 14.1 Representative case for craniotomy for management of brain metastases. hx, History.

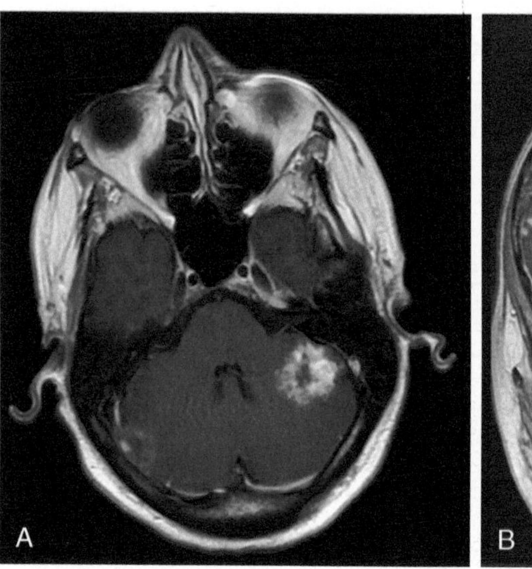

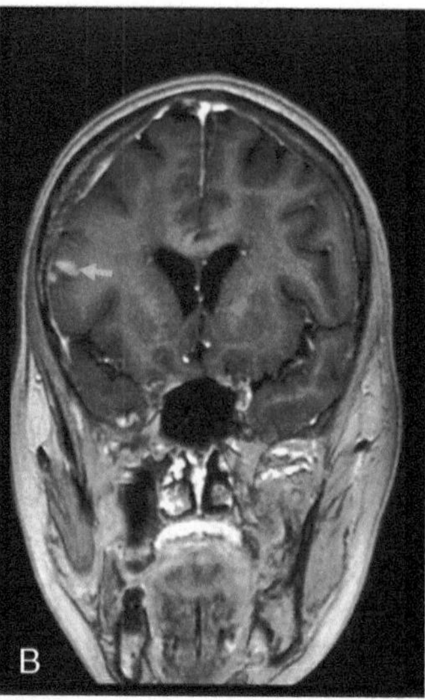

Fig. 14.2 MRI Brain of the patient in Case 14.1 including (A) axial and (B) coronal T1-weighted gadolinium enhanced MRI sequences with a large, enhancing lesion in the left cerebellum and small enhancing lesion in the right cerebellar folia (A) and a small lesion in the right frontal lobe (B, *orange arrow*).

Table 14.2 Indications and contraindications for craniotomy for management of brain metastases

CRANIOTOMY FOR BRAIN METASTASES	
Indications	**Contraindications**
No known cancer diagnosis	Eloquent area location (language centers, brainstem, occipital lobe, optic apparatus, motor cortex)
Large, symptomatic lesion with mass effect ≥3 cm	Patient health declining precipitously, unrelated to brain mass
Recurrent brain metastasis previously treated with radiosurgery	Surgery would delay urgent chemotherapy

A key concept in neuro-oncologic care is to preserve quality of life, independence, and neurologic function. In patients who are at risk of neurologic death from mass effect of a brain metastasis, surgical resection with tumor removal may rapidly alleviate symptoms. Conversely, surgery is often avoided in patients who are at risk of permanent neurologic deterioration after surgery. If the metastasis is close to an "eloquent area" of the brain, which includes the motor cortex, optic structures, occipital lobes, brainstem, or Wernicke's or Broca's areas, surgery is generally avoided.[5] Radiation therapy can treat larger lesions effectively; however, these patients are at higher risk of morbidity due to acute brain swelling. A functional MRI or diffusion tensor weighted imaging to visualize neuronal tracks may be useful to delineate neuronal fibers and reduce damage to normal anatomy.

Patients who undergo a craniotomy for brain metastases, particularly in the cerebellum, are at a higher risk of developing leptomeningeal dissemination of cancer cells.[6] The rate of leptomeningeal dissemination is approximately 20–30% in patients who undergo craniotomy, whereas it is less common in patients who are treated with SRS alone without craniotomy.[7] Patients with leptomeningeal disease may present with progressive cranial nerve deficits, severe headaches, hydrocephalus, confusion, and altered mental status. A representative radiographic image of leptomeningeal disease is demonstrated in Fig. 14.5. Lumbar puncture can confirm leptomeningeal disease, but a negative result from lumbar puncture does not exclude this etiology (see Chapter 15, Cases 15.1 and 15.2). The prognosis of patients with leptomeningeal disease is poor, measured in weeks to months.[8] There is no accepted standard treatment for leptomeningeal disease; however, whole brain radiation therapy (WBRT), SRS, intrathecal chemotherapy, high-dose methotrexate (for selected cancer histologies), or best supportive care are reasonable options based on patient and clinician preference.

The role of cavity-directed radiosurgery

Following surgery alone for brain metastasis, up to 50% of tumors will recur within the resection cavity without additional treatment.[9] Cavity-directed SRS after craniotomy reduces the rate of recurrence to approximately 10–20%.[10] Radiotherapy kills microscopic cancer cells left behind after surgery, which likely seed the tumor bed. SRS also provides an opportunity to treat other metastases during the same session of radiation

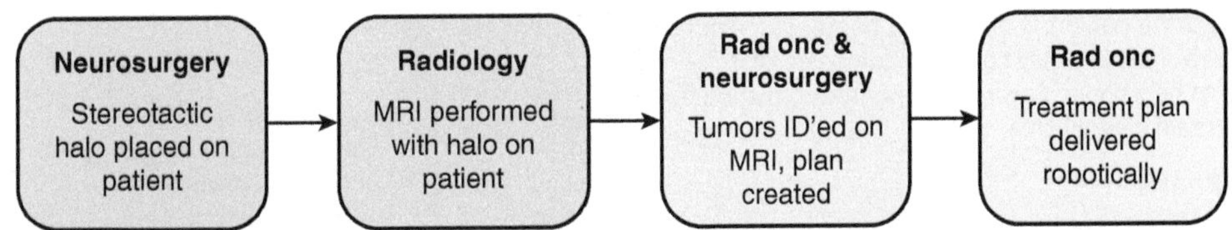

Fig. 14.3 Timeline of events for delivery of stereotactic radiosurgery. Radiation Oncology (Rad Onc), Identified (ID'ed).

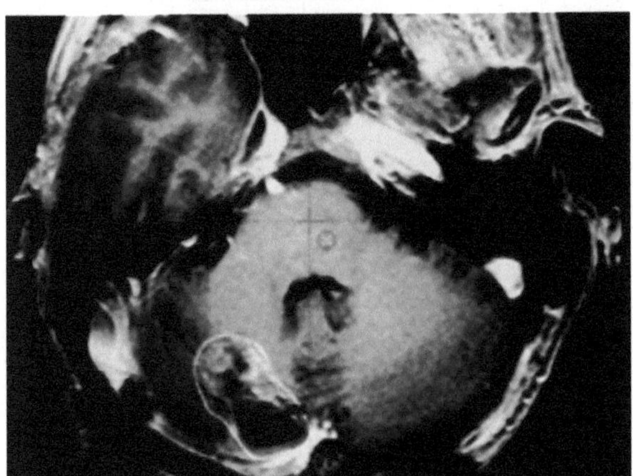

Fig. 14.4 Stereotactic radiosurgery plan for a right cerebellar postoperative cavity. The *red line* indicates the outlined surgical resection bed. The radiation field is delineated in *yellow* and encompasses the postoperative cavity.

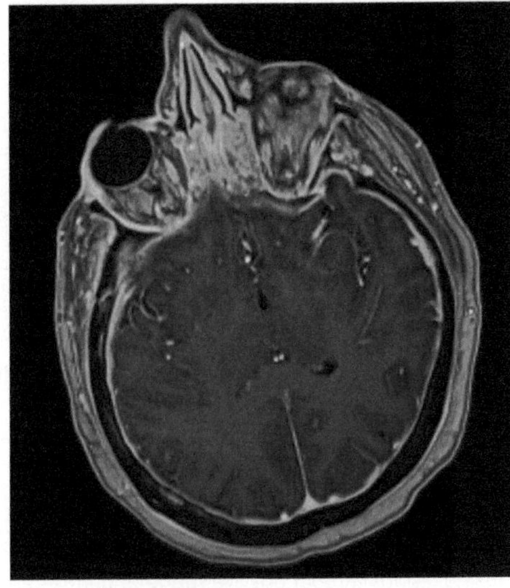

Fig. 14.5 Representative MRI of patient with leptomeningeal disease. There is flattening of the sulci, diffuse thickening of the dura, and extension into the orbit in the T1+contrast MRI.

therapy. In the case presented above, the two remaining metastases were managed during the same SRS delivery.

SRS involves several steps for treatment delivery and can be delivered with a Gamma Knife (Elekta, Stockholm, Sweden) or a specialized linear accelerator (see Chapter 3, Case 3.2 for further discussion of principles of stereotactic radiosurgery). Both emit high-energy photons, which kill cells via damage to DNA. The key differences between the two machines are that Gamma Knife uses radioactive Cobalt-60 as a photon source and treats only intracranial targets. A linear accelerator does not have radioactive material stored inside, but rather accelerates electrons, which collide with a block of tungsten. This collision of electrons and tungsten emits photons, which are directed toward the patient. Linear accelerators are more versatile than the Gamma Knife and can treat intracranial targets as well as other cancers throughout the body (i.e., gliomas, head and neck cancer, prostate cancer, breast cancer, etc.).[11]

Radiosurgery treatment planning. There are several steps involved with radiation therapy delivery (Fig. 14.3). First, the head must be immobilized so the patient cannot move during treatment. This can be accomplished with a stereotactic halo placed by neurosurgery (e.g., with Gamma Knife) or with the use of a tight-fitting mask (e.g., with linear accelerator). Then, the patient undergoes an MRI with contrast. The neurosurgeon and radiation oncologist outline the edges of the tumor on the MRI, using the T1-weighted contrast-enhanced sequences for target delineation. In the case of the stereotactic halo, this is placed during the treatment planning MRI, and clinicians can use the exact geometric coordinates to create a plan, with 0.1 mm accuracy. In the patient case presented above, the two small asymptomatic lesions were also treated and would be outlined at this point in the treatment-planning process. The radiation oncologist and neurosurgeon design a plan to effectively treat the resection bed (e.g., cavity-direct therapy), which harbors microscopic tumor cells, while minimizing the risk to normal brain parenchyma. After the radiation plan is created, the treatment is automated and delivered. In the figure (Fig. 14.4), a right cerebellar cavity has been outlined and a treatment plan created to effectively treat microscopic disease. All of the enhancing cavity bed is outlined and targeted.

Radiosurgery treatment delivery. Treatment typically lasts 30 minutes to 2–3 hours, depending on the complexity of the plan. The patient is awake, without general anesthesia and does not have to be NPO prior to the procedure. The patient does not feel the radiation, and many fall asleep during treatment. After the radiation is delivered, the stereotactic halo is removed and the patient is discharged home. For very large metastases, a short 2–3-day course of corticosteroids may be prescribed to help prevent acute swelling from radiation damage to the brain parenchyma.

Clinical Pearls

1. Brain metastases are the most common CNS malignancy with approximately 160,000 new cases per year.
2. Craniotomy is indicated for patients with large, symptomatic lesions or those without a known diagnosis of cancer.
3. Cavity-directed SRS is indicated to reduce the risk of recurrence after craniotomy for brain metastases.

CASE 14.2 APPROACH TO NUMEROUS BRAIN METASTASES WITH WHOLE BRAIN RADIATION THERAPY

Case. A 62-year-old female with an 80 pack-year history of smoking presents to the ED for new-onset seizures (Fig. 14.6). On examination, she is oriented to person and place but not time. She has cerebellar ataxia but no focal cranial nerve deficits. The patient has a history of early-stage breast cancer treated 6 years ago with lumpectomy, radiation therapy, and anti-estrogen therapy. An MRI of the brain shows 18 small enhancing lesions throughout the supra- and infra-tentorium suspicious for brain metastases (Fig. 14.7). CT of the chest reveals a large mediastinal mass and bilateral palpable supraclavicular lymph nodes.

A fine-needle aspiration (FNA) is performed on admission by pathology, and diagnosis reveals likely non–small-cell lung cancer. The patient is placed on steroids (dexamethasone 4 mg every 6 hours), levetiracetam, and omeprazole, and her symptoms improve. Following histologic confirmation of the malignancy, WBRT is recommended and the patient is treated over the next 2 weeks with 30 Gy in 10 daily fractions. Combination chemotherapy and immunotherapy is started after the patient completes whole brain radiation therapy.

Teaching Points: Indications for Whole Brain Radiation Therapy. WBRT is a useful tool for clinicians to manage patients with a high volume of intracranial disease. The use of WBRT is declining due to its deleterious side effects. The advantages of WBRT include its simple delivery, low cost, and efficacy.[12] It is effective for treating large, visible metastases within the brain *and* microscopic disease that cannot be visualized on the MRI. The disadvantage of WBRT is that it causes a delay in systemic therapy for patients with metastatic disease, diffuse alopecia, an acute short-term worsening of quality of life, and irreversible neurocognitive decline. Recently completed prospective trials have shown that one-third to one-half of patients receiving WBRT experience a 3-standard-deviation drop in cognitive testing 3 to 6 months after completion of WBRT.[13] These declines have been observed in episodic memory, executive function, processing speed, and fine motor control.[14,15]

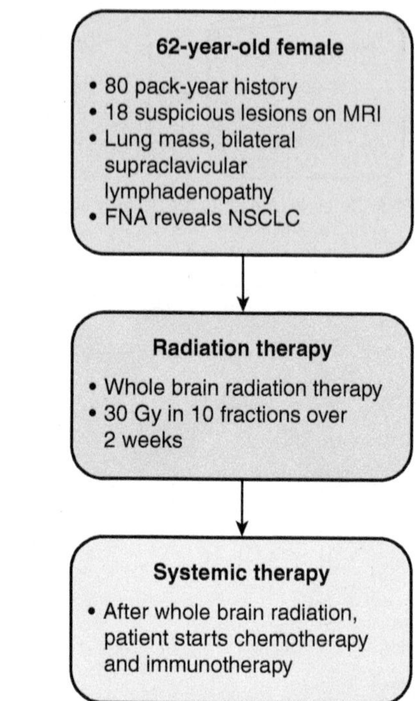

Fig. 14.6 Representative case for whole brain radiation. *FNA*, Fine-needle aspiration; *NSCLC*, non–small-cell lung cancer.

The standard WBRT field is displayed in Fig. 14.8. The field is designed to treat all of the potential cerebrospinal fluid and parenchymal spaces that could be seeded by cancer, including the cisterna magna, cribriform plate, and posterior orbital globe. The face, including the oropharynx, nasopharynx, and lens of the eye, is shielded from radiation to avoid causing radiation toxicity to these structures.

In the case outlined above, the patient presented without a known active cancer diagnosis, although a lung primary was suspected. Corticosteroids and levetiracetam effectively stabilized the patient and allowed time for pathologic confirmation of the diagnosis. Although suspicion for brain metastasis was high, it was important to avoid starting WBRT prior to a definitive pathologic diagnosis. In addition to brain metastases, the differential for multiple enhancing brain lesions includes infections (toxoplasmosis, cysticercosis), multifocal glioma, CNS lymphoma, intracranial hemangiomas, or hemangioblastomas in the setting of Von Hippel-Lindau disease. Obtaining an FNA from an easily palpable lymph node can be performed quickly by pathology to obtain a diagnosis of cancer.

Whole brain radiation therapy delivery. WBRT is typically delivered over 10 once-daily fractions at 3 Gy per fraction for a total of 30 Gy. Common indications for WBRT include (1) patients with small-cell lung cancer, (2) patients with >15 brain metasta-

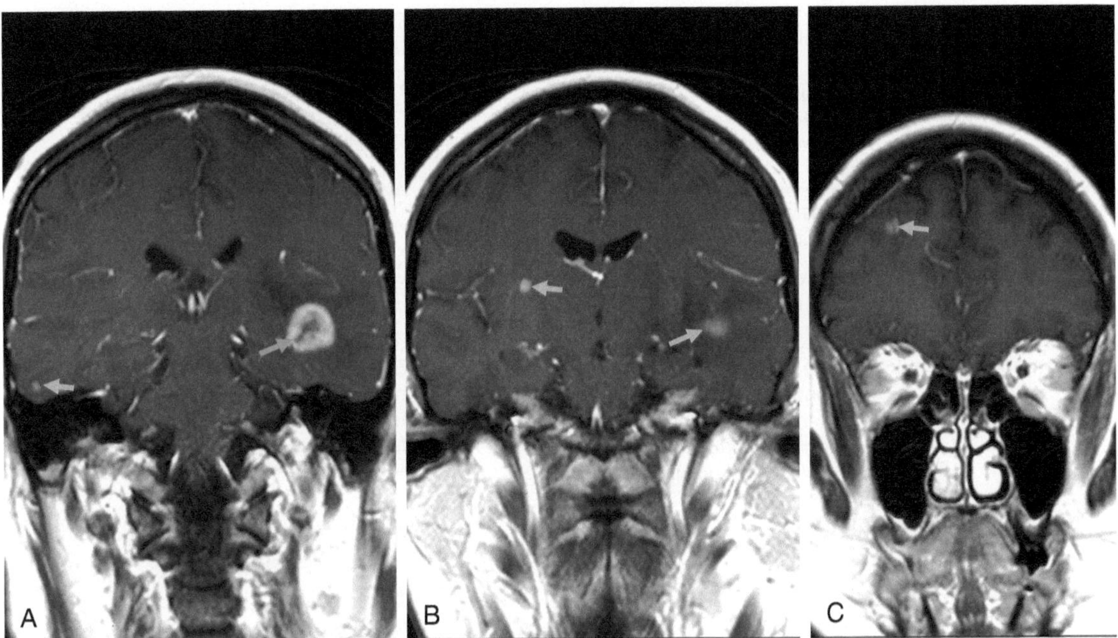

Fig. 14.7 (A–C) MRI Brain of the patient in Case 14.2 showing three representative coronal T1-weighted gadolinium-enhancing images of the brain showing multiple scattered ring-enhancing *(green arrow)* and homogeneously enhancing punctate lesion *(orange arrow)* throughout the brain with a total of 18 supra- and infratentorial lesion (not all shown).

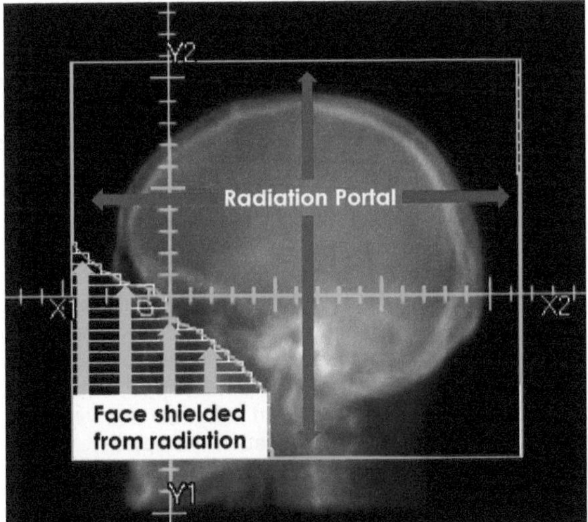

Fig. 14.8 This is a representative field or "portal" for whole brain radiation therapy. The face is shielded from radiation therapy to avoid toxicity. The entire brain and scalp are exposed to radiation therapy in order to adequately deliver radiation to all potential cerebrospinal fluid and parenchymal spaces.

ses, (3) rapidly progressive brain metastases (multiple new brain metastases within a few months) after SRS, or (4) progressive leptomeningeal disease. For patients with four or fewer brain

Table 14.3 Advantages and disadvantages of whole brain radiation therapy in the management of brain metastases

WHOLE BRAIN RADIATION THERAPY	
Advantages	**Disadvantages**
Effectively treats microscopic and macroscopic brain metastases	Worse quality of life and irreversible neuro-cognition
Low cost ($5,000–15,000 for course of treatment)	Delays chemotherapy, immunotherapy
Simple to plan and start urgently	Diffuse alopecia, acute fatigue

metastases, WBRT is avoided. For patients with 5–15 brain metastases, a choice is made between WBRT or SRS on a case-by-case basis. For patients with >15 brain metastases, WBRT is generally the treatment of choice except in extenuating circumstances (Table 14.3). The topic of hippocampal avoidance with WBRT, a technique designed to reduce the neurocognitive effects of WBRT, is discussed later in this chapter.

Contraindications to whole brain radiation therapy. There are several contraindications to WBRT. WBRT is avoided in a patient that has *already* received WBRT. This occurs in a patient who was treated with WBRT in the past, received systemic therapy, and then 1–2 years later develops a disease recurrence and the brain is reseeded with cancer. Delivering

Table 14.4 Indications and contraindications for whole brain radiation therapy

WHOLE BRAIN RADIATION THERAPY	
Indications	**Relative Contraindications**
Small-cell lung cancer	Previous whole brain radiation therapy
>15 brain metastases	Cancer with targeted agent that can cross the blood-brain barrier
Progressive leptomeningeal disease	Poor life expectancy <3 months due to the extent of extracranial disease, innumerable lung metastases, multiple liver metastases, etc.
Rapidly progressive, new brain metastases after initial stereotactic radiosurgery	Severely obtunded without improvement from corticosteroids

WBRT a second time would be deleterious and could cause significant harm to a patient with a poor prognosis. Radiosurgery or corticosteroids is preferred in this setting. WBRT is also contraindicated in patients with a very poor life expectancy due to extracranial disease. A randomized controlled trial performed in the United Kingdom randomized patients with brain metastases to oral corticosteroids versus abbreviated WBRT with steroids. There was no difference in overall survival between the two groups, suggesting that WBRT does not improve quality of life or survival in poor performance status patients.[16] Practically applied, if a patient is found to have innumerable brain metastases, is obtunded, and the confusion does not improve with corticosteroids over a 24–48 hours, then WBRT would not likely be of benefit, and best supportive care with corticosteroids is preferred (Table 14.4).

Clinical Pearls

1. WBRT is useful for patients with too many brain metastases to effectively treat with SRS.
2. WBRT contributes to decline in quality of life and neurocognitive decline, and is avoided when possible due to side effects.

CASE 14.3 APPROACH TO MULTIFOCAL LIMITED NUMBER OF BRAIN METASTASIS AMENABLE TO SRS

Case. A 72-year-old male with a history of stage III melanoma complains of intermittent episodes of left-hand weakness and numbness (Fig. 14.9). An MRI is obtained, which shows an enhancing, 1-cm lesion in the right motor cortex and two other lesions throughout the brain. Due to the recurrence of disease, a PET/CT is ordered, which shows several sites of bony metastatic disease in the lumbar spine and a liver metastasis. The patient has not received any systemic therapy. He is treated with SRS for his brain metastases and initiates immunotherapy the following week. Three months later, he returns for a follow-up MRI with radiation oncology, and one new brain metastases is discovered. He is treated again with SRS without interruption of his immunotherapy.

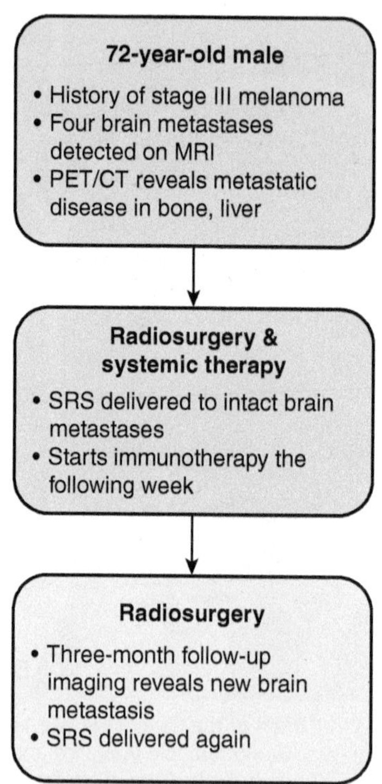

Fig. 14.9 Representative case for stereotactic radiosurgery *(SRS)*.

Teaching Points: Factors That Influence the Decision for SRS Versus Whole Brain Radiation Therapy. Several randomized trials demonstrate the efficacy of SRS alone for brain metastases. SRS hinges on its ability to deliver a very high dose of radiation sufficient to kill tumors in the brain to a small spot with <1 mm accuracy. As a result of sparing the normal brain parenchymal tissue, SRS avoids the cognitive decline in patients treated with WBRT.[15] The likelihood of eliminating a tumor treated with SRS is over 90%. Local control for SRS in treating lesions <1 cm is over 90%, although SRS is more limited in treating larger lesions, particularly ones that approach 3 cm or larger. Unlike WBRT, SRS can be used to treat new brain metastases that arise in the parenchyma, or patients who develop new brain metastases after WBRT (Table 14.5).

Table 14.5 **Advantages and disadvantages of stereotactic radiosurgery in setting of brain metastases**

STEREOTACTIC RADIOSURGERY (SRS)	
Advantages	**Disadvantages**
Effectively treats disease visualized on MRI	Will not treat microscopic disease not observed on MRI, more prone to develop new brain metastases
Avoids neurocognitive decline by sparing normal brain tissue	Can result in radiation necrosis, causing swelling and inflammation around treated brain metastasis
Avoids systemic treatment delays, typically single-day delivery	More intensive planning required, difficult to perform urgently
Able to retreat with SRS for new lesions that arise	Higher cost than whole brain radiation therapy ($50,000–100,000)

Randomized trials have proven that patients with a limited number of brain metastases have equivalent overall survival when treated with WBRT or SRS. Whereas SRS spares the patient from experiencing cognitive decline in most cases, it is also associated with a higher risk of developing new brain metastases, as observed in the patient treated above. Fortunately, new brain metastasis is easily treated with repeat SRS.

The maximum number of brain metastases that should be treated in a single setting with SRS continues to be defined. In patients with newly diagnosed brain metastasis (e.g., prior to any other brain metastasis-directed therapy), randomized trials have shown an advantage in treating up to four brain lesions with SRS compared to WBRT, with SRS patients having less cognitive decline. A large prospective trial from Japan showed that patients with 5–10 brain metastases have equivalent survival to patients with 2–4 brain metastases when treated with SRS.[17] The data from this trial suggests that SRS is reasonable in patients with up to 10 brain metastases, and WBRT could be spared in this population. The total number of brain metastases that is considered reasonable to treat with SRS continues to increase, and recent retrospective data have even shown that patients with 5–15 brain metastases have comparable survival to those with 2–4 brain metastases.[18] The Canadian Clinical Trials Group is conducting a prospective randomized trial (the CE.7 study) that will randomize patients with 5–15 brain metastases to either SRS or WBRT.[19] The results of this trial will provide randomized data to inform the proper choice between patients with 5–15 brain metastases treated with SRS or WBRT. This trial is also incorporating a formal cost-effectiveness quality analysis modeling that will likely advise insurance decisions and hopefully reduce health care–related costs for treatment of patients with brain metastases.

Clinical Pearls

1. SRS for intact brain metastases is preferred for treatment of a limited number of brain metastases, as it preserves quality of life and neuro-cognition.
2. Patients who are managed with SRS are more likely to develop new brain metastases than those with WBRT, but these can be managed with a second session of SRS.

CASE 14.3 APPROACH TO MULTIFOCAL LIMITED NUMBER OF BRAIN METASTASIS AMENABLE TO SRS

APPROACH TO SEIZURE MANAGEMENT AND CONTRAINDICATIONS TO DRIVING IN PATIENTS WITH BRAIN METASTASIS

Seizures are a common complication of brain metastasis that can affect patient quality of life and functional independence. The use of prophylactic antiepileptic drugs (AEDs) in patients with brain metastases is controversial given the lack of quality prospective evidence. Recent guidelines do not recommend routine antiepileptic prophylaxis in patients with intact brain metastasis.[20] Patients who are at higher risk for seizures include patients with tumors in the temporal lobe, those with leptomeningeal involvement, and those with metastases within or in close proximity to primary motor regions within the brain. In these circumstances, clinicians may treat prophylactically with AEDs even in the absence of prior seizures. Antiepileptic therapy in the prophylactic setting can be discontinued 3–4 weeks after SRS for brain metastasis. Moreover, some patients undergoing craniotomy are also treated with seizure prophylaxis, although recent studies suggest that this practice may not be helpful in reducing postoperative seizures.[21]

Driving recommendations. Driving restrictions are a major consideration when adjusting and determining AED therapy. In general, when patients experience a seizure related to a brain metastasis, they are instructed to refrain from driving for a period of time defined by the state Department of Motor Vehicles (e.g., often up to 6 months) in order to demonstrate an ability to remain seizure-free on AEDs. Few studies provide clear criteria to predict which patients may successfully taper off of AEDs and who will need long-term AED treatment. Clinical factors that may be considered include tumor location (e.g., temporal vs not temporal), whether the metastasis was removed or responded to treatment, and whether there is residual edema.

Visual field, cognitive deficits, and symptoms that necessitate pre-driving assessment. Patients may also suffer visual field deficits from tumors in the occipital region or visual pathway. These patients are frequently referred to an ophthalmologist to guide the objective assessment of the visual field deficit and inform the decision of whether a patient may safely operate a motor vehicle. Patients who have some degree of cognitive impairment may also present limitation to driving. In these patients, strict thresholds for driving safety can be more challenging. In these situations, our practice is to refer the patient to a neuropsychologist for dedicated neuropsychiatric testing, on-road occupational therapy driving evaluation, or similar assessment of physical, visual, and mental readiness to drive.

Clinical Pearls

1. Patients who experience a seizure due to brain metastases should be managed with brain metastases and advised to not drive an automobile for at least 6 months after last seizure.

APPROACH TO DIAGNOSING AND MANAGING RADIATION NECROSIS AFTER BRAIN METASTASIS TREATMENT

Radiation necrosis represents an inflammatory cascade of cell injury in brain parenchyma that occurs after radiotherapy. It is more common in patients treated with SRS than with conventionally fractionated radiation and occurs in approximately 10% of cases. Neuroimaging generally demonstrates an increase in the volume of enhancement as well as increasing surrounding vasogenic edema. Treatment of larger brain metastases increases the risk of radiation necrosis after SRS. Recent reports have also suggested that concurrent immunotherapy at the time of SRS may also be a risk factor for developing radiation necrosis.[22]

It can be difficult to distinguish radiation necrosis from tumor progression with noninvasive imaging alone. Conventional MRI does not reliably distinguish tumor progression from pseudoprogression, though several methods have been studied and are used variably by clinicians. The ratio of cerebral edema to volume of contrast enhancement (i.e., linear quotient and T1/T2 mismatch) have been proposed as a means of distinguishing these entities, but validation studies have been discordant. Advanced MR imaging techniques such as diffusion imaging, perfusion imaging, and spectroscopy have also been explored. Although data is suggestive that these advanced imaging techniques may hold more promise than conventional MR sequences, sensitivity and specificity are not currently sufficient for definitive noninvasive diagnosis by imaging alone. MR spectroscopy appears to have an operator dependence. MR perfusion is not ubiquitous at community centers due to the need for a power injector and extra contrast bolus. PET imaging has also been assessed, though access to tracers that can be used in the brain such as C11-methionine limit its usage.

Because imaging findings are often not definitive, close observation with serial imaging, empiric treatment with corticosteroids, and pathologic confirmation are used in cases of suspected radiation necrosis. Radiation necrosis occurs in regions of brain previously radiated and so it is imperative to determine whether new radiographic changes are in-field (i.e., in a region previously radiated) or out-of-field (i.e., outside of previously radiated brain tissue). In general, when necrosis is symptomatic and imaging reveals progressive edema, corticosteroids are a standard treatment option. If necrosis is refractory to corticosteroids, or if there is significant mass effect, resection may be needed to remove the necrosis. Removal of the focus of necrosis is thought to help stop the inflammatory cascade. Laser interstitial thermotherapy (LITT) has also been used recently to treat radiation necrosis. The advantage of this treatment is that a biopsy can be performed using the same needle trajectory as the laser therapy so that pathologic confirmation can be performed just prior to ablation of the focus of radiation necrosis. LITT can sometimes treat deeper lesions that may not be amenable to craniotomy-based resection.

Bevacizumab is a monoclonal antibody against circulated vascular endothelial growth factor. This infusion therapy has shown promise in treating radiation necrosis. Doses required to manage radiation necrosis (e.g., 5 mg/kg every 14 days) are often lower than those used for antineoplastic treatment (e.g., 10 mg/kg every 14 days). A clinical trial randomizing bevacizumab to corticosteroids for treatment of radiation necrosis recently closed. Although target accrual was not met, the results of the trial are still expected to be reported.

Clinical Pearls

1. Follow-up for brain metastases with MRI is critical in order to detect new brain metastases prior to developing symptoms and to detect radiation necrosis after SRS.

APPROACH TO DIAGNOSING AND MANAGING OTHER NEUROLOGICAL COMPLICATIONS OF TREATMENT FOR BRAIN METASTASIS

As the prognosis for patients with brain metastases has improved, there has been increasing focus on minimizing toxicity associated with treatment of brain metastasis. WBRT has long been associated with cognitive decline, particularly in the domains of memory and verbal learning. The recently published N0574 trial demonstrated that 92% of patients receiving WBRT experienced a greater than 1-standard-deviation decline from baseline in at least one cognitive test administered 3 months after treatment.[23] When a patient receives WBRT, there does not appear to be a plateau in the incidence of radiation-induced cognitive decline with time. Once cognitive decline begins, it tends to progressively worsen in severity. The likelihood of radiation-induced dementia is less common at conventional fractionation schemes for WBRT. In the N0574 study, 21% of patients receiving WBRT experienced a 2-standard-deviation drop in score on the Hopkins Verbal Learning Test (HVLT).

Several clinical trials have been reported with regards to strategies to mitigate the cognitive deficits faced by patients treated with WBRT (Chapter 25 for discussion of radiation-induced cognitive dysfunction). The use of SRS significantly decreases the likelihood of cognitive decline as compared with WBRT (64% vs 92%).[15] The sharp dose falloff of SRS leads to minimal radiation dose delivered to distant portions of the brain not treated by SRS. Future trials plan on evaluating the dose to the hippocampus delivered by SRS and if that affects cognition.

The Radiation Therapy Oncology Group (RTOG) 0614 study randomized patients receiving WBRT to memantine vs placebo.[24] Memantine is a NMDA receptor blocker used to treat Alzheimer's disease. Patients receiving memantine in the RTOG 0614 experienced a trend toward less decline on a HVLT, and had multiple other domains that were improved on cognitive testing. Use of memantine with WBRT has since been adopted as a standard treatment for clinical trials receiving WBRT and measuring cognitive decline.

Hippocampal-avoidance (HA)-WBRT is a technique developed to minimize the radiation dose to the bilateral hippocampi, structures within the mesial temporal lobe known to be critical in the function of short-term memory. The RTOG 0933 phase II trial assessing cognition in patients receiving HA-WBRT demonstrated improved HVLT scores over historical controls.[25] A subsequent randomized phase III confirmed the cognitive benefit of HA-WBRT over standard WBRT.[26] The population eligible for HA-WBRT are patients without metastases within 5 mm of either hippocampus, though some centers will consider unilateral sparing of the contralateral hippocampus in this scenario.

Clinical Pearls

1. Neurocognitive dysfunction is common after whole brain radiation therapy, with up to 90% of patients developing a decline in neurocognitive testing after WBRT.
2. In patients who do undergo WBRT, clinicians may consider strategies to avoid long-term neurocognitive dysfunction including hippocampal avoidance and prophylactic pharmacologic therapy (e.g., memantine, donepezil), though the benefits of these interventions have not been confirmed in large, randomized phase III studies.

Conclusion

Brain metastases from solid malignancies are the most common intracranial malignancy. Although patients with metastatic disease are unlikely to be cured, preserving quality of life by avoiding neurocognitive side effects from treatment as well as eliminating the brain metastases are two important goals in management. SRS effectively avoids the normal brain parenchyma and preserves cognition, but is unable to treat patients with a large number of brain metastases. WBRT is useful for treating the visible and microscopic brain metastases, but is associated with cognitive decline. Craniotomy is useful to obtain pathologic diagnosis as well as controlling large, symptomatic brain metastases >3 cm. Multidisciplinary discussion involving medical oncology, radiation oncology, neurosurgery, and neuropsychology is useful for patients with complex disease.

References

1. Ellis TL, Neal MT, Chan MD. The role of surgery, radiosurgery and whole brain radiation therapy in the management of patients with metastatic brain tumors. *Int J Surg Oncol*. 2012;2012:952345.
2. Sperduto PW, Kased N, Roberge D, et al. Summary report on the graded prognostic assessment: an accurate and facile diagnosis-specific tool to estimate survival for patients with brain metastases. *J Clin Oncol*. 2012;30(4):419–425.
3. Yu Y, El-Sayed IH, McDermott MW, et al. Dural recurrence among esthesioneuroblastoma patients presenting with intracranial extension. *Laryngoscope*. 2018;128(10):2226–2233.
4. Patchell RA, Tibbs PA, Walsh JW, et al. A randomized trial of surgery in the treatment of single metastases to the brain. *N Engl J Med*. 1990;322(8):494–500.
5. Dea N, Borduas M, Kenny B, Fortin D, Mathieu D. Safety and efficacy of Gamma Knife surgery for brain metastases in eloquent locations. *J Neurosurg*. 2010;113:79–83.
6. Huang AJ, Huang KE, Page BR, et al. Risk factors for leptomeningeal carcinomatosis in patients with brain metastases who have previously undergone stereotactic radiosurgery. *J Neurooncol*. 2014;120(1):163–169.
7. Marcrom S, Foreman PM, McDonald A, et al. Focal management of large brain metastases and risk of leptomeningeal disease. *Int J Radiat Oncol Biol Phys*. 2017;99(2):S172–S173.
8. Wang N, Bertalan MS, Brastianos PK. Leptomeningeal metastasis from systemic cancer: review and update on management. *Cancer*. 2018;124(1):21–35.
9. Patchell RA, Tibbs PA, Regine WF, et al. Postoperative radiotherapy in the treatment of single metastases to the brain: a randomized trial. *JAMA*. 1998;280(17):1485–1489.
10. Jensen CA, Chan MD, McCoy TP, et al. Cavity-directed radiosurgery as adjuvant therapy after resection of a brain metastasis. *J Neurosurg*. 2011;114(6):1585–1591.
11. Soike MH, Hughes RT, Farris M, et al. Does stereotactic radiosurgery have a role in the management of patients presenting with 4 or more brain metastases? *Neurosurgery*. 2019;84(3):558–566. https://doi.org/10.1093/neuros/nyy216.
12. Shenker R, McTyre E, Cramer C, et al. Drivers of the cost of management in patients treated with radiosurgery without whole brain radiotherapy for brain metastases. *Int J Radiat Oncol Biol Phys*. 2017;99:E414–E415.
13. Brown PD, Ahluwalia MS, Khan OH, Asher AL, Wefel JS, Gondi V. Whole-brain radiotherapy for brain metastases: evolution or revolution? *J Clin Oncol*. 2018;36:483–491.

14. Chang EL, Wefel JS, Hess KR, et al. Neurocognition in patients with brain metastases treated with radiosurgery or radiosurgery plus whole-brain irradiation: a randomised controlled trial. *Lancet Oncol.* 2009;10(11):1037–1044.
15. Brown PD, Jaeckle K, Ballman KV, et al. Effect of radiosurgery alone vs radiosurgery with whole brain radiation therapy on cognitive function in patients with 1 to 3 brain metastases: a randomized clinical trial. *JAMA.* 2016;316(4):401–409.
16. Mulvenna P, Nankivell M, Barton R, et al. Dexamethasone and supportive care with or without whole brain radiotherapy in treating patients with non-small cell lung cancer with brain metastases unsuitable for resection or stereotactic radiotherapy (QUARTZ): results from a phase 3, non-inferiority, randomised trial. *Lancet.* 2016;388(10055):2004–2014.
17. Yamamoto M, Serizawa T, Higuchi Y, et al. A multi-institutional prospective observational study of stereotactic radiosurgery for patients with multiple brain metastases (JLGK0901 study update): irradiation-related complications and long-term maintenance of mini-mental state examination scores. *Int J Radiat Oncol Biol Phys.* 2017;99(1):31–40.
18. Hughes RT, Masters AH, McTyre ER, et al. Initial SRS for patients with 5 to 15 brain metastases: results of a multi-institutional experience. *Int J Radiat Oncol Biol Phys.* 2019;104:1091–1098. https://doi.org/10.1016/j.ijrobp.2019.03.052.
19. Roberge D, Brown P, Mason W, et al. Cmet-48. Ce7 Canadian Clinical Trials Group/Alliance for Clinical Trials in Oncology. A phase III trial of stereotactic radiosurgery compared with whole brain radiotherapy (WBRT) for 5–15 brain metastases. *Neuro Oncol.* 2017;19(suppl 6):vi49.
20. Chang SM, Messersmith H, Ahluwalia M, et al. Anticonvulsant prophylaxis and steroid use in adults with metastatic brain tumors: summary of SNO and ASCO endorsement of the Congress of Neurological Surgeons guidelines. *Neuro Oncol.* 2019;21(4):424–427.
21. Lockney DT, Vaziri S, Walch F, et al. Prophylactic antiepileptic drug use in patients with brain tumors undergoing craniotomy. *World Neurosurg.* 2017;98:28–33.
22. Lanier CM, Hughes R, Ahmed T, et al. Immunotherapy is associated with improved survival and decreased neurologic death after SRS for brain metastases from lung and melanoma primaries. *Neurooncol Pract.* 2019;6:402–409. https://doi.org/10.1093/nop/npz004.
23. Brown PD, Asher AL, Ballman KV, et al. NCCTG N0574 (Alliance): a phase III randomized trial of whole brain radiation therapy (WBRT) in addition to radiosurgery (SRS) in patients with 1 to 3 brain metastases. *J Clin Orthod.* 2015;33(18 suppl). LBA4–LBA4.
24. Brown PD, Pugh S, Laack NN, et al. Memantine for the prevention of cognitive dysfunction in patients receiving whole-brain radiotherapy: a randomized, double-blind, placebo-controlled trial. *Neuro Oncol.* 2013;15(10):1429–1437.
25. Gondi V, Tolakanahalli R, Mehta MP, et al. Hippocampal-sparing whole-brain radiotherapy: a "How-To" technique using helical tomotherapy and linear accelerator–based intensity-modulated radiotherapy. *Int J Radiat Oncol Biol Phys.* 2010;78(4):1244–1252. https://doi.org/10.1016/j.ijrobp.2010.01.039.
26. Gondi V, Pugh SL, Tome WA, et al. Preservation of memory with conformal avoidance of the hippocampal neural stem-cell compartment during whole-brain radiotherapy for brain metastases (RTOG 0933): a phase II multi-institutional trial. *J Clin Oncol.* 2014;32(34):3810–3816.

Chapter 15

Approach to the patient with leptomeningeal metastases

Jigisha Thakkar and Priya Kumthekar

CHAPTER OUTLINE

Introduction

Leptomeningeal spread occurs in both solid tumors and hematologic malignancies. Leptomeningeal disease (LMD) for all primary cancer types portends a very poor prognosis, with survival measured in weeks if left untreated and an average of only 3.5 months with maximal therapy. The gold standard for diagnosing LMD is the presence of malignant cells observed on cerebrospinal fluid (CSF) cytology, though in a patient with known malignancy supportive radiologic findings in the setting of new neurological signs and symptoms is highly suggestive. Treatment is individualized based on various factors including the patient's performance status, the type and status of systemic cancer, burden of LMD, and clinical symptoms. Management is best conducted by a multidisciplinary team with involvement of palliative care for symptom management, radiation oncology, hematology or oncology, neuro-oncology, neurology, and neurosurgery. In this chapter we begin with a review of the common clinical principles for understanding LMD, including the clinical presentation, diagnostic tools, and therapeutic options. We then provide a case-based review with three cases (Cases 15.1–15.3) that focus on the approach to diagnosing LMD and two cases (Cases 15.4 and 15.5) that highlight the approach to treatment.

General principles for understanding leptomeningeal disease

Central nervous system (CNS) metastases from systemic cancers involve metastases to the brain parenchyma, dura, and leptomeninges (pia, subarachnoid space, and arachnoid mater). LMD is also known as neoplastic meningitis and carcinomatous meningitis. Leptomeningeal spread occurs in both solid tumors and hematologic malignancies via hematogenous dissemination, direct extension from solid brain lesions, as well as endoneural, perineural, and perivascular spread.[1]

Common solid tumors that metastasize to the leptomeninges include melanoma, breast cancer, small-cell lung cancer, and non–small-cell lung cancer.[2,3] Higher prevalence is seen in breast cancer, followed by lung cancer and melanoma.[4] In patients with breast cancer, HER2-positive and triple-negative breast cancers are associated with increased risk of CNS metastases including both brain parenchymal disease and LMD.[5,6] LMD occurs in 10–30% of acute leukemias (acute myelogenous leukemia more than acute lymphoblastic leukemia at diagnosis) and is rare in chronic leukemias. It is more common in non-Hodgkin's lymphoma (5–30%; 5% in diffuse large B-cell and peripheral T-cell lymphoma and 24% in Burkitt and lymphoblastic leukemia) and is rare in Hodgkin's lymphoma.[3,7] Median time from systemic cancer diagnosis to the diagnosis of LMD ranges from 11 months in hematologic malignancies to 2 years in solid tumors.[4,8]

The diagnosis of LMD for all primary cancer types portends a very poor prognosis with average survival of 4–6 weeks post diagnosis if left untreated and an average of 3.5 months if treated.[9–12] In those with breast cancer, patients with triple-negative breast cancer have the poorest survival, HER2-positive patients have the longest survival, and hormone receptor–positive patients have the longest time to the development of LMD.[10,13,14] A multidisciplinary approach to management is optimal with involvement of palliative care for symptom management, radiation oncology, and hemato-oncology in conjunction with neuro-oncology for systemic and intra-CSF therapies, and neurosurgery for placement of Ommaya and ventriculoperitoneal (VP) shunt when appropriate.

Patient presentation

LMD can clinically manifest in a variety of ways including focal neurologic symptoms and generalized neurologic decline from hydrocephalus as well as cranial nerve and spinal nerve findings. These various clinical manifestations occur from tumor infiltration of the leptomeninges, cranial nerves, spinal nerves, and cortical surfaces.

Infiltration of leptomeninges with cancer cells can cause clogging of arachnoid granulations causing increased intracranial pressure (ICP) and hydrocephalus.[1] This can lead to morning headaches, nausea, vision decline, cranial nerve palsy, unsteadiness of gait, urinary incontinence, and even mental status changes. There can also be dysfunction from cortical irritation particularly in the setting of bulky or nodular disease-causing seizures, headache, and encephalopathy.

Focal symptoms occur with involvement of different areas of the neuro-axis.[3] Tumor cells can invade spinal and cranial nerves (CN) passing through the subarachnoid space, at first producing demyelination and finally destroying the axons of those nerves.[4] Involvement of CN causes ptosis, extra-ocular movement abnormalities, diplopia, facial droop, changes in facial sensation, difficulty swallowing, dysarthria, and hearing difficulty. Multiple CN deficits without crossed motor or sensory deficits suggests involvement of the subarachnoid space. The ventral root containing the motor axons and the dorsal root containing the sensory axons exit the spinal cord into the subarachnoid space to form spinal nerves. Spinal nerves then enter the neural foramen and exit the vertebral column. Infiltration of the nerve roots and spinal nerves causes lower motor weakness, hypoesthesia, paresthesia, and neuropathic pain, as well as cauda equina syndrome (saddle anesthesia, urinary incontinence, fecal incontinence and constipation from parasympathetic denervation of the rectum, and sigmoid and anal sphincters).[4,15]

Diagnosis

Per National Comprehensive Cancer Network (NCCN) guidelines, LMD can be diagnosed in patients who have: (1) CSF cytology showing malignant cells; (2) positive radiologic findings with supportive clinical findings or signs and symptoms suggestive of CSF involvement in a patient with known malignancy.[16]

Approach to Diagnosis. Clinical symptoms and signs are critical for recognizing involvement of the leptomeningeal compartment. Clinicians should have a high suspicion for the possibility of leptomeningeal dissemination in a patient with metastatic cancer and should prompt further workup. LMD can be diagnosed in asymptomatic patients who are diagnosed incidentally during follow-up staging imaging. When evaluating a patient with possible leptomeningeal disease, clinicians should consider the following:

1. Symptomatic versus asymptomatic disease: is the patient symptomatic for LMD or asymptomatic?
2. Burden of disease: is there diffuse leptomeningeal involvement or focal disease?
3. Bulky disease: is there bulky, nodular disease (e.g., >2 mm thickness on imaging) or non-bulky disease?
4. Location of leptomeningeal metastasis: is there cranial disease, spinal disease, or a combination?
5. State of systemic disease: is there progressive systemic disease, controlled systemic disease on treatment, or no evidence of systemic disease?
6. CSF flow: is there patency of CSF flow to ensure uniform distribution of intrathecal chemotherapy?

Diagnostic tests. Workup of LMD may include the following investigations: (1) CSF sampling (gold standard) with at least CSF cell count, glucose, protein, cytology, and, in hematologic malignancies, CSF flow cytometry; (2) neuroimaging with MRI Brain and total spine with and without contrast or CT Brain and Spine with and without contrast if MRI is contraindicated; (3) CSF flow study via radionuclide cisternogram; and/or (4) CT or PET for systemic staging.

Treatment

The following treatment modalities may be used either alone or in combination and are reviewed further in the following cases.

1. Radiation therapy (e.g., stereotactic radiosurgery, conventional fractionated radiation therapy, or whole brain radiation therapy)
2. Systemic therapy (e.g., chemotherapy, targeted treatment, and immunotherapy)
3. Intrathecal therapy (e.g., Ommaya placement and intrathecal agents)

Clinical cases

CASE 15.1 DIAGNOSIS OF LMD IN A PATIENT WITH METASTATIC LUNG CANCER

Case. A 49-year-old female with history of progressive metastatic epidermal growth factor receptor (EGFR)-mutated non–small-cell lung cancer (NSCLC) received three lines of treatment with carboplatin, pemetrexed, afatinib, and osimertinib as well as radiation to symptomatic bony metastases. Three years after diagnosis she presented with progressive lower extremity weakness and numbness of 4 weeks, duration followed by urinary and fecal incontinence for 2 weeks. Neurological examination showed 3+/5 strength in bilateral lower extremities, saddle anesthesia, decreased proprioception, allodynia in bilateral lower extremities, hyporeflexia, and decreased rectal tone. MRI Brain and Spine did not reveal evidence of LMD. Initial lumbar puncture was performed with negative CSF cytology. Repeat CSF sampling showed elevated protein at 65 mg/dL, normal glucose, mild leukocytosis (largely lymphocytosis), and CSF cytology was positive for malignant cells.

Teaching Points: Serial Spinal Taps May Be Needed in Highly Suspected Cases Where Initial CSF Cytology Is Negative. This case highlights the importance of serial CSF sampling in patients with high suspicion of disease but negative initial CSF cytology. As was the case for this patient, a negative MRI and a single negative cytology does not rule out LMD. CSF testing is the gold standard for diagnosing LMD.[1] CSF cytology helps establish the diagnosis and monitor treatment response. CSF sampling should include measurement of the opening pressure, cell count, protein, and glucose. CSF cytology should be performed to assess for malignant cells, and flow cytometry should be included when evaluating patients with known or suspected hematologic malignancies.[3] Indicators of CSF involvement include elevated opening pressure and elevated protein.[4]

In patients where there is high clinical suspicion for LMD based on clinical signs and symptoms, a second CSF analysis or third CSF sample may be needed to confirm the diagnosis. Shedding of malignant cells into the CSF likely occurs intermittently, and thus there is a high false-negative rate with initial CSF sampling in patients with active leptomeningeal dissemination. Prior studies suggest that, in patients with active LMD, CSF cytology will be positive in 45% of patients with first spinal tap. This increases to 86% with the second and >90% with third.[4] Factors that increase the diagnostic yield include the volume of CSF sampled, speed of processing CSF for cytology, obtaining CSF in close proximity to a site of active disease, and increasing the number of spinal taps. To increase the diagnostic yield, at least 10.5 mL is generally recommended to be sent for CSF cytology, as the likelihood of capturing malignant cells increases with higher volume. CSF should be processed immediately to reduce cell death. Delay in CSF processing results in 50% of the cells being viable after 30 minutes and only 10% after 90 minutes.[17] Clinicians should be aware that sampling from lumbar dural puncture is more likely to be positive in patients with spinal than intracranial disease. These patients may need repeat sampling.

Clinical Pearls

1. CSF cytology is the gold standard for diagnosing leptomeningeal disease.
2. Common solid tumors that metastasize to the leptomeninges include melanoma, breast cancer, small-cell lung cancer, and non–small-cell lung cancer.
3. CSF cytology has a high false-negative rate; in patients with a high index of suspicion for LMD, a second or third dural puncture may be needed if CSF cytology is negative after the first spinal tap.

CASE 15.2 DIAGNOSIS OF LMD IN A PATIENT WITH HEMATOLOGIC MALIGNANCY

Case. A 67-year-old male with a 1-year history of progressive anemia and drenching night sweats underwent further workup that revealed abdominal lymphadenopathy. Laparoscopic biopsy of an abdominal lymph node revealed marginal zone lymphoma. Bone marrow biopsy showed bone marrow involvement. He was treated with six cycles of bendamustine and rituximab, followed by maintenance rituximab, which he self-discontinued after a year. Five years after his diagnosis, he developed recurrence of symptoms including night sweats, fatigue, and weight loss. Work-up including repeat bone marrow biopsy revealed recurrent marginal zone lymphoma, and PET-CT showed positive paratracheal lymphadenopathy with minimal bone marrow involvement. He was re-challenged with rituximab monotherapy and, after 2 months of treatment, developed new-onset headaches and suffered a seizure. Neuroimaging with MRI Brain and Total Spine showed no evidence of CNS metastases. Lumbar puncture was performed, showing CSF leukocytosis at 44/UL (85% lymphocytes), protein 284 mg/dL, glucose 40 mg/dL. Flow cytometry with immunophenotyping revealed predominantly T cells and a small population of kappa-restricted CD5-, CD10-, CD20+ B cells (3.2% of total cellular events) consistent with low-level involvement by the patient's previously diagnosed lymphoplasmacytic lymphoma. Cytology was negative for malignancy. The patient underwent Ommaya placement, and intrathecal chemotherapy was initiated with thiotepa as well as high-dose methotrexate (HD-MTX) and systemic ibrutinib. He had clearance of CSF after four rounds of intrathecal chemotherapy. After 2 months, thiotepa was switched to intrathecal MTX monotherapy due to toxicity. He developed encephalopathy after two doses of intrathecal MTX, and intrathecal therapy was discontinued. He continues to have good performance status 7 months after diagnosis of LMD.

Teaching Points: Flow Cytometry Should Be Included in CSF Sampling for Patients With Hematologic Malignancies. This case demonstrates the role of CSF flow cytometry in evaluating LMD for patients with hematologic malignancies. For hematologic malignancies, flow cytometry is more sensitive than cytology. CSF studies in patients with LMD from any cancer frequently show lymphocytic pleocytosis with increased protein and, in more severe cases, hypoglycorrhachia (i.e., reduced CSF glucose). The differential diagnosis of hypoglycorrhachia includes neoplastic meningitis, bacterial or fungal meningitis, or, in rare cases, noninfectious inflammatory etiologies.

Flow cytometry and DNA single-cell cytometry are two techniques that measure the chromosomal content of cells. Flow cytometry is two to three times more sensitive than cytology for the detection of hematologic malignant cells in the CSF.[18,19] In leukemic or lymphomatous meningitis (e.g., LMD in patients with hematologic malignancies), nonspecific markers of LMD include elevation of β-glucoronidase, β-microglobulin, and isoenzyme V of lactate dehydogenase. Epithelial cell adhesion molecule (EpCAM) is expressed by solid tumors of epithelial origin like non–small-cell lung cancer, breast cancer, or ovarium cancer. EpCAM-based flow cytometry assay is superior to CSF cytology for the diagnosis of LMD in patients with epithelial tumors.[20]

Clinical Pearls

1. In patients with suspected LMD, CSF studies should include cell count, glucose, protein, and cytology.
2. In patients with known or suspected hematologic malignancies, CSF flow cytometry should be performed, as it is two to three times more sensitive than cytology for the detection of leukemic or lymphomatous meningitis.

CASE 15.3 RADIOGRAPHIC DIAGNOSIS OF LMD IN A BREAST CANCER PATIENT WITH CRANIAL NEUROPATHY

Case. A 51-year-old female was diagnosed with left breast invasive lobular carcinoma, tumor >5 cm, involvement of one to three axillary lymph nodes, and no distant metastases (pT3N1M0), grade 2, estrogen receptor 100%, progesterone receptor 10%, HER2 negative. She underwent bilateral mastectomies followed by two lines of chemotherapy and hormonal therapy including adriamycin plus cyclophosphamide, followed by taxol, tamoxifen, and anastrozole. Six years later, she developed widespread skeletal metastases involving the entire spine. Treatment was switched to fulvestrant and palbociclib followed by capecitabine and navelbine. Two years later, she presented with morning headaches, diplopia, dysarthria, difficulty swallowing, neck pain, and paresthesia in bilateral lower extremities. On examination, she had hypoesthesia and decreased strength (4/5) in bilateral lower extremities and cranial nerve XII palsy. Her Karnofsky performance status (KPS) was 80%. MRI Brain and Spine revealed enhancement along the cerebral sulci, cerebellar folia, and brainstem as well as spinal cord (Fig. 15.1). She received systemic treatment with exemestane and underwent Ommaya placement. CSF from Ommaya was positive for malignancy. She underwent whole brain radiation treatment (WBRT) and subsequently received intrathecal chemotherapy with topotecan. CSF cleared after two doses of topotecan. Treatment was complicated by chemical meningitis after cycle three and bacterial meningitis after cycle four. Intrathecal treatment was discontinued. She had progression of her systemic disease, gallstone pancreatitis, and significant deterioration in performance status. She was transitioned to hospice care 3 months post-diagnosis of LMD and succumbed to disease 5 months after her LMD diagnosis.

Teaching Points: MRI plays an important role in diagnosing leptomeningeal disease and evaluating for extent of bulky, nodular disease that guides therapy decisions. This case highlights the role of the clinical examination and imaging in diagnosing LMD in patients with cancer and the multimodality therapeutic options available for treating LMD. Positive radiologic findings in a patient with supportive clinical signs and symptoms are suggestive of CSF involvement in patients with known malignancy.[16] In this case, there was high suspicion for LMD based on the clinical presentation. This was confirmed by MRI Brain, which showed findings consistent with a diagnosis of LMD. Due to the clinical and unequivocal radiographic evidence of LMD, CSF analysis was deferred, as the outcome was not going to impact management. That is, regardless of whether CSF cytology was negative or positive for malignant cells, the patient was planned for treatment as presumed LMD.

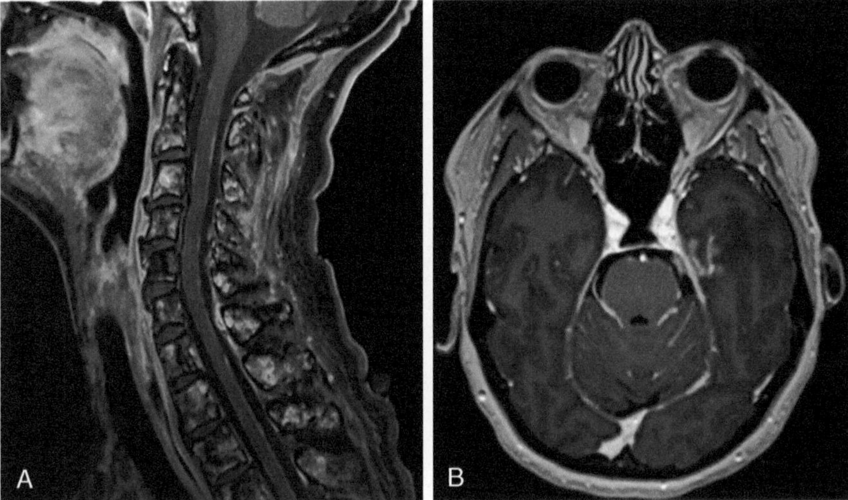

Fig. 15.1 (A) MRI of the cervical spine: T1-weighted gadolinium enhanced sagittal view with abnormal linear enhancement of leptomeninges along the anterior and posterior aspects of the cervical and thoracic spine. (B) MRI of the brain: T1-weighted gadolinium enhanced axial view with abnormal enhancement along the cerebral sulci and cerebellar folia and brain stem.

Utility of imaging for diagnosing LMD. MRI Brain and Spine with and without contrast is not the gold standard for diagnosis of LMD. MRI can be negative in patients with active leptomeningeal malignancy. However, MRI helps identify location, evaluate for bulky or nodular disease (>2 mm in thickness) that may not respond well to intrathecal therapy, and helps guide treatment.[21,22] If cranial nerve involvement is suspected, thin cuts through the brainstem should also be performed. The most frequent MRI findings include focal or diffuse enhancement of leptomeninges along the sulci, cranial nerves and spinal nerve roots, linear or nodular enhancement of the cord, and thickening of lumbosacral roots. If MRI Brain is contraindicated, then CT Brain and Spine with and without contrast can be performed.

CSF flow study. For patients who may undergo intrathecal chemotherapy, the patency of CSF pathways and normal CSF flow is imperative to ensure adequate circulation of intra-CSF chemotherapy. A radionuclide cisternogram is a nuclear medicine test that evaluates CSF flow and determines the patency of the ventricular and cerebrospinal pathways. This study involves dural puncture and injection into the CSF of the radionuclide tracer DPTA tagged with Indium-111. Repeat imaging is performed at 48–72 hours. Abnormal CSF flow interferes with uniform distribution of intrathecal chemotherapy and can lead to excess build-up of chemotherapy causing toxicity and limiting therapeutic efficacy.[23] In these clinical cases, intrathecal therapy would not be advised. In patients, particularly those with bulky or nodular meningeal disease, CSF flow may be disrupted. In these patients, radiation therapy may have the ability to restore CSF outflow, which helps facilitate administration of intrathecal chemotherapy.

Approach to managing patients with LMD

This case also highlights the approach to managing patients with LMD. Treatment of these patients is complex and is best guided by a multidisciplinary team. Radiation (focal or WBRT), intrathecal chemotherapy, and systemic treatments may all be utilized for cancer-directed therapy. In patients for whom treatment is contraindicated due to poor performance status, supportive care is often the most reasonable option. Risk stratification can help to guide decision making, and in general, patients can be divided into high-risk or low-risk.[24] High-risk patients are those with poor performance status (KPS <60%), progressive systemic disease with minimal or no treatment options, and bulky LMD with major neurological deficits. Low-risk patients are those with good performance status (KPS >60%), minimal or well-controlled systemic disease with favorable treatment options, and minor neurological deficits.[24]

Factors affecting approach to treatment. Several factors influence treatment of LMD including: (1) solid versus hematologic malignancy, (2) the state of systemic cancer (stable versus progressive disease), (3) the presence of bulky versus non-bulky LMD metastasis, (4) patient performance status, and (5) clinical symptom burden. In general, the goals of treatment are to improve patient symptoms and treat the cancer (Fig. 15.2).

Symptomatic Treatment

For patients with high-risk disease, supportive care alone is typically preferred. Palliative and hospice care should be considered and a primary goal of managing patient symptoms should be pursued. Symptomatic treatments may involve management of elevated ICP or management of localized symptoms from infiltration at specific regions of the neuroaxis.

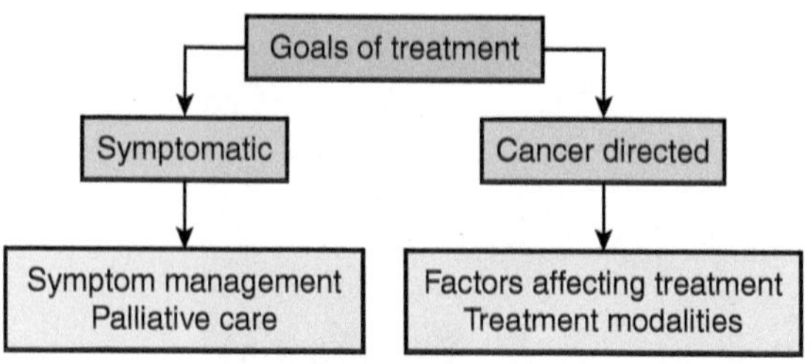

Fig. 15.2 Goals of treatment for LMD. Both cancer-directed and palliative/symptomatic treatments may coexist in LMD management. Exclusive symptomatic treatment is opted in cases where patients cannot tolerate cancer-directed treatment. *LMD*, Leptomeningeal disease.

Management of elevated ICP. Symptoms of elevated ICP and hydrocephalus (communicating and noncommunicating) include headache, gait unsteadiness, and nausea/vomiting. These symptoms are managed by pharmacologically or mechanically lowering ICP. Communicating hydrocephalus is typically due to malignant cells in the subarachnoid space that obstruct normal CSF reabsorption pathways. Pharmacologic lowering of ICP includes administration of diamox (decreases CSF production), mannitol (osmotic agent that decreases cerebral blood volume), and corticosteroids (decreases vasogenic edema and reduces resistance to CSF outflow).[25] Mechanical lowering of ICP is achieved by CSF diversion through placement of an external ventricular drain (temporary) or VP shunt (permanent). At times WBRT may also be considered for treating bulky meningeal disease, allowing CSF reabsorption and lowering ICP. VP shunt remains a valid option for cancer patients with low KPS, as it improves the quality of life. Although intraperitoneal seeding remains a possibility, it has not been encountered or reported in studies.[26,27] Noncommunicating hydrocephalus (e.g., obstructive hydrocephalus) is due to focal lesions obstructing CSF flow. Obstructive hydrocephalus is managed by removing the obstruction, either through focal radiotherapy (RT) to an obstructing lesion or, in rare cases, surgical intervention. Corticosteroids can be temporarily used for treating elevated ICP. Dexamethasone is the corticosteroid of choice and is frequently administered at doses of 16 mg/day and tapered over 1–2 weeks until definitive treatment is performed.[28,29]

Seizure management. Patients with LMD who do not have a history of seizures do not require empiric seizure prophylaxis. If seizures do occur, patients are treated with antiepileptic drugs that are similar to those used for primary brain tumors, metastatic brain tumors, and other lesional epilepsies. Clinicians may consider agents such as levetiracetam, lacosamide, zonisamide, topiramate, or other agents. In general, agents that are known to strongly induce or inhibit cytochrome P450 (CYP) enzymes, including carbamazepine, phenytoin, and phenobarbital, are avoided, as these can interact with chemotherapies used to treat systemic disease.

Other symptomatic managements. Patients may also suffer from symptoms due to cranial neuropathy, cauda equina involvement, and other sites of disease. When present, paresthesias and neuropathic pain may be treated with gabapentin, pregabalin, duloxetine, or amitriptyline. New-onset radicular pain in a cancer patient should raise strong suspicion for LMD and responds well to corticosteroids and/or focal radiation. Radiation to focal lesions along the neuro-axis may alleviate various symptoms including radicular pain, extremity weakness, cranial nerve deficits, urinary incontinence, and constipation. Patients with cranial neuropathies may require supportive measures due to involvement of oculomotor cranial nerves III, IV, VI, and cranial nerve VII. This may include an eye patch for diplopia, and eye drops or corneal lubrication for patients with peripheral facial nerve palsy who are unable to completely close their eye. Other interventions include implementing scheduled voiding or catheterization for urinary incontinence. Antidepressants may be beneficial for patients suffering from depression. Neurologic stimulants may be considered for patients with cancer- and/or treatment-associated fatigue (i.e., modafinil, methylphenidate).

Cancer-directed treatment

For patients with reasonable performance status, aggressive treatments aimed at decreasing the number of circulating cancer cells in the CSF and decreasing the burden of disease are considered. Historically, radiation therapy was the mainstay to treatment, but systemic and intrathecal therapies are also utilized. Treatment must be individualized based on patient- and tumor-specific factors to achieve the best results.

Clinical Pearls

1. The most frequent MRI findings of LMD are focal or diffuse enhancement of leptomeninges along the sulci, cranial nerves and spinal nerve roots, linear or nodular enhancement of the cord, and thickening of lumbosacral roots.
2. Neuroimaging also helps define the extent of disease and the presence of bulky/nodular disease that may require radiation or selected high-dose systemic therapies.
3. Cancer-directed treatment is individualized based on various factors including the type of malignancy (e.g., solid versus hematologic malignancy), performance status, type and state of systemic cancer, burden of leptomeningeal disease, and clinical symptoms.
4. Symptomatic treatments include management of elevated intracranial pressure, seizure treatment, supportive care for cranial neuropathies, and pain control.

CASE 15.4 MANAGEMENT OF LMD IN PATIENTS WITH SYMPTOMATIC BULKY DISEASE

Case. A 58-year-old female with triple-negative breast cancer received neoadjuvant therapy with doxorubicin, cyclophosphamide, and paclitaxel. She then underwent left mastectomy and radiation to left chest wall. One year later, she was

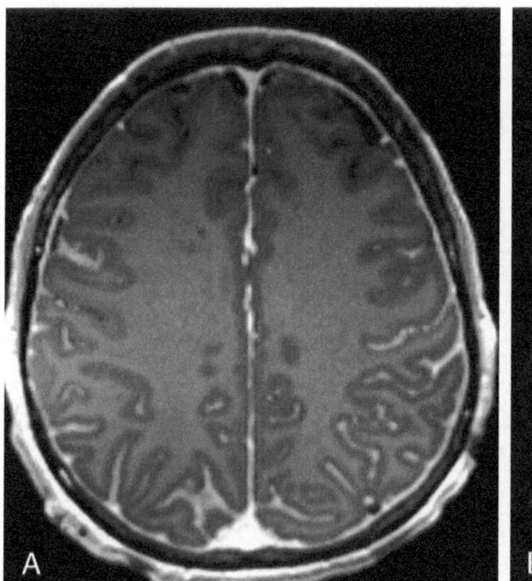

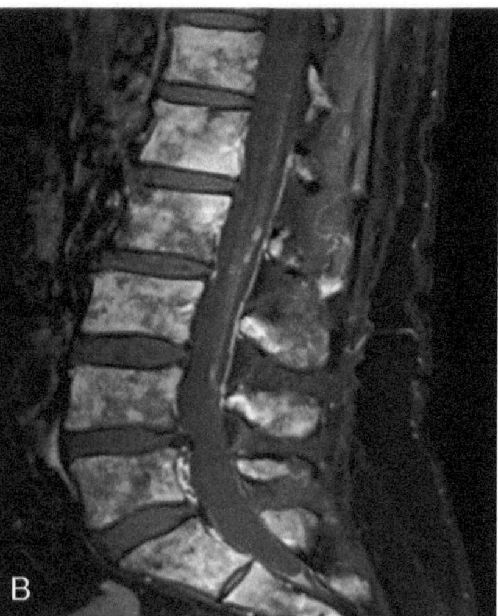

Fig. 15.3 (A) MRI of the brain: T1-weighted gadolinium-enhanced axial view with abnormal diffuse bulky leptomeningeal enhancement along bilateral cerebral hemispheres. (B) MRI of the lumbar spine: T1-weighted gadolinium-enhanced sagittal view with abnormal nodular enhancement of leptomeninges along the cauda equina nerve roots.

diagnosed with intraparenchymal metastases and received resection of a large right frontoparietal mass and stereotactic radiosurgery to the remaining lesions (e.g., surgical cavity, R parietal, R temporal). Approximately 1.5 years following her initial diagnosis of breast cancer, she presented with progressive headache, nausea, vomiting, photophobia, urinary incontinence, radicular pain in bilateral upper and lower extremities, and anorexia. On examination, she was in moderate distress due to pain and was cachectic with decreased alertness. She was able to follow simple commands and noted to have a left CN VI and VII palsy and 3+/5 strength in bilateral lower extremities. KPS was 50%. CT Head demonstrated ventriculomegaly. CSF profile was notable for xanthochromic appearance, pleocytosis (48% neutrophils, 14% lymphocytes), elevated protein to 247 mg/dL, normal glucose. CSF cytology was positive for malignant cells. MRI revealed diffuse bulky leptomeningeal enhancement along the bilateral cerebral hemispheres, cerebellar folia, and spinal cord (Fig. 15.3). She refused further cancer-directed treatment. She was treated with palliative focal radiation to symptomatic metastases in the cauda equine and underwent placement of a VP shunt for communicating hydrocephalus. Gabapentin was used to manage neuropathic pain. She was transitioned to hospice care. She succumbed to the disease 6 weeks after the diagnosis of LMD.

Teaching Points: Treatment of Bulky Leptomeningeal Metastasis. Intrathecal chemotherapy has limited value in treating bulky meningeal disease, as it penetrates only a monolayer of cells adjacent to the CSF and has a diffusion capacity of 1–2 mm.[21,22] Hence, for bulky metastasis, radiation therapy or systemic therapy are favored. Asymptomatic patients may be first treated with radiation to sites of bulky disease to aid penetration of intrathecal drugs. In symptomatic patients, radiation is a favored treatment. In the case of this patient, she had imaging evidence of bulky, nodular disease that had disseminated to both the spinal cord and intracranial compartments. Her performance status was poor. Thus, symptomatic therapies were performed including CSF diversion for headaches, radiation to symptomatic sites of disease, and supportive care. In patients with active systemic disease, systemic therapies with good CNS penetration may also be considered, as bulkier areas of disease rely on neovascularization for continued growth.[30]

The role of radiation therapy

Radiation is the mainstay of treatment for symptom palliation. Radiation may also help improve penetration of systemic treatments by mechanical disruption of the blood-brain barrier (BBB) and blood-CSF barrier (BCSFB). Radiotherapy options include stereotactic radiosurgery, conventionally fractionated radiation therapy, and whole brain radiation (see Chapter 3 for principles of radiotherapy in neuro-oncology). Patients commonly receive WBRT and, to a lesser extent, focal radiation or, in rare cases, cranio-spinal radiation (whole brain and spinal RT). WBRT is used for diffuse LMD with symptoms of high ICP to improve CSF flow. Focal radiation may be used for symptomatic bulky lesions that impair CSF flow (noncommunicating hydrocephalus) and can improve delivery

Table 15.1 Systemic agents used in the treatment of leptomeningeal disease

Agent	Dose	Mechanism	Use
HD-MTX[37]	Up to 8 gm/m^2	Antifolate metabolite	Breast
Temozolomide[38,39]	75 mg/m^2 with RT 150–200 mg/m^2 without RT 50 mg/m^2 per day (metronomic)	Alkylating	Breast Lung
Gefitinib[40]	250 mg QD	First-generation EGFR TKI	NSCLC-EGFR mutated
Erlotinib[41,42]	1000–2000 mg weekly	First-generation EGFR-TKI	NSCLC-EGFR mutated
Afatinib[43]	40 mg QD	Second-generation EGFR-TKI	NSCLC-EGFR mutated
Osimertinib[44]	160 mg QD	Third-generation EGFR-TKI	NSCLC-EGFR mutated
Ceretinib[45]	750 mg QD	ALK TKI	ALK-positive NSCLC
Alectinib[46]	300–900 mg BID	ALK TKI	ALK-positive NSCLC
Dabrafeninb[47]	150 mg BID	BRAF inhibitor	Melanoma
Vemurafinib[48–52]	960 mg BID	BRAF inhibitor	Melanoma
Trametinib[49]	2 mg QD	MEK inhibitor	Melanoma

ALK, Anaplastic lymphoma kinase; BID, twice daily; EGFR, epidermal growth factor receptor; HD-MTX, high-dose methotrexate; NSCLC, non–small-cell lung cancer; RT, radiotherapy; QD, once daily; TKI, tyrosine kinase inhibitor.

of intrathecal drugs. Focal radiation is also favored for palliating symptomatic cranial neuropathies and painful nerve root lesions.[31,32] Craniospinal irradiation (CSI) is used in rare cases of hematologic malignancies and primary brain tumors like medulloblastoma and CNS germinoma. In the majority of patients with advanced systemic cancers (e.g., breast cancer, lung, melanoma) who have received prior myelosuppressive chemotherapy and have osseous metastatic disease, CSI is not well tolerated due to severe myelosuppression.[33]

Coadministration of radiation with systemic or intrathecal drugs may increase radiation-associated side effects and is avoided. Common side effects of brain radiation are asthenia, myelosuppression, mucositis, esophagitis (e.g., with cervical spine radiation), and delayed leukoencephalopathy (higher incidence with the combination of radiation and MTX[34]). Leukoencephalopathy has been reported with various agents including intrathecal cytarabine and MTX.[35] MTX can cause direct toxic damage of the axons and myelin sheath.[36]

The role of systemic therapy

Systemic therapy includes chemotherapeutic and targeted agents (Table 15.1). Most chemotherapy regimens fail to penetrate the CSF at therapeutic concentrations. However, some agents do achieve therapeutic concentrations in the CSF, often when given in higher than typical doses. Systemic therapy is favored when agents are available that have favorable BBB-penetrating properties. If such agents are not available, both systemic and CSF-directed therapies are combined rationally. CNS-penetrating systemic treatments are particularly helpful for patients with simultaneous leptomeningeal and progressive systemic disease, as both CNS and extra-CNS disease can be targeted with a single agent or regimen. Systemic therapy may also be effective in bulky disease, which relies on neovascularization for continued growth.

Immune therapies. Immune therapies including both anti-PD1 and anti-CTLA4 (i.e., immune checkpoint inhibitors, see Chapter 29) have shown safety and activity in brain metastases, and are also being evaluated in LMD. A phase 2 study of pembrolizumab (PD1 Ab) in LMD patients, with more than 80% breast cancer patients, reported that this agent was well tolerated and 44% of patients survived 3 months after enrollment.[53] Other immune therapies including nivolumab (PD1 Ab), ipilimumab (anti-CTLA4/cytotoxic T-lymphocyte antigen), and atezolizumab (anti–PD-L1 monoclonal antibody) have shown activity in brain metastases but patients with LMD have been excluded from these studies.[54–60]

Clinical Pearls

1. Whole brain radiotherapy is used for treating diffuse leptomeningeal disease in patients with symptoms of high ICP to improve CSF flow.
2. Focal conformal radiation therapy or stereotactic radiosurgery are used for treating bulky lesions that impair CSF flow (noncommunicating hydrocephalus) or symptomatic nodules that result in impaired neurological function.
3. In LMD patients with active systemic therapy, clinicians should explore systemic chemotherapy or targeted therapies with favorable blood-brain barrier penetrating properties.

CASE 15.5 MANAGEMENT OF LMD IN PATIENTS WITHOUT BULKY DISEASE

Case. A 48-year-old female was initially diagnosed with limited-stage small-cell carcinoma arising from the thyroid. She underwent treatment with four cycles of carboplatin and etoposide with complete response and remained disease free until a paratracheal mass was discovered 1 year from diagnosis. She underwent resection followed by radiation therapy. She declined concurrent chemotherapy and remained disease free for 2 years. She developed sudden onset of right hemisensory loss and suffered a seizure and was found to have a large, 7.2 cm × 6.1 cm left parietal lesion (Fig. 15.4A, measured with green lines) and underwent resection showing metastatic small-cell carcinoma and WBRT (37.50 Gy in 15 fractions). She remained disease free systemically and did well for 16 months until surveillance imaging showed a marginal failure that was treated with Gamma Knife stereotactic radiosurgery followed by four cycles of carboplatin and etoposide. She remained disease free for 12 months until she developed new headaches and neuroimaging showed new multifocal enhancing nodules along the ependymal surface of the ventricles (Fig. 15.4B, orange arrows) and an enhancing lesion in the cauda equine (Fig. 15.4D, red circle) consistent with LMD. An Ommaya reservoir was placed and she was treated with intrathecal etoposide (0.5 mg daily × 5 days every 14 days) based on her repeated systemic responses to this agent. After two cycles of treatment, she was found to have a mixed response with complete response of intracranial disease (Fig. 15.4C, blue arrows) but progression of bulky nodular disease in the cauda equine (Fig. 15.4E, red circle). After conformal radiation therapy to the spine was performed (30 Gy in 5 fractions), intrathecal chemotherapy was resumed with intrathecal MTX 12 mg twice weekly for 4 weeks. Repeat imaging showed continued progressive disease. She was treated with three cycles of nivolumab without response, transitioned to hospice, and, after 2 months, died from progressive disease.

Teaching Points: Treatment of Non-Bulky, Diffuse Leptomeningeal Metastasis. In patients with low-risk LMD, an aggressive approach to treatment is reasonable. This may involve systemic therapy, intrathecal treatment, symptom palliation with radiation, or any combination of these. The patient in this case highlights the use of each of these treatment options and the ability to combine various therapies to maximize tumor-directed therapy and symptom management. The first step in evaluation and management of these patients is to determine the status of systemic disease. This patient had stable systemic disease, and treatment was directed to the CSF compartment alone. Radiation therapy was favored for management of bulky disease. Highly radiosensitive tumors include lymphoma, multiple myeloma, and small-cell carcinoma. Small-cell carcinoma has a predilection for seeding the brain, and thus, at the time of the initial brain tumor, WBRT was performed and she had a very nice response. At the time of leptomeningeal dissemination, her systemic disease was well controlled and bulky disease was minimal, thus intrathecal chemotherapy was favored; however, the largest lesion in the cauda equina did not respond, perhaps related to the inability of intrathecal treatment to penetrate this lesion. When intrathecal therapy failed, systemic treatment with nivolumab was attempted.

The superiority of systemic versus intrathecal chemotherapy has not been established. Like in this case, intrathecal therapy is considered in non-bulky disease without evidence of obstruction to CSF outflow. Intrathecal therapy may also be generally preferred for selected hematologic malignancies that show a more favorable response (e.g., lymphoma) as compared with solid tumors that may not.

The role of intrathecal therapy

Intrathecal chemotherapy overcomes the poor penetration of systemic drugs due to the BCSFB. Intrathecal therapy Eliminated IT has lower toxicity and helps achieve higher CSF concentration of drugs without systemic administration. It is administered via an intrathecal route either through lumbar puncture or intraventricular administration through an Ommaya reservoir. The intraventricular route helps to achieve uniform distribution and steady therapeutic levels in the CSF.[61] For this treatment, an Ommaya reservoir is placed, frequently in the right frontal horn of the lateral ventricle. The Ommaya is a surgically implanted subcutaneous subgeal device that provides access to the ventricular system through a catheter terminating in the lateral ventricle. VP shunts with on-off valves have also been used in administering intraventricular therapy.

Intrathecal chemotherapy treats only a monolayer of cells adjacent to the CSF, hence it is preferred in non-bulky LMD or post-radiation in bulky disease.[21,22] Various intrathecal drugs have been shown to be effective in hematologic malignancies and limited solid tumors (Table 15.2). These include MTX, cytarabine, thiotepa, topotecan, etoposide, trastuzumab, and rituximab, among others.

Complications of intrathecal therapy include infectious meningitis, encephalopathy, and ascending myelopathy. Aseptic meningitis occurs in up to 20% of patients and presents as abrupt onset of headache, stiff neck, nausea, vomiting, lethargy, and fever several hours after the injection. This typically lasts for 12 to 72 hours. Delayed leukoencephalopathy can also be seen but presents later, often months to years after treatment.[1]

Clinical Pearls

1. In LMD patients without bulky, nodular disease, intrathecal chemotherapy is a treatment consideration, particularly for patients without active systemic disease.
2. Intrathecal chemotherapy is administered either by lumbar puncture or intraventricular administration via a surgically implanted Ommaya reservoir.
3. Intrathecal chemotherapy is generally well tolerated, though up to 20% of patients will develop aseptic meningitis and present with abrupt onset of headache, stiff neck, nausea, vomiting, lethargy, and fever several hours after the injection.

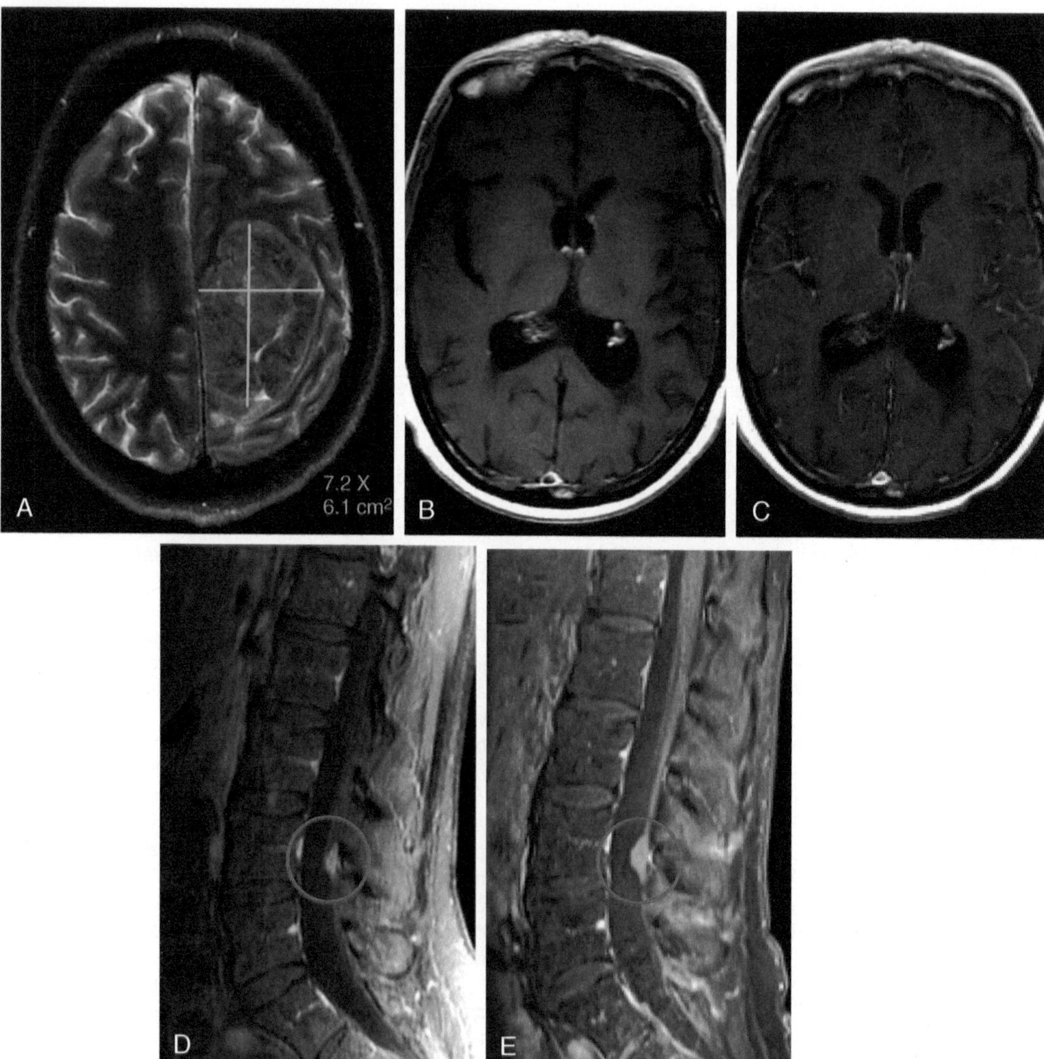

Fig. 15.4 (A) MRI of the brain: T2-weighted axial view showing a large 7.2 cm × 6.1 cm lesion in the left posterior frontal and parietal lobe. (B) Pre-treatment MRI of the brain: T1-weighted axial gadolinium enhanced view showing three multifocal enhancing nodules lining the ependymal surface *(orange arrows)* consistent with leptomeningeal disease. (C) Post-treatment MRI of the brain: T1-weighted axial gadolinium enhanced view performed 1 month after the MRI in (B) showing complete resolution of the three multifocal enhancing nodules lining the ependymal surface *(blue arrows)* consistent with complete response. (D) Pre-treatment MRI of the spine: T1-weighted sagittal gadolinium enhanced view showing an enhancing nodule along the cauda equina *(red circle)* consistent with leptomeningeal disease. (E) Post-treatment MRI of the spine: T1-weighted sagittal gadolinium enhanced view performed 1 month after the MRI in (D) showing enlargement of the enhancing nodule along the cauda equina *(red circle)* consistent with disease progression.

Table 15.2 Intrathecal agents for the treatment of leptomeningeal disease

Intrathecal Agent	Mechanism	Regimen
Methotrexate[2,62]	Cell cycle specific folate-antimetabolite	10–15 mg twice weekly for 4 weeks, then 10–15 mg once weekly for 4 weeks, then 10–15 mg once monthly
Cytarabine[2,63]	Cell-cycle specific Pyrimidine nucleoside analogue	25–100 mg twice weekly for 4 weeks, 25–100 mg once weekly for 4 weeks, then 25–100 mg once monthly
Thiotepa[2,64]	Alkylating ethyleneimine compound	10 mg twice weekly for 4 weeks, then 10 mg once weekly for 4 weeks, then 10 mg once a month
Topotecan[65,66]	Camptothecin analog	0.4 mg twice weekly × 6 weeks followed by weekly for 6 weeks then twice monthly × 4 months then monthly
Etoposide[67,68]	Cytotoxic effect through inhibition of DNA topoisomerase II	0.5 mg once daily for 5 days, repeat course Q3 weeks
Trastuzumab[69]	Monoclonal antibody against HER2	12.5 to 25 mg increase to 100 mg weekly
Rituximab[69,70]	Monoclonal antibody against CD20 antigen	10–25 mg. Once a week for week 1, then twice a week for 4 weeks

Conclusions

Leptomeningeal disease is a devastating complication of cancer. Diagnosis is challenging given the high rate of false-negative test results. Therefore, clinicians must have a high index of suspicion in cancer patients who present with new neurological symptoms. Diagnostic testing includes a comprehensive neurological examination, neuroimaging of the brain and total spine, and dural puncture for CSF analysis and cytology with flow cytometry for hematologic malignancies. Treatment options include radiation therapy, intrathecal chemotherapy, and systemic therapy along with supportive care for patients with poor performance. There is ongoing research to optimize diagnostic strategies as well as to develop new drugs with better CSF bioavailability. Novel treatments including proton radiation to the entire craniospinal axis (NCT03520504), immunotherapy including pembrolizumab (NCT02939300) and the combination of nivolumab and ipilimumab (NCT03091478) for LMD with solid tumors, as well as paclitaxel trevatide for HER2-negative breast with newly diagnosed LMD (NCT03613181) are under investigation.[71] These novel therapies are the hope to ideally extend the life of patients with this challenging disease while still maintaining an appropriate quality of life.

References

1. Chang EL, Lo S. Diagnosis and management of central nervous system metastases from breast cancer. *Oncol*. 2003;8(5): 398–410.
2. Taillibert S, Chamberlain MC. Leptomeningeal metastasis. *Handb Clin Neurol*. 2018;149:169–204.
3. Leal T, Chang JE, Mehta M, Robins HI. Leptomeningeal metastasis: challenges in diagnosis and treatment. *Curr Cancer Ther Rev*. 2011;7(4):319–327.
4. Wasserstrom WR, Glass JP, Posner JB. Diagnosis and treatment of leptomeningeal metastases from solid tumors: experience with 90 patients. *Cancer*. 1982;49(4):759–772.
5. Slimane K, Andre F, Delaloge S, et al. Risk factors for brain relapse in patients with metastatic breast cancer. *Ann Oncol*. 2004;15(11):1640–1644.
6. Maurer C, Tulpin L, Moreau M, et al. Risk factors for the development of brain metastases in patients with HER2-positive breast cancer. *ESMO Open*. 2018;3(6):e000440.
7. Enting RH. Leptomeningeal neoplasia: epidemiology, clinical presentation, CSF analysis and diagnostic imaging. *Cancer Treat Res*. 2005;125:17–30.
8. Waki F, Ando M, Takashima A, et al. Prognostic factors and clinical outcomes in patients with leptomeningeal metastasis from solid tumors. *J Neuro Oncol*. 2009;93(2):205–212.
9. Ferguson SD, Bindal S, Bassett Jr RL, et al. Predictors of survival in metastatic melanoma patients with leptomeningeal disease (LMD). *J Neuro Oncol*. 2019;142(3):499–509.
10. Kingston B, Kayhanian H, Brooks C, et al. Treatment and prognosis of leptomeningeal disease secondary to metastatic breast cancer: a single-centre experience. *Breast*. 2017;36:54–59.
11. Li YS, Jiang BY, Yang JJ, et al. Leptomeningeal metastases in patients with NSCLC with EGFR mutations. *J Thorac Oncol*. 2016;11(11):1962–1969.
12. Remon J, Le Rhun E, Besse B. Leptomeningeal carcinomatosis in non-small cell lung cancer patients: a continuing challenge in

the personalized treatment era. *Cancer Treat Rev*. 2017;53: 128–137.
13. Yust-Katz S, Garciarena P, Liu D, et al. Breast cancer and leptomeningeal disease (LMD): hormone receptor status influences time to development of LMD and survival from LMD diagnosis. *J Neuro Oncol*. 2013;114(2):229–235.
14. Abouharb S, Ensor J, Loghin ME, et al. Leptomeningeal disease and breast cancer: the importance of tumor subtype. *Breast Cancer Res Treat*. 2014;146(3):477–486.
15. Winge K, Rasmussen D, Werdelin LM. Constipation in neurological diseases. *J Neurol Neurosurg Psychiatry*. 2003;74(1):13–19.
16. Guidelines N. *National Comprehensive Cancer Network*; 2020. Version 2, April 2020. Available at: https://www.nccn.org/professionals/physician_gls/pdf/cns.pdf
17. Dux R, Kindler-Röhrborn A, Annas M, Faustmann P, Lennartz K, Zimmermann CW. A standardized protocol for flow cytometric analysis of cells isolated from cerebrospinal fluid. *J Neurol Sci*. 1994;121(1):74–78.
18. Hegde U, Filie A, Little RF, et al. High incidence of occult leptomeningeal disease detected by flow cytometry in newly diagnosed aggressive B-cell lymphomas at risk for central nervous system involvement: the role of flow cytometry versus cytology. *Blood*. 2005;105(2):496–502.
19. French CA, Dorfman DM, Shaheen G, Cibas ES. Diagnosing lymphoproliferative disorders involving the cerebrospinal fluid: increased sensitivity using flow cytometric analysis. *Diagn Cytopathol*. 2000;23(6):369–374.
20. Milojkovic Kerklaan B, Pluim D, Bol M, et al. EpCAM-based flow cytometry in cerebrospinal fluid greatly improves diagnostic accuracy of leptomeningeal metastases from epithelial tumors. *Neuro Oncol*. 2016;18(6):855–862.
21. Burch PA, Grossman SA, Reinhard CS. Spinal cord penetration of intrathecally administered cytarabine and methotrexate: a quantitative autoradiographic study. *J Natl Cancer Inst*. 1988;80(15):1211–1216.
22. Benjamin JC, Moss T, Moseley RP, Maxwell R, Coakham HB. Cerebral distribution of immunoconjugate after treatment for neoplastic meningitis using an intrathecal radiolabeled monoclonal antibody. *Neurosurgery*. 1989;25(2):253–258.
23. Siegal T. Toxicity of treatment for neoplastic meningitis. *Curr Oncol Rep*. 2003;5(1):41–49.
24. Chamberlain MC, Tsao-Wei D, Groshen S. Neoplastic meningitis-related encephalopathy: prognostic significance. *Neurology*. 2004;63(11):2159–2161.
25. Diringer MN, Scalfani MT, Zazulia AR, Videen TO, Dhar R, Powers WJ. Effect of mannitol on cerebral blood volume in patients with head injury. *Neurosurgery*. 2012;70(5):1215–1218. discussion 1219.
26. Nigim F, Critchlow JF, Kasper EM. Role of ventriculoperitoneal shunting in patients with neoplasms of the central nervous system: an analysis of 59 cases. *Mol Clin Oncol*. 2015;3(6):1381–1386.
27. Berger MS, Baumeister B, Geyer JR, Milstein J, Kanev PM, LeRoux PD. The risks of metastases from shunting in children with primary central nervous system tumors. *J Neurosurg*. 1991;74(6):872–877.
28. Brainin M, Barnes M, Baron JC, et al. Guidance for the preparation of neurological management guidelines by EFNS scientific task forces--revised recommendations 2004. *Eur J Neurol*. 2004;11(9):577–581.
29. Ryken TC, McDermott M, Robinson PD, et al. The role of steroids in the management of brain metastases: a systematic review and evidence-based clinical practice guideline. *J Neuro Oncol*. 2010;96(1):103–114.
30. Omar AIMW. *Neurologic Complications of Cancer*. 2nd ed. New York, NY: Oxford University Press; 2009.
31. Posner JB. *Neurologic Complications of Cancer*. Philadelphia, PA: FA Davis; 1995.
32. Mehta M, Bradley K. Radiation therapy for leptomeningeal cancer. *Cancer Treat Res*. 2005;125:147–158.
33. Hermann B, Hültenschmidt B, Sautter-Bihl ML. Radiotherapy of the neuroaxis for palliative treatment of leptomeningeal carcinomatosis. *Strahlenther Onkol*. 2001;177(4):195–199.
34. Correa DD, Shi W, Abrey LE, et al. Cognitive functions in primary CNS lymphoma after single or combined modality regimens. *Neuro Oncol*. 2011;14(1):101–108.
35. Colamaria V, Caraballo R, Borgna-Pignatti C, et al. Transient focal leukoencephalopathy following intraventricular methotrexate and cytarabine. A complication of the Ommaya reservoir: case report and review of the literature. *Childs Nerv Syst*. 1990;6(4):231–235.
36. Ozutemiz C, Roshan SK, Kroll NJ, et al. Acute toxic leukoencephalopathy: etiologies, imaging findings, and outcomes in 101 patients. *AJNR Am J Neuroradiol*. 2019;40(2):267–275.
37. Glantz MJ, Cole BF, Recht L, et al. High-dose intravenous methotrexate for patients with nonleukemic leptomeningeal cancer: is intrathecal chemotherapy necessary? *J Clin Oncol*. 1998;16(4):1561–1567.
38. Addeo R, De Rosa C, Faiola V, et al. Phase 2 trial of temozolomide using protracted low-dose and whole-brain radiotherapy for nonsmall cell lung cancer and breast cancer patients with brain metastases. *Cancer*. 2008;113(9):2524–2531.
39. Ostermann S, Csajka C, Buclin T, et al. Plasma and cerebrospinal fluid population pharmacokinetics of temozolomide in malignant glioma patients. *Clin Cancer Res*. 2004;10(11):3728–3736.
40. Togashi Y, Masago K, Masuda S, et al. Cerebrospinal fluid concentration of gefitinib and erlotinib in patients with non-small cell lung cancer. *Cancer Chemother Pharmacol*. 2012;70(3):399–405.
41. Clarke JL, Pao W, Wu N, Miller VA, Lassman AB. High dose weekly erlotinib achieves therapeutic concentrations in CSF and is effective in leptomeningeal metastases from epidermal growth factor receptor mutant lung cancer. *J Neuro Oncol*. 2010;99(2):283–286.
42. Milton DT, Azzoli CG, Heelan RT, et al. A phase I/II study of weekly high-dose erlotinib in previously treated patients with nonsmall cell lung cancer. *Cancer*. 2006;107(5):1034–1041.
43. Lin CH, Lin MT, Kuo YW, Ho CC. Afatinib combined with cetuximab for lung adenocarcinoma with leptomeningeal carcinomatosis. *Lung Canc*. 2014;85(3):479–480.
44. Yang JC-H, Cho BC, Kim D-W, et al. Osimertinib for patients (pts) with leptomeningeal metastases (LM) from EGFR-mutant non-small cell lung cancer (NSCLC): updated results from the BLOOM study. *J Clin Oncol*. 2017;35(suppl 15):2020.
45. Crino L, Ahn MJ, De Marinis F, et al. Multicenter phase II study of whole-body and intracranial activity with ceritinib in patients with ALK-rearranged non-small-cell lung cancer previously treated with chemotherapy and crizotinib: results from ASCEND-2. *J Clin Oncol*. 2016;34(24):2866–2873.
46. Gadgeel SM, Gandhi L, Riely GJ, et al. Safety and activity of alectinib against systemic disease and brain metastases in patients with crizotinib-resistant ALK-rearranged non-small-cell lung cancer (AF-002JG): results from the dose-finding portion of a phase 1/2 study. *Lancet Oncol*. 2014;15(10):1119–1128.
47. Wilgenhof S, Neyns B. Complete cytologic remission of V600E BRAF-mutant melanoma-associated leptomeningeal carcinomatosis upon treatment with Dabrafenib. *J Clin Oncol*. 2015;33(28):e109–e111.

48. McArthur GA, Maio M, Arance A, et al. Vemurafenib in metastatic melanoma patients with brain metastases: an open-label, single-arm, phase 2, multicentre study. *Ann Oncol.* 2017;28(3):634–641.
49. Kim DW, Barcena E, Mehta UN, et al. Prolonged survival of a patient with metastatic leptomeningeal melanoma treated with BRAF inhibition-based therapy: a case report. *BMC Canc.* 2015;15:400.
50. Floudas CS, Chandra AB, Xu Y. Vemurafenib in leptomeningeal carcinomatosis from melanoma: a case report of near-complete response and prolonged survival. *Melanoma Res.* 2016;26(3):312–315.
51. Schafer N, Scheffler B, Stuplich M, et al. Vemurafenib for leptomeningeal melanomatosis. *J Clin Oncol.* 2013;31(11):e173–174.
52. Lee JM, Mehta UN, Dsouza LH, Guadagnolo BA, Sanders DL, Kim KB. Long-term stabilization of leptomeningeal disease with whole-brain radiation therapy in a patient with metastatic melanoma treated with vemurafenib: a case report. *Melanoma Res.* 2013;23(2):175–178.
53. Brastianos PK, Prakadan S, Alvarez-Breckenridge C, et al. Phase II study of pembrolizumab in leptomeningeal carcinomatosis. *J Clin Oncol.* 2018;36(suppl 15):2007.
54. Goldberg SB, Gettinger SN, Mahajan A, et al. Pembrolizumab for patients with melanoma or non-small-cell lung cancer and untreated brain metastases: early analysis of a non-randomised, open-label, phase 2 trial. *Lancet Oncol.* 2016;17(7):976–983.
55. Margolin K, Ernstoff MS, Hamid O, et al. Ipilimumab in patients with melanoma and brain metastases: an open-label, phase 2 trial. *Lancet Oncol.* 2012;13(5):459–465.
56. Geukes Foppen MH, Brandsma D, Blank CU, van Thienen JV, Haanen JB, Boogerd W. Targeted treatment and immunotherapy in leptomeningeal metastases from melanoma. *Ann Oncol.* 2016;27(6):1138–1142.
57. Tawbi HA, Forsyth PA, Algazi A, et al. Combined nivolumab and ipilimumab in melanoma metastatic to the brain. *N Engl J Med.* 2018;379(8):722–730.
58. Long GV, Atkinson V, Lo S, et al. Combination nivolumab and ipilimumab or nivolumab alone in melanoma brain metastases: a multicentre randomised phase 2 study. *Lancet Oncol.* 2018;19(5):672–681.
59. Lukas RV, Gandhi M, O'Hear C, Hu S, Lai C, Patel JD. Safety and efficacy analyses of atezolizumab in advanced non-small cell lung cancer (NSCLC) patients with or without baseline brain metastases. *Ann Oncol.* 2017;28(suppl 2):21–29.
60. Gadgeel SM, Lukas RV, Goldschmidt J, et al. Atezolizumab in patients with advanced non-small cell lung cancer and history of asymptomatic, treated brain metastases: exploratory analyses of the phase III OAK study. *Lung Canc.* 2019;128:105–112.
61. Shapiro WR, Young DF, Mehta BM. Methotrexate: distribution in cerebrospinal fluid after intravenous, ventricular and lumbar injections. *N Engl J Med.* 1975;293(4):161–166.
62. Bleyer WA, Dedrick RL. Clinical pharmacology of intrathecal methotrexate. I. Pharmacokinetics in nontoxic patients after lumbar injection. *Cancer Treat Rep.* 1977;61(4):703–708.
63. Zimm S, Collins JM, Miser J, Chatterji D, Poplack DG. Cytosine arabinoside cerebrospinal fluid kinetics. *Clin Pharmacol Ther.* 1984;35(6):826–830.
64. Le Rhun E, Taillibert S, Chamberlain MC. Neoplastic meningitis due to lung, breast, and melanoma metastases. *Cancer Control.* 2017;24(1):22–32.
65. Groves MD, Glantz MJ, Chamberlain MC, et al. A multicenter phase II trial of intrathecal topotecan in patients with meningeal malignancies. *Neuro Oncol.* 2008;10(2):208–215.
66. Blaney SM, Heideman R, Berg S, et al. Phase I clinical trial of intrathecal topotecan in patients with neoplastic meningitis. *J Clin Oncol.* 2003;21(1):143–147.
67. van der Gaast A, Sonneveld P, Mans DR, Splinter TA. Intrathecal administration of etoposide in the treatment of malignant meningitis: feasibility and pharmacokinetic data. *Cancer Chemother Pharmacol.* 1992;29(4):335–337.
68. Chamberlain MC, Tsao-Wei DD, Groshen S. Phase II trial of intracerebrospinal fluid etoposide in the treatment of neoplastic meningitis. *Cancer.* 2006;106(9):2021–2027.
69. Gabay MP, Thakkar JP, Stachnik JM, Woelich SK, Villano JL. Intra-CSF administration of chemotherapy medications. *Cancer Chemother Pharmacol.* 2012;70(1):1–15.
70. Rubenstein JL, Fridlyand J, Abrey L, et al. Phase I study of intraventricular administration of rituximab in patients with recurrent CNS and intraocular lymphoma. *J Clin Oncol.* 2007;25(11):1350–1356.
71. Kumthekar P, Tang S-C, Brenner AJ, et al. ANG1005, a novel brain-penetrant taxane derivative, for the treatment of recurrent brain metastases and leptomeningeal carcinomatosis from breast cancer. *J Clin Oncol.* 2016;34(suppl 15):2004.

Chapter | 16 |

Approach to patients with the neoplasms associated with neurofibromatosis type 1, neurofibromatosis type 2, and schwannomatosis

Jaishri Blakeley, Shannon Langmead and Peter de Blank

CHAPTER OUTLINE

Introduction

Neurofibromatosis type 1 (NF1), neurofibromatosis type 2 (NF2), and schwannomatosis (SWN) are rare tumor suppressor conditions with estimated incidences of 1:3,000, 1:60,000, and 1:100,000, respectively.[1–3] Although all three conditions are autosomal dominant and predispose to tumors throughout the central and peripheral nervous systems, the natural history for all of these conditions is highly variable both across and within families (Table 16.1).

For example, NF1 manifests with skin findings, peripheral nerve tumors (e.g., neurofibromas), and, in some cases, malignancy. Skin findings include café-au-lait macules (CALMs) and axillary or inguinal freckling. Tumors may involve the skin (e.g., cutaneous neurofibroma [cNF]), superficial and deep nerves (e.g., diffuse infiltrating, nodular, and [pNFs]), or astrocytes (e.g., optic pathway gliomas [OPGs]). Malignant cancers include malignant peripheral nerve sheath tumor (MPNST), malignant glioma, gastrointestinal stromal tumor (GIST), and juvenile myelomonocytic leukemia (JMML).[4–6] There is a remarkable range in the frequency of each of these manifestations. It is estimated that up to 99% of adults with NF1 will have cNF, but less than 1% of children with NF1 develop JMML.[7,8] There is also variability in presentation and manifestations experienced across and within families such that one family member may have a heavy burden of cNF and another may have a paucity of skin findings. Differences even exist in manifestations across stages of development within a given person with NF1.

Like NF1, in NF2 there is variability in the frequency and severity of manifestations; however, there is more consistency within families and more consistent genotype-phenotype relationships. For example, the full complement of tumors seen in NF2 including bilateral vestibular schwannoma (VS), intracranial and spinal meningioma, and spinal schwannomas are found in 77%, 52%, and 65%, respectively, in children with a constitutional truncating mutation in exon 2–13 of the *NF2* gene in population studies in England. This was compared with bilateral VS in only 52% of children with "mild" mutations (including certain splice site mutations, small in-frame deletions, and missense mutations) and only 4% having meningioma or paraspinal schwannomas.[9]

Schwannomatosis (SWN) is the most recently identified and least well defined of these tumor predisposition syndromes. SWN is defined by multiple schwannomas throughout the peripheral nervous system most often associated with regional and generalized pain. Importantly, the pain may or may not be associated with a particular neoplasm and the pain is far more prominent than any other neurologic symptoms.[10] People with SWN may have unilateral VS, nonvestibular cranial schwannomas, and meningiomas, but not bilateral VS or ependymomas. By far the most common presentation is paraspinal and peripheral schwannomas. The predominance of peripheral schwannomas, some intracranial schwannomas, and meningiomas can create diagnostic confusion due to the clinical overlap with NF2; however, there are distinct genes associated with SWN (e.g., *LZTR1* and *SMARCB1*) and germline *NF2* testing is negative in people with SWN.[11]

The high frequency of these conditions as well as the common, progressive, and often severe neurologic and oncologic disability that results from pathognomonic tumors (e.g., gliomas, schwannomas, meningiomas) warrants awareness from neurologists, neurosurgeons, oncologists, and related clinical communities (Table 16.1).

Genetics

NF1, NF2, and SWN are all genetic conditions with autosomal dominant transmission. NF1 is by far the most common of the three syndromes. The condition NF1 is due to a germline mutation in one of the two alleles of the tumor suppressor gene *NF1* on chromosome 17q11.2.[12,13] NF1 is a true tumor predisposition syndrome—germline mutation in *NF1* is sufficient to cause the condition, and a "second hit" resulting in loss of function in the second *NF1* allele is required for tumor formation. The protein product, neurofibromin, is a regulator of Ras.[14] In the absence of normal neurofibromin, the proto-oncogene Ras is dysregulated and contributes to excessive cell growth. Roughly 50% of people with NF1 have inherited the gene from an affected parent; in the other 50% of patients, the germline mutation is *de novo*.[1] There is complete penetrance such that all people who have a germline *NF1* mutation have the condition NF1. However, the manifestations can vary dramatically even among family members with the same mutation (e.g., variable expressivity).

NF2 is similar to NF1 in that: (1) it is autosomal dominant; (2) heterozygous loss of *NF2* results in the condition, but biallelic mutations are required for tumor formation; (3) roughly 50% of people with NF2 have a familial mutation and 50% have a *de novo* mutation; (4) the location of the *NF2* gene (chromosome 22q12.2) and protein product (merlin) are known; and (5) there is complete penetrance but variable expression. Important differences in the genetics of NF1 and NF2 are that NF2 is comparatively rare and the existence of a genotype-phenotype correlation in NF2. Specifically, the type of mutation in the *NF2* gene is associated with disease severity to a degree that influences clinical management as detailed above. Hence, genetic testing is warranted if feasible in people who meet the clinical criteria for NF2, as the type of mutation influences management.

SWN is unique from both NF1 and NF2, as the genetic condition can be caused by at least two different genes on chromosome 22q11: *LZTR1* and *SMARCB1*.[15–17] It is known that there are people and families who meet the clinical criteria for SWN who test negative for germline mutations or deletions in *NF2*, *LZTR1*, and *SMARCB1* indicating that additional genes are likely involved in SWN.[18]

Importantly, only roughly 86% of people who meet the clinical criteria for familial SWN test positive for a *LZTR1* gene mutation and 48% of people with the familial form of *SMARCB1* SWN test positive for the germline mutation.[11] Far fewer people with the *de novo* form of SWN test positive for a germline mutation of *LZTR1* or *SMARCB1* mutation. Also unique from NF1 and NF2, there appears to be incomplete penetrance and germline mosaicism with SWN.[11,19,20]

Adding to the complexity is that there is significant overlap between NF2 and schwannomatosis in the types of tumors seen in each condition (e.g., schwannomas and meningiomas; ependymomas are not known to occur in schwannomatosis) and the mutations found within the tumor.[20,21,22] Specifically, the schwannomas in SWN commonly have either three or four molecular losses underlying the tumor including biallelic NF2 loss of function (hits 1 and 2) with loss of function in one or both *LZTR1* or *SMARCB1* alleles.[23] However, schwannomas in people with NF2 may also have loss of *LZTR1* or SMARCB1.[17,18,19,23–26]

Pathophysiology

Neurofibromatosis type 1. NF1 is the most common neurocutaneous tumor predisposition condition. In fact, it is one of the most common autosomal dominant diseases of the nervous system, with estimates of incidence as high as 1:2600 people, affecting all races, ethnicities, and both sexes equally.[1–3] The protein product of *NF1*, neurofibromin, is a large protein that is a GTPase-activating protein (GAP).[27,28] The GAP-related domain is the most intensely studied portion of the protein, as this is the portion that acts as a tumor suppressor via reduction of Ras activity.[29] Ras is an oncogene, and in the absence of neurofibromin, it is constitutively activated resulting in excessive stimulation of multiple pro-growth pathways.[30] There are additional important functional regions of the Ras protein including a portion that regulates cyclic adenosine monophosphate (cAMP). cAMP is a ubiquitous mediator of intracellular signaling activated by a wide variety of pathways via the G protein–coupled receptor. Intracellular cAMP activity has been linked to both tumor growth and senescence in NF1.[31]

As a result of abnormal cellular regulation, people with NF1 are prone to multiple tumors. The most common tumors are peripheral nerve sheath tumors (PNSTs), including cNFs that involve the skin and soft tissue or nodular and pNF that originate from deeper nerves. An estimated 30–50% of patients with NF1 develop pNFs.[6,32,33] These tumors can both cause significant neurologic disability and transform into malignant sarcomas (MPNST).[34,35] Hallmark cutaneous findings include CALMs, skinfold freckling, and cNFs. Additional common manifestations of NF1 include central nervous system (CNS) tumors such as gliomas, which frequently occur along the optic track (OPGs) or in the posterior fossa. Many patients with NF1 have cognitive deficits, bone dysplasias including scoliosis, and ophthalmologic abnormalities. There is also an increased risk of vascular abnormalities and non–nervous system malignancies, such as GISTs, leukemia, and neuroendocrine tumors including pheochromocytomas (Table 16.1).[7,36–38]

Neurofibromatosis type 2. NF2 is caused by mutations in the *NF2* gene on chromosome 22q11. The *NF2* gene encodes the protein Merlin (moesin-ezrin-radixin-like protein) that is best known for its activity as a membrane-cytoskeleton scaffolding protein that operates as a tumor suppressor.[39] In the absence of normal Merlin, there is a predisposition to development of multiple nervous system tumors. The pathognomonic presentation for NF2 is bilateral VS. This is present in the vast majority of people with NF2 by the age of 30 years and often results in hearing loss by early adulthood.

Schwannomas of cranial nerves are not unique to NF2 and can happen sporadically or as part of other conditions such as schwannomatosis. It is when schwannomas involve the bilateral vestibular nerves that NF2 is considered. That said, bilateral VS can be seen in people >60 years old as a matter of chance occurrence of two unique schwannomas given the frequency of sporadic VS in the general population.[40] Furthermore, in some cases, lesions seen involving the vestibular nerve are secondary to other processes such as the sequelae of prior radiation therapy or related to leptomeningeal disease.[41] Hence, a full history and examination is needed before confirming that bilateral VS are due to NF2. In addition to schwannomas of the cranial nerves, people with NF2 have a propensity for schwannomas throughout the peripheral nervous system including the spinal nerves and involvement of more distal peripheral nerves. Intracranial and paraspinal meningiomas are also common in people with NF2. Meningiomas are the most common tumor of the cranium in all populations and can be seen in other conditions such as schwannomatosis and forms of meningiomatosis that are independent, but phenotypically overlap with NF2. Finally, ependymomas, most commonly of the spinal cord, are common in NF2. No one of these tumors is particularly challenging in terms of sequelae or management options in and of itself. However, the multiplicity of the schwannomas, meningiomas, and ependymomas and their progressive nature across a lifetime in NF2 result in dire consequences including progressive severe neurologic disability and ultimately death secondary to the complications of these tumors.[42,43]

Schwannomatosis. As mentioned earlier, there is significant overlap between schwannomatosis and NF2 in that multiple schwannomas are part of the diagnostic criteria and presentation of both conditions.[44–47] Furthermore, it has been recently shown that people with confirmed schwannomatosis can develop unilateral VS as well as meningiomas.[19,21,22] Hence, the presence of these lesions is no longer an accurate reason to conclude that a person has NF2 versus schwannomatosis.[48] Increasing evidence indicates that mosaic NF2 is more common than previously suspected and can be very suggestive of schwannomatosis clinically.[49] Finally, although pain is the most common manifestation of schwannomatosis, pain can be a part of NF2 as well.[10,50] Indeed, there is so much overlap in clinical presentation between these conditions that the diagnostic criteria has undergone revision and clarification many times in the last several years and is currently under review in the hopes of improving clarity about the diagnostic criteria for each condition. However, as above, given that there are people who fulfill current clinical diagnostic criteria who test negative for *NF2*, *SMARCB1*, and *LZTR1*, additional criteria are likely to be needed in the future as additional genes associated with schwannomatosis are discovered.[17,18,24,25]

Chromosome 22q11. What is shared across NF1, NF2, and schwannomatosis is that the tenants of Knudson's two-hit hypothesis are met: there is a germline mutation that serves as the "first hit," but neoplasms form when there is a "second hit" causing loss of heterozygosity.[51] As discussed above, in the case of SWN, there is an additional requirement for somatic loss of both alleles of *NF2*, so there is a three or four hit hypothesis for schwannomatosis.[23] Given this clinical and molecular overlap, molecular testing on at least two independent tumors and blood is the ideal approach for confirming the diagnosis of either mosaic or germline NF2 or schwannomatosis.[47]

Clinical cases

The diagnoses of NF1, NF2, and SWN can very often be made clinically, although as there is greater data available about the genotype-phenotype relationships that may influence clinical management and given the increasingly recognized overlap between NF2 and SWN, molecular testing is playing an increasingly important role. In this chapter, we present a series of cases that highlight some of the most common clinical scenarios encountered in the care of people with NF1, NF2, and SWN including management of symptomatic and growing pNF in an adult with NF1, OPG in a child with NF1, non-OPG in a child with NF1, bilateral VS with variable hearing loss in a young adult with NF2, and the diagnosis and management of painful tumors in adults with SWN.

CASE 16.1 APPROACH TO AN ADULT WITH NF1 ASSOCIATED PLEXIFORM NEUROFIBROMA

Case. A 21-year-old man with NF1 presented to clinic with increasing pain-limiting activities of daily living. He was diagnosed with NF1 at age 13 based on the presence of >6 CALMs and >10 cNFs. He was subsequently confirmed to have Lisch nodules (i.e., iris hamartomas) and several deep lesions consistent with neurofibroma of the right forearm, bilateral neck, back, and jaw on imaging as well as some lesions palpable on examination beneath the skin (Fig. 16.1C,D). By the age of 19 years, he developed progressive pain in the neck, bilateral upper extremities, head, abdomen/pelvis, and at sites of his cNFs and felt that there had been visible growth of several of the deep nodular and cNF. The increased pain had prompted two emergency room visits and the addition of gabapentin and oxycodone as needed for severe breakthrough pain not adequate to manage the multifocal pain. In addition, he reported new symptoms of urinary frequency and hesitancy. On examination, there were no signs of myelopathy or radiculopathy with normal motor, sensory, and reflex examinations. There were many palpable nodules deep to the cutaneous and subcutaneous regions in the extremities, some of which were tender to palpation. There were also >100 skin lesions consistent with cNFs. In the setting of known pNFs and the clinical presentation of increasing pain prompting acute care visits despite daily medication for neuropathic pain, fluorodeoxyglucose positron emission tomography (FDG-PET) was ordered to assess for any evidence of malignant conversion.

FDG-PET showed an area with standardized uptake value maximum (SUVmax) of 4.3 in a lesion within the left neck (Fig. 16.1A,B). Whole body MRI (WBMRI) was also recommended, as there were no localizing signs on examination, increasing size of palpable lesions on examination, and the FDG-PET was suggestive but not specific for potential conversion to MPNST.[52] WBMRI is an MRI technique that encompasses head, neck, chest, abdomen, pelvis, and lower extremities MRI (e.g., to the lower leg, Fig. 16.1D).[53] It allows key anatomic and functional sequences to be performed across a large body area in a single acquisition session. The WBMRI showed extensive replacement of the right masseter muscle by pNF, masses in bilateral foramen at every level of the cervical spine, in the prevertebral space narrowing the airway, throughout bilateral brachial plexi, within the mediastinum, along the intercostal neurovascular bundles, within the retroperitoneum, mesentery, throughout the paraspinal soft tissues, within every visualized sacral neural foramen, extensive intrapelvic plexiform tumor burden particularly along the lumbosacral plexus and smaller pelvic nerves that encompasses the rectum, bladder, and cervix with displacement of the urinary bladder, and the rectosigmoid (Fig. 16.1D). Throughout all of these lesions, the target sign was maintained, there was no distinct nodular lesion or suspicious imaging features such as restricted diffusion to indicate malignant degeneration.[54,55] He was ultimately referred for needle biopsy of the neck lesion with the highest SUVmax on FDG-PET with conscious sedation and MRI-guided biopsy. Pathology confirmed pNF. Based on this reassuring pathology, but ongoing pain despite multiple pain medications and radiographic progression, he was enrolled on a clinical trial with a mitogen-activated protein kinase inhibitor (MEKi). Within 1 month of starting drug, he developed extensive acneiform rash and erythema nodosum-type rash. Oral doxycycline and topical clindamycin and topical corticosteroids were started and the dose of the MEKi was reduced by 25%. Rash was manageable thereafter. Within 2 months of starting the MEKi, the diffuse sites of pain reduced from roughly 8/10 to 3/10 based on self-report. By 8 months of starting the MEKi, MRI showed reduction in size of many of the lesions and no evidence of progression.

Teaching Points. This case highlights several important aspects of NF1 including that (1) new unexplained pain should prompt evaluation for malignant degeneration of a pNF; (2) in patients where MRI with diffusion-weighted sequences and FDG-PET are inconclusive, biopsy may be needed to confirm pathology; and (3) new systemic treatments are being studied and currently under review by the Food and Drug Administration for treating progressive pNF in NF1.

Plexiform neurofibromas. pNFs are common in people with NF1 and may be congenital or start growth early in life, but grow rapidly in childhood.[56,57] Although they are histologically benign, these tumors often result in disfigurement, pain, and focal and diffuse loss of motor and sensory function, as well as compression of organs, great vessels, and the airway.[6,58] These functional consequences can be associated with severe morbidity and even mortality.[59] Furthermore, they carry a risk of transformation into MPNSTs for which there is no cure outside of aggressive resection, which is rarely feasible given the deep and infiltrative nature of these tumors. Because of this, MPNST are the leading cause of death for people with NF1.[60] There is an association between burden of neurofibroma and MPNST, and hence, people with a high burden of neurofibroma (as in this case) warrant close clinical and radiographic monitoring.[61,62] Clinically, changes in the severity or nature of pain or rapid growth warrants evaluation for possible malignant conversion with imaging and biopsy.[63]

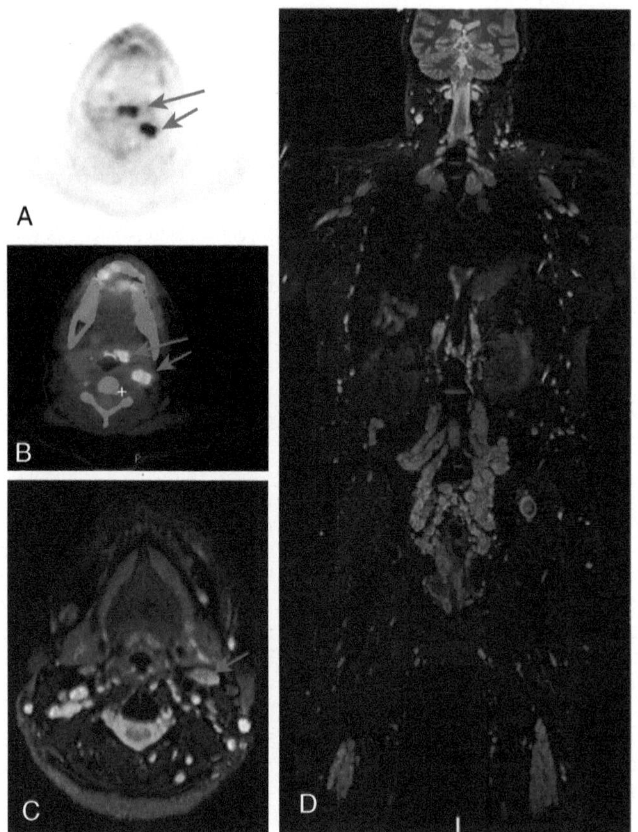

Fig. 16.1 Many plexiform neurofibromas seen on imaging in a patient with neurofibromatosis 1. (A, B) Fluorodeoxyglucose positron emission tomography (FDG-PET) showing two regions of elevated SUVmax *(green arrows)* ultimately determined to be pathologically consistent with neurofibroma. (C) Axial T2-weighted MRI showing that this lesion was nonspecific on MRI *(green arrow)*. (D) Whole body MRI with T2-weighted images showing multiple plexiform neurofibromas *(orange arrows)* involving bilateral brachial plexi, nerve roots at every level of the spinal cord, and in the distal nerves.

As illustrated in this case, pain is one of the most common symptoms associated with pNFs, although progressive neurologic dysfunction or compression of critical organs or regions (i.e., airway) related to the tumor location are also indications for treatment.[64–66] The approach to pain management is multifaceted and includes medications for neuropathic pain, antiinflammatories, and nonpharmacologic approaches.[6,38,67]

Neuroimaging of pNF. MRI is the recommended imaging modality for the diagnosis and surveillance of pNFs.[53] Biologic sequences such as apparent diffusion coefficient (ADC) and diffusion-weighted imaging are increasingly used to distinguish between benign and malignant peripheral nerve sheath tumors.[54] FDG-PET has been the imaging modality recommended for distinguishing between pNF and MPNST; however, there is a relatively high false-positive rate as indicated in this case in which there is high SUVmax (i.e., SUVmax >3) seen in a tumor that is histologically proven to be a be benign neurofibroma.[52]

Classification of benign, atypical, and malignant pNF. There is a recently recognized entity of atypical neurofibroma or atypical neurofibromatous neoplasms of uncertain biologic potential (ANNUBP) that may account for some of the imaging heterogeneity seen in NF1-associated PNSTs.[68,69] Neurofibromas are notoriously heterogeneous and may have multiple different histologic regions and somatic mutations within a given tumor.[70] There is an increasing understanding of an evolution of benign to malignant neurofibroma that can be occurring within different regions of a single tumor or across different tumors within a given patient with NF1.[63,64,65,71] Hence, atypical neurofibromas or ANNUBPs are considered to be precursors to MPNST and, although clear standards for management have not yet been set for these tumors, they warrant consideration of surgical resection when feasible or at the very least close surveillance for rapid growth.[38,53,66,72] It is possible that atypical neurofibromas are represented on MRI as distinct nodular lesions with a round/ovoid and well

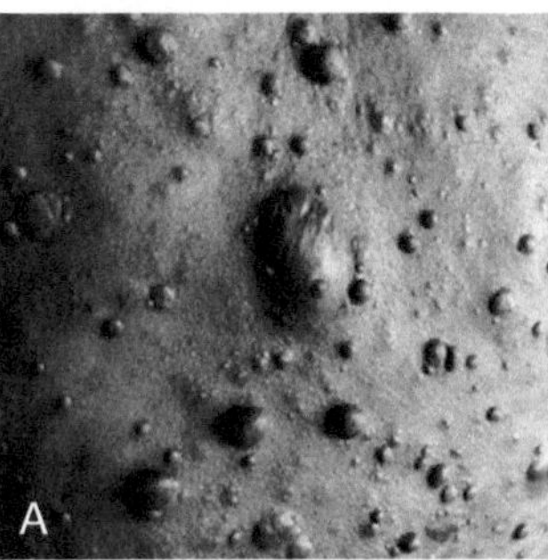

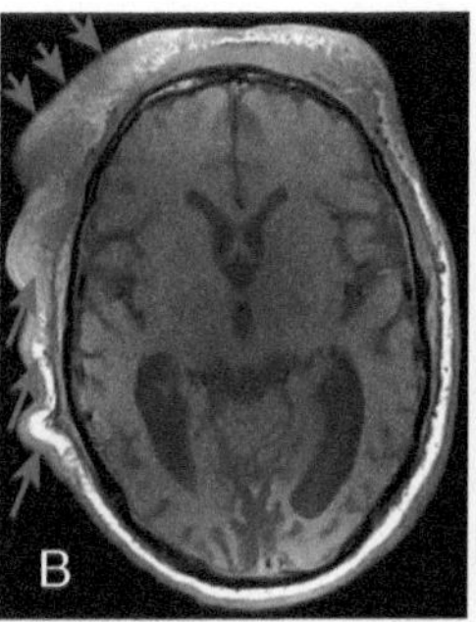

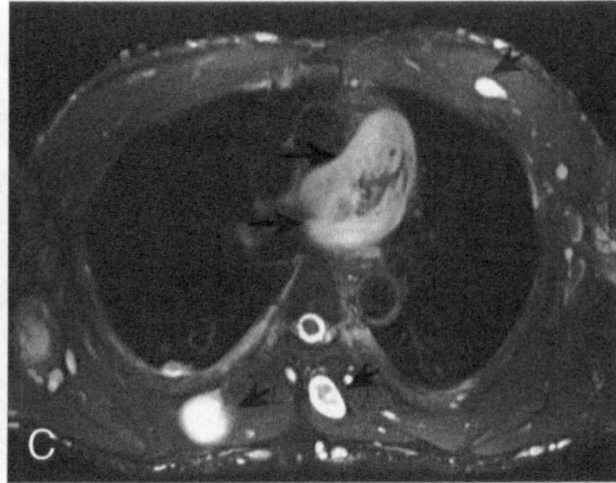

Fig. 16.2 Images of cutaneous and plexiform neurofibromas. (A) Picture of a patch of skin with multiple cutaneous neurofibromas and a diffuse superficial neurofibroma. (B) Shows axial T1-weighted images with a diffuse infiltrating neurofibroma of the scalp *(green arrows)* and (C) shows axial T2-weighted MRI images with a deep nodular *(orange arrow)* and plexiform neurofibromas *(red arrows)*.

demarcated margin that is distinct from the surrounding pNF; however, work is ongoing to validate this observation. Currently, in a person with NF1 with a growing pNF that is increasingly symptomatic and has findings that could be consistent with malignant degeneration based on a distinct nodular appearance on anatomical MRI, low ADC on diffusion MRI, and elevated SUVmax on FDG-PET, biopsy of the most atypical region on imaging should be pursued if feasible.[54,66,73]

Plexiform vs cutaneous neurofibromas. It is important to distinguish pNF from cutaneous and subcutaneous neurofibromas that can involve the skin. The majority of adults, and many children, with NF1 will develop cNFs (Fig. 16.2).[7] These are tumors that are limited to the skin and, unlike pNFs, have virtually no chance of becoming malignant. As such, cNFs do not require regular surveillance; however, given that they are a major cause of poor quality of life and affect almost all adults with NF1, there are major research efforts underway to identify the most effective currently available therapies and develop new therapies for these tumors.[74–77]

Treatment options for pNF. The standard of care for symptomatic or growing pNFs has long been surgical resection as this can result in complete resection for some tumors and resolution of symptoms even with minor debulking in others.[38] However, due to the intrinsic involvement of nerve, diffuse infiltration, deep locations, and excessive perfusion, surgery is often challenging or not feasible. There is also no defined role for radiation therapy for these tumors and it is avoided due to concern for secondary malignancies.[78] As such, there is a long history of preclinical and clinical efforts to develop promising medical therapies for pNFs.[64,79] There are several clinical trials that are showing early signs of reducing tumor volume and potentially improving tumor-associated symptoms for both children and adults with morbid pNFs (NCT03962543, NCT03231306, NCT02407405, NCT02101736, NCT03326388).[80] Given these early successes, there has been enthusiasm by many patients for enrollment on clinical trials and off-label use of various targeted therapies for pNFs. This is reasonable in the right clinical context, and there are increasingly good medical options for both adults and children with pNF. However, each of these agents carries with it potentially serious complications and many low-grade toxicities that require close surveillance and management to make these therapies feasible—as was the case with this patient.[81,82] We also do not have data about the long-term safety and consequences of these therapies at this time. Furthermore, there is no evidence to date that the drugs developed for pNF are effective for sporadic PNSTs.

Clinical Pearls

1. In NF1 patients with pNF, changes in the severity or nature of pain or rapid growth warrants evaluation with imaging for possible malignant conversion.
2. Imaging findings that suggest malignant degeneration include a distinct nodular appearance on anatomical MRI, low ADC on diffusion MRI, and elevated SUVmax on FDG-PET; in such lesions, biopsy of the most atypical region should be pursued if feasible.
3. It is important to distinguish pNF from cutaneous and subcutaneous neurofibromas that can involve the skin; cNFs have no malignant potential and do not require regular surveillance.
4. Increasingly, medical options are being investigated for both adults and children with pNF but neurofibroma specialty care centers are recommended for these considerations.

CASE 16.2 DIAGNOSIS AND MANAGEMENT OF NF1 ASSOCIATED OPTIC PATHWAY GLIOMA

Case. A 17-month-old girl with NF1 underwent an MRI of brain and spine for evaluation of motor developmental delay. Although no cause for motor delay was found, evaluation of

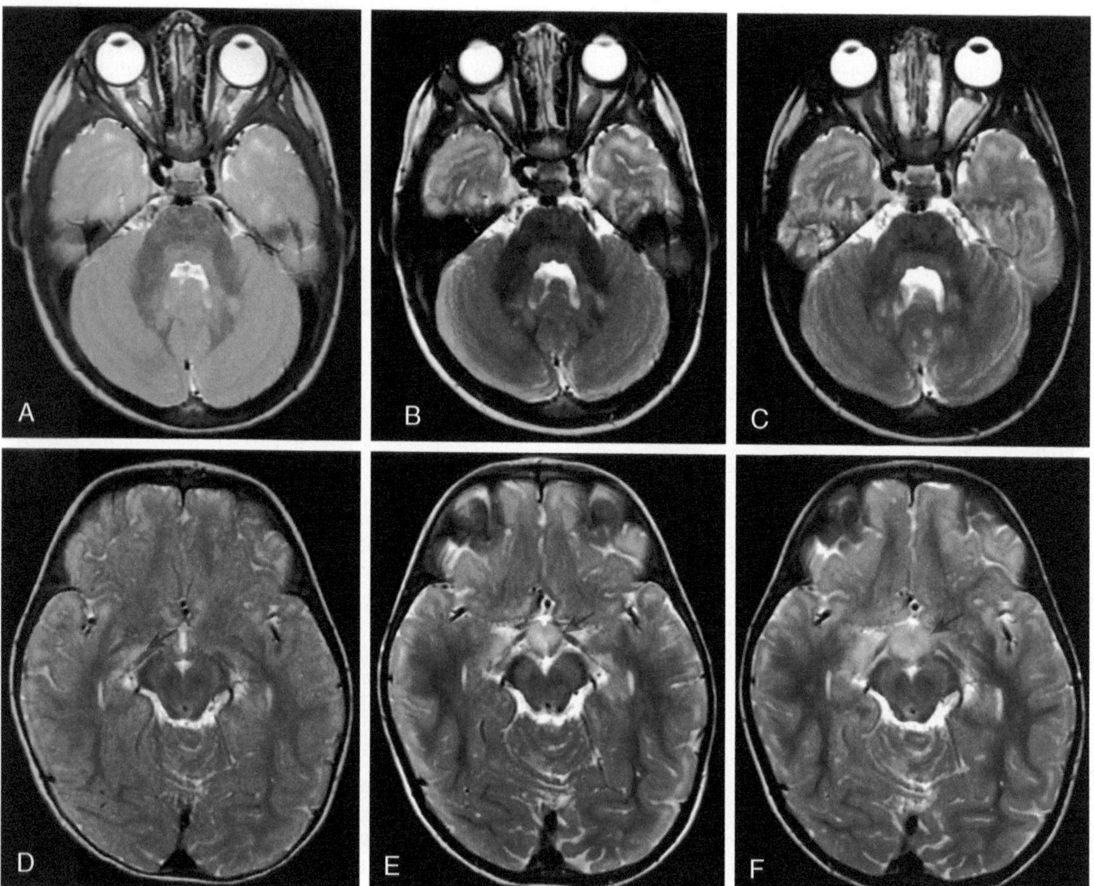

Fig. 16.3 Serial axial T2-weighted MRI sequences of the optic nerves *(top row)* and chiasm/hypothalamus *(bottom row)* in a young girl with NF1 showing progressive enlargement of the optic nerves *(green arrows)*, chiasm, and optic tracts *(orange arrows)* at diagnosis (A, D), 3 months (B, E) and 6 months (C, F).

her orbits showed tortuosity of bilateral optic nerves, asymmetric enlargement of the intraorbital optic nerves (right greater than left), and bilateral optic tracts along with contrast enhancement in the optic nerves (Fig. 16.3A, D). Laboratory evaluation for endocrinopathy (e.g., thyroid stimulating hormone, free thyroxine, growth hormone evaluation) revealed no abnormalities, and a vision test using Teller Acuity Cards showed normal visual acuity for age (20/94 right eye, 20/130 left eye). No surgeries were performed and no therapies undertaken. Three months later, a repeat MRI showed tumor growth in the left optic nerve and chiasm/hypothalamus (Fig. 16.3B, E) but vision had improved (visual acuity: 20/63 right eye, 20/94 left eye). At the latest follow-up, 6 months from initial examination, the tumor had continued to grow in the left optic nerve and chiasm/hypothalamus (Fig. 16.3C, F) but vision was unaffected (visual acuity: 20/63 right eye, 20/63 left eye). Motor delays improved with physical therapy. Despite tumor growth, she remains unaffected by her tumor and has not started therapy for her OPG, although she remains under close surveillance.

Teaching Points. This case highlights the management options and natural history of OPGs in children with NF1, including the importance of clinical assessment to guide treatment decisions. OPGs are common tumors that threaten vision in NF1. Many of these tumors remain asymptomatic, and routine screening with MRI is not recommended because early identification of tumor does not appear to affect outcomes and may serve only to heighten parental anxiety.[83,84] Instead, annual surveillance with ophthalmology in children with NF1 is important to identify symptomatic OPG.[85] Once they are identified, children with OPG should be followed closely for tumor growth and new symptoms with MRI and ophthalmology evaluations. Careful surveillance with both MRI and vision testing is imperative to reduce the functional impact of these tumors. Decisions to treat are complex and should be undertaken by a team of experts including oncologists and ophthalmologists with expertise in NF1.

Principles of NF1-associated OPG

General description. OPGs are low-grade gliomas (LGGs) that occur in the pre-cortical visual pathway, commonly involving the optic nerves and chiasm and sometimes including the optic tracts and optic radiations (as in this case). OPGs occur in 15–20% of children with NF1 and are the most common brain tumor in children with NF1.[86–88] Most symptomatic tumors are discovered by 6 years of age,[89] but rarely tumors may present in older children and adults.[90] Optic nerve tortuosity is common in children with NF1 and does not necessarily indicate the presence of an OPG, but enlargement and enhancement in the optic pathway should be considered to be a tumor.[91]

Presentation and clinical assessment. Although NF1-associated OPG may cause vision loss, proptosis, and hypothalamic dysfunction, the majority of these tumors remain asymptomatic.[87,93] Tumors are often slow growing and may undergo long periods of quiescence. However, individual tumors may show significant variability in growth rate, and careful surveillance with paired MRI and comprehensive ophthalmology assessment is critical to evaluate the impact of these tumors and determine the need for treatment. Vision testing in young children may be challenging due to age and inattention, but preferential looking tests such as Teller Acuity Cards can be reliably performed in children as young as 6 months of age.[94] As visual acuity improves with age in young children, best-corrected visual acuity should be compared with age-based norms.[95] A decrease in best-corrected visual acuity of two lines or more in one or both eyes is cause for concern and potentially an indication for treatment.[85] Although an increase in tumor dimensions should increase vigilance for vision changes, change in tumor size does not always correlate with changes in visual acuity, as was the case for the patient presented here.[96]

Treatment of OPG in NF1. Chemotherapy is considered first-line therapy for NF1-associated OPG that are symptomatic. Diagnostic biopsy is unnecessary for lesions with characteristic imaging features. Surgical resection is rarely possible without significant visual deficits. Because NF1 is a tumor predisposition syndrome, radiotherapy is rarely used due to concern for second malignancies, as well as cognitive and vascular complications of this therapy.[78,97,98] Carboplatin-based therapies are frequently used as a first-line therapy in NF1-associated OPG. In one multicenter retrospective study of previously untreated children with NF1-associated OPG, carboplatin-based therapy resulted in improved visual acuity in approximately one-third, stable vision in one-third, and progressive vision loss in one-third.[96] Recently developed targeted agents such as MEK inhibitors have demonstrated dramatic responses in NF1-associated tumors, but functional outcomes such as vision are poorly studied.[99,100] A study developed by the Children's Oncology Group (COG) and the European Society for Paediatric Oncology (SIOPE) will compare radiographic and functional outcomes after treatment with carboplatin/vincristine versus selumetinib (a MEK inhibitor) in NF1-associated LGGs.

Treatment indications for NF1-associated OPG are complex and nuanced, and treatment decisions should involve a team of NF1 experts.[85] Although this patient's tumor has grown significantly in the past 6 months, her vision remains stable or improving. A reduction in visual acuity or further tumor growth may prompt treatment, and it is important to follow her MRI and ophthalmology surveillance closely.

Clinical Pearls

1. Optic pathway gliomas are seen in 15–20% of NF1 patients.
2. Vision should be followed with yearly eye examination in all NF1 children and, if vision deficits are observed, MRI imaging and regular ophthalmology examination should be performed to follow patients found to have an OPG.
3. Changes in imaging often do not correlate with changes in vision, and treatment decisions should involve clinicians experienced in NF1.

CASE 16.3 MANAGEMENT OF BRAIN LESIONS IN CHILDREN WITH NF1

Case. A 9-year-old boy with NF1, paraspinal pNF, and associated scoliosis presented with increasing headaches for 2 months. Pain was rated between 3 and 9 out of 10, occasionally radiated to his neck, and was infrequently associated with vomiting. His headaches did not wake him from sleep and were not associated with photophobia or phonophobia. An MRI of the brain demonstrated non-enhancing T2 hyperintense lesions in the globus palladus, bilateral thalami, pons, and midbrain, as well as an enhancing lesion with mass effect in the right middle cerebellar peduncle (Fig. 16.4A, B). Edema surrounding the enhancing cerebellar lesion extended to the superior cerebellar peduncle and superolateral right cerebellar hemisphere. A repeat scan 6 weeks later demonstrated that the cerebellar tumor had increased in size and associated edema, and a subtotal resection of this lesion was performed. Pathology was consistent with pilocytic astrocytoma (WHO grade I) with intravascular thrombosis and chronic inflammation. Because of residual tumor and recent aggressive growth, he was started on carboplatin and vincristine. After 3 months of this regimen, his residual tumor decreased in size, but he developed an allergic reaction to carboplatin, and he was switched to trametinib (a MEK inhibitor). Persistent paronychia that was not responsive to typical care necessitated a dose reduction; however, his residual cerebellar tumor continued to decrease in size. He remains on trametinib currently.

Teaching Points. This case demonstrates the range of neuroimaging findings of the brain that are seen in patients with NF1 including benign focal areas of T2-weighted hyperintensity (Fig. 16.4C, D) and tumors (Fig. 16.4A, B). Children with NF1 are predisposed to brain tumors, especially LGG. It is important to distinguish tumors from areas of T2-weighted hyperintensity commonly seen in children with NF1. Lesions

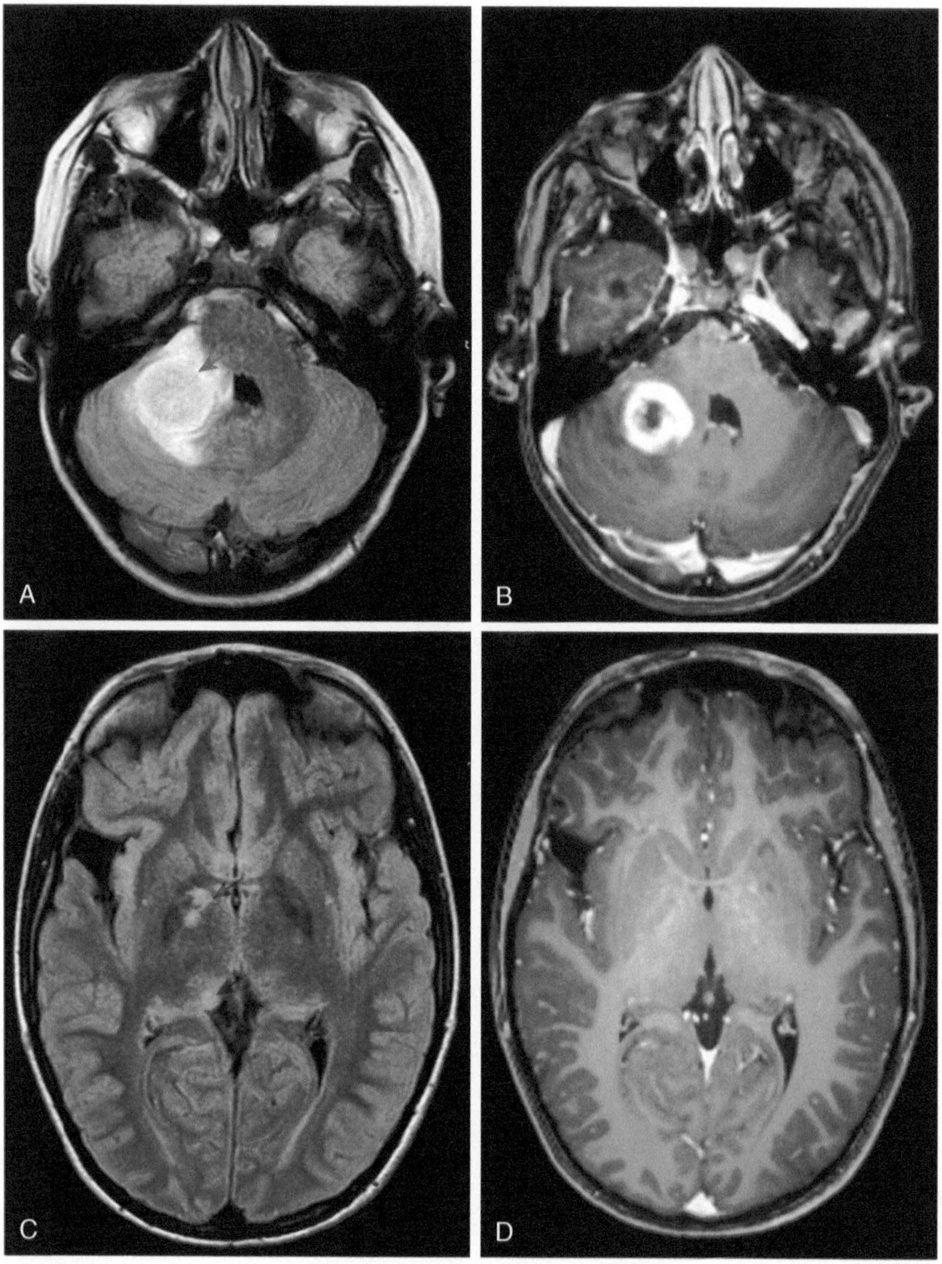

Fig. 16.4 Imaging from a 9-year-old boy with neurofibromatosis 1 and progressive headaches including axial fluid-attenuated inversion recovery MRI imaging (A, C) and post-gadolinium T1-weighted sequences (B, D) showing a cerebellar low-grade glioma "(A, B, *green arrow*)," as well as typical focal areas of signal intensity "(FASI; C, D, *orange arrows*)."

that demonstrate mass effect or enhancement are concerning for tumor and should be followed closely. Many tumors will remain asymptomatic but should be evaluated by an oncologist. Although many NF1-associated LGGs are slow growing, treatment should be considered for tumors that grow or cause symptoms. Chemotherapy regimens used for LGG are frequently more effective in children with NF1 than in sporadic cases, and recent targeted agents such as MEK inhibitors may offer new approaches to the treatment of brain tumors in children with NF1.

Principles of brain lesions in NF1

Focal areas of signal abnormality (FASI). Children with NF1 frequently exhibit areas of non-enhancing T2-weighted signal abnormality on brain MRI that regress with age.[101–103] These focal areas of signal abnormality (FASI), previously referred to as unidentified bright objects[104,105] or spongiotic/spongiform change,[106] may be found throughout the CNS,[107] but are frequently found in the globus pallidus, cerebellum, and midbrain in up to two-thirds of children with NF1.[108] Pathologic characterization of these lesions is uncommon[106] because they are considered benign and largely asymptomatic.[109–111] It is important to distinguish FASI from LGG, which may cause symptoms with continued growth and should be followed with surveillance imaging. Prior studies have distinguished tumor from FASI based on any of three tumor characteristics: contrast enhancement, mass effect on surrounding tissue, or T1-weighted hypointensity relative to gray matter.[103,112]

Low-grade glioma in NF1. NF1 is one of the most common tumor predisposition syndromes, and brain tumors, particularly LGG, are frequently seen in children. The product of the *NF1* gene is a tumor suppressor and negative regulator of RAS activity.[113] A second hit in the mitogen-activated protein (MAP) kinase pathway results in RAS activation and MAP kinase pathway hyperactivation, which is a common feature in most pediatric LGG.[114] Although NF1 and sporadic LGG share a common activated pathway, NF1-associated LGG are more often located in the optic pathway (see prior case) and are frequently less aggressive than their non-NF1 counterparts.[115] Many NF1-associated LGGs may be asymptomatic at presentation and demonstrate minimal or no growth over time. Spontaneous regression of NF1-associated LGG has also been reported.[116]

Management of brain lesions in NF1. Lesions concerning for tumor should be followed by an oncologist familiar with NF1. Asymptomatic lesions identified in the brainstem or optic pathway where biopsy or resection may be challenging are frequently followed by observation alone. Tumors outside the optic pathway that are symptomatic or demonstrate consistent growth merit consideration of biopsy and/or resection. The majority of NF1-associated brain tumors are LGG, but high-grade glioma and other brain tumors may also be seen. For NF1-associated LGG, surgical resection is the mainstay of therapy. Tumors that have been completely or nearly resected often require no further therapy. If tumor progression is seen following resection, adjuvant therapy with or without a second resection is often required. As in NF1-associated OPG (see prior case), radiation is frequently avoided in NF1 due to the risk of late complications such as second malignancy, cognitive deficits, and vasculopathy. Chemotherapy with carboplatin and vincristine has been associated with 5-year progression-free survival of 69% in children with NF1-associated LGG.[115] Recently, a variety of MEK inhibitors have also shown significant tumor response for previously treated NF1-associated LGG. In a recent trial of selumetinib for recurrent/progressive NF1-associated LGG, 40% of pediatric patients demonstrated a sustained reduction in tumor dimensions by at least half.[99] Among 25 patients with progressive NF1-associated LGG, the 2-year progression free survival was 96%. Common side effects include rash, paronychia, and creatine phosphokinase elevation, although surveillance must be performed for other serious complications. It is unclear how long patients should remain on MEK inhibitor therapy and what the long-term complications and outcomes may be. A phase III study is currently investigating MEK inhibitor therapy in children with newly diagnosed NF1-associated LGG.

Clinical Pearls

1. Three imaging characteristics favor that a brain lesion in an NF1 patient is low-grade glioma (LGG) and not a benign focal area of signal abnormality (FASI) including: contrast enhancement, mass effect on surrounding tissue, or T1-weighted hypointensity relative to gray matter.
2. Lesions concerning for tumor should be followed by an oncologist familiar with NF1.
3. For NF1-associated LGG, surgical resection is the mainstay of therapy. Tumors that have been completely or nearly resected often require no further therapy. Subtotally resected or recurrent tumors are treated with chemotherapy or targeted systemic therapies.

CASE 16.4 APPROACH TO MANAGEMENT OF BILATERAL VESTIBULAR SCHWANNOMAS

Case. A 24-year-old woman presents to an otolaryngologist for evaluation after 6 months of progressive tinnitus and new hearing loss. On clinical examination, there was no evidence of deficits outside of word recognition scores (WRS) of 70% on the right and 10% on the left. Based on this, she was referred for MRI Brain, and this showed a complex tumor involving the right skull base (Fig. 16.5A). There were also two additional small lesions in the left frontal and parafalcine region consistent with meningiomas. She was subsequently referred for MRI of the entire spine, which showed a small intramedullary lesion at the intersection of the cervical and thoracic spine consistent with ependymoma, and additional extramedullary, intradural lesions that could be consistent with meningioma or schwannoma (Fig. 16.5B,C). Her examination showed relative hearing loss on the left, intermittent fasciculations in the right face, and slight sensory loss in cranial nerve V2 and V3 on the right, but was otherwise normal. Based on her presentation indicating profound hearing loss on the side of the smaller lesion (left) and functional hearing on the right side, she was recommended for short-interval follow-up with repeat MRI Brain with thin cuts through the internal auditory canals to optimally evaluate the skull base, obtained in a fashion that allowed volumetric analysis and repeat audiometry for WRS. At the time of the follow-up imaging 4 months later, she had volumetric MRI progression of the right complex tumor, but no change in hearing, and the neurologic examination was

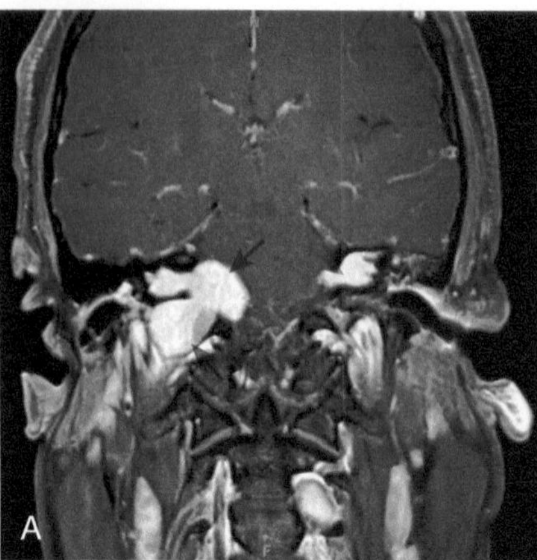

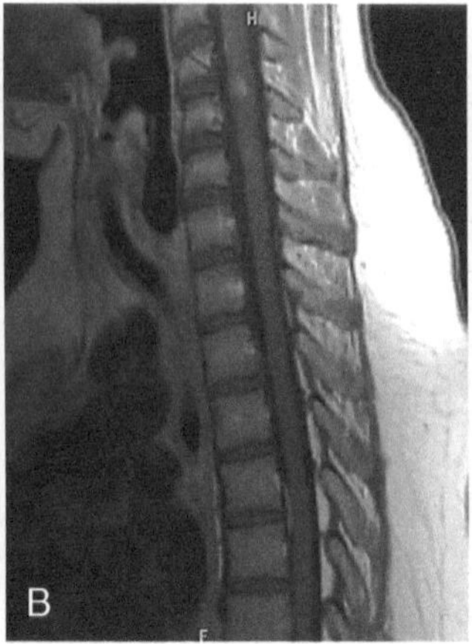

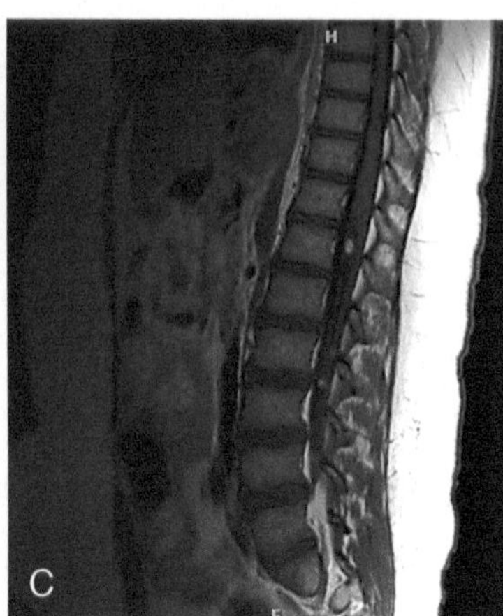

Fig. 16.5 MRI images from a patient with neurofibromatosis 2. (A) Shows coronal T1-weighted gadolinium enhanced MRI Brain with a collision tumor on the right with a presumed vestibular schwannoma *(orange arrow)* and a meningioma *(red arrow)* causing some compression on the brainstem and a more classic vestibular schwannoma on the left *(green arrow)*; (B) sagittal T1-weighted gadolinium enhanced spine MRI shows an enhancing lesion with imaging characteristics consistent with ependymoma *(green arrow)*; and (C) sagittal T1-weighted gadolinium enhanced spine MRI showing an enhancing intradural, extramedullary lesion with imaging features consistent with schwannoma *(green arrow)*.

stable. Monitoring was continued until she had decline in her right WRS to 50%. Based on the persistent increased growth of the complex skull-base tumor on the right, ultimately associated with hearing decline, she was started on bevacizumab 7.5 mg/kg intravenously every 3 weeks. Follow-up MRI and audiometry at 4 months showed improvement in WRS to 75% but no significant improvement in tumor volume. Based on improved hearing, she stayed on bevacizumab and, at 12 months of treatment, she did have a 15% reduction in tumor volume. Bevacizumab had to be withheld for 3 months for severe menorrhagia. Once adequately controlled, bevacizumab was restarted. Hearing benefit was maintained even when off drug for 3 months. Ultimately, the interval between bevacizumab was increased to every 8 weeks in an effort to reduce the risk of proteinuria. There was no increase in size of the skull-based tumors or loss of hearing benefit on serial evaluations with this dosing interval.

Teaching Points. This case highlights a number of important principles of NF2 including (1) new hearing loss in an adult should prompt evaluation with imaging and, if bilateral VS are observed, is sufficient to establish a diagnosis of NF2, (2) the importance of monitoring hearing function and patient symptoms in patients with multiple tumors to guide treatment decisions as tumor size and function are not strongly correlated, and (3) the role of bevacizumab in the management of patients with NF2-associated VS that cause hearing loss.

Principles of VS management in patients with NF2

As stated, NF2 is far rarer than NF1, and hence seen less frequently, but should be considered when a young person presents with hearing loss, a VS at an early age, or whenever there are bilateral VS. Bilateral VS are the most common presentation of NF2. VS cause sensorineural hearing loss, tinnitus, facial nerve palsy, and balance difficulty, but in people with NF2, the bilateral nature of these tumors ultimately causes deafness and possible brainstem compression.[117]

Presentation of NF2. The average onset of symptoms is early 20s and the most common symptoms are hearing loss, tinnitus, imbalance, and multifocal motor neuropathy. Hearing loss in adults is by far the most common initial presentation, but this can be missed for extended periods of time due to variable loss across both ears.[117,118] Furthermore, there is not a direct correlation between tumor size and hearing function. This can result in people coming to diagnosis after they have large tumors as illustrated in this case. Finally, as mentioned above, there is increasing recognition of genotype-phenotype correlations that influence how people with NF2 may present to clinical care.[9] Specifically, people with a truncating exon 2–13 pathogenic variant are more likely to present early in life (<10 years old) and have focal neurologic deficits as their presenting symptoms with a higher tumor burden.[9,119]

Monitoring recommendations in NF2. Monitoring includes MRI of the brain with thin cuts through the internal auditory canal to best investigate the position and size of the VS and whether there are any collision tumors (confluence of tumor from schwannomas and meningiomas), as these are more complicated to treat. This is recommended at least annually; however, if there is any evidence of rapid growth of tumor, shorter interval imaging (between 3–6 months) is warranted depending on symptoms and growth pattern. In addition, audiology with WRS assessment is recommended every 6–12 months depending on the degree and rate of hearing loss.[120] WRS is the best metric to assess the ability to hear and discern speech and therefore is the most accurate assessment for conversational hearing.[121]

Retrospective natural history studies suggest an average growth rate for VS of 1 mm/year.[122] Another natural history study evaluated both the rate of hearing loss and VS growth by volume (with growth defined as >20% in size) and showed that the mean rate of hearing decline as assessed by WRS was 16% decline 3 years from diagnosis with a VS growth rate of 79% at 3 years.[123] Cumulatively, the available data indicate that NF2-associated VS are progressive tumors over time, and will cause progressive hearing loss over time, but that each person and each tumor has its own natural history that must be established to determine the optimal surveillance for that tumor.

Management of VS in NF2. Sporadic VS are one of the most common brain tumors and are treated with either surgical resection or radiation therapy.[124] These two modalities remain the standard of care in the setting of NF2, but with caveats given the multiplicity of tumors that need treatment over time with this condition. Specifically, surgical resection carries the risk of hearing loss, facial nerve weakness, swallowing dysfunction, and brainstem injury.[125] In addition, both surgical resection and radiation therapy have lower rates of efficacy in the setting of NF2 than with sporadic VS.[125] Finally, there are reports that there are both early and late complications of radiation therapy, including an enhanced risk of malignant conversion in people with NF2.[126] Hence, there is an effort to defer radiation therapy for as long as possible more so than surgery in people with NF2. Given the fact that the tumors associated with NF2 continue to grow and that there is a desire to minimize surgery and radiation therapy, there have been great efforts to develop drug therapies to manage NF2 associated VS.[118] To date, the drug that is most effective has been bevacizumab.[127,128] Bevacizumab is an inhibitor of the protein VEGF and has been shown to both improve hearing and reduce VS size in roughly 40% of adults.[127,128] Importantly, the data available indicates that there is a lower rate of response to bevacizumab in children versus adults.[127] Furthermore, there is an increasing risk of side effects such as proteinuria, hypertension, and irregular menstruation with prolonged dosing that may limit dosing.[129] In an effort to reduce the risk of toxicity in people who are having a good response, the dosing interval is increased or the dose reduced.

Clinical Pearls

1. Bilateral vestibular schwannomas (VS) are pathognomonic for NF2 and typically present with hearing loss, tinnitus, balance difficulty, and, rarely, vertigo.
2. NF2 patients should initially be monitored with neuroimaging of suspicious lesions and audiometry at 6-month intervals to establish a trajectory of tumor growth and functional impact.
3. Removal of every tumor in NF2 is frequently not feasible or clinically necessary. Treatment should focus on the preservation of function and maximizing quality of life.
4. Bevacizumab has been studied at multiple dose frequencies and schedules, each showing a hearing improvement rate of around 40–50% and radiographic response rate of 30–50% in NF2 patients.

CASE 16.5 DIAGNOSIS OF SCHWANNOMATOSIS

Case. A 58-year-old man presented with a 1.5-year history of pain in the left lower extremity and progressive weakness. Evaluation for these concerns included MRI of the pelvis and lumbar spine, which revealed multiple lesions in the paraspinal region consistent with nerve sheath tumors. His history was significant for resection of painful right thigh and left upper extremity tumors (5 and 8 years ago, respectively) at which time he was told only that the lesions were "benign." He also reported a family history of father with multiple "benign tumors" removed, but did not have any genetic testing or histologic diagnoses for these tumors. Based on this information, he was given the diagnosis of NF1. Upon presentation to a specialty center, examination revealed one CALM, no skinfold freckling, no bone abnormalities, no Lisch nodules, and a single, 1 cm, mobile, nodular subcutaneous lesion in the right calf with pain on palpation. His neurologic examination was normal with the exception of bilateral lower extremity hyperreflexia. MRI of the brain with thin cuts through the internal auditory canal was without intracranial masses. MRI of the entire spine revealed intradural, extramedullary lesions throughout the cervical, thoracic, and lumbar spine consistent with nerve sheath tumor (Fig. 16.6). Outside pathology samples were requested from his prior two surgeries and revealed diffusely positive for S-100 and negative for desmin, consistent with schwannomas. Based on this pathology, as well as the exam and imaging findings (e.g., absence of clinical findings consistent with NF1 or intracranial lesions to support a diagnosis of NF2), he met the clinical criteria for diagnosis of schwannomatosis, although the specific subtype is not known until molecular testing is performed.

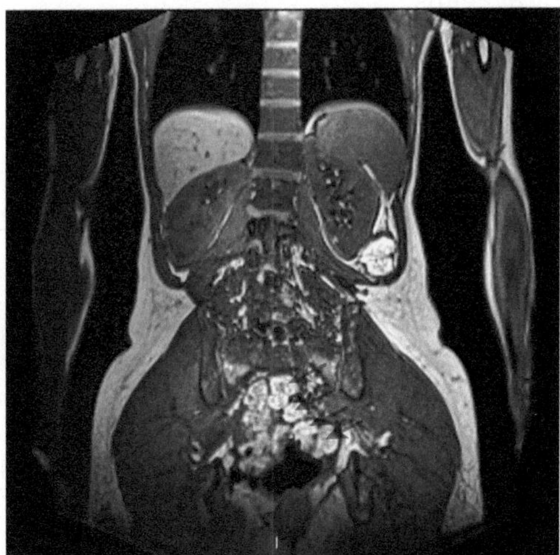

Fig. 16.6 Coronal short T1 inversion recover MRI showing extensive schwannomas throughout the pelvis *(orange arrows)*.

Teaching Points. This case demonstrates a typical presentation and approach to the diagnosis of schwannomatosis. The presence of lesions consistent with nerve sheath tumors should prompt consideration of underlying tumor predisposition syndrome, such as NF1, NF2, and SWN. Although NF1 is the most common of these three conditions, diagnosis can often be made or excluded with proper physical examination, as was the case for this patient. The presence of multiple peripheral nerve schwannomas and no evidence of VS on MRI Brain by the age of 30 years is consistent with SWN.

Clinical evaluation of SWN. Imaging also plays an important role in evaluating suspected schwannomatosis. Schwannomatosis patients should have brain MRI scans with contrast and thin cuts through the internal auditory canal to identify schwannomas and meningiomas.[10] MRI of the entire spine should be performed to identify spinal tumors. MRI of the body should be performed to investigate unexplained neurologic symptoms or pain that could be related to peripheral schwannomas. Pathology is the most helpful and critical for fulfilling the clinical criteria of SWN, but does have limitations.[26] Specifically, schwannoma and neurofibroma can appear similar pathologically, since they are both nerve tumors that are predominantly composed of Schwann cells.[23] Depending on the amount of tissue available, the pathologic interpretation can be incorrect.

Older age at presentation and prominent neuropathic or radiculopathic pain at presentation are most often seen in the setting of SWN and can assist in sorting SWN from NF1 and NF2, but are not official diagnostic criteria, as pain can be a manifestation of all three conditions.[47] Molecular testing is particularly important when feasible for the diagnosis of SWN, as there is considerable overlap in presentation between mosaic NF2 and SWN and there are distinct molecular subtypes of SWN that may have different natural histories and therefore require different management.[47]

Clinical Pearls

1. Genetically, schwannomatosis is characterized by germline pathogenic variants in *SMARCB1* or *LZTR1* genes; additional unidentified genes also likely exist.
2. Tumor formation in schwannomatosis is caused by concomitant mutational inactivation of two genes including the *NF2* gene as well as either *SMARCB1* or *LZTR1*.

CASE 16.6 MANAGEMENT OF PAIN IN ADULTS WITH SCHWANNOMATOSIS

Case. A 36-year-old woman with schwannomatosis of the left upper extremity, with diagnosis based on age (>30 years old), multiple lesions seen on imaging with pathology from two revealing schwannoma, negative family history, and negative MRI of the brain with thin cuts through the internal auditory canal. She developed a painful mass in her left upper extremity in her early teen years that was associated with weakness. The mass was removed, and pathology revealed schwannoma. Pain was improved following surgery. Later imaging revealed multiple nerve sheath tumors throughout the peripheral nervous system tumors; however, they were not always anatomically related to the area in which she experienced the greatest pain. Over the years, she developed multiple additional painful (and not painful) masses. The pain was refractory to multiple therapies including gabapentin, pregabalin, duloxetine, amitriptyline, meloxicam, naproxen, oxycodone, morphine, and tramadol. She was seen by multiple providers before being seen at a specialty center and given the diagnosis of schwannomatosis. She had developed a distrust of the medical system due to repeatedly having her pain symptoms dismissed or being treated as if she were drug seeking. Her pain progressed to the point it was affecting her sleep and making her feel irritable and thus impacting her relationships. The pain was widespread and, therefore, without a clear surgical target. Hence, nonsurgical pain management approaches were maximized. Her best response was with combination of gabapentin and naproxen addressing both neuropathic and inflammatory elements of pain. This approach "took the edge off" and allowed her to sleep; however, she still had significant pain that impacted her ability to exercise and perform activities of daily living. She tried marijuana, which provided some benefit but was not logistically feasible. Physical therapy and occupational therapy helped maintain strength but did not improve pain. She was then evaluated for possible neuromodulation and underwent temporary spinal cord stimulator trial. After a few days, she reported almost complete resolution in pain and was able to return to multiple activities of daily living. She went on to have a permanent, MRI-compatible stimulator implanted (to allow for continued monitoring of tumors). She was able to wean off her nonsteroidal antiinflammatory drug and gabapentin following placement of her stimulator.

Teaching Points. Pain is one of the key features of SWN and the pain can be disproportionate to the size of tumor or even independent of tumor.[11] For example, very tiny tumors can produce severe pain and there can be pain that is tumor independent. Conversely, tumors of all sizes can be clinically silent. Due to this lack of correlation between tumor size and pain experience, patients with schwannomatosis often see many providers before obtaining a diagnosis and can be stigmatized as "drug seeking" when that is not the case.[10] Treatment of pain in schwannomatosis can be difficult and can require multiple modalities. Medications effective at addressing neuropathic pain are often the most effective. In some cases, addressing both neuropathic and inflammatory contributors to pain is effective. Notably, narcotic medications are not often effective and are generally avoided. Unfortunately, often times, multiple medications or combinations of medications are not effective at managing pain. As a result, patients with schwannomatosis-associated chronic pain also often develop sleep disturbance and mood changes related to living with chronic pain and these must also be treated. Continued evaluation of all possible modalities for pain management including devices, clinical trials, and, if a clear correlation between tumor and pain localization can be made, surgery, is necessary to maximize pain control across the lifes pan for people with schwannomatosis.

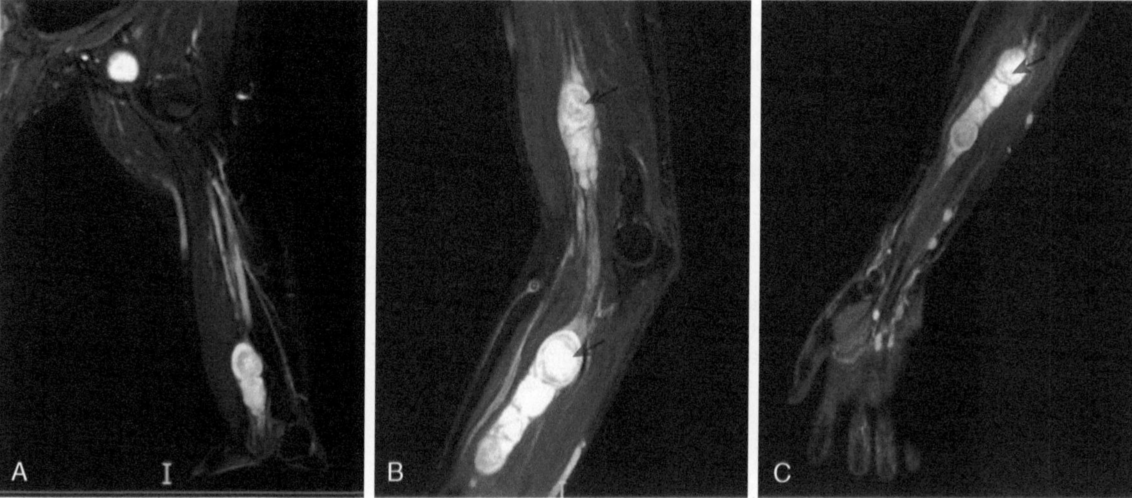

Fig. 16.7 Coronal views of complex, multi-nodular schwannomas involving the left lower extremity and the left forearm *(orange arrows)*. The multifocal lesions seen in panel B demonstrate schwannomas that are unlikely to benefit from surgical resection due to the multifocality.

Principles of schwannomatosis associated pain

Surgical treatment options. Surgery is the gold-standard treatment for painful schwannomas; however, in schwannomatosis, patients often have many solitary or plexiform tumors (Fig. 16.7 A–C) that can be contributing to symptoms. Thus, there is not a single surgical target, and removal of all tumors would produce severe neurologic deficits.[130] Hence, although surgical resection of schwannomas may relieve pain, it is not always advisable depending on the type and localization of pain and the features of the schwannoma.

Nonsurgical treatment options. Nonsurgical management often includes medications for neuropathic pain medications as well as antiinflammatory medications, but very rarely opioid-based medications.[10] Often, combinations of medications work better than single agents and, in some situations, consideration of off-label medication is also appropriate. Complementary alternative medicine therapies can also be therapeutic and provide additional benefits in pain, sleep, and mood. Specifically, physical and occupational therapy, yoga, mindfulness, tai chi, biofeedback, scrambler therapy, and acupuncture have demonstrated improvement in neuropathy, chronic musculoskeletal pain, sleep, and mood symptoms. Neuromodulation via devices can also be considered, especially in patients with symptoms in specific nerve distributions and the development of MRI-compatible devices allows for both tumor surveillance and pain control.

Clinical Pearls

1. The most common symptom reported by patients with schwannomatosis is chronic pain, which is reported in over 65% of patients.
2. Management of chronic pain is challenging as no class of pain medication has been associated with consistent benefit.
3. Referral to pain specialists for comprehensive management may be helpful, and management of concomitant anxiety and depression is strongly recommended.

Conclusion

Hereditary nervous system tumor syndromes are uncommon but important causes of tumors of the central and peripheral nervous system. NF1, NF2, and SWN are among the most commonly encountered and clinically relevant of these syndromes for clinical providers. Over the past decade, major therapeutic advances have, for the first time, provided systemic treatment options for patients with NF2. Emerging, targeted therapies are likely to become available for patients with NF1. Given that each of these conditions is characterized by a unique constellation of clinical symptoms that are used to establish the diagnosis and monitored serially, neurologists should be familiar with these conditions, recommendations for surveillance imaging, indications for treatment, and therapeutic options.

Table 16.1 Current diagnostic criteria and common clinical features of NF1, NF2, and Schwannomatosis

	NF1	NF2	SWN
Diagnostic criteria	At least two of the following: 1) >6 café au lait macules 2) >2 solitary neurofibromas or 1 plexiform neurofibroma 3) Axillary or inguinal freckling 4) Optic pathway glioma 5) >2 Lisch nodules 6) A distinctive bony abnormality such as sphenoid dysplasia, pseudarthrosis, or thinning of the long bone cortex 7) A first-degree relative (FDR) with NF1	Main criteria: 1) Bilateral vestibular schwannomas (VS) OR 2) FDR with NF2 and a. Unilateral VS *or* b. any two other tumors typically associated with NF2 Additional criteria: 3) Unilateral VS and any two other tumors typically associated with NF2 OR 4) ≥2 meningiomas and a. Unilateral VS or b. Any two other tumors typically associated with NF2	Molecular diagnosis: 1) >2 pathologically proved schwannomas or meningiomas AND genetic studies 2) One pathologically proved schwannoma or meningioma AND germline *SMARCB1* pathogenic mutation Clinical diagnosis: 1) ≥2 non-intradermal schwannomas, one with pathologic confirmation, and no bilateral VS 2) One pathologically confirmed schwannoma or intracranial meningioma AND affected FDR 3) Possible SWN: >2 non-intradermal tumors without pathology Exclusion criteria: 1) Fulfill diagnostic criteria for NF2 (FDR with NF2 or germline NF2 mutation) 2) Schwannomas only in previous field of radiation therapy
Most common tumor	Neurofibroma (cutaneous, nodular or plexiform)	Bilateral VS	Multiple peripheral schwannomas
Central nervous system tumors	• Optic pathway glioma • Astrocytoma (pilocytic, anaplastic astrocytoma, glioblastoma)	• Intracranial and paraspinal meningioma • Cranial nerve schwannoma • Spinal ependymoma	• Meningioma • Cranial nerve schwannoma including unilateral VS
Other tumors and cancers	• Malignant peripheral nerve sheath tumor (MPNST) • Gastrointestinal stromal tumor • Pheochromocytoma • Glomus tumors • Neuroendocrine tumor • Rhabdomyosarcoma • Breast cancer • Juvenile myelomonocytic leukemia • Non-ossifying fibroma	• Peripheral nerve schwannoma	• Possible malignancies, incidence not known
Common Symptoms	• Pain • Disfigurement due to cutaneous and plexiform neurofibromas • Cognitive difficulties • Gastrointestinal complaints • Itching	• Hearing loss • Vision loss or alteration • Facial wezakness • Swallowing and speech difficulty • Elevated intracranial pressure • Myelopathy • Pain • Multifocal motor and sensory neuropathy • Tumor associated seizures	• Pain (often severe, chronic, multifocal) • Sensory and motor neuropathy

NF, Neurofibromatosis, *SWN*, schwannomatosis.

References

1. Evans DG, Howard E, Giblin C, et al. Birth incidence and prevalence of tumor-prone syndromes: estimates from a UK family genetic register service. *Am J Med Genet.* 2010;152A(2):327–332.
2. Kallionpaa RA, Uusitalo E, Leppavirta J, Pöyhönen M, Peltonen S, Peltonen J. Prevalence of neurofibromatosis type 1 in the Finnish population. *Genet Med.* 2018;20(9):1082–1086.
3. Uusitalo E, Leppävirta J, Koffert A, et al. Incidence and mortality of neurofibromatosis: a total population study in Finland. *J Invest Dermatol.* 2015;135(3):904–906.
4. Peltonen S, Kallionpää RA, Rantanen M, et al. Pediatric malignancies in neurofibromatosis type 1: a population-based cohort study. *Int J Cancer.* 2019;145(11):2926–2932.
5. Uusitalo E, Rantanen M, Kallionpää RA, et al. Distinctive cancer associations in patients with neurofibromatosis type 1. *J Clin Oncol.* 2016;34(17):1978–1986.
6. Ly KI, Blakeley JO. The diagnosis and management of neurofibromatosis type 1. *Med Clin North Am.* 2019;103(6):1035–1054.
7. Ortonne N, Wolkenstein P, Blakeley JO, et al. Cutaneous neurofibromas: current clinical and pathologic issues. *Neurology.* 2018;91(2 suppl 1):S5–S13.
8. Zvulunov A, Barak Y, Metzker A. Juvenile xanthogranuloma, neurofibromatosis and juvenile chronic myelogenous leukemia. World statistical analysis. *Arch Dermatol.* 1995;131:904–908.
9. Halliday D, Emmanouil B, Vassallo G, et al. Trends in phenotype in the English paediatric neurofibromatosis type 2 cohort stratified by genetic severity. *Clin Genet.* 2019;96(2):151–162.
10. Merker VL, Esparza S, Smith MJ, Stemmer-Rachamimov A, Plotkin SR. Clinical features of schwannomatosis: a retrospective analysis of 87 patients. *Oncol.* 2012;17(10):1317–1322. https://doi.org/10.1634/theoncologist.2012-0162.
11. Evans DG, Bowers NL, Tobi S, et al. Schwannomatosis: a genetic and epidemiological study. *J Neurol Neurosurg Psychiatry.* 2018;89(11):1215–1219.
12. Messiaen LM, Callens T, Mortier G, et al. Exhaustive mutation analysis of the NF1 gene allows identification of 95% of mutations and reveals a high frequency of unusual splicing defects. *Hum Mutat.* 2000;15(6):541–555.
13. Skuse GR, Kosciolek BA, Rowley PT. Molecular genetic analysis of tumors in von Recklinghausen neurofibromatosis: loss of heterozygosity for chromosome 17. *Genes Chromosomes Cancer.* 1989;1(1):36–41.
14. Weiss B, Bollag G, Shannon K. Hyperactive Ras as a therapeutic target in neurofibromatosis type 1. *Am J Med Genet.* 1999;89(1):14–22.
15. Smith MJ, Isidor B, Beetz C, et al. Mutations in LZTR1 add to the complex heterogeneity of schwannomatosis. *Neurology.* 2015;84(2):141–147.
16. Piotrowski A, Xie J, Liu YF, et al. Germline loss-of-function mutations in LZTR1 predispose to an inherited disorder of multiple schwannomas. *Nat Genet.* 2014;46(2):182–187. https://doi.org/10.1038/ng.2855.
17. Hulsebos TJ, Plomp AS, Wolterman RA, Robanus-Maandag EC, Baas F, Wesseling P. Germline mutation of INI1/SMARCB1 in familial schwannomatosis. *Am J Hum Genet.* 2007;80(4):805–810.
18. Hutter S, Piro RM, Reuss DE, et al. Whole exome sequencing reveals that the majority of schwannomatosis cases remain unexplained after excluding SMARCB1 and LZTR1 germline variants. *Acta Neuropathol.* 2014;128(3):449–452.
19. van den Munckhof P, Christiaans I, Kenter SB, Baas F, Hulsebos TJ. Germline SMARCB1 mutation predisposes to multiple meningiomas and schwannomas with preferential location of cranial meningiomas at the falx cerebri. *Neurogenetics.* 2012;13(1):1–7.
20. Hulsebos TJ, Kenter SB, Jakobs ME, Baas F, Chong B, Delatycki MB. SMARCB1/INI1 maternal germ line mosaicism in schwannomatosis. *Clin Genet.* 2010;77(1):86–91.
21. Kehrer-Sawatzki H, Kluwe L, Friedrich RE, et al. Phenotypic and genotypic overlap between mosaic NF2 and schwannomatosis in patients with multiple non-intradermal schwannomas. *Hum Genet.* 2018;137(6–7):543–552.
22. Smith MJ, Bowers NL, Bulman M, et al. Revisiting neurofibromatosis type 2 diagnostic criteria to exclude LZTR1-related schwannomatosis. *Neurology.* 2017;88(1):87–92.
23. Sestini R, Bacci C, Provenzano A, Genuardi M, Papi L. Evidence of a four-hit mechanism involving SMARCB1 and NF2 in schwannomatosis-associated schwannomas. *Hum Mutat.* 2008;29(2):227–231.
24. Halliday D, Parry A, Evans DG. Neurofibromatosis type 2 and related disorders. *Curr Opin Oncol.* 2019;31(6):562–567.
25. Smith MJ, Wallace AJ, Bowers NL, et al. Frequency of SMARCB1 mutations in familial and sporadic schwannomatosis. *Neurogenetics.* 2012;13(2):141–145.
26. Hadfield KD, Newman WG, Bowers NL, et al. Molecular characterisation of SMARCB1 and NF2 in familial and sporadic schwannomatosis. *J Med Genet.* 2008;45(6):332–339.
27. Scheffzek K, Welti S. Neurofibromin: protein domains and functional characteristics. In: Upadhyaya M, Cooper D, eds. *Neurofibromatosis Type 1.* Berlin, Heidelberg: Springer; 2012:305326. 2012.
28. Li Y, O'Connell P, Breidenbach HH, et al. Genomic organization of the neurofibromatosis 1 gene (NF1). *Genomics.* 1995;25:9–18.
29. Upadhyaya M, Cooper DN, eds. *Neurofibromatosis Type 1: Molecular and Cellular Biology.* Berlin, Heidelberg: Springer; 2012.
30. Le LQ, Parada LF. Tumor microenvironment and neurofibromatosis type I: connecting the GAPs. *Oncogene.* 2007;26:4609–4616.
31. Warrington NM, Gianino SM, Jackson E, et al. Cyclic AMP suppression is sufficient to induce gliomagenesis in a mouse model of neurofibromatosis-1. *Cancer Res.* 2010;70:5717–5727.
32. Ferner RE, Huson SM, Thomas N, et al. Guidelines for the diagnosis and management of individuals with neurofibromatosis 1. *J Med Genet.* 2007;44:81–88.
33. McGaughran JM, Harris DI, Donnai D, et al. A clinical study of type 1 neurofibromatosis in North West England. *J Med Genet.* 1999;36:197–203.
34. Evans DG, Baser ME, McGaughran J, Sharif S, Howard E, Moran A. Malignant peripheral nerve sheath tumours in neurofibromatosis. *J Med Genet.* 2002;39:311–314.
35. Huson SM, Harper PS, Compston DA. Von Recklinghausen neurofibromatosis. A clinical and population study in South-East Wales. *Brain.* 1988;111(Pt 6):1355–1381.

36. Wang X, Teer JK, Tousignant RN, et al. Breast cancer risk and germline genomic profiling of women with neurofibromatosis type 1 who developed breast cancer. Genes Chromosomes Cancer. 2018;57(1):19–27 .doi:10.1002/gcc.22503.
37. Miller DT, Freedenberg D, Schorry E, et al. Health supervision for children with neurofibromatosis type 1. *Pediatrics*. 2019;143(5):e20190660.
38. Stewart DR, Korf BR, Nathanson KL, Stevenson DA, Yohay K. Care of adults with neurofibromatosis type 1: a clinical practice resource of the American College of Medical Genetics and Genomics (ACMG). *Genet Med*. 2018;20(7):671–682.
39. Trofatter JA, MacCollin MM, Rutter JL, et al. A novel moesin-, ezrin-, radixin-like gene is a candidate for the neurofibromatosis 2 tumor suppressor. *Cell*. 1993;75(4):826.
40. Evans DG, Freeman S, Gokhale C, et al. Bilateral vestibular schwannomas in older patients: NF2 or chance? *J Med Genet*. 2015;52(6):422–424.
41. Bokstein F, Dubov T, Toledano-Alhadef H, et al. Cranial irradiation in childhood mimicking neurofibromatosis type II. *Am J Med Genet*. 2017;173(6):1635–1639.
42. Evans DG, Stivaros SM. Multifocality in neurofibromatosis type 2. *Neuro Oncol*. 2015;17(4):481–482.
43. Hexter A, Jones A, Joe H, et al. Clinical and molecular predictors of mortality in neurofibromatosis 2: a UK national analysis of 1192 patients. *J Med Genet*. 2015;52(10):699–705.
44. Baser ME, Friedman JM, Aeschliman D, et al. Predictors of the risk of mortality in neurofibromatosis 2. *Am J Hum Genet*. 2002;71:715–723.
45. MacCollin M, Chiocca EA, Evans DG, et al. Diagnostic criteria for schwannomatosis. *Neurology*. 2005;64(11):1838–1845.
46. MacCollin M, Willett C, Heinrich B, et al. Familial schwannomatosis: exclusion of the NF2 locus as the germline event. *Neurology*. 2003;60(12):1968–1974.
47. Plotkin SR, Blakeley JO, Evans DG, et al. Update from the 2011 International schwannomatosis Workshop: from genetics to diagnostic criteria. *Am J Med Genet*. 2013;161A(3):405–416.
48. Smith MJ, Kulkarni A, Rustad C, et al. Vestibular schwannomas occur in schwannomatosis and should not be considered an exclusion criterion for clinical diagnosis. *Am J Med Genet*. 2012;158A(1):215–219.
49. Evans DG, Hartley CL, Smith PT, et al. Incidence of mosaicism in 1055 de novo NF2 cases: much higher than previous estimates with high utility of next-generation sequencing. *Genet Med*. 2020;22:53–59.
50. Merker VL, Bergner AL, Vranceanu AM, Muzikansky A, Slattery III W, Plotkin SR. Health-related quality of life of individuals with neurofibromatosis type 2: results from the NF2 natural history study. *Otol Neurotol*. 2016;37(5):574–579.
51. Knudson Jr AG. Mutation and cancer: statistical study of retinoblastoma. *Proc Natl Acad Sci U S A*. 1971;68(4):820–823.
52. Ferner RE, Golding JF, Smith M, et al. [18F]2-fluoro-2-deoxy-D-glucose positron emission tomography (FDG PET) as a diagnostic tool for neurofibromatosis 1 (NF1) associated malignant peripheral nerve sheath tumours (MPNSTs): a long-term clinical study. *Ann Oncol*. 2008;19(2):390–394.
53. Ahlawat S, Blakeley JO, Langmead S, Belzberg AJ, Fayad LM. Current status and recommendations for imaging in neurofibromatosis type 1, neurofibromatosis type 2, and schwannomatosis. *Skeletal Radiol*. 2020;49(2):199–219.
54. Ahlawat S, Blakeley JO, Rodriguez FJ, Fayad LM. Imaging biomarkers for malignant peripheral nerve sheath tumors in neurofibromatosis type 1. *Neurology*. 2019;93(11):e1076–e1084.
55. Ahlawat S, Fayad LM, Khan MS, et al. Current whole-body MRI applications in the neurofibromatoses: NF1, NF2, and schwannomatosis. *Neurology*. 2016;87(7 suppl 1):S31–S39.
56. Nguyen R, Dombi E, Widemann BC, et al. Growth dynamics of plexiform neurofibromas: a retrospective cohort study of 201 patients with neurofibromatosis 1. *Orphanet J Rare Dis*. 2012;7:75.
57. Plotkin SR, Bredella MA, Cai W, et al. Quantitative assessment of whole-body tumor burden in adult patients with neurofibromatosis. *PloS One*. 2012;7(4):e35711.
58. Mautner VF, Hartmann M, Kluwe L, Friedrich RE, Fünsterer C. MRI growth patterns of plexiform neurofibromas in patients with neurofibromatosis type 1. *Neuroradiology*. 2006;48(3):160–165.
59. Gross AM, Singh G, Akshintala S, et al. Association of plexiform neurofibroma volume changes and development of clinical morbidities in neurofibromatosis 1. *Neuro Oncol*. 2018;20(12):1643–1651.
60. Farid M, Demicco EG, Garcia R, et al. Malignant peripheral nerve sheath tumors. *Oncol*. 2014;19(2):193–201.
61. Nguyen R, Jett K, Harris GJ, Cai W, Friedman JM, Mautner VF. Benign whole body tumor volume is a risk factor for malignant peripheral nerve sheath tumors in neurofibromatosis type 1. *J Neuro Oncol*. 2014;116(2):307–313.
62. Tucker T, Wolkenstein P, Revuz J, Zeller J, Friedman JM. Association between benign and malignant peripheral nerve sheath tumors in NF1. *Neurology*. 2005;65(2):205–211.
63. King AA, Debaun MR, Riccardi VM, Gutmann DH. Malignant peripheral nerve sheath tumors in neurofibromatosis 1. *Am J Med Genet*. 2000;93(5):388–392.
64. Kim A, Gillespie A, Dombi E, et al. Characteristics of children enrolled in treatment trials for NF1-related plexiform neurofibromas. *Neurology*. 2009;73(16):1273–1279.
65. Prada CE, Rangwala FA, Martin LJ, et al. Pediatric plexiform neurofibromas: impact on morbidity and mortality in neurofibromatosis type 1. *J Pediatr*. 2012;160(3):461–467.
66. Wolters PL, Burns KM, Martin S, et al. Pain interference in youth with neurofibromatosis type 1 and plexiform neurofibromas and relation to disease severity, social-emotional functioning, and quality of life. *Am J Med Genet*. 2015;167A(9):2103–2113.
67. Allen TM, Struemph KL, Toledo-Tamula MA, et al. The relationship between heart rate variability, psychological flexibility, and pain in neurofibromatosis Type 1. *Pain Pract*. 2018;18(8):969–978.
68. Beert E, Brems H, Daniels B, et al. Atypical neurofibromas in neurofibromatosis type 1 are premalignant tumors. *Genes Chromosomes Cancer*. 2011;50(12):1021–1032.
69. Miettinen MM, Antonescu CR, Fletcher CDM, et al. Histopathologic evaluation of atypical neurofibromatous tumors and their transformation into malignant peripheral nerve sheath tumor in patients with neurofibromatosis 1: a consensus overview. *Hum Pathol*. 2017;67:1–10.
70. Carrió M, Gel B, Terribas E, et al. Analysis of intratumor heterogeneity in neurofibromatosis type 1 plexiform neurofibromas and neurofibromas with atypical features: correlating histological and genomic findings. *Hum Mutat*. 2018;39(8):1112–1125.
71. Higham CS, Dombi E, Rogiers A, et al. The characteristics of 76 atypical neurofibromas as precursors to neurofibromatosis 1 associated malignant peripheral nerve sheath tumors. *Neuro Oncol*. 2018;20(6):818–825.

72. Nelson CN, Dombi E, Rosenblum JS, et al. Safe marginal resection of atypical neurofibromas in neurofibromatosis type 1. *J Neurosurg.* 2019:1–11.
73. Meany H, Dombi E, Reynolds J, et al. 18-fluorodeoxyglucose-positron emission tomography (FDG-PET) evaluation of nodular lesions in patients with neurofibromatosis type 1 and plexiform neurofibromas (PN) or malignant peripheral nerve sheath tumors (MPNST). *Pediatr Blood Cancer.* 2013;60(1):59–64.
74. Guiraud M, Bouroubi A, Beauchamp R, et al. Cutaneous neurofibromas: patients' medical burden, current management and therapeutic expectations: results from an online European patient community survey. *Orphanet J Rare Dis.* 2019;14(1):286.
75. Brosseau JP, Pichard DC, Legius EH, et al. The biology of cutaneous neurofibromas: consensus recommendations for setting research priorities. *Neurology.* 2018;91(2 suppl 1):S14–S20.
76. Slopis JM, Arevalo O, Bell CS, et al. Treatment of disfiguring cutaneous lesions in neurofibromatosis-1 with everolimus: a phase II, open-label, single-arm trial. *Drugs R.* 2018;18(4):295–302.
77. Blakeley JO, Wolkenstein P, Widemann BC, et al. Creating a comprehensive research strategy for cutaneous neurofibromas. *Neurology.* 2018;91(2 suppl 1):S1–S4.
78. Bhatia S, Chen Y, Wong FL, et al. Subsequent neoplasms after a primary tumor in individuals with neurofibromatosis type 1. *J Clin Oncol.* 2019;37(32):3050–3058.
79. Maertens O, McCurrach ME, Braun BS, et al. A collaborative model for accelerating the discovery and translation of cancer therapies. *Cancer Res.* 2017;77(21):5706–5711.
80. Dombi E, Baldwin A, Marcus LJ, et al. Activity of selumetinib in neurofibromatosis type 1-related plexiform neurofibromas. *N Engl J Med.* 2016;375(26):2550–2560.
81. Tyagi P, Santiago C. New features in MEK retinopathy. *BMC Ophthalmol.* 2018;18(suppl 1):221.
82. Livingstone E, Zimmer L, Vaubel J, Schadendorf D. BRAF, MEK and KIT inhibitors for melanoma: adverse events and their management. *Chin Clin Oncol.* 2014;3(3):29.
83. Listernick R, Charrow J. Knowledge without truth: screening for complications of neurofibromatosis type 1 in childhood. *Am J Med Genet.* 2004;127A(3):221–223.
84. Trevisson E, Cassina M, Opocher E, et al. Natural history of optic pathway gliomas in a cohort of unselected patients affected by neurofibromatosis 1. *J Neuro Oncol.* 2017;134(2):279–287.
85. de Blank PMK, Fisher MJ, Liu GT, et al. Optic pathway gliomas in neurofibromatosis type 1: an update: surveillance, treatment indications, and biomarkers of vision. *J Neuro Ophthalmol.* 2017;37(suppl 1):S23–S32.
86. Blanchard G, Lafforgue MP, Lion-Francois L, et al. Systematic MRI in NF1 children under six years of age for the diagnosis of optic pathway gliomas. Study and outcome of a French cohort. *Eur J Paediatr Neurol.* 2016;20(2):275–281.
87. Prada CE, Hufnagel RB, Hummel TR, et al. The use of magnetic resonance imaging screening for optic pathway gliomas in children with neurofibromatosis type 1. *J Pediatr.* 2015;167(4):851–856. e851.
88. Albers AC, Gutmann DH. Gliomas in patients with neurofibromatosis type 1. *Expert Rev Neurother.* 2009;9(4):535–539.
89. Listernick R, Charrow J, Greenwald M, Mets M. Natural history of optic pathway tumors in children with neurofibromatosis type 1: a longitudinal study. *J Pediatr.* 1994;125:63–66.
90. Listernick R, Ferner RE, Piersall L, Sharif S, Gutmann DH, Charrow J. Late-onset optic pathway tumors in children with neurofibromatosis 1. *Neurology.* 2004;63(10):1944–1946.
91. Levin MH, Armstrong GT, Broad JH, et al. Risk of optic pathway glioma in children with neurofibromatosis type 1 and optic nerve tortuosity or nerve sheath thickening. *Br J Ophthalmol.* 2016;100(4):510–514.
92. Azizi AA, Walker DA, Liu JF, et al. NF1 optic pathway glioma. Analysing risk factors for visual outcome and indications to treat [published online ahead of print, 2020 Jul 6]. Neuro Oncol. 2020;noaa153. doi:10.1093/neuonc/noaa153.
93. Balcer LJ, Liu GT, Heller G, et al. Visual loss in children with neurofibromatosis type 1 and optic pathway gliomas: relation to tumor location by magnetic resonance imaging. *Am J Ophthalmol.* 2001;131:442–445.
94. Fisher MJ, Avery RA, Allen JC, et al. Functional outcome measures for NF1-associated optic pathway glioma clinical trials. *Neurology.* 2013;81(21 suppl 1):S15–S24.
95. Avery RA, Ferner RE, Listernick R, Fisher MJ, Gutmann DH, Liu GT. Visual acuity in children with low grade gliomas of the visual pathway: implications for patient care and clinical research. *J Neuro Oncol.* 2012;110(1):1–7.
96. Fisher MJ, Loguidice M, Gutmann DH, et al. Visual outcomes in children with neurofibromatosis type 1-associated optic pathway glioma following chemotherapy: a multicenter retrospective analysis. *Neuro Oncol.* 2012;14(6):790–797.
97. Cappelli C, Grill J, Raquin M, et al. Long-term follow up of 69 patients treated for optic pathway tumours before the chemotherapy era. *Arch Dis Child.* 1998;79(4):334.
98. Ullrich NJ, Robertson R, Kinnamon DD, et al. Moyamoya following cranial irradiation for primary brain tumors in children. *Neurology.* 2007;68(12):932–938.
99. Fangusaro J, Onar-Thomas A, Young Poussaint T, et al. Selumetinib in paediatric patients with BRAF-aberrant or neurofibromatosis type 1-associated recurrent, refractory, or progressive low-grade glioma: a multicentre, phase 2 trial. *Lancet Oncol.* 2019;20(7):1011–1022.
100. de Blank P, Bandopadhayay P, Haas-Kogan D, Fouladi M, Fangusaro J. Management of pediatric low-grade glioma. *Curr Opin Pediatr.* 2019;31(1):21–27.
101. Parmeggiani A, Boiani F, Capponi S, et al. Neuropsychological profile in Italian children with neurofibromatosis type 1 (NF1) and their relationships with neuroradiological data: preliminary results. *Eur J Paediatr Neurol.* 2018;22(5):822–830.
102. Griffith JL, Morris SM, Mahdi J, Goyal MS, Hershey T, Gutmann DH. Increased prevalence of brain tumors classified as T2 hyperintensities in neurofibromatosis 1. *Neurol Clin Pract.* 2018;8(4):283–291.
103. Castillo M, Green C, Kwock L, et al. Proton MR spectroscopy in patients with neurofibromatosis type 1: evaluation of hamartomas and clinical correlation. *AJNR Am J Neuroradiol.* 1995;16(1):141–147.
104. DeBella K, Poskitt K, Szudek J, Friedman JM. Use of "unidentified bright objects" on MRI for diagnosis of neurofibromatosis 1 in children. *Neurology.* 2000;54(8):1646–1651.

105. Friedrich RE, Nuding MA. Optic pathway glioma and cerebral focal abnormal signal intensity in patients with neurofibromatosis type 1: characteristics, treatment choices and follow-up in 134 affected individuals and a brief review of the literature. *Anticancer Res.* 2016;36(8):4095–4121.
106. DiPaolo DP, Zimmerman RA, Rorke LB, Zackai EH, Bilaniuk LT, Yachnis AT. Neurofibromatosis type 1: pathologic substrate of high-signal-intensity foci in the brain. *Radiology.* 1995;195(3):721–724.
107. Ruegger AD, Coleman L, Hansford JR, McLean N, Dabscheck G. Spinal cord hyperintensities in neurofibromatosis type 1: are they the cord equivalent of unidentified bright objects in the brain? *Pediatr Neurol.* 2018;86:63–65.
108. Goldstein SM, Curless RG, Donovan Post MJ, Quencer RM. A new sign of neurofibromatosis on magnetic resonance imaging of children. *Arch Neurol.* 1989;46(11):1222–1224.
109. Goh WH, Khong PL, Leung CS, Wong VC. T2-weighted hyperintensities (unidentified bright objects) in children with neurofibromatosis 1: their impact on cognitive function. *J Child Neurol.* 2004;19(11):853–858.
110. Hyman SL, Gill DS, Shores EA, et al. Natural history of cognitive deficits and their relationship to MRI T2-hyperintensities in NF1. *Neurology.* 2003;60(7):1139–1145.
111. Payne JM, Moharir MD, Webster R, North KN. Brain structure and function in neurofibromatosis type 1: current concepts and future directions. *J Neurol Neurosurg Psychiatry.* 2010;81(3):304–309.
112. Mahdi J, Shah AC, Sato A, et al. A multi-institutional study of brainstem gliomas in children with neurofibromatosis type 1. *Neurology.* 2017;88(16):1584–1589.
113. Dasgupta B, Li W, Perry A, Gutmann DH. Glioma formation in neurofibromatosis 1 reflects preferential activation of K-RAS in astrocytes. *Cancer Res.* 2005;65(1):236–245.
114. Dougherty MJ, Santi M, Brose MS, et al. Activating mutations in BRAF characterize a spectrum of pediatric low-grade gliomas. *Neuro Oncol.* 2010;12(7):621–630.
115. Ater JL, Xia C, Mazewski CM, et al. Nonrandomized comparison of neurofibromatosis type 1 and non-neurofibromatosis type 1 children who received carboplatin and vincristine for progressive low-grade glioma: a report from the Children's Oncology Group. *Cancer.* 2016;122(12):1928–1936.
116. Piccirilli M, Lenzi J, Delfinis C, Trasimeni G, Salvati M, Raco A. Spontaneous regression of optic pathways gliomas in three patients with neurofibromatosis type I and critical review of the literature. *Child's Nerv Syst.* 2006;22(10):1332–1337.
117. Ferner RE, Shaw A, Evans DG, et al. Longitudinal evaluation of quality of life in 288 patients with neurofibromatosis 2. *J Neurol.* 2014;261(5):963–969.
118. Blakeley JO, Plotkin SR. Therapeutic advances for the tumors associated with neurofibromatosis type 1, type 2, and schwannomatosis. *Neuro Oncol.* 2016;18(5):624–638.
119. Halliday D, Emmanouil B, Pretorius P, et al. Genetic severity score predicts clinical phenotype in NF2. *J Med Genet.* 2017;54(10):657–664.
120. Shukla A, Hsu FC, Slobogean B, et al. Association between patient-reported outcomes and objective disease indices in people with NF2. *Neurol Clin Pract.* 2019;9(4):322–329.
121. Huang V, Bergner AL, Halpin C, et al. Improvement in patient-reported hearing after treatment with bevacizumab in people with neurofibromatosis type 2. *Otol Neurotol.* 2018;39(5):632–638.
122. Plotkin SR, Merker VL, Muzikansky A, Barker II FG, Slattery III W. Natural history of vestibular schwannoma growth and hearing decline in newly diagnosed neurofibromatosis type 2 patients. *Otol Neurotol.* 2014;35(1):e50–e56.
123. Peyre M, Goutagny S, Bah A, et al. Conservative management of bilateral vestibular schwannomas in neurofibromatosis type 2 patients: hearing and tumor growth results. *Neurosurgery.* 2013;72(6):907–913. discussion 914, quiz 914.
124. Rowe JG, Radatz MW, Walton L, Hampshire A, Seaman S, Kemeny AA. Gamma knife stereotactic radiosurgery for unilateral acoustic neuromas. *J Neurol Neurosurg Psychiatry.* 2003;74(11):1536–1542.
125. Evans DG, Baser ME, O'Reilly B, et al. Management of the patient and family with neurofibromatosis 2: a consensus conference statement. *Br J Neurosurg.* 2005;19(1):5–12.
126. King AT, Rutherford SA, Hammerbeck-Ward C, et al. High-grade glioma is not a feature of neurofibromatosis type 2 in the unirradiated patient. *Neurosurgery.* 2018;83(2):193–196.
127. Plotkin SR, Duda DG, Muzikansky A, et al. Multicenter, prospective, phase II and biomarker study of high-dose bevacizumab as induction therapy in patients with neurofibromatosis type 2 and progressive vestibular schwannoma. *J Clin Oncol.* 2019;37(35):3446–3454.
128. Blakeley JO, Ye X, Duda DG, et al. Efficacy and biomarker study of bevacizumab for hearing loss resulting from neurofibromatosis type 2-associated vestibular schwannomas. *J Clin Oncol.* 2016;34(14):1669–1675.
129. Slusarz KM, Merker VL, Muzikansky A, Francis SA, Plotkin SR. Long-term toxicity of bevacizumab therapy in neurofibromatosis 2 patients. *Cancer Chemother Pharmacol.* 2014;73(6):1197–1204.
130. Li P, Zhao F, Zhang J, et al. Clinical features of spinal schwannomas in 65 patients with schwannomatosis compared with 831 with solitary schwannomas and 102 with neurofibromatosis type 2: a retrospective study at a single institution. *J Neurosurg Spine.* 2016;24(1):145–154.

Chapter 17

Approach to the patient with tuberous sclerosis

Mary Silvia and Roy E. Strowd, III

CHAPTER OUTLINE

Introduction

Tuberous sclerosis complex (TSC) is an autosomal dominant neurocutaneous condition characterized by a predisposition to hamartomas in the brain, heart, kidney, skin, eye, and other organs. TSC is the second most common neurogenetic tumor syndrome affecting approximately 1 in 5500 to 10,000 live births, making it less common than neurofibromatosis (NF) 1 but more common than NF2.[1–5] There is no racial, ethnic, or sex predilection.[6,7] Neurologic and neurooncologic manifestations feature prominently. The majority of patients experience seizures, many have refractory epilepsy, and neuroimaging reveals cortical tubers which are the hallmark of the disease along with subependymal nodules and, in some cases, subependymal giant cell astrocytomas (SEGAs). Any organ can be affected with common extranervous system manifestations including renal angiomyolipomas (AMLs), pulmonary lymphangioleiomyomatosis (LAM), cardiac rhabdomyomas, facial angiofibromas, and neurocognitive or neuropsychiatric symptoms (e.g., TSC-associated neuropsychiatric disorder, TAND).

Genetics

TSC is a genetic syndrome that results from mutation in one of two TSC tumor suppressor genes, *TSC1* or *TSC2*. Much of the genetic principles underlying other tumor suppressor syndromes reviewed in prior chapters (e.g., NF1 and NF2) also apply to TSC. Inheritance follows an autosomal dominant pattern; however, *de novo* mutations occur in up to 70% of patients, meaning that these affected individuals harbor a new germline mutation without a prior family history.[8] *TSC1* encodes the protein hamartin which is located on chromosome 9q34.[9] *TSC2* encodes the protein tubulin on chromosome 16p13.[10] Original estimates suggested an equal prevalence of *TSC1* and *TSC2*[9]; however, recent reports suggest that this may only be true for familial inherited cases. There is complete penetrance, meaning that all patients with a TSC genotype will express phenotypic manifestations. There is variable expressivity, meaning that symptoms vary from individual to individual and the severity of disease in one family member cannot be used to predict disease burden in another.

Pathophysiology

TSC is a tumor suppressor syndrome that results from abnormal signaling within the mammalian target of rapamycin (mTOR) pathway. In the cell, hamartin and tuberin heterodimerize and act as a tumor suppressor GTPase of Rheb.[11–20] Dephosphorylation of Rheb-GTP to Rheb-GDP inhibits the activation of mTOR complex 1 (mTORC1) and may also independently inactivate mTORC2. The end result is reduced mTORC activity. In the diseased state, loss of hamartin-tuberin function leads to increased mTORC activity, which promotes cell proliferation, growth, and hamartoma formation.[12] Like most other tumor suppressor syndromes, tumors form according to Knudson's two-hit hypothesis. An inactivating germline mutation causes a "first hit," which increases susceptibility to a "second" somatic loss of heterozygosity, which results in tumor formation and many of the major manifestations of this syndrome (Table 17.1). In addition, one functioning TSC allele is, in many cases, insufficient to maintain normal cell function, a process termed *haploinsufficiency*, and may contribute to many of the minor manifestations of the disease.

Like NF1 and NF2, which were reviewed in the previous chapter, the diagnosis of TSC is made by clinical criteria that have been established by consensus conference. In this chapter, we first review the clinical criteria that are most frequently used to establish a diagnosis of TSC for pediatric and adult patients (Cases 17.1 and 17.2). The following cases review common neurological manifestations including seizures and neuroimaging findings (Cases 17.3 and 17.4). The last case reviews the diagnosis and management of the renal AMLs (Case 17.5). This is followed by a general discussion of other common manifestations and a discussion of clinically relevant take-home points for TSC patients undergoing targeted therapy with mTOR inhibition.

Clinical cases

CASE 17.1 DIAGNOSING TSC IN A PEDIATRIC PATIENT

Case. A patient is referred after a prenatal diagnosis of TSC based on the presence of cardiac rhabdomyomas and postnatal MRI Brain with multiple subependymal nodules

Table 17.1 Clinical diagnostic criteria for tuberous sclerosis complex (TSC)

Major features	Hypomelanotic macules (e.g., *Ash leaf spots*)	- 3 or more - 5 mm or more in diameter
	Angiofibromas or fibrous cephalic plaque	- 3 or more angiofibromas - 1 or more fibrous cephalic plaque
	Ungual fibromas	- 2 or more
	Shagreen patch	
	Retinal hamartomas	- 2 or more
	Cortical tubers *(or other cortical dysplasias, i.e., whiter matter radial migration lines)*	
	Subependymal nodules	
	Cardiac rhabdomyoma	
	Pulmonary lymphangioleiomyoma (LAM)[a]	
	Angiomyolipomas[a]	- 2 or more
Minor features	Confetti Lesions	
	Dental enamel pits	- Three or more
	Intraoral fibromas	- 2 or more
	Retinal achromatic patch	
	Multiple renal cysts	
	Nonretinal hamartoma	

[a]If LAM and angiomyolipomas co-occur, they count as one major feature, not two.
Clinical criteria for the diagnosis of TSC, including major manifestations and minor manifestations. A definitive diagnosis requires two major criteria are met or one major and two minor criteria.

including at the bilateral foramen of Munro, cortical tubers, and radial migration lines. The mother and brother also have TSC. The patient was brought to the emergency room at age 2 months due to parental concern for infantile spasms and evidence of multiple hypopigmented macules consistent with Ash leaf spots. He was evaluated with continuous EEG and did not have infantile spasms or hypsarrhythmia. He was sent home without treatment. Given that her other son had infantile spasms, the mother remained vigilant and returned at 5 months old for similar concerns. Continuous EEG was consistent with infantile spasms, and the patient was started on hormonal (steroid) therapy. Although it was partially effective, he still had spasm clusters. When changed to vigabatrin, he had a remarkable response and was spasm free. He was weaned off and did not have return of spasms or other seizures.

Teaching Points. This case highlights (1) the clinical diagnostic criteria used to establish a diagnosis of TSC, and (2) common cutaneous manifestations used to establish a TSC diagnosis. Guidelines for making a diagnosis of TSC were first published in 1998 and revised by the International Tuberous Sclerosis Complex Consensus Conference in 2012.[21] The criteria can be divided into major and minor manifestations of the disease, with the following being required to establish the diagnosis (Table 17.1):

1. Definitive TSC diagnosis:
   a. Two major criteria OR
   b. One major criteria and two or more minor criteria
2. Possible TSC diagnosis:
   a. One major criteria OR
   b. Two or more minor criteria

Principles of TSC Diagnosis. One of the earliest manifestations of TSC are cardiac rhabdomyomas, which can be detected with prenatal ultrasound screening.[22] Seizures may begin during infancy and often initially manifest as infantile spasms, though multiple seizure types are not uncommon including generalized tonic-clonic, tonic, clonic, atonic, and others. Cutaneous findings are present in approximately 90% of TSC patients.[23] The first cutaneous sign is often hypopigmented macules called Ash leaf spots (Fig. 17.1A), which are first apparent in infancy. These and the major cutaneous findings reviewed below should be assessed in all children presenting with a new diagnosis of infantile spasms.

Hypomelanotic macules: These lesions look like an Ash leaf, often with a rounded appearance on one side and tapering to a sharp edge on the contralateral side. They are the most common cutaneous finding in TSC and occur in 90% of affected patients compared with only 1–4% of healthy children.[24] The presence of three or more hypopigmented lesions >5 mm in diameter is one of the most specific diagnostic findings and should strongly suggest a diagnosis of TSC.[25] A woods lamp examination may be useful in accentuating the appearance of these macules, particularly in individuals with light-colored skin. Though TSC is one of the more common conditions characterized by Ash leaf macules, other conditions can mimic TSC, including MEN-1, Birt-Hogg Dube syndrome, acne vulgaris, trichoepitheliomas, idiopathic guttate hypomelanosis, and congenital hypopigmented macules, and should be considered in patients without other TSC manifestations.[21]

Shagreen patch: Shagreen patches are collagenoma-like lesions that typically occur in the lumbosacral region often with an "orange peel" appearance that may by hypopigmented, hyperpigmented, or skin-colored. A shagreen patch is the second most common cutaneous finding estimated to be present in up to 50% of TSC patients in the first decade of life.[25] In patients who present with multiple hypopigmented macules (e.g., Ash leaf spots), a detailed skin examination should be performed to evaluate for the presence of a shagreen patch, fibrous cephalic plaque, or confetti lesions (see below).

Angiofibromas: Angiofibromas are facial cutaneous lesions occurring in the malar region across the nasal bridge, nasolabial folds, forehead, chin, and cheek (Fig. 17.1E).[6,26] They are rarely present at birth, often develop during the first decade of life, and can increase in number during adolescence and even into adulthood.[27] Ungual fibromas are identical lesions that occur in the periungual and subungual nailfold regions (Fig. 17.1D). Intraoral fibromas are similar in appearance and are located in the gingiva, buccal mucosa, labial mucosa, or tongue, and may be seen in 20–70% of TSC patients (Fig. 17.1C).[28,29] One or two fibromas are common in the general healthy population; however, three or more is rare and fulfills a major diagnostic criterion. Topical mTOR inhibitors have shown benefit for angiofibroma, fibrous plaques, and hypomelanotic macules.

Fibrous cephalic plaque: Fibrous cephalic plaques are a variant of facial angiofibromas that occur on the forehead, scalp, and face. They have the appearance of a firm, yellow or brown slow-growing lesion on the forehead and are found in 20–36% of TSC patients.[30]

Clinical Pearls

1. Cutaneous findings are present in approximately 90% of TSC patients.
2. The first cutaneous sign is often hypopigmented macules called Ash leaf spots which are first apparent in infancy.

CASE 17.2 DIAGNOSIS OF TSC IN AN ADULT PATIENT

Case 17.2a. A 27-year-old female presented for new evaluation of long-standing TSC with a history of intractable seizures, aggressive behavior, mood irritability, and developmental delay (e.g., nonverbal). She was diagnosed with TSC around 18 months of age due to new-onset seizures and the presence of cortical tubers on neuroimaging. Genetic testing was not performed and she developed intractable epilepsy with multiple seizures types, including generalized tonic-clonic, and stereotyped laughing

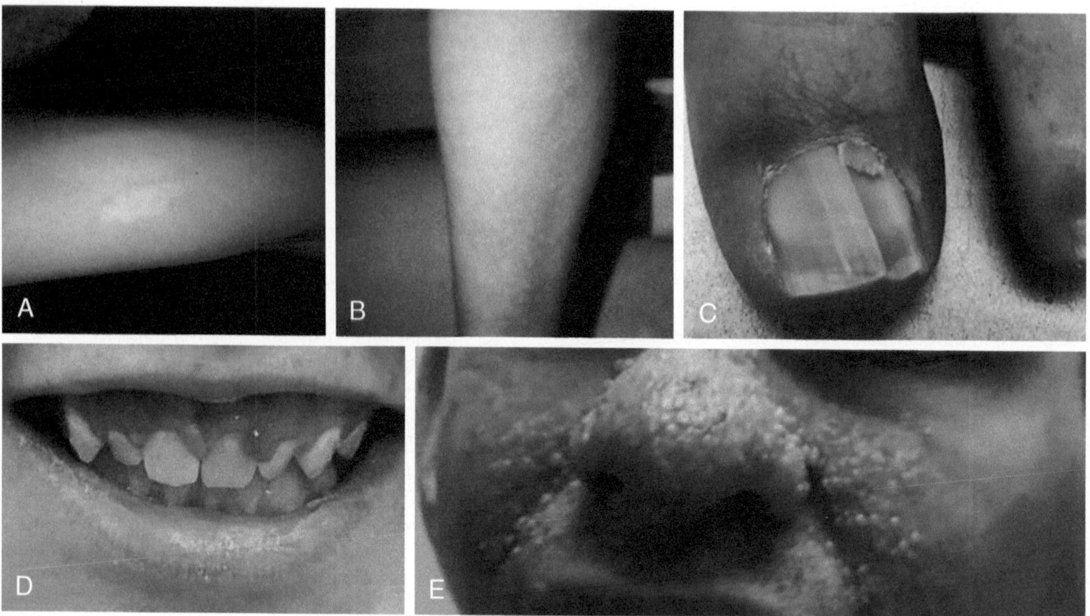

Fig. 17.1 Common cutaneous findings in patients with tuberous sclerosis including hypopigmented macule or Ash leaf spot (A), confetti lesions (B), ungual fibroma (C), gingival fibromas (D), and facial angiofibromas (E).

episodes followed by behavioral arrest previously treated with rufinamide, brivaracetam, and topiramate and currently taking clobazam and valproic acid. At the time of her first referral evaluation, her mother was found to have multiple facial angiofibromas (Fig. 17.1E), subtle neurocognitive complaints, two periungual fibromas, and shagreen patch consistent with a diagnosis of TSC.

Case 17.2b. A 41-year-old female presented for new evaluation of TSC. She was diagnosed 5 years ago when she had a brain MRI for evaluation of migrainous headaches. Her imaging had shown two small cortically based hyperintensities consistent with cortical tubers. She had no prior history of seizures or genetic testing. Skin examination showed mild facial angiofibromas and periungual fibromas. Further imaging revealed an asymptomatic renal AML measuring 3.3 cm in greatest dimension.

Teaching Points. A new diagnosis of TSC in an adult patient is uncommon. The majority of patients will develop recognizable manifestations sufficient to establish a diagnosis in childhood. However, these adult cases underscore the benefit of recognizing the clinical features of TSC even in adult patients who do not carry a known diagnosis. Several important TSC findings manifest later in life including pulmonary LAM, which occurs more commonly in adult women. In one study, nearly half of adult-diagnosed TSC patients presented with symptoms of LAM, all of whom were women.[31] Clinicians should be aware that, although adult-onset presentations are less common, such diagnoses when made are important for patient counseling and surveillance imaging.

Principles of TSC Diagnosis. Clinical examination is critical to establishing a TSC diagnosis and should not be replaced with genetic testing alone. Identification of a pathogenic mutation in *TSC1* or *TSC2* from blood or biopsy of normal tissue is sufficient to establish a definitive diagnosis of TSC. However, it is important to note that between 10% and 25% of patients who fulfill the clinical criteria for TSC will have no identified mutation on genetic testing.

Minor cutaneous manifestations include the following (Table 17.1)[32,33]:

Confetti lesions: These hypomelanotic lesions are smaller in size to Ash leaf spots and often appear in groups or clusters (Fig. 17.1B). They are common in the first decade of life and can help contribute to the diagnosis of TSC, fulfilling a minor diagnosis criterion.

Oral lesions: Other than the intraoral fibroma, the most common oral lesion is dental enamel pitting. This is present in virtually all people with TSC but may also occur in between 7% and 70% of healthy persons and thus may be less helpful in isolation to establish a possible clinical diagnosis of TSC but are important to monitor.[34,35] Current guidelines recommend dental examinations every 6 months (Table 17.2).

Clinical Pearls

1. Between 10% and 25% of patients who fulfill the clinical criteria for TSC will have no identified mutation on genetic testing.
2. Several important TSC findings manifest later in life including pulmonary lymphangioleiomyomatosis (LAM), which occurs more commonly in adult women.

Table 17.2 Surveillance recommendations for monitoring patients with tuberous sclerosis complex (TSC)

Dental	Dental examination *(e.g., oral fibroma and dental enamel pits)*	Every 6 months *(same as general population)*
Neuropsychiatric	Screen for behavior problems and intellectual disability *(i.e., TSC-associated neuropsychiatric disorder, TAND)*	Annually
	Comprehensive neuropsychiatric screening	Once during following age ranges (years): 0–3, 3–6, 6–9, 12–16, 18–25
Neurological	EEG *(for interictal epileptiform activity or subclinical seizures)*	At time of diagnosis 24-hour monitoring as needed after suspected seizure activity, behavioral change, or positive comprehensive neuropsychiatric screening
	Brain MRI with and without contrast *(for cortical tubers, subependymal nodules, and SEGA)*	At time of diagnosis; repeat every 1–3 years until age 25 years
Cardiovascular	Echocardiogram *(for rhabdomyoma)*	At time of diagnosis if less than 3 years old; repeat for asymptomatic lesions every 1–3 years until regression Referral to cardiology if symptomatic
	EKG *(for arrhythmia)*	At time of diagnosis
	Blood pressure monitoring	Annually
Pulmonary	High resolution CT scan 6-minute walk test, pulmonary function testing *(for Lymphangioleiomyomatosis)*	At time of diagnosis if symptomatic or if a woman >18 years old Repeat every 5–10 years if asymptomatic Repeat every 2–3 years if symptomatic
Renal	Abdominal MRI (renal ultrasound or CT abdomen, less sensitive); *for angiomyolipoma and renal cysts*	At time of diagnosis Repeat every 1–3 years
	Glomerular filtration rate	Annually
Dermatologic	Complete skin examination *(for hypomelanotic macules, shagreen patches, angiofibromas, fibrous cephalic plaques, confetti lesions, etc.)*	At time of diagnosis and annually
Ophthalmologic	Dilated fundoscopic examination *(for retinal hamartomas or eye lesion)*	At time of diagnosis Annually if known lesion

Recommendation for surveillance in those with tuberous sclerosis complex, organized by organ system. *EKG*, Electocardiogram; *SEGA*, subependymal giant cell astrocytoma.

CASE 17.3 DIAGNOSIS AND MANAGEMENT OF TSC-ASSOCIATED EPILEPSY

Case. A now 10-year-old with gene test negative tuberous sclerosis was initially diagnosed at age 4 months when she had her first seizure. She quickly became intractable to multiple medications, and at age 8 months, a presurgical evaluation was initiated. In addition to her numerous tubers, subependymal nodules, she also had a rather large right parietal brain malformation. The decision was made to defer surgery. She remained intractable to polypharmacy, even to everolimus. At age 7 years, a vagal nerve stimulator (VNS) was placed, with modest results. As her seizures appeared to have a consistent clinical semiology, she was evaluated for epilepsy surgery a second time. After prolonged EEG, MRI, and PET scan, the findings were similar, with likely correlation to the large right parietal cortical malformation. Due to the patient's autism and developmental delay, it was again decided to defer resective surgery for now, as she would have difficulty tolerating more invasive monitoring for such a large lesion.

Teaching Points. Epilepsy is the most common and clinically challenging manifestation of TSC. Seizures occur in approximately 85% of TSC patients, often beginning as infantile spasms and progressing to include multiple seizures types. Management of seizures is best led by an epileptologist familiar with TSC and this case highlights the importance of a multidisciplinary team approach considering all options, including antiepileptic drugs (AEDs), surgical therapies (e.g., seizure focus resection, VNS), and targeted therapy (e.g., mTOR inhibitors—everolimus). Vigabatrin is the only AED with TSC-specific data supporting its efficacy in TSC. As a result, vigabatrin is the recommended first-line agent for monotherapy treatment in TSC children with infantile spasms or focal seizures presenting at <1 year of age. Monitoring for vigabatrin-associated retinal toxicity is required given the risk of retinal damage.[36] ACTH is effective for infantile spasms and is considered second-line therapy. Combination therapy is recommended when initial monotherapy has failed.

Principles of TSC-Associated Epilepsy. Outcomes for TSC patients with seizures varies and tends to follow one of two clinical courses. Within the first year of life, up to 60% of TSC patients will present with new-onset seizures. Of these patients, approximately two-thirds will develop refractory epilepsy and often suffer long-term neurocognitive and neurodevelopmental abnormalities, with many remaining nonverbal. The other one-third of patients will achieve seizure remission and nearly 40% of these patients will be able to discontinue antiepileptic therapy.[37–39] Neurodevelopmental outcomes in these patients are significantly more favorable, though some patients may manifest minor neurocognitive dysfunction. As a result, the goal of epilepsy treatment in children with TSC is to control or prevent seizures as soon as possible in hopes of preventing long-term neurocognitive disability.

In TSC adults who do not have a prior seizure history, new epilepsy can still occur in up to 12% of patients, underscoring the need for lifelong evaluation of stereotypic events.[31,40] Current guidelines recommend screening electroencephalography at diagnosis and 24-hour monitoring as needed for suspected new seizures, behavioral change, or positive neuropsychiatric screening to evaluate for subclinical seizures (Table 17.2).

Targeted therapy with mTOR inhibitors (e.g., everolimus) has been shown to be effective in reducing seizure frequency and is considered as an early adjunct in patients with refractory seizures on combination AED therapy. The EXIST-3 trial evaluated the efficacy and safety of everolimus as an adjunctive treatment for seizures in TSC. In this study, low-dose and higher-dose everolimus treatment led to sustained reductions in seizure frequency that was time- and dose-dependent. Longer duration of therapy was associated with higher response rates: 30% achieving >50% seizure reduction at 6 months, 40% at 1 year, and 50% at 2 years. Higher drug exposure was also associated with significantly higher responses, with 28% achieving >50% seizure reduction in the low-exposure group compared with 40% in the high-exposure group.[41] For additional review of targeted therapy with everolimus including common side effects and monitoring, see the last section of this chapter on mTOR Inhibition.

Other treatment options include epilepsy surgery, ketogenic diet, and VNS. Recently, alternatives to open surgical resection, including minimally invasive approaches with laser interstitial thermal therapy, have been reported to be safe in small series of TSC patients and may provide a minimally invasive alternative.[42] These options should be considered by a multidisciplinary team familiar with the management of TSC-associated epilepsy and these treatment modalities.

Clinical Pearls

1. Seizures occur in approximately 85% of TSC patients, often beginning as infantile spasms and progressing to include multiple seizures types.
2. Vigabatrin is the only AED with TSC-specific data supporting its efficacy in TSC.
3. In the EXIST-3 study, treatment with the oral mTOR inhibitor everolimus resulted in improvement in seizures in 50% of patients at 2 years.

CASE 17.4 DIAGNOSIS AND MANAGEMENT OF SUBEPENDYMAL GIANT CELL ASTROCYTOMA

Case. A 25-year-old patient with existing TSC diagnosed at 3 months due to infantile spasms, cortical tubers, subependymal nodule, and SEGA was managed with multiple AEDs for refractory epilepsy and SEGA was monitored with serial neuroimaging performed every 1–3 years. At age 25, surveillance imaging showed growth over the preceding 3 years with concern for impending obstruction at the foramen of Munro due to tumor location, and initiation of everolimus was recommended. The patient tolerated daily everolimus 7.5 mg/day for 2 years with imaging response but developed unexplained chronic cough and recurrent pneumonia requiring hospitalization, and everolimus was discontinued. Over the subsequent 2 years, slow regrowth occurred but did not reach the pretreatment size, and the patient remained symptom free without everolimus or other intervention (Fig. 17.2).

Teaching Points. This case highlights (1) the major neuroimaging findings in TSC, (2) the natural history of SEGA, and (3) treatment options for managing growing SEGAs. The three most common neuroimaging findings in TSC are cortical tubers (Fig. 17.3A, orange arrows), subependymal nodules (Fig. 17.3A, C, blue arrowhead), and subependymal giant cell astrocytomas (SEGAs, Fig. 17.3A, B, green arrow), which occur almost exclusively in TSC. Cortical tubers are the neuropathologic hallmark of the disease and represent glioneuronal hamartomas or dysplastic neural proliferation that forms during fetal development and may occur in the cortex or subcortex. These lesions occur in 90% of TSC patients and have no malignant potential, but

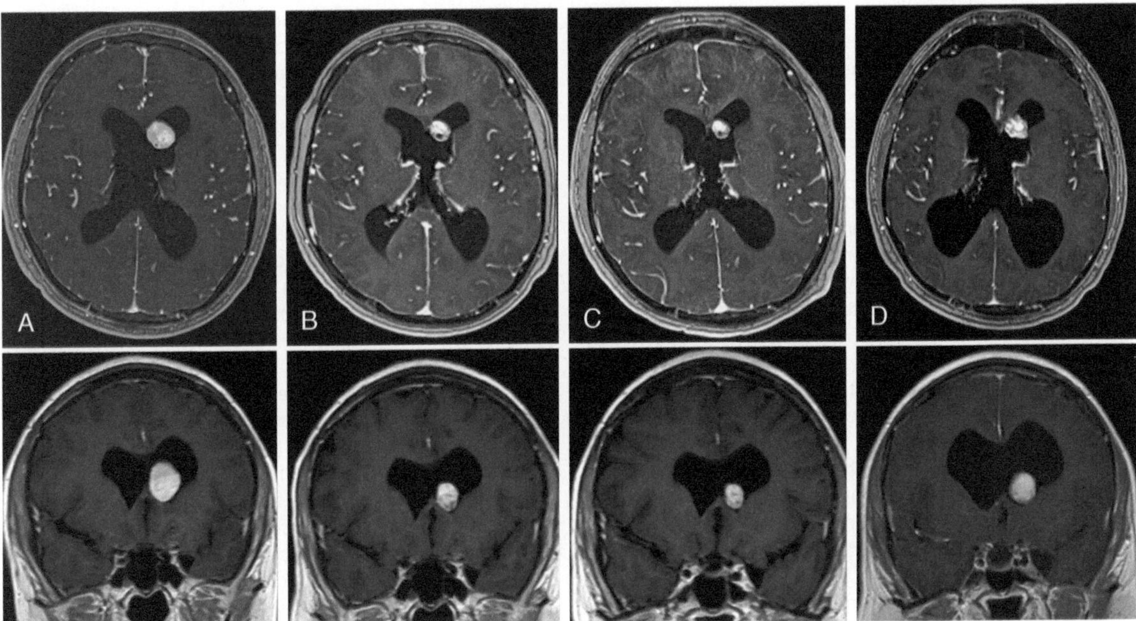

Fig. 17.2 Brain MRI including T1-weighted post-gadolinium infused axial *(top row)* and coronal *(bottom row)* images showing subependymal giant cell astrocytoma (SEGA) in the left lateral ventricle adjacent to the foramen of Munro prior to everolimus (A), 1 year after initiation of everolimus (B), at the time of discontinuation of everolimus (C), and 3 years after discontinuation of everolimus (D) showing interval treatment response and slight regrowth after drug discontinuation, with stable but worse ventriculomegaly at that time (D).

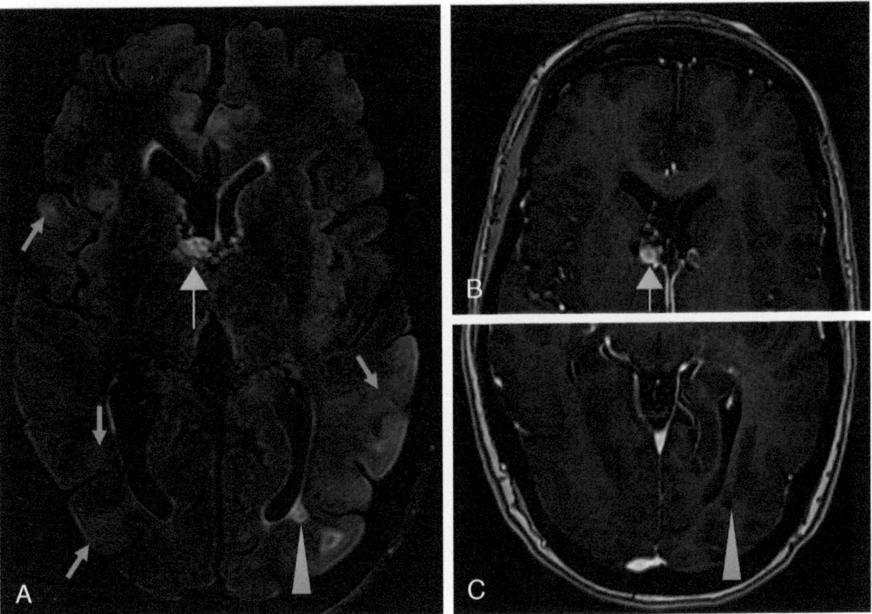

Fig. 17.3 Characteristic neuroimaging findings of tuberous sclerosis including fluid-attenuated inversion recovery (FLAIR) imaging (A) and axial post-gadolinium enhanced T1-weighted images (B, C). Imaging shows the three characteristics brain findings including cortical tubers (orange arrows), subependymal nodules (blue arrowheads), and a subependymal giant cell astrocytoma (green arrows).

can contribute to epilepsy and neurocognitive dysfunction.[43–46] Subependymal nodules are hyperintense lesions adjacent to the ventricular surface that do not enhance with gadolinium contrast. They can be calcified, do not grow or enlarge, and, when enhancement is present, consideration of transformation to SEGA should be entertained. SEGAs typically occur within the lateral ventricle and often at the caudothalamic grove adjacent to the foramen of Munro. In contrast to subependymal nodules, they can grow over time and may obstruct cerebrospinal fluid outflow from the lateral ventricles, resulting in ventriculomegaly or noncommunicating hydrocephalus.

Principles of SEGA Treatment. Screening brain MRI is recommended until age 25 as new occurrence of SEGA in an asymptomatic individual is rare in adults (Table 17.2). Children with known asymptomatic SEGAs should be imaged periodically throughout adulthood. Risk of growth is higher for patients with tumors >2 cm, younger age, and *TSC2* genotype.[47] Historically, surgery has been the mainstay for treating symptomatic SEGAs. Indications for surgery including acute hydrocephalus, increased seizure burden that coincides with SEGA growth, or rapid asymptomatic growth with concern for impending hydrocephalus. Stereotactic radiosurgery has typically been reserved for recurrent SEGA.

Targeted therapy with mTOR inhibitors is first-line for treatment of SEGA, particularly in those for whom total resection is not possible or when there is a contraindication to surgery.[48] Like treatment of TSC-associated epilepsy, response to everolimus is time- and dose-dependent. Although early tumor shrinkage occurs, in prospective studies median time to response was 3.5 months and overall response rate was 50%, with 27% responding at 3 months, 37% at 6 months, 46% at 1 year, and 47% at 2 years.[49,50] Recently, minimally invasive surgical approaches have also proved to be increasingly valuable with several reports demonstrating success of laser-interstitial thermal therapy for the minimally invasive surgical treatment.[44,51–58]

Clinical Pearls

1. Cortical tubers occur in 90% of TSC patients, have no malignant potential, but can contribute to epilepsy.
2. Subependymal nodules are hyperintense lesions adjacent to the ventricular surface that do not enhance with gadolinium contrast.
3. Subependymal giant cell astrocytomas (SEGAs) are a WHO grade 1 glioma that occur within the ventricular system, often around the foramen of Munro and enhance with gadolinium contrast.

CASE 17.5 DIAGNOSIS AND MANAGEMENT OF RENAL ANGIOMYOLIPOMA

Case. A 38-year-old male with a long history of TSC diagnosed in infancy based on presentation of infantile spasms and characteristics skin lesions. Seizure types included focal seizures, tonic seizures, atonic seizures, tonic-clonic seizures, clonic seizures, and "absences"-type seizures. He also had pulmonary hamartomas, facial angiofibromas, and innumerable bilateral angiomyolipomas in the kidneys with the largest growing by 15% over the past 2 years (Fig. 17.4A, B and 17,4C, D). He had been previously treated with over five AEDs, including cannabidiol, without significant benefit. Everolimus was initiated and titrated to 8 ng/mL. After 15 months of therapy, clinical examination confirmed improvement in seizure frequency and repeat imaging showed interval response of the renal AMLs (Fig. 17.4E, F).

Key Considerations. This case highlights that (1) renal angiomyolipomas (AMLs) are a major manifestation of TSC, (2) their common presentation as large asymptomatic lesions, and (3) the role of targeted therapy in treating AMLs in TSC. AMLs are benign tumors composed of vascular cells, immature smooth muscle, and adipose tissue. The presence of two AMLs fulfills a major diagnostic criterion for TSC and is present in up to 80% of patients with TSC (Table 17.1). AMLs commonly present as asymptomatic lesions but can present with hematuria or reduced kidney function. The feared complication is renal hemorrhage, which is rare. Recent reports suggest that the prevalence of renal hemorrhage in TSC AMLs is low, is most common between ages 20–30 years, and can be managed conservatively.[59]

Principles of Evaluating and Managing Renal Angiomyolipomas in TSC. AMLs tend to develop during childhood and slowly enlarge until early adulthood. Growth ceases in up to 30% of TSC adults. Current recommendations for surveillance are for renal imaging with either MR Abdomen, renal ultrasound, or CT of the abdomen every 1–3 years (Table 17.2).[60,61] Historically, treatment of AMLs was reserved to those whose size was >3 cm in diameter due to the perceived risk of hemorrhage, though recent reports caution against use of size alone in treatment determinations, and consultation with a multidisciplinary team familiar with TSC should be performed. When treatment is indicated, mTOR inhibitors are first-line therapy with an overall response rate of 58%.[62,63] Second-line treatments include embolization, followed by kidney sparing resection, or robotic partial nephrectomy. When surveillance imaging shows growth >0.5 cm per year, then biopsy should be considered to rule out renal cell carcinoma (RCC). RCC is more common in TSC than the general population, though the overall prevalence remains low.

Clinical Pearls

1. Angiomyolipomas (AMLs) are benign kidney tumors that are present in up to 80% of patients with TSC.
2. AMLs rarely develop into renal cell carcinoma but can be complicated by renal hemorrhage, which is rare.
3. When treatment of an AML is indicated, mTOR inhibitors (e.g., everolimus) are first-line therapy with an overall response rate of 58%.

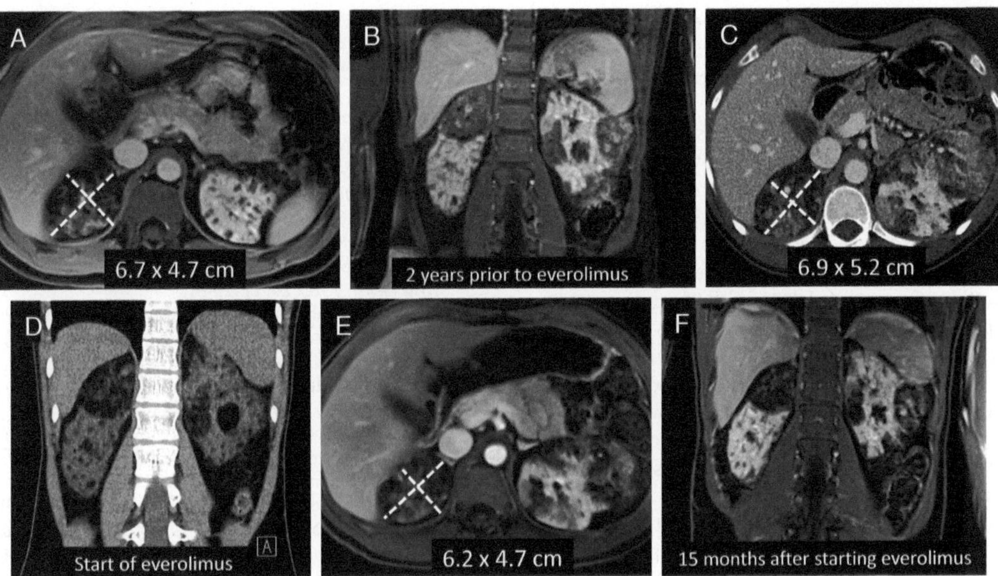

Fig. 17.4 TSC-associated renal angiomyolipomas (AML) in a patient treated with everolimus showing axial (A) and coronal (B) T1-weighted MRI images 2 years prior to starting everolimus; axial (C) and coronal (D) CT at the time of initiation of everolimus showing 15% increase in the size of target AML; and axial (E) and coronal (F) T1-weighted MRI images 15 months after initiation of everolimus showing a 19% reduction in lesion size.

Other extra-nervous and non-oncologic manifestations of TSC

TSC can affect any organ in the body. Other common extra-nervous system sites of disease include retinal hamartomas in the eye, cardiac rhabdomyomas in the heart, and pulmonary LAM.

Retinal: Retinal hamartomas are flat translucent or mulberry-like lesions seen in 30–50% of individuals with TSC and are rarely symptomatic but should be evaluated at the time of diagnosis in all patients (Table 17.2).[64]

Rhabdomyomas: Rhabdomyoma, or benign tumors of the cardiac muscle, can be an early sign of TSC when discovered within the cardiac ventricle on prenatal echocardiogram, often after the 20th week of gestation.[65] The presence of multiple cardiac rhabdomyomas at birth confers a 75–80% chance of subsequent TSC diagnosis.[22,66,67] Although usually asymptomatic, manifestations may range from ventricular dysfunction, valvular dysfunction, cardiomegaly, arrhythmia, non-immune hydrops fetalis, and death. Cardiac rhabdomyomas can resolve spontaneously with age.[68]

Lymphangioleiomyomatosis: LAM is a condition of the lung that arises from benign interstitial expansion of the smooth muscle cells of the lung. Unlike other TSC manifestations, there is a female predominance, with LAM occurring in 30–80% of females and only 10–12% of males with TSC.[69–72] LAM typically presents in the third to fourth decade, with symptoms of worsening dyspnea and recurrent pneumothoraces. High-resolution CT shows cystic pulmonary lesions.[71] Confirmation by pathological examination can be necessary when other clinical diagnostic features are not present. Noninvasive diagnostic criteria using high-resolution CT have been proposed by the European Respiratory Society and include: (1) more than four cysts, no confounding comorbidities or exposures, and at least one other major or two minor criteria for TSC (outside of angiomyolipoma); or (2) one of the following: abdominal or thoracic LAM, chylous pleural effusion, or chylous ascites. In patients with LAM who have abnormal or declining lung function, consensus recommendation is for treatment with mTOR inhibition.[73,74] LAM should not be confused with multifocal micronodular pneumocyte hyperplasia, which is characterized by nodular proliferation of type II pneumocytes and can occur in the presence or absence of LAM.

Treatment with mTOR inhibition: clinical efficacy and side effects

mTOR inhibitors (e.g., everolimus, sirolimus) have revolutionized the treatment of TSC and expanded the options for managing clinically challenging manifestations such as epilepsy, SEGA, and AMLs, as well as treating manifestations that previously had few options such as LAM. Three large randomized phase 3 studies have been performed evaluating the role of everolimus in patients with TSC:

- EXIST-1 assessed the efficacy and safety of everolimus versus placebo for treatment of TSC-related SEGA.[49,50] Of the 111 evaluable patients, the overall response rate was 50% with 27% responding at 3 months, 37% at 6 months, 46% at 1 year, and 47% at 2 years.
- EXIST-2 assessed the efficacy of everolimus versus placebo for TSC-associated AMLs.[62,63] The response rate at 3 months was 42% compared with 0% in the placebo group with 95% of patients in the everolimus-treated arm having tumor shrinkage and no reported hemorrhage. Median time to AML response was 2.9 months with an overall response rate of 58%, including 44% responding at 3 months, 55% at 6 months, 62% at 1 year, and 63% at 2 years.
- EXIST-3 assessed the efficacy and safety of low-exposure (trough 3–7 ng/mL) and high-exposure (trough 9–15 ng/mL) everolimus versus placebo for treatment-resistant focal epilepsy.[41,75] Response rate at 3 months was 15.1% with placebo, 28.2% with low exposure, and 40.0% with high exposure. Following 1 year of treatment, 49% of patients had responded to everolimus with a median percent reduction in seizures of 48%.[75]
- In these studies, improvement in other TSC manifestations has also been reported, including 58–68% of patients with partial response of skin lesions.[76]

The most common side effects include stomatitis (40–70%), nasopharyngitis, acne-like skin lesions, and, uncommonly, hyperlipidemia or hypertriglyceridemia, and, in rare cases, pneumonia. Prophylactic use of corticosteroid-containing mouthwash can be considered on an "as needed" basis; full blood count, renal and liver function, blood pressure, and fasting lipid monitoring including triglycerides and cholesterol should be performed every 3–6 months.[77]

Conclusion

In summary, tuberous sclerosis is characterized by tumors of the brain, eye, heart, and kidney as well as cutaneous findings and, in some cases, abnormalities in the lung. Brain findings in tuberous sclerosis include cortical tubers, subependymal nodules, and subependymal giant cell astrocytomas (SEGAs) which predispose patients to seizures. In addition to surgical treatments, mTOR inhibitors such as everolimus reduce SEGA size and improve seizure frequency in >50% of tuberous sclerosis patients who are treated with long-term therapy.

References

1. Osborne JP, Fryer A, Webb D. Epidemiology of tuberous sclerosis. *Ann N Y Acad Sci*. 1991;615:125–127.
2. Curatolo P, Bombardieri R, Jozwiak S. Tuberous sclerosis. *Lancet*. 2008;372(9639):657–668. https://doi.org/10.1016/S0140-6736(08)61279-9.
3. Sampson JR, Scahill SJ, Stephenson JB, Mann L, Connor JM. Genetic aspects of tuberous sclerosis in the west of Scotland. *J Med Genet*. 1989;26(1):28–31.
4. Morrison PJ, Shepherd CH, Stewart FJ, Nevin NC. Prevalence of tuberous sclerosis in UK. *Lancet*. 1998;352(9124):318–319.
5. Wiederholt WC, Gomez MR, Kurland LT. Incidence and prevalence of tuberous sclerosis in Rochester, Minnesota, 1950 through 1982. *Neurology*. 1985;35(4):600–603.
6. Sadowski K, Kotulska K, Schwartz RA, Jozwiak S. Systemic effects of treatment with mTOR inhibitors in tuberous sclerosis complex: a comprehensive review. *J Eur Acad Dermatol Venereol*. 2016;30(4):586–594. https://doi.org/10.1111/jdv.13356.
7. DiMario FJJ, Sahin M, Ebrahimi-Fakhari D. Tuberous sclerosis complex. *Pediatr Clin North Am*. 2015;62(3):633–648. https://doi.org/10.1016/j.pcl.2015.03.005.
8. Nevin NC, Pearce WG. Diagnostic and genetical aspects of tuberous sclerosis. *J Med Genet*. 1968;5(4):273–280.
9. Povey S, Burley MW, Attwood J, et al. Two loci for tuberous sclerosis: one on 9q34 and one on 16p13. *Ann Hum Genet*. 1994;58(2):107–127.
10. Kandt RS, Haines JL, Smith M, et al. Linkage of an important gene locus for tuberous sclerosis to a chromosome 16 marker for polycystic kidney disease. *Nat Genet*. 1992;2(1):37–41. https://doi.org/10.1038/ng0992-37.
11. Huang J, Dibble CC, Matsuzaki M, Manning BD. The TSC1-TSC2 complex is required for proper activation of mTOR complex 2. *Mol Cell Biol*. 2008;28(12):4104–4115. https://doi.org/10.1128/MCB.00289-08.
12. Tee AR, Fingar DC, Manning BD, Kwiatkowski DJ, Cantley LC, Blenis J. Tuberous sclerosis complex-1 and -2 gene products function together to inhibit mammalian target of rapamycin (mTOR)-mediated downstream signaling. *Proc Natl Acad Sci U S A*. 2002;99(21):13571–13576. https://doi.org/10.1073/pnas.202476899.
13. Lamb RF, Roy C, Diefenbach TJ, et al. The TSC1 tumour suppressor hamartin regulates cell adhesion through ERM proteins and the GTPase Rho. *Nat Cell Biol*. 2000;2(5):281–287. https://doi.org/10.1038/35010550.
14. Zhang Y, Gao X, Saucedo LJ, Ru B, Edgar BA, Pan D. Rheb is a direct target of the tuberous sclerosis tumour suppressor proteins. *Nat Cell Biol*. 2003;5(6):578–581. https://doi.org/10.1038/ncb999.
15. Tee AR, Manning BD, Roux PP, Cantley LC, Blenis J. Tuberous sclerosis complex gene products, tuberin and hamartin, control mTOR signaling by acting as a GTPase-activating protein complex toward Rheb. *Curr Biol*. 2003;13(15):1259–1268.
16. Stocker H, Radimerski T, Schindelholz B, et al. Rheb is an essential regulator of S6K in controlling cell growth in Drosophila. *Nat Cell Biol*. 2003;5(6):559–565. https://doi.org/10.1038/ncb995.
17. Manning BD, Cantley LC. AKT/PKB signaling: navigating downstream. *Cell*. 2007;129(7):1261–1274. https://doi.org/10.1016/j.cell.2007.06.009.

18. Inoki K, Li Y, Xu T, Guan K-L. Rheb GTPase is a direct target of TSC2 GAP activity and regulates mTOR signaling. *Genes Dev.* 2003;17(15):1829–1834. https://doi.org/10.1101/gad.1110003.
19. Garami A, Zwartkruis FJT, Nobukuni T, et al. Insulin activation of Rheb, a mediator of mTOR/S6K/4E-BP signaling, is inhibited by TSC1 and 2. *Mol Cell.* 2003;11(6):1457–1466.
20. van Slegtenhorst M, Nellist M, Nagelkerken B, et al. Interaction between hamartin and tuberin, the TSC1 and TSC2 gene products. *Hum Mol Genet.* 1998;7(6):1053–1057.
21. Northrup H, Krueger DA, International Tuberous Sclerosis Complex Consensus Group. Tuberous sclerosis complex diagnostic criteria update: recommendations of the 2012 International Tuberous Sclerosis Complex Consensus conference. *Changes.* 2012;29(6):997–1003.
22. Holley DG, Martin GR, Brenner JI, et al. Diagnosis and management of fetal cardiac tumors: a multicenter experience and review of published reports. *J Am Coll Cardiol.* 1995;26(2):516–520.
23. Jacks SK, Witman PM. Tuberous sclerosis complex: an update for dermatologists. *Pediatr Dermatol.* 2015;32(5):563–570. https://doi.org/10.1111/pde.12567.
24. Strowd RE, Strowd LC, Blakeley JO. Cutaneous manifestations in neuro-oncology: clinically relevant tumor and treatment associated dermatologic findings. *Semin Oncol.* 2016;43(3): 401–407. https://doi.org/10.1053/j.seminoncol.2016.02.029.
25. Jóźwiak S, Schwartz R a, Janniger CK, Michałowicz R, Chmielik J. Skin lesions in children with tuberous sclerosis complex: their prevalence, natural course, and diagnostic significance. *Int J Dermatol.* 1998;37(12):911–917.
26. Haemel AK, O'Brian AL, Teng JM. Topical rapamycin: a novel approach to facial angiofibromas in tuberous sclerosis. *Arch Dermatol.* 2010;146(7):715–718. https://doi.org/10.1001/archdermatol.2010.125.
27. Jozwiak S, Schwartz RA, Janniger CK, Bielicka-Cymerman J. Usefulness of diagnostic criteria of tuberous sclerosis complex in pediatric patients. *J Child Neurol.* 2000;15(10):652–659. https://doi.org/10.1177/088307380001501003.
28. Sparling JD, Hong C-H, Brahim JS, Moss J, Darling TN. Oral findings in 58 adults with tuberous sclerosis complex. *J Am Acad Dermatol.* 2007;56(5):786–790. https://doi.org/10.1016/j.jaad.2006.11.019.
29. Lygidakis NA, Lindenbaum RH. Oral fibromatosis in tuberous sclerosis. *Oral Surg Oral Med Oral Pathol.* 1989;68(6):725–728.
30. Oyerinde O, Buccine D, Treichel A, et al. Fibrous cephalic plaques in tuberous sclerosis complex. *J Am Acad Dermatol.* 2018;78(4):717–724. https://doi.org/10.1016/j.jaad.2017.12.027.
31. Seibert D, Hong C-H, Takeuchi F, et al. Recognition of tuberous sclerosis in adult women: delayed presentation with life-threatening consequences. *Ann Intern Med.* 2011;154(12):806–813. https://doi.org/10.7326/0003-4819-154-12-201106210-00008. W-294.
32. Au KS, Williams AT, Roach ES, et al. Genotype/phenotype correlation in 325 individuals referred for a diagnosis of tuberous sclerosis complex in the United States. *Genet Med.* 2007;9(2):88–100. https://doi.org/10.1097/GIM.0b013e31803068c7.
33. Sancak O, Nellist M, Goedbloed M, et al. Mutational analysis of the TSC1 and TSC2 genes in a diagnostic setting: genotype--phenotype correlations and comparison of diagnostic DNA techniques in tuberous sclerosis complex. *Eur J Hum Genet.* 2005;13(6):731–741. https://doi.org/10.1038/sj.ejhg.5201402.
34. Flanagan N, O'Connor WJ, McCartan B, Miller S, McMenamin J, Watson R. Developmental enamel defects in tuberous sclerosis: a clinical genetic marker? *J Med Genet.* 1997;34(8): 637–639.
35. Mlynarczyk G. Enamel pitting: a common symptom of tuberous sclerosis. *Oral Surg Oral Med Oral Pathol.* 1991;71(1): 63–67.
36. Camposano SE, Major P, Halpern E, Thiele EA. Vigabatrin in the treatment of childhood epilepsy: a retrospective chart review of efficacy and safety profile. *Epilepsia.* 2008;49(7): 1186–1191. https://doi.org/10.1111/j.1528-1167.2008.01589.x.
37. Bombardieri R, Pinci M, Moavero R, Cerminara C, Curatolo P. Early control of seizures improves long-term outcome in children with tuberous sclerosis complex. *Eur J Paediatr Neurol.* 2010;14(2):146–149. https://doi.org/10.1016/j.ejpn.2009.03.003.
38. Curatolo P, Jozwiak S, Nabbout R. Management of epilepsy associated with tuberous sclerosis complex (TSC): clinical recommendations. *Eur J Paediatr Neurol.* 2012;16(6):582–586. https://doi.org/10.1016/j.ejpn.2012.05.004.
39. Curatolo P, Nabbout R, Lagae L, et al. Management of epilepsy associated with tuberous sclerosis complex: updated clinical recommendations. *Eur J Paediatr Neurol.* 2018;22(5):738–748. https://doi.org/10.1016/j.ejpn.2018.05.006.
40. Chu-Shore CJ, Major P, Camposano S, Muzykewicz D, Thiele EA. The natural history of epilepsy in tuberous sclerosis complex. *Epilepsia.* 2010;51(7):1236–1241. https://doi.org/10.1111/j.1528-1167.2009.02474.x.
41. French JA, Lawson JA, Yapici Z, et al. Adjunctive everolimus therapy for treatment-resistant focal-onset seizures associated with tuberous sclerosis (EXIST-3): a phase 3, randomised, double-blind, placebo-controlled study. *Lancet.* 2016;388(10056):2153–2163. https://doi.org/10.1016/S0140-6736(16)31419-2.
42. Tovar-spinoza Z, Ziechmann R, Zyck S. Single and staged laser interstitial thermal therapy ablation for cortical tubers causing refractory epilepsy in pediatric patients. *Neurosurg Focus.* 2018;45:E9. https://doi.org/10.3171/2018.6.FOCUS18228.
43. Frerebeau P, Benezech J, Segnarbieux F, Harbi H, Desy A, Marty-Double C. Intraventricular tumors in tuberous sclerosis. *Childs Nerv Syst.* 1985;1(1):45–48.
44. Jiang T, Jia G, Ma Z, Luo S, Zhang Y. The diagnosis and treatment of subependymal giant cell astrocytoma combined with tuberous sclerosis. *Childs Nerv Syst.* 2011;27(1):55–62. https://doi.org/10.1007/s00381-010-1159-1.
45. Cuccia V, Zuccaro G, Sosa F, Monges J, Lubienieky F, Taratuto AL. Subependymal giant cell astrocytoma in children with tuberous sclerosis. *Childs Nerv Syst.* 2003;19(4):232–243. https://doi.org/10.1007/s00381-002-0700-2.
46. Kingswood JC, d'Augères GB, Belousova E, et al. TuberOus SClerosis registry to increase disease Awareness (TOSCA) - baseline data on 2093 patients. *Orphanet J Rare Dis.* 2017;12(1):2. https://doi.org/10.1186/s13023-016-0553-5.
47. Jóźwiak S, Mandera M, Młynarski W. Natural history and current treatment options for subependymal giant cell astrocytoma in tuberous sclerosis complex. *Semin Pediatr Neurol.* 2015;22(4):274–281. https://doi.org/10.1016/j.spen.2015.10.003.
48. Franz DN, Belousova E, Sparagana S, et al. Long-term use of everolimus in patients with tuberous sclerosis complex: final results from the EXIST-1 study. *PLoS One.* 2016;11(6):e0158476. https://doi.org/10.1371/journal.pone.0158476.

49. Franz DN, Belousova E, Sparagana S, et al. Efficacy and safety of everolimus for subependymal giant cell astrocytomas associated with tuberous sclerosis complex (EXIST-1): a multicentre, randomised, placebo-controlled phase 3 trial. *Lancet*. 2013;381(9861):125–132. https://doi.org/10.1016/S0140-6736(12)61134-9.
50. Franz DN, Belousova E, Sparagana S, et al. Everolimus for subependymal giant cell astrocytoma in patients with tuberous sclerosis complex: 2-year open-label extension of the randomised EXIST-1 study. *Lancet Oncol*. 2014;15(13):1513–1520. https://doi.org/10.1016/S1470-2045(14)70489-9.
51. Campen CJ, Porter BE. Subependymal giant cell astrocytoma (SEGA) treatment update. *Curr Treat Options Neurol*. 2011;13(4):380–385. https://doi.org/10.1007/s11940-011-0123-z.
52. Krueger DA, Care MM, Holland K, et al. Everolimus for subependymal giant-cell astrocytomas in tuberous sclerosis. *N Engl J Med*. 2010;363(19):1801–1811. https://doi.org/10.1056/NEJMoa1001671.
53. Matsumura H, Takimoto H, Shimada N, Hirata M, Ohnishi T, Hayakawa T. Glioblastoma following radiotherapy in a patient with tuberous sclerosis. *Neurol Med Chir (Tokyo)*. 1998;38(5):287–291.
54. Park KJ, Kano H, Kondziolka D, Niranjan A, Flickinger JC, Lunsford LD. Gamma Knife surgery for subependymal giant cell astrocytomas. Clinical article. *J Neurosurg*. 2011;114(3):808–813. https://doi.org/10.3171/2010.9.JNS10816.
55. de Ribaupierre S, Dorfmüller G, Bulteau C, et al. Subependymal giant-cell astrocytomas in pediatric tuberous sclerosis disease: when should we operate? *Neurosurgery*. 2007;60(1):83–90. https://doi.org/10.1227/01.NEU.0000249216.19591.5D.
56. Goh S, Butler W, Thiele EA. Subependymal giant cell tumors in tuberous sclerosis complex. *Neurology*. 2004;63(8):1457–1461.
57. Berhouma M. Management of subependymal giant cell tumors in tuberous sclerosis complex: the neurosurgeon's perspective. *World J Pediatr*. 2010;6(2):103–110. https://doi.org/10.1007/s12519-010-0025-2.
58. Moavero R, Pinci M, Bombardieri R, Curatolo P. The management of subependymal giant cell tumors in tuberous sclerosis: a clinician's perspective. *Childs Nerv Syst*. 2011;27(8):1203–1210. https://doi.org/10.1007/s00381-011-1406-0.
59. Cockerell I, Guenin M, Heimdal K, Bjørnvold M, Selmer KK, Rouvière O. Prevalence of renal angiomyolipomas and spontaneous bleeding related to angiomyolipomas in tuberous sclerosis complex patients in France and Norway—a questionnaire study. *Urology*. 2017;104:70–76. https://doi.org/10.1016/J.UROLOGY.2017.02.023.
60. Bissler JJ, Kingswood JC. Optimal treatment of tuberous sclerosis complex associated renal angiomyolipomata: a systematic review. *Ther Adv Urol*. 2016;8(4):279–290. https://doi.org/10.1177/1756287216641353.
61. Yates JRW, Maclean C, Higgins JNP, et al. The Tuberous Sclerosis 2000 Study: presentation, initial assessments and implications for diagnosis and management. *Arch Dis Child*. 2011;96(11):1020–1025. https://doi.org/10.1136/adc.2011.211995.
62. Bissler JJ, Kingswood JC, Radzikowska E, et al. Everolimus for angiomyolipoma associated with tuberous sclerosis complex or sporadic lymphangioleiomyomatosis (EXIST-2): a multicentre, randomised, double-blind, placebo-controlled trial. *Lancet*. 2013;381(9869):817–824. https://doi.org/10.1016/S0140-6736(12)61767-X.
63. Bissler JJ, Kingswood JC, Radzikowska E, et al. Everolimus long-term use in patients with tuberous sclerosis complex: four-year update of the EXIST-2 study. *PLoS One*. 2017;12(8):e0180939. https://doi.org/10.1371/journal.pone.0180939.
64. Dabora SL, Jozwiak S, Franz DN, et al. Mutational analysis in a cohort of 224 tuberous sclerosis patients indicates increased severity of TSC2, compared with TSC1, disease in multiple organs. *Am J Hum Genet*. 2001;68(1):64–80. https://doi.org/10.1086/316951.
65. Ng KH, Ng SM, Parker A. Annual review of children with tuberous sclerosis. *Arch Dis Child Educ Pract Ed*. 2015;100(3):114–121. https://doi.org/10.1136/archdischild-2013-304948.
66. Harding CO, Pagon RA. Incidence of tuberous sclerosis in patients with cardiac rhabdomyoma. *Am J Med Genet*. 1990;37(4):443–446. https://doi.org/10.1002/ajmg.1320370402.
67. Beghetti M, Gow RM, Haney I, Mawson J, Williams WG, Freedom RM. Pediatric primary benign cardiac tumors: a 15-year review. *Am Heart J*. 1997;134(6):1107–1114.
68. Sciacca P, Giacchi V, Mattia C, et al. Rhabdomyomas and tuberous sclerosis complex: our experience in 33 cases. *BMC Cardiovasc Disord*. 2014;14(1):66. https://doi.org/10.1186/1471-2261-14-66.
69. Johnson SR, Cordier JF, Lazor R, et al. European Respiratory Society guidelines for the diagnosis and management of lymphangioleiomyomatosis. *Eur Respir J*. 2010;35(1):14–26. https://doi.org/10.1183/09031936.00076209.
70. Cudzilo CJ, Szczesniak RD, Brody AS, et al. Lymphangioleiomyomatosis screening in women with tuberous sclerosis. *Chest*. 2013;144(2):578–585. https://doi.org/10.1378/chest.12-2813.
71. Adriaensen MEAPM, Schaefer-Prokop CM, Duyndam DAC, Zonnenberg BA, Prokop M. Radiological evidence of lymphangioleiomyomatosis in female and male patients with tuberous sclerosis complex. *Clin Radiol*. 2011;66(7):625–628. https://doi.org/10.1016/j.crad.2011.02.009.
72. Moss J, Avila NA, Barnes PM, et al. Prevalence and clinical characteristics of lymphangioleiomyomatosis (LAM) in patients with tuberous sclerosis complex. *Am J Respir Crit Care Med*. 2001;164(4):669–671. https://doi.org/10.1164/ajrccm.164.4.2101154.
73. McCormack FX, Gupta N, Finlay GR, et al. Official American Thoracic Society/Japanese Respiratory Society Clinical Practice Guidelines: lymphangioleiomyomatosis diagnosis and management. *Am J Respir Crit Care Med*. 2016;194(6):748–761. https://doi.org/10.1164/rccm.201607-1384ST.
74. Goldberg HJ, Harari S, Cottin V, et al. Everolimus for the treatment of lymphangioleiomyomatosis: a phase II study. *Eur Respir J*. 2015;46(3):783–794. https://doi.org/10.1183/09031936.00210714.
75. Curatolo P, Franz DN, Lawson JA, et al. Adjunctive everolimus for children and adolescents with treatment-refractory seizures associated with tuberous sclerosis complex: post-hoc analysis of the phase 3 EXIST-3 trial. *Lancet Child Adolesc Health*. 2018;2(7):495–504. https://doi.org/10.1016/S2352-4642(18)30099-3.

76. Franz DN, Budde K, Kingswood JC, et al. Effect of everolimus on skin lesions in patients treated for subependymal giant cell astrocytoma and renal angiomyolipoma: final 4-year results from the randomized EXIST-1 and EXIST-2 studies. *J Eur Acad Dermatol Venereol*. 2018;32(10):1796–1803. https://doi.org/10.1111/jdv.14964.

77. Davies M, Saxena A, Kingswood JC. Management of everolimus-associated adverse events in patients with tuberous sclerosis complex: a practical guide. *Orphanet J Rare Dis*. 2017;12(1):35. https://doi.org/10.1186/s13023-017-0581-9.

Chapter 18

Approach to von Hippel Lindau, Cowden disease, and other inherited conditions

Sapna Pathak, Thuy M. Vu, and Roy E. Strowd, III

CHAPTER OUTLINE

Introduction

Although neurofibromatosis and tuberous sclerosis comprise some of the most common inherited tumor syndromes in neuro-oncology, clinicians will encounter patients with other, less common syndromes who could present with a range of neurologic and extranervous manifestations of their disease. Awareness of these syndromes, understanding of the common neurological manifestations, and familiarity of the associated nonnervous features will aid the clinician in evaluating, managing, and counseling patients with these conditions.

In this chapter, we review several of the less common but clinically relevant inherited syndromes for which brain or spinal cord lesions are a common feature including von Hippel Lindau syndrome (vHL), Cowden syndrome, Li-Fraumeni syndrome, and Lynch syndrome.

Clinical cases

CASE 18.1 VON HIPPEL LINDAU DISEASE

Case. An adult female presents on referral for gait instability. She was diagnosed with vHL disease as a teenager. Her mother also had vHL but she has no other siblings with the disease. She has multiple hemangioblastomas of the central nervous system (CNS) including both the brain and spinal cord. Over the years, she has undergone multiple craniotomies including suboccipital craniotomy and spinal laminectomies, as well as Gamma Knife stereotactic radiation treatments, for management of these hemangioblastomas. In addition, she has had renal lesions and undergone bilateral radiofrequency ablations for multiple renal cell carcinomas. Several years ago she was found to have an enlarging pancreatic cyst that required a distal pancreatectomy and splenectomy. She is blind in the right eye due to complications from a retinal hemangioblastoma. After spinal surgery for tumor resection at T11 1 year ago, she reports that she has never regained full feeling in her legs and has persistent gait imbalance, near falls, and reduced sensation in her lower extremities. Imaging of her cerebellar and spinal cord shows stable residual hemangioblastomas without fourth ventricular compression or evidence of radiographic progression.

Teaching Points. vHL is tumor-predisposition syndrome characterized by neoplasms of the nervous system, kidneys, and other organs. This case highlights a number of key features of vHL including the (1) neurological manifestations which include hemangioblastomas of the cerebellum, spinal cord, and retina; (2) that management of vHL-associated tumors requires coordination across a multidisciplinary treatment team; and (3) that neurological complications of these tumors and their treatment contribute to patient morbidity.

Cerebellar, spinal, and retinal hemangioblastomas are the most common nervous system manifestations. Extranervous features including renal cysts, clear-cell renal cell carcinoma (RCC), pheochromocytoma, endolymphatic sac tumors, epididymal cystadenomas, and broad ligament cystadenomas. Cerebellar hemangioblastomas are benign, slow-growing, highly vascular, cystic WHO grade I neoplasms. They rarely occur sporadically, and approximately 30% of patients who present with such a lesion will have vHL. In vHL, cerebellar hemangioblastomas tend to be multiple and present at a younger age (mean age 33 years) compared to sporadic cerebellar hemangioblastomas (mean age 43 years).

As in this case, management of vHL-associated tumors is best conducted by a multidisciplinary team familiar with this condition including a neurosurgeon, radiation oncologist, geneticist, urologist, gastrointestinal or general surgeon, and ophthalmologist among others. When CNS lesions are symptomatic or growing rapidly, surgery is the treatment of choice. Lesions that cannot be completely resected or are not amenable to surgery are often treated with radiation therapy. Research on the efficacy of nonsurgical interventions such as systemic therapy (e.g., vascular endothelial growth factor [VEGF] and fibroblast growth factor receptor inhibitors) is promising; however, these treatments are not currently approved for use.[1,2]

Neurological complications of these tumors and their treatment are not uncommon and may include symptoms arising from (1) direct compression of the tumor on surrounding structures (e.g., myelopathy, cerebellar dysfunction, increased intracranial pressure, or vision loss), (2) side effects of treatment (e.g., stroke, intracranial hemorrhage, CNS infection), or (3) a combination of these. Fortunately, the risk of spontaneous intracranial hemorrhage from the cerebellar tumor is low.

Von Hippel Lindau Disease. vHL is an autosomal dominant tumor syndrome affecting 1 in 31,000 live births. Patients are predisposed to multiorgan cystic and neoplastic lesions of the kidneys, spinal, cerebellum, and other organs. Both benign and malignant tumors may occur. The *VHL* gene is a tumor suppressor gene located on chromosome 3p25. This gene encodes the von Hippel Lindau protein (pVHL), which is a chaperone protein that ushers two important cytoplasmic transcription factors, hypoxia-inducible factors 1 alpha and 2 alpha (HIF1a and HIF2a) to the proteasome for degradation. HIF1a and HIF2a participate in the cellular response to hypoxia. When active, they increase expression of genes involved in cell proliferation and angiogenesis including transforming growth factor (TGF)-alpha, VEGF, and platelet-derived growth factor (PDGF)-beta.[3–5] HIF1a and HIF2a also play an important role in erythropoietin (EPO) regulation. In vHL patients, loss of pVHL results in the inability to degrade HIF1a and HIF2a, which leads to activation of pro-growth pathways and tumor formation.

Neurologic Manifestations

Hemangioblastomas are the most common tumor in patients with vHL and are seen in 60–84% of cases.[6] These are benign, highly vascular tumors that do not metastasize or invade surrounding tissue. On neuroimaging, they appear as cystic enhancing lesions often with a cyst with mural nodule appearance on T1-weighted gadolinium enhanced sequences (Fig. 18.1A). Tumors are frequently scattered throughout the cerebellar cortex. In the spine, spinal hemangioblastomas avidly enhance but may lack a clear cystic component (Fig. 18.1B). These lesions can hemorrhage or compress neighboring structures resulting in morbidity and rarely mortality. Although they commonly occur in the cerebellum and spinal cord, clinicians should be aware that they may also develop in the retina and contribute to vision loss.

Retinal capillary hemangioblastomas in vHL are often multiple, bilateral, and can cause vision impairment or blindness due to retinal traction and/or detachment, retinal edema, and glaucoma.[7] They are present in up to 70% of vHL patients by age 60 years. Because of the high prevalence, any patient presenting with a retinal capillary hemangioblastoma should receive genetic testing for vHL germline mutations, and patients with vHL should undergo routine ophthalmologic examination for surveillance. First-line treatment for these lesions includes laser photocoagulation and cryotherapy. Typically, these lesions require only one treatment, as the success rate is approximately 70%.[8] Other treatment options include photodynamic therapy, external beam radiotherapy, and surgical resection.

Evaluation of hemangioblastomas is best conducted by a team familiar with this syndrome. Studies have shown that about half of hemangioblastomas do not grow during a patient's lifetime and can be observed with surveillance imaging. Asymptomatic patients are often followed clinically and with brain MRI with and without contrast every 2–3 years. In the remaining patients, growth can be step-wise, linearly, or exponential, and thus monitoring with imaging is important to determine the growth trajectory to guide treatment decisions.[9]

Extraneurologic Manifestations

Renal cell carcinoma (usually clear-cell tumors) and renal cysts occur in approximately two-thirds of patients with vHL disease. One study demonstrated that 69% of vHL patients who were at least 60 years old had developed RCC, with a mean age of onset of 44 years.[6] RCC often occurs bilaterally with multiple lesions as for the patient in this case (Fig. 18.1C, D). RCC may occur alongside benign renal cysts or develop from malignant transformation of atypical cells within a renal cyst. The management of RCC in patients with vHL disease focuses on nephron-sparing therapies that aim at maintaining as much healthy renal parenchyma as possible. These include observation, partial nephrectomy, cryotherapy, and radiofrequency ablation which are more conservative than the historic standard of care—radical nephrectomy.[10,11] Several systemic approaches, such as anti-VEGF and anti-angiogenic therapies (e.g., axitinib, cabozantinib, sorafenib, sunitinib, and pazopanib), have utility in metastatic disease, as well as in tumors that are not amenable to surgical resection.

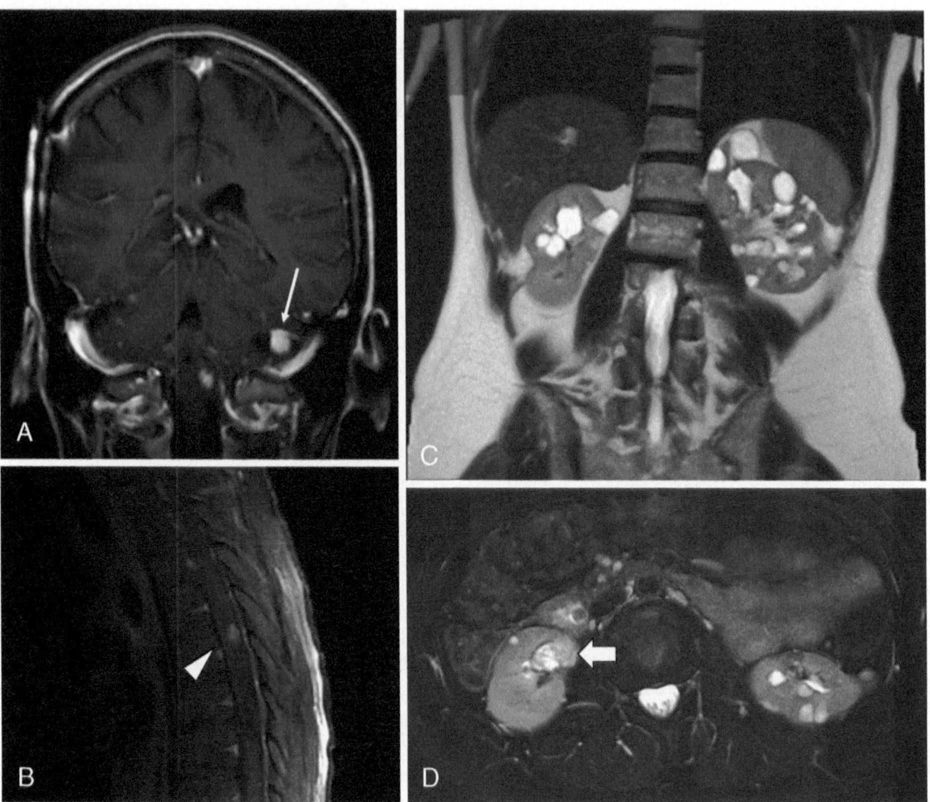

Fig. 18.1 Imaging findings in patients with von Hippel Lindau. (A) T1-weighted gadolinium enhanced MRI with several scattered homogeneously enhancing lesions with surrounding cyst *(white arrow)* consistent with a cyst with mural nodule lesion consistent with cerebellar hemangioblastoma alongside with an enhancing medullary lesion. (B) T1-weighted gadolinium enhanced MRI of the spine showing an enhancing thoracic spine lesion *(arrowhead)* consistent with a spinal cord hemangioblastoma. (C) T2-weighted MR of the kidneys showing numerous renal cysts; and (D) an irregular appearing lesion with bulbous outgrowth in the right upper renal pole *(large white arrow)* concerning for renal cell carcinoma that was subsequently ablated.

Pheochromocytomas occur either sporadically or as a part of a genetic tumor syndrome such as vHL, multiple endocrine neoplasia type 2 (MEN2), and neurofibromatosis type 1 (NF1). Patients with vHL disease who develop pheochromocytomas are usually younger in age and less likely to manifest typical symptoms of catecholamine production (e.g., hypertension, tachycardia, diaphoresis, headaches).[12,13] Measures of plasma and/or urine metanephrines and normetanephrines can aid in the diagnosis. NF1 patients may have higher normetanephrine-to-metanephrine ratio compared to patients with sporadic pheochromocytomas.[14] Management involves resection of the tumor; however, it is essential that alpha-blockers are given prior to surgery, as unopposed alpha receptor stimulation can lead to significant vasoconstriction and even death.

Pancreatic tumors, cysts, and neuroendocrine tumors are common in up to 77% of patients with vHL disease.[15] Pancreatic cysts and serous cystadenomas can either be asymptomatic or present with epigastric pain, change in stools, or abdominal discomfort.[16] Patients with vHL disease have *not* been found to be at increased risk of pancreatic adenocarcinoma. Pancreatic neuroendocrine tumors such as VIPomas (vasoactive intestinal peptide tumors) and insulinomas may produce symptoms such as diarrhea and hypoglycemia. Typically, management involves surgical resection.

Other nonneurologic manifestations of VHL disease include endolymphatic tumors of the middle ear and papillary cystadenomas of the epididymis and broad ligament.

Diagnosis

Diagnosis of vHL is made clinically and often supported by genetic testing. Patients with a first-degree family member with vHL disease or those who have manifestations of at least one vHL-associated tumor should undergo genetic testing for the *VHL* gene. Next-generation sequencing (NGS) has become one of the mainstays of genetic testing for vHL, as well as for many other genetic tumor syndromes. Clinical criteria have been defined (Table 18.1). Patients fulfill clinical criteria for a diagnosis of VHL if one of the following are met:

1. For patients *with* a family history of VHL
   a. One CNS hemangioblastoma OR pheochromocytoma OR clear-cell renal carcinoma
2. For patients *without* a family history of VHL
   a. Two or more CNS hemangioblastomas or one CNS hemangioblastoma and a visceral tumor (excluding epididymal or renal cysts)

Somatic mosaicism, which describes a mutation that occurs *after* fertilization and during embryogenesis, should be considered in patients who present with vHL-associated tumors but have negative genetic tests.

Management

For patients newly diagnosed with vHL, genetic counseling is essential. Although the *VHL* gene followed an autosomal dominant inheritance, sporadic de novo mutations occur as in neurofibromatosis and tuberous sclerosis. All patients with a CNS or retinal hemangioblastoma should be tested for *VHL* germline mutation. Routine screening with MRI of the brain and spinal cord with and without contrast should be performed in patients with vHL disease who are older than 8 years of age. Neuroimaging is typically performed every 1–3 years depending on growth trajectory. Screening for RCC in patients with vHL disease should start at age 10 years.

Table 18.1 Clinical Criteria for von Hippel Lindau Disease

Clinical diagnostic criteria for von Hippel Lindau disease (vHL)
1. Any blood relative of a person diagnosed with vHL disease who has a: a. Central nervous system (CNS) hemangioblastoma OR b. Pheochromocytoma OR c. Clear-cell renal cell carcinoma (RCC)
2. Any person without a family history of vHL who has two vHL-associated tumors including: a. Hemangioblastoma b. RCC c. Pheochromocytoma d. Endolymphatic sac tumor of the middle ear e. Epididymal or adnexal papillary cystadenoma f. Pancreatic cystadenoma g. Pancreatic neuroendocrine tumor
Patients who should undergo genetic testing for vHL
1. Any person with one or more of the following: a. CNS hemangioblastoma b. Pheochromocytoma or paraganglioma c. Endolymphatic sac tumor d. Epididymal papillary cystadenoma
2. Any person with: a. Clear-cell RCC diagnosed <40 years old b. RCC that is bilateral or has multiple lesions c. >1 pancreatic serous cystadenoma d. >1 pancreatic neuroendocrine tumor e. Multiple pancreatic cysts AND any other vHL-associated lesion

For patients with a family history of vHL, a clinical diagnosis of vHL can be made if the patient has one CNS hemangioblastoma OR pheochromocytoma OR clear-cell renal carcinoma. For patients without a family history of vHL, a clinical diagnosis of vHL can be made if the patient has two or more CNS hemangioblastomas or one CNS hemangioblastoma and a visceral tumor (excluding epididymal or renal cysts).

CASE 18.2 COWDEN SYNDROME

Case. A healthy woman presents for evaluation of 1 year of progressively worsening headaches. She was initially diagnosed with a ganglioneuroblastoma of the spine and base of the brain as a child and treated with chemotherapy. Later, she was found to have a thyroid goiter and diagnosed with Graves disease, for which she underwent a thyroidectomy. Additional cancers include prior diagnosis of endometrial cancer, for which she underwent a total abdominal hysterectomy and bilateral salpingo-oophorectomy. About 1 month ago she underwent a colonoscopy for abdominal pain and was found to have multiple polyps in the proximal transverse colon. Biopsy was negative for adenomatous epithelium. There is a strong family history of early-onset cancer, including breast cancer in her mother and grandmother and colon cancer in an uncle, all prior to age 40 years. She was recently referred to genetic counseling and underwent genetic testing showing a pathogenic mutation in the PTEN gene, and she was diagnosed with Cowden syndrome/PTEN hamartoma tumor syndrome. Following evaluation, the patient was referred for brain MRI with and without contrast, which revealed a hyperintense lesion on T2-weighted and fluid-attenuated inversion recovery (FLAIR) sequences that was consistent with a dysplastic gangliocytoma of the cerebellum.

Teaching Points. Cowden syndrome is a rare autosomal dominant disorder affecting 1 in 250,000 live births.[17] The syndrome results from germline mutation in the phosphatase and tensin homolog (*PTEN*) gene on chromosome 10 (10q22-23). This case highlights several important principles for clinicians who encounter patients with Cowden syndrome including: (1) the importance of being familiar with tumors associated with this syndrome so that prompt genetic counseling referral can be made, and (2) the association with dysplastic gangliocytoma of the cerebellum.

Cowden syndrome is associated with a variety of benign and malignant tumors. Neurologic manifestations in Cowden syndrome frequently include benign CNS tumors such as men-

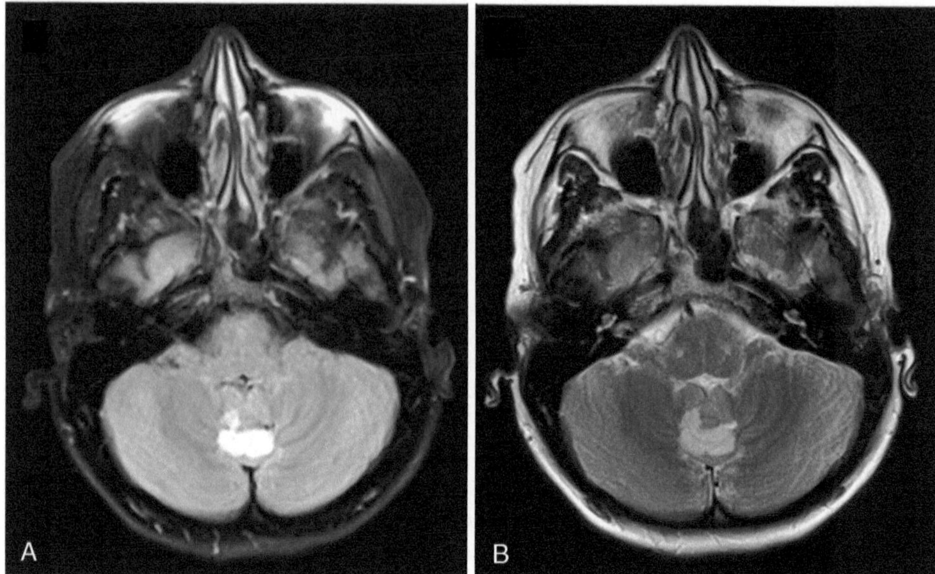

Fig. 18.2 Imaging findings in an atypical case of Lhermite-Duclos disease (LDD). MRI showing a fluid-attenuated inversion recovery sequence (A) and a T2-weighted sequence (B) with a hyperintense lesion in the cerebellar vermis that was resected and consistent with dysplastic gangliocytoma of the cerebellum in this patient with Cowden syndrome. Typically, these lesions occur within the folia of the lateral cerebellar cortex.

ingiomas, macrocephaly, heterotopias, vascular abnormalities, and developmental delay. Extranervous manifestations include tumors of the skin and mucous membranes, breast, thyroid, genitourinary tract, gastrointestinal tract (including tumors and polyps in the stomach and colon), and defects in immune function.

The most common CNS neoplasm is the dysplastic gangliocytoma of the cerebellum which, when present, is known as *Lhermitte-Duclos disease* (LDD). In adults, LDD is pathognomonic for Cowden syndrome. LDD is characterized by the presence of benign, slow-growing hamartomatous enlargement of the cerebellar folia. The majority of patients present with slowly progressive cerebellar ataxia, elevated intracranial pressure due to fourth ventricular compression, or headache, as was present in this patient's case. Imaging shows nonenhancing enlargement of the cerebellar cortex that often has a striated or tiger-striped appearance on T2-weighted imaging sequences. Given the progressive nature of this lesion, asymptomatic patients should be followed with serial imaging. Symptomatic patients are considered for surgical resection. Radiotherapy is often delayed until recurrence.

Overview

Like the other inherited syndromes reviewed here, Cowden syndrome follows an autosomal dominant pattern of inheritance, though sporadic mutations occur up to one-third of cases.[18] The *PTEN* protein is an important tumor suppressor in the PI3-K-AKT-mTOR cell proliferation pathway. Patients may present at any age with symptoms of tumor growth from nearly any organ system.

Neurologic Manifestations

The prototypical CNS manifestation is the dysplastic cerebellar gangliocytoma that occurs in up to 32% of patients with Cowden syndrome and indicates a diagnosis of LDD.[19] Although typically occurring in the cerebellar folia, tumors can rarely occur within the cerebellar vermis (Fig. 18.2) and appear as nonenhancing hyperintense lesions on T2-weighted and FLAIR sequences. Other brain tumors have also been reported including gliomas and meningiomas; however, in many cases it is unclear whether this is a sequelae of the disease or a coincidental finding.[20,21] In about one-third of patients, venous and cavernous angiomas are observed, though they are rarely symptomatic and often discovered incidentally on surveillance neuroimaging.[21]

Macrocephaly, which is defined as a head circumference that exceeds the 98th percentile for a chronological age, sex, and gestational age, has been reported in 21–38% of patients with Cowden syndrome.[22] Often macrocephaly occurs in combination with symptoms of autism and developmental delay.

Extraneurologic Manifestations

Mucocutaneous lesions are some of the most common clinical manifestations of the disease and include trichilemmomas (benign tumors found on hair follicles or other skin surfaces of the face and neck), facial/oral papules, and acral keratoses (commonly seen on the feet, hands, and wrists). Many of these mucocutaneous findings are also characteristic of other genetic syndromes such as NF1, tuberous sclerosis, Gardner syndrome, and Brooke-Spiegler syndrome; thus, it is important to differentiate the underlying disease process through identification of other clinical manifestations and genetic testing.[23]

Breast cancer is the most common malignancy reported in patients with Cowden syndrome.[24] Mean age at diagnosis is 38–46 years, with this cancer following a more aggressive course than for breast cancer patients in the general population.[25] *Thyroid disease*, which includes both benign (i.e., adenomas, Hashimoto thyroiditis, multinodular goiters) and malignant conditions (i.e., papillary and follicular thyroid cancer), are seen in about one-half of patients.[26] *Genitourinary cancers*, such as endometrial cancer and RCC occur at increased frequency in Cowden syndrome patients.[27] Bilateral lipomatosis of the testes, which is benign, has also been reported. Four main *gastrointestinal manifestations* occur in Cowden syndrome including: (1) esophageal glycogen acanthosis, (2) gastric and duodenal polyps, (3) colonic polyps, and (4) colorectal cancer. Patients are also predisposed to a higher prevalence of immune dysregulation.

Diagnosis

Genetic testing is useful in the diagnosis of Cowden syndrome. The clinical diagnosis requires at least three major clinical criteria including one which must be a neurologic manifestation or two major *and* three minor criteria (Table 18.2).

Management

Cowden syndrome affects multiple organ systems to varying degrees, so it is important to have a multidisciplinary approach to management and treatment, including genetic counseling for families. Cancer surveillance is extremely important. Specific recommendations regarding cancer screening include annual breast and thyroid examinations, annual thyroid ultrasound starting at the time of diagnosis, and colonoscopy every 5 years starting at age 35 (or earlier if suspicious lesions are detected). In selected patients, renal ultrasound, annual dermatologic examinations, and/or brain MRI can be performed based on clinical symptoms. For women with Cowden syndrome, annual screening mammography and breast MRI can be considered starting at age 35 (or 5–10 years before a family member was diagnosed), as well as annual transvaginal ultrasound and/or endometrial biopsies.

Treatment of the benign and malignant tumors is typically similar to those in sporadically occurring patients. Tumors that are routinely surgically resected include gangliocytomas of the cerebellum to prevent development of hydrocephalus and GI polyps to avoid progression to cancer. For cerebellar gangliocytomas, complete resection is often not possible given the indistinct margins. Given the slowly progressive nature, these lesions are typically observed with surveillance neuroimaging annually. Systemic therapies that target cell cycle dysregulation and gene mutations are being studied; however, currently these are not routinely used for treatment.

Table 18.2 Clinical Criteria for Cowden Syndrome

Major criteria	Minor criteria
Macrocephaly	Mental retardation (IQ ≤75)
Lhermitte-Duclos disease in an adult	Autism spectrum disorder
At least three gastrointestinal hamartomas	Colon cancer
Breast cancer	At least three esophageal glycogenic acanthosis
Follicular thyroid cancer	At least three lipomas
Endometrial cancer	Papillary (or follicular variant of papillary) thyroid cancer
Hyperpigmentation of the glans penis	Benign thyroid disease
Multiple mucocutaneous lesions (including but not limited to at least three trichilemmomas, oral papillomas, mucocutaneous neuromas, or acral keratoses)	Renal cell carcinoma
	Testicular lipomatosis
	Intracranial vascular abnormalities

CASE 18.3 LI-FRAUMENI SYNDROME

Case. A young woman was referred from her primary physician for consideration of brain MRI due to a strong family history of cancer, including brain tumors. The patient's child died from a sarcoma at age 2 years. One sibling died from breast cancer in her twenties and another died from complications of a malignant brain tumor and a sarcoma. The patient's mother along with three other second-degree relatives were diagnosed with breast cancer prior to age 35 years. Other maternal relatives died of lung cancer prior to age 40 years, leukemia prior to age 30 years, and colon cancer prior to age 40 years. The patient reported a mild headache, which had previously been attributed to sinus headaches or allergies. She had no other neurological symptoms. Referral to genetic counseling had been placed previously and when blood testing revealed a germline mutation in *TP53*, she was referred for consideration of neuroimaging.

Teaching Points. Li-Fraumeni is a rare autosomal dominant disease that results from inactivating mutation in the *TP53* gene, which predisposes patients to a wide array of neoplasms including breast cancer, osteosarcoma, soft tissue sarcomas, leukemia, adrenal cortex tumors, and brain tumors. This case highlights the role of neurological evaluation for these patients and the controversy regarding surveillance neuroimaging.

CNS neoplasms occur in approximately 10% of patients with Li-Fraumeni syndrome prior to the age of 45 years. These include supratentorial tumors, neuroectodermal tumors, choroid plexus carcinomas, and medulloblastoma. Management is similar to those that occur with sporadic CNS tumors including surgery, radiation, chemotherapy, or a combination. Surveillance imaging is controversial given that the majority of these tumors do not exist in situ prior to detection and are not slow growing to allow sufficient lag time for imaging detection.

Overview

Li-Fraumeni syndrome is estimated to affect 1 in 10,000 to 1 in 25,000 individuals worldwide. The lifetime cancer risk in patients born with a mutated *TP53* is extremely high, nearing 100% in women[28,29] and 73% in men.[30] Studies have demonstrated that once an affected individual develops one type of malignancy, his/her risk of developing a second malignancy substantially increases compared to the general population. In one study of 200 Li-Fraumeni syndrome patients, 57% had developed a second malignancy within 30 years of their initial cancer diagnosis.[31]

Neurologic Manifestations

High-grade gliomas and medulloblastomas, along with various other brain tumors, including choroid plexus carcinomas, have been associated with Li-Fraumeni syndrome.[32,33] Patients are often diagnosed at a younger age than those in the general population.

Extraneurologic Manifestations

The most common tumor seen in Li-Fraumeni syndrome is a **sarcoma**, which accounts for 25% of all tumors in these patients. The median age of diagnosis is 15 years,[34] which is significantly different than with spontaneously occurring sarcomas. Osteosarcomas are common as well as rhabdomyosarcomas, which are typically seen in children less than 5 years old. Compared to the general population, women are more likely to develop **breast cancer**, which often occurs at an earlier age (median age of diagnosis is 30–33 years).[32] **Adrenocortical carcinoma** is a rare malignancy with an incidence of 0.5–2 cases per million individuals each year, which is also more common in patients with Li-Fraumeni syndrome. Diagnosis and Management

Genetic testing for the *TP53* mutation is currently the most definitive diagnostic tool available. Patients should be screened if they have the following:

- A sarcoma diagnosed before age 45 AND
- A first-degree family member with any malignancy diagnosed before age 45 AND
- A first- or second-degree family member with any malignancy diagnosed before age 45 or a sarcoma during his/her lifetime

Routine cancer screening is of paramount importance for patients with Li-Fraumeni syndrome. When cancers occur, the management is largely the same as those in the general population with the exception of breast cancer. Due to the risk of developing a second breast cancer, mastectomy plus radiation therapy is often favored over lumpectomy.

CASE 18.4 LYNCH SYNDROME

Case. A young female with a family history of Lynch syndrome presented with headaches, nausea, anorexia, weight loss, altered mental status, and focal seizure. Imaging revealed a ring-enhancing lesion in the right parietal lobe with surrounding cerebral edema concerning for high-grade glioma. She underwent a gross total resection, and pathology was read as glioblastoma, WHO grade IV. Family history was notable for several family members with early onset cancer, including four family members with colon cancer occurring before age 40 years. One family member had previously undergone genetic testing that had revealed germline mutation in the *MLH1* mismatch repair (MMR) gene consistent with a family history of Lynch syndrome.

Teaching Points. This case highlights the association genetic link between colorectal cancer and brain tumors in patients with MMR gene mutation. This has been termed Lynch syndrome (e.g., hereditary nonpolyposis colorectal cancer syndrome) and is a multitumor syndrome caused by germline mutation in DNA MMR genes *MLH1*, *MSH2*, *MSH6*, and *PMS2*. Lynch syndrome is characterized by a significantly increased risk of colorectal and endometrial cancer along with a fourfold higher risk of brain tumors, primarily glioblastoma, as in this case. As in this case, patients with a strong family history of early onset colorectal cancer and childhood-onset glioblastoma should be referred for genetic counseling evaluation to consider MMR deficiency syndrome.

Lynch Syndrome and MMR Deficiency Syndromes

Lynch syndrome is characterized by the predisposition to colorectal and endometrial cancers as well as a number of other tumors including gastric, ovarian, breast, sarcoma, and brain tumors, primarily glioblastoma and medulloblastoma. Historically, several Lynch syndrome variants have also been described, including Turcot syndrome, Muir-Torre syndrome, and constitutional MMR deficiency syndrome. Turcot syndrome refers to individuals with a pathogenic variant in one of the MMR genes and presentation with colorectal cancer and a CNS astrocytoma. Muir-Torre syndrome is primarily linked to mutations in *MSH2* gene and presents with sebaceous skin tumors, glioblastoma, and Lynch syndrome tumors. Constitutional MMR deficiency (e.g., bi-allelic MMR deficiency syndrome) is a unique variant in which individuals are homozygous for the pathogenic variant in an MMR gene often reported as a result of consanguinity. Children with this variant present with hematologic malignancies, brain tumors, colorectal cancer, and intestinal polyps in childhood.

Neurologic Manifestations

Primary CNS tumors are identified in approximately 1–14% of patients with Lynch syndrome. The median age of onset is nearly 10 years younger than that of sporadic CNS tumors. Mutations in the *MSH2* gene are most common, followed by *MLH1*, *MSH6*, and *PMS2*. Glioblastoma is the most frequent histologic type of CNS tumor, though diffuse astrocytomas, oligodendrogliomas, and medulloblastomas may occur. The presence of colorectal cancer can precede or occur simultaneous to the brain tumor diagnosis.

Diagnosis and Management

A diagnosis of Lynch syndrome should be considered in an individual presenting with one or more of the following:

- Colorectal or endometrial cancer diagnosed before age 50 years
- Synchronous or metachronous Lynch syndrome–related cancers (e.g., colorectal, endometrial, gastric, small intestinal, hepatobiliary, renal, ureteral, brain)
- Colorectal or endometrial tumor tissue with microsatellite instability (MSI)-high histology or loss of expression of one or more MMR gene products
- First-degree relative with any Lynch syndrome–related cancer diagnosed before age 50 years or two first-degree relatives with any Lynch syndrome–related cancer at any age

Gene testing is the diagnostic method of choice by identifying a heterozygous germline pathogenic variant in one of the MMR genes *MLH1*, *MSH2*, *MSH6*, *PMS2*, or *EPCAM*. Patients with an established diagnosis are at increased risk for colorectal (50–80% lifetime risk), endometrial (40–60% risk), gastric (7–10%), ovarian (5–8%), urinary (2–5%), small bowel (1–4%), pancreas (1%), and brain cancers (1–14%). Cancer surveillance is vital and should include colonoscopy every 1–2 years in addition to other routine cancer screening. Surveillance imaging for brain tumors is not typically performed in asymptomatic individuals.

Like the other syndromes discussed in this chapter, management typically follows guidelines similar to that for sporadically occurring tumors. However, growing evidence indicates that tumors harboring MMR defects are associated with increased density of tumor infiltrating lymphocytes and may be more amenable to immune-mediated elimination with immunotherapy. Ongoing studies will define the role of early targeted and immunotherapy approaches to these cancers.

Conclusion

Although the most common inherited tumor syndromes associated with brain tumors are neurofibromatosis and tuberous sclerosis, other rare genetic syndromes also contribute to an increased risk of brain tumor formation. A familiarity with these syndromes and with the neurological and extranervous manifestations can help in guiding individuals to genetic counseling, advise on appropriate surveillance imaging, and support management of tumors and their complications. Clinicians should be aware of these rare but important inherited syndromes when evaluating patients in neuro-oncology.

References

1. Jonasch E, McCutcheon IE, Waguespack SG, et al. Pilot trial of sunitinib therapy in patients with von Hippel-Lindau disease. *Ann Oncol*. 2011;22(12):2661–2666.
2. Kim BY, Jonasch E, McCutcheon IE. Pazopanib therapy for cerebellar hemangioblastomas in von Hippel-Lindau disease: case report. *Target Oncol*. 2012;7(2):145–149.
3. Kim WY, Kaelin WG. Role of VHL gene mutation in human cancer. *J Clin Oncol*. 2004;22(24):4991–5004.
4. Sufan RI, Jewett MA, Ohh M. The role of von Hippel-Lindau tumor suppressor protein and hypoxia in renal clear cell carcinoma. *Am J Physiol Renal Physiol*. 2004;287(1):F1–F6.
5. Barry RE, Krek W. The von Hippel-Lindau tumour suppressor: a multi-faceted inhibitor of tumourigenesis. *Trends Mol Med*. 2004;10(9):466–472.
6. Maher ER, Yates JR, Harries R, et al. Clinical features and natural history of von Hippel-Lindau disease. *Q J Med*. 1990;77(283):1151–1163.
7. Singh AD, Shields CL, Shields JA. von Hippel-Lindau disease. *Surv Ophthalmol*. 2001;46(2):117–142.
8. Singh AD, Nouri M, Shields CL, Shields JA, Perez N. Treatment of retinal capillary hemangioma. *Ophthalmology*. 2002;109(10):1799–1806.
9. Lonser RR, Butman JA, Huntoon K, et al. Prospective natural history study of central nervous system hemangioblastomas in von Hippel-Lindau disease. *J Neurosurg*. 2014;120(5):1055–1062.
10. Steinbach F, Novick AC, Zincke H, et al. Treatment of renal cell carcinoma in von Hippel-Lindau disease: a multicenter study. *J Urol*. 1995;153:1812–1816.
11. Bratslavsky G, Liu JJ, Johnson AD, et al. Salvage partial nephrectomy for hereditary renal cancer: feasibility and outcomes. *J Urol*. 2008;179:67–70.
12. Eisenhofer G, Walther MM, Huynh TT, et al. Pheochromocytomas in von Hippel-Lindau syndrome and multiple endocrine neoplasia type 2 display distinct biochemical and clinical phenotypes. *J Clin Endocrinol Metab*. 2001;86:1999–2008.
13. Walther MM, Reiter R, Keiser HR, et al. Clinical and genetic characterization of pheochromocytoma in von Hippel-Lindau families: comparison with sporadic pheochromocytoma gives insight into natural history of pheochromocytoma. *J Urol*. 1999;162:659–664.
14. Eisenhofer G, Lenders JW, Linehan WM, Walther MM, Goldstein DS, Keiser HR. Plasma normetanephrine and metanephrine for detecting pheochromocytoma in von Hippel-Lindau disease and multiple endocrine neoplasia type 2. *N Engl J Med*. 1999;340:1872–1879.
15. Hammel PR, Vilgrain V, Terris B, et al. Pancreatic involvement in von Hippel-Lindau disease. The Groupe Francophone d'Etude de la Maladie de von Hippel-Lindau. *Gastroenterology*. 2000;119:1087–1095.
16. Neumann HP, Dinkel E, Brambs H, et al. Pancreatic lesions in the von Hippel-Lindau syndrome. *Gastroenterology*. 1991;101:465–471.
17. Nelen MR, Kremer H, Konings IB, et al. Novel PTEN mutations in patients with Cowden disease: absence of clear genotype-phenotype correlations. *Eur J Hum Genet*. 1999;7:267–273.
18. Mester J, Eng C. Estimate of de novo mutation frequency in probands with PTEN hamartoma tumor syndrome. *Genet Med*. 2012;14:819–822.

19. Zhou XP, Marsh DJ, Morrison CD, et al. Germline inactivation of PTEN and dysregulation of the phosphoinositol-3-kinase/Akt pathway cause human Lhermitte-Duclos disease in adults. *Am J Hum Genet*. 2003;73:1191–1198.
20. Pilarski R. Cowden syndrome: a critical review of the clinical literature. *J Genet Couns*. 2009;18:13–27.
21. Lok C, Viseux V, Avril MF, et al. Brain magnetic resonance imaging in patients with Cowden syndrome. *Medicine (Baltim)*. 2005;84:129–136.
22. Hanssen AM, Werquin H, Suys E, Fryns JP. Cowden syndrome: report of a large family with macrocephaly and increased severity of signs in subsequent generations. *Clin Genet*. 1993;44:281–286.
23. Ponti G, Nasti S, Losi L, et al. Brooke-Spiegler syndrome: report of two cases not associated with a mutation in the CYLD and PTCH tumor-suppressor genes. *J Cutan Pathol*. 2012;39:366–371.
24. FitzGerald MG, Marsh DJ, Wahrer D, et al. Germline mutations in PTEN are an infrequent cause of genetic predisposition to breast cancer. *Oncogene*. 1998;17:727–731.
25. Schrager CA, Schneider D, Gruener AC, Tsou HC, Peacocke M. Clinical and pathological features of breast disease in Cowden's syndrome: an underrecognized syndrome with an increased risk of breast cancer. *Hum Pathol*. 1998;29:47–53.
26. Hall JE, Abdollahian DJ, Sinard RJ. Thyroid disease associated with Cowden syndrome: a meta-analysis. *Head Neck*. 2013;35:1189–1194.
27. Tan MH, Mester JL, Ngeow J, Rybicki LA, Orloff MS, Eng C. Lifetime cancer risks in individuals with germline PTEN mutations. *Clin Cancer Res*. 2012;18:400–407.
28. Chompret A, Brugières L, Ronsin M, et al. P53 germline mutations in childhood cancers and cancer risk for carrier individuals. *Br J Cancer*. 2000;82:1932–1937.
29. Mai PL, Best AF, Peters JA, et al. Risks of first and subsequent cancers among TP53 mutation carriers in the National Cancer Institute Li-Fraumeni syndrome cohort. *Cancer*. 2016;122:3673–3681.
30. Wu CC, Shete S, Amos CI, Strong LC. Joint effects of germ-line p53 mutation and sex on cancer risk in Li-Fraumeni syndrome. *Cancer Res*. 2006;66:8287–8292.
31. Hisada M, Garber JE, Fung CY, Fraumeni Jr JF, Li FP. Multiple primary cancers in families with Li-Fraumeni syndrome. *J Natl Cancer Inst*. 1998;90:606–611.
32. Olivier M, Goldgar DE, Sodha N, et al. Li-Fraumeni and related syndromes: correlation between tumor type, family structure, and TP53 genotype. *Cancer Res*. 2003;63:6643–6650.
33. Waszak SM, Northcott PA, Buchhalter I, et al. Spectrum and prevalence of genetic predisposition in medulloblastoma: a retrospective genetic study and prospective validation in a clinical trial cohort. *Lancet Oncol*. 2018;19:785–798.
34. Olivier M, Goldgar DE, Sodha N, et al. Li-Fraumeni and related syndromes: correlation between tumor type, family structure, and TP53 genotype. *Cancer Res*. 2003;63:6643–6650.

Chapter | 19 |

Neurologic complications of cancer

Andrea Wasilewski and Nimish Mohile

CHAPTER OUTLINE

Introduction to medical complications of brain tumors

Patients with brain tumors are at risk of many complications from their cancer. Complications may result from direct effects of the tumor itself due to infiltration of the brain parenchyma or mass effect, often manifesting as focal neurologic deficits. Non-focal symptoms such as headache, nausea, vomiting, and mental status changes may occur as a result of increased intracranial pressure or endocrinopathy. Brain tumors and associated cerebral edema may compress blood vessels or cerebrospinal fluid (CSF) outflow, resulting in ischemic or hemorrhagic stroke or hydrocephalus. Irritation of the cerebral cortex or cortical networks by either tumor or cerebral edema may result in tumor-associated epilepsy. Indirect effects of brain tumors occur due to disruption of neuronal networks and can present as cognitive dysfunction, memory loss, fatigue, and sleep disturbances. Additionally, patients with brain tumors are at risk for venous thromboembolic events due to hypercoagulability from their malignancy and have a high prevalence of limb paresis and limited mobility. Providers should maintain a high level of suspicion for medical complications, as these are common in brain tumor patients and require urgent evaluation and management.

When evaluating a brain tumor patient with new onset of symptoms, a detailed history and physical examination are imperative. The onset and temporal evolution of symptoms can provide valuable information to guide further workup. For example, acute onset of headache and lethargy favors intracerebral hemorrhage, whereas the same symptoms presenting as gradual worsening over several weeks may suggest obstructive hydrocephalus. In this chapter, we will discuss the presentation, evaluation, management, and treatment of common medical complications of brain tumors.

Clinical cases

CASE 19.1 DIRECT EFFECTS OF BRAIN TUMORS

Case. A 45-year-old woman with a history of glioblastoma presents to the Emergency Department with confusion and a progressively worsening headache over the past 2 weeks. She also complains of nausea and vomiting during this time. She appears to be visibly in pain. On examination, she is disoriented to time and place and has difficulty answering simple questions. Her metabolic and hematologic laboratory values are within normal limits. CT Head shows dilation of the lateral ventricles with near obstruction of the fourth ventricle, consistent with obstructive hydrocephalus. MRI Brain shows dilated ventricles with transependymal flow of cerebrospinal fluid (Fig. 19.1). Neurosurgery was emergently consulted, and an external ventricular drain was placed with rapid improvement of her symptoms.

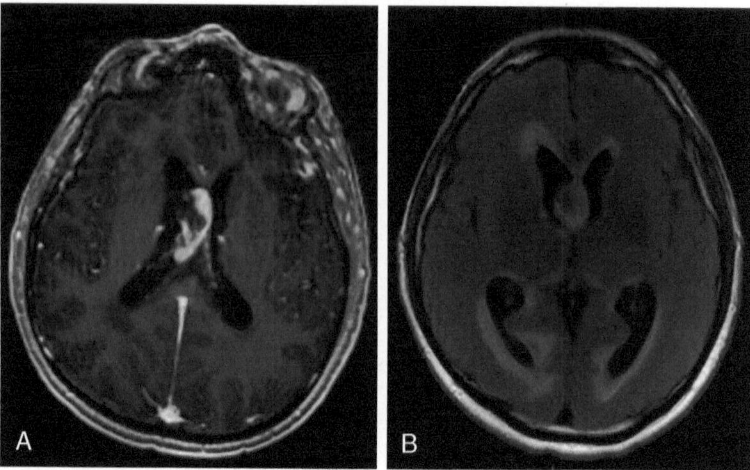

Fig. 19.1 MRI of the patient in Case 19.1. (A) Axial fluid-attenuated inversion recover image showing dilation of the lateral ventricles with obstructive hydrocephalus and trans-ependymal flow of cerebrospinal fluid. (B) Axial post-contrast T1-weighted image reveals a contrast-enhancing mass of the septum pellucidum.

Teaching Points: Managing Obstructive Hydrocephalus, Vasogenic Edema, Tumor-Associated Epilepsy and Cerebrovascular Complications. This case underscores some of the complications of brain tumors that develop as a result of the direct effects of the tumor, including obstructive hydrocephalus, vasogenic edema, tumor-associated epilepsy, hemorrhagic or ischemic stroke, and endocrinopathy. In particular, this case highlights the evaluation and management of patients with obstructive hydrocephalus.

Hydrocephalus is a potentially life-threatening complication of brain tumors and the associated cerebral edema that occurs due to obstruction of CSF flow. It commonly presents with symptoms of raised intracranial pressure such as headache, mental status changes, nausea, and vomiting. Evaluation with CT of the head can quickly evaluate for the presence and degree of hydrocephalus. Neurosurgical intervention by external ventricular drainage of CSF is often required to relieve the elevated intracranial pressure by diverting CSF from the ventricles. External ventricular drainage is a temporary solution to emergently relieve increased intracranial pressure. If obstruction is unable to be relieved with surgery or corticosteroids, conversion to a cerebral shunt may be required.

Approach to tumor-induced vasogenic edema

Tumor-induced vasogenic edema occurs due to disruption of the blood-brain barrier, preferentially affecting white matter.[1] The type and severity of neurologic symptoms are affected by the degree of edema and location of edema. Evaluation of cerebral edema is best accomplished with MRI of the brain using T2 fluid-attenuated inversion recovery (FLAIR sequences). Edema appears as T2 hyperintensity. The decision to treat cerebral edema should be based on clinical findings and neurologic symptoms. Asymptomatic patients with cerebral edema seen on imaging do not require treatment. Corticosteroids, particularly dexamethasone, are the primary treatment for clinically symptomatic cerebral edema. Dexamethasone is preferred due to its minimal mineralocorticoid activity. By decreasing blood-brain barrier permeability, corticosteroids can effectively reduce intracranial pressure, improving cerebral edema and neurologic symptoms within days.[2]

Dexamethasone. Dosing of dexamethasone is largely dependent on symptoms. Severe symptomatic cerebral edema can be treated with intravenous dexamethasone 10–24 mg followed by oral dexamethasone. Doses of 2–4 mg of oral dexamethasone administered two to four times per day are commonly used. In the outpatient setting, twice-daily dosing is often sufficient, with the second dose administered in the afternoon to prevent insomnia. Although corticosteroids can quickly improve neurologic symptoms and function, their acute and long-term use is associated with many side effects. Acutely, patients may experience hyperglycemia, insomnia, and mood disturbances such as anxiety or mania. Chronic corticosteroid use is associated with a host of complications including weight gain, Cushing syndrome, and steroid myopathy. Endocrine and neuropsychiatric effects of corticosteroids are discussed later in this chapter.

Given the side effect profile, patients should be maintained on the lowest effective dose of dexamethasone. Tapering or discontinuing corticosteroids should be considered at every patient encounter, although some patients may be unable to safely taper off steroids due to re-emergence of focal neurologic symptoms or seizures. Additionally, patients with chronic corticosteroid use may have difficulty tapering off steroids secondary to adrenal insufficiency. The risks of corticosteroid treatment must be weighed against their symptomatic benefit, as their effects can have profound medical and functional implications. Anti-angiogenic agents such as beva-

Table 19.1 Non–enzyme-inducing antiepileptic drugs commonly used in brain tumor patients

Drug	Route	Common Side Effects	Primary Metabolism
Brivaracetam	Oral, IV	Sedation, fatigue, psychiatric disturbance	Unknown
Lacosamide	Oral, IV	Dizziness	Mixed
Lamotrigine	Oral	Rash, Steven-Johnson syndrome	Hepatic
Levetiracetam	Oral, IV	Agitation, psychosis, fatigue	Unknown
Pregabalin	Oral	Weight gain, sedation, thrombocytopenia	Renal
Topiramate	Oral	Dizziness, paresthesia, nephrolithiasis, metabolic acidosis, weight loss, cognitive impairment	Mixed
Valproic acid[a]	Oral, IV	Thrombocytopenia, hair loss, tremor, hyperammonemia, weight gain, pancreatitis	Hepatic
Zonisamide	Oral	Paresthesia, nephrolithiasis, metabolic acidosis, anorexia	Renal

[a]Valproic acid is an enzyme inhibitor.
IV, Intravenous.

cizumab, a monoclonal antibody against vascular endothelial growth factor, can be used in recurrent malignant gliomas to reduce cerebral edema and corticosteroid dependence.[3]

Approach to tumor-associated epilepsy

Seizures are among the most common complications of brain tumors. The likelihood of developing seizures from a brain tumor is variable and influenced by tumor location, histology, and rate of growth. Tumors involving the cortex, temporal lobe, and insula are associated with higher rates of epilepsy, whereas tumors involving the posterior fossa or deep structures rarely cause seziures.[4] Tumor histology is also associated with increased rates of epilepsy. Dysembryoplastic neuroepithelial tumors and oligodendrogliomas are associated with epilepsy in up to 90% of cases.[5,6] In such epileptogenic tumors, gross-total surgical resection is strongly associated with seizure freedom.[5,7] High-grade glioma patients experience rates of tumor-associated epilepsy of 30–50% and may experience seizures at any point during their disease course.[8,9] Therefore, if a brain tumor patient presents with paroxysmal or fluctuating symptoms, seizure activity should be high on the differential. Electroencephalography may be helpful to characterize episodes that are not clinically consistent with seizure activity.

There is some evidence to suggest that brain tumor–directed treatment, including radiation and chemotherapy, may improve seizure control, although cancer-specific treatments are not considered first line for managing tumor-associated epilepsy.[10,11] Current standard of care practices involve treating brain tumor patients who present with seizures with antiepileptic drugs (AEDs).[12] No data exists to support the efficacy of one AED compared with another. Given the increasing number of available AEDs, the drug chosen should take into account a patient's epilepsy syndrome, medical comorbidities, desired speed of titration, and side effect profile of the drug. It is recommended to avoid enzyme-inducing drugs, as these may interact with the metabolism of corticosteroids and cancer-directed treatments such as chemotherapy. Common enzyme-inducing AEDs include phenytoin, phenobarbital, carbamazepine, and oxcarbazepine. Table 19.1 shows non–enzyme- inducing AEDs that are commonly used in brain tumor patients. For example, levetiracetam is an AED frequently used to treat tumor-associated epilepsy. It has no known drug interactions, minimal hepatic metabolism, requires no specific monitoring, and can be administered orally or intravenously. It is generally well tolerated by patients, with the most common adverse effects being agitation and aggression. Enzyme inhibiting AEDs such as valproic acid should be used with caution, especially in patients treated with hepatically cleared chemotherapeutic agents, as it may increase toxicity of these drugs.

AEDs are associated with many adverse effects and nearly 25% of patients will experience side effects of AED therapy requiring drug discontinuation.[13] Common side effects of AEDs include symptoms of central nervous system depression such as fatigue, cognitive slowing, ataxia, and dizziness. Other specific adverse effects that can be seen are drug dependent and are listed in Table 19.1. When patients present with these symptoms, a thorough history, metabolic workup, and AED serum levels may be used to distinguish whether symptoms are due to adverse effects from the drug rather than direct effects of the tumor itself. Although appropriate treatment of tumor-associated epilepsy may lead to a decrease or cessation of seizures, all patients and their caregivers should be educated on seizure safety and home management of acute, symptomatic seizures. Driving restrictions should be discussed with all patients who have experienced seizures with loss of awareness or consciousness. Driving restrictions are variable by region, therefore patients and physicians should familiarize themselves with local regulations and procedures.

The American Academy of Neurology Quality Standards Subcommittee performed a meta-analysis of randomized studies assessing the benefit of prophylactic AED treatment in brain tumor patients. Prophylactic treatment was found to have an increased burden of side effects without an improvement in rates of tumor-associated epilepsy when compared with placebo or no treatment. This led to a recommendation against administration of prophylactic AEDs in patients with brain tumors.[13] Although this recommendation was based on results from studies utilizing first- or second-generation AEDs, more recent reviews have shown similar findings with newer non–enzyme-inducing AEDs.[14] As such, it is currently recommended to only treat brain tumor patients who have experienced a seizure with AEDs.

Approach to stroke in brain tumor patients

Mechanisms of ischemic and hemorrhagic stroke. Patients with brain tumors are at risk of ischemic or hemorrhagic stroke from a variety of mechanisms including direct tumor effects and side effects of treatment. Ischemia can occur as a result of direct compression of cerebral vasculature either by tumor or associated edema. Brain tumor patients are also at risk of ischemic stroke from other mechanisms including hypercoagulability from malignancy, paroxysmal embolism from a deep venous thrombosis through a patent foramen ovale, and late effects of treatment including radiation induced vasculopathy. Cardiovascular risk factors such as hypertension, hyperlipidemia, diabetes, and smoking may also increase risk of both ischemic and hemorrhagic stroke. Certain drugs used in the management of malignant gliomas, such as bevacizumab, a monoclonal antibody against vascular endothelial growth factor, also increase the risk of arterial stroke.[15] Patients with brain tumors are also at risk for hemorrhagic stroke, with intra-tumoral hemorrhage being the most common presentation in this population. Brain tumor patients may also be at risk for cerebral hemorrhage due to thrombocytopenia or coagulopathy from chemotherapeutic treatments.

Evaluation and management of ischemic stroke in brain tumor patients. Evaluation of stroke in brain tumor patients should occur no differently than in other stroke patients. Emergent evaluation is recommended in a hospital setting. CT head should be obtained without delay to assess for hemorrhage or large vessel occlusion. Very little data exists for the use of acute interventions such as tissue-plasminogen activator (tPA) and thrombectomy in patients with brain tumors presenting with ischemic stroke,[16] which are relatively contraindicated in brain tumor patients.[17] The risk of acute interventions should be weighed with the potential benefit and life expectancy of the patient. All patients should have an MRI Brain with and without contrast to better evaluate the extent of the infarct and assess for tumor growth. In cases where tumor growth or edema have caused direct vascular compression, treatment with corticosteroids and neurosurgical tumor debulking should be considered. Vascular imaging of the head and neck vessels and echocardiogram may be indicated based on the stroke mechanism. If acute management is not appropriate, aggressive risk factor modification should be considered in all brain tumor patients, as they are at particular risk of recurrent thromboembolic strokes.[18] Risk factor modification should include correction of coagulopathy, anticoagulation when appropriate, in addition to blood pressure, cholesterol, and glucose control.

Management of hemorrhagic stroke in brain tumor patients. Patients with hemorrhagic stroke should have all antiplatelet and anticoagulant medications withheld. Aggressive blood pressure management to keep systolic blood pressure <140 mmHg is recommended.[19] In hemorrhages due to thrombocytopenia, patients should be treated with emergent platelet transfusions. In cases of a large volume or expanding hemorrhage, neurosurgical hematoma evacuation should be considered. All brain tumor patients with stroke should be considered for rehabilitation with physical and occupational therapy.

Approach to tumor-induced hydrocephalus

Etiology, presentation, and evaluation of hydrocephalus. Some brain tumors based on their location can cause intraventricular obstruction of cerebral spinal fluid flow, leading to a non-communicating or obstructive hydrocephalus. This occurs from direct obstruction from intraventricular tumors such as subependymoma, meningioma, and central neurocytoma or from extrinsic compression of the ventricle from ependymoma, astrocytoma, and metastases.[20] Hydrocephalus is most commonly seen with tumors of the posterior fossa or deep structures of the brain such as the thalamus. Patients typically present with symptoms of progressive headache, lethargy, ataxia, impaired vision, and cognitive decline, although symptoms can be acute in onset. Neurologic examination should include fundoscopy to assess for papilledema. The patient described in Case 19.1 is a classic clinical and radiographic example of obstructive hydrocephalus.

Management and treatment of obstructive hydrocephalus. All patients with concern for hydrocephalus should have urgent imaging with CT Head without contrast. Classically, imaging will show enlarged lateral ventricles with transependymal flow of CSF and obstruction of the third and fourth ventricle.[20] MRI can be used to better elucidate tumor volume, extent of edema, and aid in surgical planning. Patients with acute non-communicating hydrocephalus should be emergently evaluated, as early detection and treatment can be lifesaving. Corticosteroids are generally administered for acute symptom management. Emergent neurosurgical consultation should be obtained. Treatment of obstructive hydrocephalus depends on the level of obstruction and in the acute setting is focused on reducing elevated intracerebral pressure and diverting CSF flow, often with an extraventricular drain. Definitive treatment may involve endoscopic ventriculostomy or placement or ventriculoperitoneal shunting.[21] Urgent radiotherapy may also be appropriate in certain situations.

Approach to SIADH

Syndrome of inappropriate antidiuretic hormone in brain tumor patients. Patients with any central nervous system disorder, particularly patients with brain tumors, can develop inappropriate release of antidiuretic hormone (ADH). ADH secretion results in water retention and loss of sodium in the urine. The syndrome of inappropriate antidiuretic hormone (SIADH) is characterized by plasma hyponatremia, plasma hypoosmolality, and concentrated urine in the setting of normovolemia, normal blood pressure, and adequate renal, hepatic, adrenal, and thyroid function.[22] Patients with SIADH can present with a myriad of symptoms including weakness, lethargy, fatigue, encephalopathy, seizures, and, in severe cases, coma.[23] SIADH can occur at any point during the disease course and can occur irrespective of brain tumor progression.

Providers should have a high index of suspicion for SIADH in the setting of poorly localizing, progressive neurologic symptoms and polyuria. Initial workup should include serum chemistries to evaluate electrolytes and renal function and urinalysis with urine electrolytes and urine osmolality. Diagnosis is made in the setting of serum hyponatremia and urine hyperosmolality (>100 mosmol/kg).[24] Hyponatremia can induce brain swelling, which can be fatal for patients with brain tumors. Consultation with a nephrologist is recommended, and patients frequently require hospital admission for treatment and close monitoring of sodium levels.

Treatment of hyponatremia. Treatment of hyponatremia depends on the severity of symptoms and degree of hyponatremia. All symptomatic patients should be urgently treated. Mild symptomatic hyponatremia with serum sodium >125 mEq/L is treated with fluid restriction of less than 800 mL of fluid per day. Other treatment options for mild to moderate hyponatremia include oral salt tablets, starting at a dose of 9 g daily, or administration of loop diuretics. These treatments will correct serum sodium levels in 3–10 days. Patients with severe symptomatic hyponatremia should be considered for admission to an intensive care unit and may require administration of hypertonic saline to rapidly raise serum sodium.[25]

Approach to endocrinopathy

Endocrinopathies from tumor involvement. Endocrinopathies occur in patients with brain tumors via involvement or invasion of the hypothalamic-pituitary axis or secondarily as a consequence of radiation to the hypothalamus or pituitary gland. Tumors of the region of the sella turcica, the saddle-shaped midline bony depression in the skull, include pituitary tumors and, less commonly, craniopharyngiomas, or rarely granular cell tumors, pituicytomas, and spindle cell oncocytomas. Pituitary tumors are the most common of these tumors and one of the most common benign brain tumors (e.g., behind meningioma). Neurologists should be generally aware of the clinical presentation, imaging findings, laboratory assessment, and treatment options. Presenting symptoms result from local compression against surrounding structures such as the optic chiasm (e.g., bitemporal hemianopsia) or disruption of pituitary hormone secretion. Pituitary tumors are neoplasms that arise from the neuroendocrine cells in the pituitary gland. They can be classified histologically, radiographically, and biochemically. Histologically, they can be classified as adenomas (most common), carcinomas, and atypical adenomas with benign adenomas. On imaging, pituitary tumors are classified as microadenomas for tumors less than 10 mm in largest cross-sectional diameter, or macroadenomas for tumors larger than 10 mm. Biochemically, about two-thirds of pituitary adenomas are hormonally functional, with prolactinomas being the most common. Treatment involves replacement of hormone function and definitive tumor-directed therapy. Indications for surgery include symptomatic mass effect, vision loss, or inability to achieve hormone stability.

Post-treatment endocrinopathies in brain tumor patients. Children and young adults are most prone to radiation-induced endocrinopathies, which tend to develop several years after treatment.[26] Symptoms vary depending on the deficient hormone. Growth hormone is the most sensitive to treatment-related effects, and its deficiency results in small stature and decreased bone density. Patients with prolactinoma may present with galactorrhea, amenorrhea, hypogonadism, and erectile dysfunction. Other endocrinopathies such as gonadotropic deficiency or adrenocorticotropic hormone deficiency are less common. Cushing syndrome and hyperglycemia often occur in brain tumor patients after prolonged exposure to corticosteroids. Evaluation of endocrinopathy begins with obtaining serum hormone levels. Referral to an endocrinologist is recommended. Some patients will require treatment with hormone replacement therapy or cortico steroids. In patients with hormone-producing macroadenomas, medical treatment with agents such a bromocriptine (for prolactin secreting adenomas) may be considered. Neurosurgical resection of a pituitary mass is recommended for large tumors causing compressive neurologic symptoms and tumors refractory to medical treatment.

Clinical Pearls

1. Dexamethasone is the preferred corticosteroid for treating cerebral edema. Treatment decisions should be based on the degree of neurologic symptoms and not on imaging findings.
2. Patients should be managed on the lowest dose of dexamethasone that controls their symptoms. Given the long-term side effects, efforts should continually be made to taper or discontinue corticosteroids when symptomatically possible.
3. Brain tumor patients presenting with a seizure should be treated with an antiepileptic medication. Enzyme-inducing antiepileptic drugs should be avoided due to interactions with chemotherapy and corticosteroids.
4. There is no evidence to support the use of prophylactic anticonvulsants in brain tumor patients.
5. Brain tumor patients are at increased risk for hemorrhagic and ischemic stroke. Patients with acute onset of neurologic symptoms should be urgently evaluated for stroke.

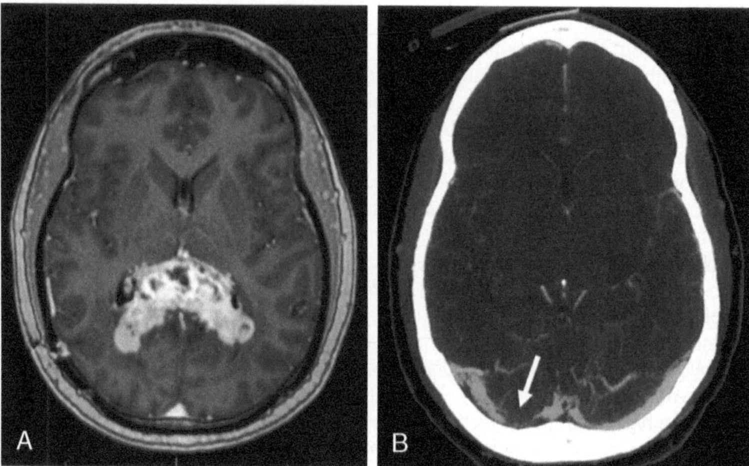

Fig. 19.2 MRI of the patient in Case 19.2. (A) Axial post-contrast T1-weighted image showing an expansile, enhancing mass involving the corpus callosum. (B) CT angiography showing a nonocclusive thrombus of the right transverse sinus indicated by the white arrow.

6. Endocrinologic complications are common in brain tumor patients and can present with variable symptoms. Hypopituitarism and SIADH should be considered in the differential of fatigue and encephalopathy.

CASE 19.2 INDIRECT MEDICAL COMPLICATIONS OF BRAIN TUMORS

Case. A 50-year-old man with an anaplastic astrocytoma currently being treated with temozolomide presented to the hospital with severe headaches, visual obscurations, nausea, and vomiting. While in the Emergency Department he was witnessed to have a generalized seizure. CT of the head showed no evidence of hemorrhage and stable tumor size when compared with prior imaging. CT angiography showed obstruction of the left transverse venous sinus consistent with cerebral venous sinus thrombosis (Fig. 19.2). He was emergently anticoagulated with intravenous unfractionated heparin and over the next 1–2 days was transitioned to low-molecular-weight heparin (LMWH) with symptomatic improvement over the following week.

Teaching Points: Managing Venous Thromboembolism, Fatigue, Sleep Dysfunction, and Neurocognitive Deficits in Brain Tumor Patients. This patient presented with an acute cerebral venous sinus thrombosis (VST). Symptoms of VST, such as increased intracranial pressure, headaches, seizures, or focal neurologic deficits, are often misattributed to the tumor itself resulting in delayed diagnosis. CT or MR angiography or venography are the preferred diagnostic imaging modalities. Treatment requires therapeutic anticoagulation to prevent thrombus propagation and venous infarction. Unfractionated heparin may be used when urgent anticoagulation is desired or when risk of intracranial hemorrhage is high. LMWH should be used for anticoagulation in the outpatient setting. This case highlights the potential indirect effects that can occur and complicate management in brain tumor patients including venous thromboembolism (VTE), fatigue, sleep dysfunction, neurocognitive deficits, mood changes, and depression.

Venous thromboembolism and hypercoagulability

Patients with brain tumors are at high risk for venous thromboembolic disease from a number of mechanisms, and this increased risk persists after the perioperative period. VTE includes deep venous thrombosis (DVT), pulmonary embolism (PE), and VST and occurs in up to 20% of patients with malignant gliomas (also see Chapter 12, Case 12.3c for approach to patients with VTE).[27] Important risk factors for VTE development include the postoperative setting, patient age over 75, prior history of VTE, limb paresis, obesity, higher grade of glioma at diagnosis, large tumor size, anti–vascular endothelial growth factor treatment (such as bevacizumab), and use of hormonal therapy.[28] Given its frequency in brain tumors patients, the provider must maintain a high index of suspicion for VTE. Any brain tumor patient presenting with new or worsening lower extremity edema, calf pain, shortness of breath, chest pain, or tachycardia should be evaluated for VTE. These conditions may be life-threatening, and patients require urgent evaluation with lower extremity venous ultrasound and contrasted CT-angiography of the chest. Additionally, in brain tumor patients presenting with new or worsening headaches not explained by routine head imaging, VST should be considered and evaluated for with CT or MR venography.

VTE is treated with systemic anticoagulation, although there are special considerations when anticoagulating brain tumor patients who may be at increased risk of intracranial hemorrhage. Large case series have demonstrated the efficacy

Table 19.2 Neuro-oncologic emergencies in brain tumor patients

Clinical Syndrome	Diagnostic Test	Emergent Treatment
Status epilepticus	EEG	Seizure termination with benzodiazepines and antiepileptic drug, adjust antiepileptic drug regimen (increase dose or add additional drugs)
Intracranial hemorrhage	CT Head without contrast	Stop or reverse anticoagulation, correct coagulopathy, blood pressure management (SBP <140 mmHg)
Stroke	MR Head with diffusion-weighted imaging	Cardiovascular risk factor modification, tPA, and thrombectomy are relatively contraindicated, stop bevacizumab
Obstructive hydrocephalus	CT Head without contrast	Neurosurgical resection of obstructing lesion or placement of external ventricular drain
SIADH	Serum and urine electrolytes and osmolality	Fluid restriction, salt tablets
Deep vein thrombosis	Lower extremity venous ultrasound	Anticoagulation with LMWH, vena cava filter if strong contraindication to anticoagulation
Pulmonary embolism	CT angiogram Chest	Anticoagulation with LMWH, unstable patients may require IV heparin
Cerebral venous thrombosis	MR venography	Anticoagulation

CT, Computed tomography; *EEG,* electroencephalography, *IV,* intravenous, *LMWH,* low-molecular-weight heparin; *MR,* magnetic resonance imaging; *SBP,* systolic blood pressure; *SIADH,* syndrome of inappropriate antidiuretic hormone secretion.

and safety of systemic anticoagulation in patients with brain metastases and high-grade gliomas.[29,30] Certain brain tumor types with a predisposition to hemorrhage such as metastatic melanoma or renal cell carcinoma pose a therapeutic challenge. These patients may be able to be safely anticoagulated, although a non-contrasted CT Head to evaluate for intracranial hemorrhage is recommended prior to initiation of treatment. In patients with a known DVT who cannot be safely anticoagulated due to recent intracranial surgery or hemorrhage, placement of an inferior vena cava filter should be considered.

Acute anticoagulation for VTE in brain tumor patients is done with LMWHs such as enoxaparin and unfractionated heparin. LMWH is the preferred agent of choice but unfractionated heparin should be used in patients with symptomatic PE, renal insufficiency, or high hemorrhage risk.[31] Oral anticoagulants such as warfarin are typically avoided in brain tumor patients due to the high risk of drug-drug interactions (especially with chemotherapy, antiepileptic medications, and antibiotics) and need for frequent laboratory monitoring. The newer oral anticoagulants, such as the factor Xa inhibitors rivaroxaban and apixaban, have not been well studied in the brain tumor population, and should be used with caution. The duration of anticoagulation should be determined on an individual basis with patients completing a minimum 6-month course of therapeutic anticoagulation. Many patients with brain tumors will require lifelong anticoagulation. Perioperative prophylactic anticoagulation has been shown to significantly decrease VTE risk without increasing risk of hemorrhage, thus it is recommended in the immediate postoperative setting.[32] Long-term prophylactic anticoagulation is not currently recommended in brain tumor patients.

Table 19.2 highlights significant neuro-oncologic emergencies experienced by brain tumor patients and their associated diagnostic testing and treatment.

Fatigue, cognitive dysfunction, and sleep disturbances in brain tumor patients

Fatigue. Fatigue is one of the most common symptoms experienced by brain tumor patients occurring in over 40–70% of patients.[33] There are many factors that lead to fatigue in brain tumor patients, including treatment with cranial irradiation and chemotherapy, adverse effects from antiepileptic and pain medications, hematologic and metabolic toxicities, mood disorders, and sleep disturbances. Fatigue is assessed by patient and caregiver report and should be addressed at every encounter with a brain tumor patient. A thorough evaluation of all cancer-directed treatments, medications, laboratory values, nutritional status, psychiatric symptoms, and sleep patterns should be completed in any brain tumor patient reporting fatigue. Efforts should be made to eliminate sedating medications, correct underlying metabolic and endocrinologic abnormalities, and treatment of underlying depression or mood disorders should be considered.

Lifestyle changes should be addressed with all patients, and they should be educated on sleep hygiene. Aerobic exercise should also be recommended to all patients, as this has been demonstrated to reduce cancer-associated fatigue.[34] Many patients with brain tumors may experience improvement in energy as a side effect from corticosteroids (which are often used for the management of cerebral edema), although these should not be used as a treatment for fatigue alone. Several studies have assessed the use of neuro-stimulating medications and have demonstrated variable responses to modafinil and armodafinil.[35,36] Patients with continued moderate to severe fatigue following the medical and lifestyle modifications may be candidates for a trial of a neuro-stimulant. Currently, there is no class I evidence to support the use of these medications in brain tumors patients, and the choice of a particular neuro-stimulant is patient specific.

Cognitive dysfunction (also see Chapter 25). Cognitive dysfunction in common in brain tumor patients. The etiology of this impairment is multifactorial and occurs due to the direct effects of the tumor and associated cerebral edema and consequences of tumor treatments, particularly radiation. Cognitive dysfunction in brain tumor patients often manifests as impairments in attention, memory, or executive function. Radiation has been shown to induce cerebral inflammation, impair neuronal function, and decrease hippocampal neurogenesis, resulting in a leukoencephalopathy and associated cognitive deficits.[37] Additionally, use of certain chemotherapeutic agents may contribute to neurocognitive impairment. It is imperative to complete a thorough assessment of a patient's medications, metabolic status, mood, and fatigue to determine whether these factors are contributing to cognitive dysfunction. Mood disorders, especially major depressive disorder, commonly occur in brain tumor patients throughout their disease course and may contribute to cognitive dysfunction.[38] It is recommended to screen all brain tumor patients for depression and provide treatment in the appropriate cases. Antidepressants can be safely used in brain tumor patients, although bupropion should be avoided, as this can lower the seizure threshold. These patients may also benefit from neuropsychiatric testing to better assess domains of impairment.

There is minimal evidence supporting the use of medications such as memantine or donepezil (commonly used to in the treatment of dementia) in patients with brain tumors. Memantine has been shown to decrease the rate of decline in memory, processing speed, and executive function in patients with brain metastases receiving whole brain radiation.[39] Donepezil has shown similar findings when studied in irradiated brain tumor patients.[40] Although the use of such medications is not standard practice, they may be considered in select patients. Cognitive rehabilitation and occupational therapy may also be considered depending on the degree and domains of cognitive impairment. Lastly, all brain tumor patients with cognitive impairment should be evaluated for social supports, driving abilities, and home safety.

Sleep disturbance syndrome cluster. Sleep dysregulation is a frequent occurrence and an important contributor to fatigue in cancer patients.[41] Sleep disturbances in this population range from hypersomnia to insomnia and may be due to effects of the tumor itself, cancer-directed treatments, and supportive care medications. Any patient presenting with sleep disturbance should be counselled on sleep hygiene and lifestyle interventions to improve sleep quality. Such interventions include establishing a restful sleep environment, setting a sleep schedule, limiting naps or caffeine intake during the day, and limiting stimuli prior to sleep.

Screening for daytime sleepiness can be done using the Epworth Sleepiness Scale or patient reported sleep diaries.[42] Patients with hypersomnia should be evaluated in a similar fashion as those with fatigue, including assessment and management of sedating medications, metabolic or endocrine abnormalities, and underlying psychiatric conditions. When these factors are appropriately managed, consideration should be given to primary sleep disorders such as obstructive sleep apnea. Some patients may benefit from polysomnography and consultation with a sleep specialist.

Insomnia is often reported by brain tumor patients, particularly in patients taking corticosteroids. To manage corticosteroid-induced insomnia, patients should be treated with the lowest possible dose of corticosteroids and evening doses should be avoided. Cognitive behavioral therapy in conjunction with sleep hygiene interventions should be considered when nonpharmacologic treatment is desired. Few studies have assessed pharmacologic treatment of insomnia in brain cancer patients. Over-the-counter medications and supplements such as melatonin or antihistamines have been used with mixed results. Hypnotic medications including benzodiazepines can be considered in severe cases and should be used at the lowest effective dose. Long-term use of benzodiazepines should be avoided.[42]

Clinical Pearls

1. Venous thromboembolism is common in brain tumor patients. Patients with new lower extremity swelling, shortness of breath, or hypoxia should be urgently evaluated for DVT or PE with lower extremity ultrasound or CT angiogram of the chest.
2. Prophylactic anticoagulation is only indicated for brain tumor patients in the perioperative setting.
3. Therapeutic anticoagulation with LMWH is preferred for prevention of recurrent venous thromboembolism in cancer patients.
4. The etiology of fatigue and cognitive dysfunction in brain tumor patients is multifactorial. Assessment includes evaluation of antitumor treatments, supportive care medications, metabolic and endocrine abnormalities, mood disturbance, and sleep dysregulation.

5. All patients should be screened for depression throughout their disease course and treated when appropriate.

Conclusions

Brain tumor patients are at an increased risk of a multitude of medical complications secondary to direct effects of the tumor itself, indirect effects such as hypercoagulability, and toxicities of treatment. New medical or neurologic symptoms in these patients should be urgently and thoroughly evaluated. The risk of such complications will likely increase as the treatment of brain tumors becomes more sophisticated and complex. A high index of suspicion and systematic approach to evaluating new medical problems are crucial for appropriately diagnosing and treating these conditions. Appropriate treatment of these complications can positively affect patient independence, quality of life, and survival.

References

1. Machein MR, Kullmer J, Fiebich BL, Plate KH, Warnke PC. Vascular endothelial growth factor expression, vascular volume and capillary permeability in human brain tumors. *Neurosurgery*. 1999;44(4):732–740.
2. Dietrich J, Rao K, Pastorino D, Kesari D. Corticosteroids in brain cancer patients: benefits and pitfalls. *Expert Rev Clin Pharmacol*. 2011;4(2):233–242.
3. Gerstner ER, Duda DG, di Tomaso E, et al. VEGF inhibitors in the treatment of cerebral edema in patients with brain cancer. *Nat Rev Clin Oncol*. 2009;6(4):229–236.
4. Hurwitz S, Drappatz J, Kesari S, et al. Morphological characteristics of brain tumors causing seizures. *Arch Neurol*. 2010;67(3):336–342.
5. Kerkhof M, Vecht CJ. Seizure characteristics and prognostic factors of gliomas. *Epilepsia*. 2013;54(suppl 9):12–17.
6. Pallud J, Audureau E, Blonski M, et al. Epileptic seizures in diffuse low-grade gliomas in adults. *Brain*. 2014;137(2):449–462.
7. Englot DJ, Berger MS, Barbaro NM, Chang EF. Predictors of seizure freedom after resection of supratentorial low-grade gliomas. a review. *J Neurosurg*. 2011;115(2):240–244.
8. Van Breemen MS, Wilms EB, Vecht CJ. Epilepsy in patients with brain tumors: epidemiology, mechanisms and management. *Lancet Neurol*. 2007;6(5):421–430.
9. Bromfileld EB. Epilepsy in patients with brain tumors and other cancers. *Rev Neurol Dis*. 2004;1(suppl 1):S27–S33.
10. Ruda R, Magliola U, Bertero L, et al. Seizure control following radiotherapy in patients with diffuse gliomas: a retrospective study. *Neuro Oncol*. 2013;15(12):1739–1749.
11. Sherman JH, Moldovan K, Yeoh HK, et al. Impact of temozolomide chemotherapy on seizure frequency in patients with low-grade gliomas. *J Neurosurg*. 2011;114(6):1617–1621.
12. Rossetti AO, Stupp R. Epilepsy in brain tumor patients. *Curr Opin Neurol*. 2010;23(6):603–609.
13. Glantz MJ, Cole BF, Forsyth PA, et al. Practice parameter: anticonvulsant prophylaxis in patients with newly diagnosed brain tumors. report of the quality standard subcommittee of the american academy of neurology. *Neurology*. 2000;54(10):1886.
14. Perry J, Zinman L, Chambers A, et al. The use of prophylactic anticonvulsants in patients with brain tumors- a systematic review. *Curr Oncol*. 2006;13(6):222–229.
15. Friedman HS, Prados MD, Wen PY, et al. Bevacizumab alone and in combination with irinotecan in recurrent glioblastoma. *J Clin Oncol*. 2009;27(28):4733–4740.
16. Etgen T, Steinich I, Gsottschneider L. Thrombolysis for ischemic stroke in patients with brain tumors. *J Stroke Cerebrovasc Dis*. 2014;23(2):361–366.
17. Fugate JE, Rabinstein A. Absolute and relative contraindications to IV rt-PA for acute ischemic stroke. *Neurohospitalist*. 2015;5(3):110–121.
18. Parikh NS, Burch JE, Kamel H, DeAngelis LM, Navi BB. Recurrent thromboembolic events after ischemic stroke in patients with primary brain tumors. *J Stroke Cerebrovasc Dis*. 2017;26(10):2396–2403.
19. Rabinstein A. Optimal blood pressure after intracerebral hemorrhage: still a moving target. *Stroke*. 2018;49:275–276.
20. Maller VV, Gray RI. Noncommunicating hydrocephalus. *Semin Ultrasound CT MR*. 2016;37(2):109–119.
21. Roux A, Botella C, Still M, et al. Posterior fossa metastasis-associated obstructive hydrocephalus in adult patients: literature review and practical considerations from the euro-oncology club of the french society of neurosurgery. *World Neurosurg*. 2018;117:271–279.
22. Velasco Cano MV, Runkle de la Vega I. Current considerations in syndrome of inappropriate secretion of antidiuretic hormone/syndrome of inappropriate antidiuresis. *Endocrinol Nutr*. 2010;57(suppl 2):22–29.
23. Flounders JA. Continuing education: oncology emergency modules: syndrome of inappropriate antidiuretic hormone. *Oncol Nurs Forum*. 2003;30(3):E63–E70.
24. Adrogue HJ, Madias NE. Hyopnatremia. *N Engl J Med*. 2000;342:1581–1589.
25. Sterns RH, Nigwekar SU, Hix JK. The treatment of hyponatremia. *Semin Nephrol*. 2009;29(3):282–299.
26. Sathyapalan T, Dixit S. Radiotherapy-induced hypopituitarism: a review. *Expert Rev Anticancer Ther*. 2012;12(5):669–683.
27. Perry JR. Thromboembolic disease in patients with high-grade glioma. *Neuro Oncol*. 2012;14(suppl 4):iv73–iv80.
28. Schiff D, Lee EQ, Nayak L, Norden AD, Reardon DA, Wen PY. Medical management of brain tumors. *Neuro Oncol*. 2015;17(4):488–504.
29. Choucair AK, Silver P, Levin VA. Risk of intracranial hemorrhage in glioma patients receiving anticoagulant therapy for venous thromboembolism. *J Neurosurg*. 1987;66(3):357–358.
30. Schiff D, DeAngelia LM. Therapy of venous thromboembolism in patients with brain metastases. *Cancer*. 1994;73(2):493–498.
31. Jenkins EO, Schiff D, Mackman N, Key NS. Venous thromboembolism in malignant gliomas. *J Thromb Haemost*. 2010;8(2):221–227.
32. Agnelli G, Piovella F, Buoncristiani P, et al. Enoxaparin plus compression stockings compared to compression stockings alone in the prevention of venous throm-

boembolism after elective neurosurgery. *N Engl J Med.* 1998;339(2):80–85.
33. Armstong TS, Gilbert MR. Practical strategies for management of fatigue and sleep disorders in people with brain tumors. *Neuro Oncol.* 2012;13(suppl 4):iv65–iv72.
34. Cramp F, Byron-Daniel J. Exercise for the management of cancer-associated fatigue in adults. *Cochrane Database Syst Rev.* 2012;11:CD006145.
35. Lee EQ, Muzikansky A, Kesari S, et al. A randomized placebo-controlled pilot trial of armodafinil for fatigue in patients with gliomas undergoing radiotherapy. *J Clin Oncol.* 2014;32(suppl 5s). abstr 2004.
36. Shaw EG, Case D, Bryant D, et al. Phase II double-blind placebo-controlled study of armodafinil for brain radiation induced fatigue. *J Clin Oncol.* 2013;31:9505.
37. Greene-Schloesser D, Moore E, Robbins ME. Molecular pathways: radiation-induced cognitive impairment. *Clin Cancer Res.* 2013;19(9):2294–2300.
38. Rooney AG, Carson A, Grant R. Depression in cerebral glioma patients: a systematic review of observational studies. *J Natl Cancer Inst.* 2011;103(1):61–76.
39. Brown PD, Pugh S, Laack NN, et al. Memantine for the prevention of cognitive dysfunction in patients receiving whole brain radiotherapy: a randomized, double-blind, placebo-controlled trial. *Neuro Oncol.* 2013;15(10):1429–1437.
40. Shaw EG, Rosdhal R, D'Agostino Jr RB, et al. Phase II study of donepezil in irradiated brain tumor patients: effect on cognitive function, mood and quality of life. *J Clin Oncol.* 2006;24(9):1415–1420.
41. National Comprehensive Cancer Network. *Cancer-Related Fatigue (Version 2.2015)*; 2015. Available at: https://jnccn.org/abstract/journals/jnccn/13/8/article-p1012.xml. Accessed May 14, 2019.
42. Armstrong TS, Gilbert MR. Practical strategies for managing fatigue and sleep disorders in people with brain tumors. *Neuro Oncol.* 2012;14(suppl 4):iv65–iv72.

Chapter 20

Paraneoplastic neurological disorder syndromes

Luisa A. Diaz-Arias and John C. Probasco

CHAPTER OUTLINE

Introduction

Paraneoplastic neurological disorder (PND) syndromes are immune-mediated disorders that affect the central, peripheral, or autonomic nervous system in the setting of a cancer.[1] These disorders are not caused by a direct tissue invasion of cancer; instead, they are associated with cancer-induced immune responses directed toward neuronal proteins.[2] They are extremely rare, estimated to affect less than 0.1% of patients with cancer.[3] This, however, is likely an underestimate. The recognition of PND syndromes is crucial given that they often occur before the diagnosis of a cancer or a cancer recurrence, offering an opportunity to diagnose and treat cancer earlier and with associated improved outcomes.

PND syndromes may be related to benign tumors, such as thymoma, or malignant tumors, such as small-cell carcinoma of the lung (SCLC) and breast cancer.[4] SCLC is the most frequent malignancy associated with PND syndromes.[5] The most commonly accepted theory is that the immune system reacts against proteins expressed by tumors, which are similar to neuronal proteins, allowing for a response to cancer as well as a mistaken response against the brain, spinal cord, nerves, neuromuscular junction, or muscle individually as well as in combination. Several antibodies have been described since the first report in 1949 (e.g., anti-Hu, anti-CV2/collapsing response mediator protein 5 [CRMP5/CV2], anti-*N*-methyl-D-aspartate receptor [NMDAR] and anti-Yo).[6,7] These antibodies can recognize intracellular as well as cell-surface antigens, and their associated syndromes differ in terms of clinical profile, pathogenesis, and outcome.

In this chapter, we will present case-based discussions of the classic PND syndromes as well as paraneoplastic mononeuritis multiplex (MM), with special attention paid to their respective clinical presentations, treatments, and prognoses. We begin with a brief discussion of the classification, pathophysiology, clinical presentation, general diagnostic approach, and treatments. This is followed by a case-based presentation of the common and clinically relevant PND syndromes.

Classification

Broadly, PND syndromes can be classified by the location of the antibody target and, specifically, whether the target is an intracellular antigen or an antigen found on the neuronal cell surface.

Intracellular antigen syndromes. Antibodies to intracellular antigens are associated with subacute onset, progressive illness, and poor outcomes, given that they result from rapid and irreversible neuronal damage.[8] These antibodies can recognize any area of the neuroaxis in isolation or combination, leading to characteristic syndromes such as paraneoplastic cerebellar degeneration (PCD), limbic encephalitis, and sensory neuronopathy. PND syndromes have been associated with anti-Hu, anti-Yo, anti-CRMP5/CV2, anti-Ri, anti-Ma1, anti-Ma2, anti-amphiphysin, anti-Purkinje cell antibody type 2 (PCA-2), and anti-neuronal nuclear antibody type 3 (ANNA-3), among others.[9] Detection of these antibodies should be followed by screening for an occult neoplasm. Their pathophysiology is thought to be primarily mediated by CD8+ T lymphocytes that induce cell death through cytotoxic activity. As a consequence, motor and sensory functions are markedly affected in these patients.[10,11] For instance, in anti-Yo PCD, 90% of patients become non-ambulatory.[12,13] Tumor treatment is related to the stabilization of neurological syndrome, rather than improvement.[14]

Cell surface antigen syndromes. There are also syndromes associated with antibodies against cell-surface antigens targeting membrane receptors, ion channels, and synaptic proteins that occur less commonly in the setting of cancer (Table 20.1).[15] The past decade has seen a rise in the number of newly described syndromes. They are typically associated with better response to immunotherapy and thus better outcomes. Some of these antibodies include anti-α-amino-3-hydroxy-5-methyl-4-isoxazolepropionic acid receptor (AMPAR), anti-gamma-aminobutyric acid type B receptor ($GABA_B$), anti-$GABA_A$ receptor, anti-NMDAR, anti-dipeptidyl-peptidase-like protein 6 (DPPX), anti-voltage gated calcium channel (VGCC; associated with malignant tumors), anti-leucine-rich glioma inactivated 1 (LGI1), and anti-contactin-associated protein 2 (CASPR2).[16] In some instances, the antibodies against cell-surface proteins appear to be related directly with the disease pathophysiology. For instance, antibodies to the NMDA receptor crosslink the receptor, leading to receptor internalization, whereas antibodies against LGI1 interfere with protein-protein interactions.[17,18] Clinical presentation varies from limbic encephalitis to, more rarely, cerebellar ataxia and dysautonomia.

Pathophysiology

Although the pathophysiology of PND syndromes is incompletely understood, autoimmune responses are believed to be involved, with patients developing T-cells and antibodies that are directed against antigens of the central nervous system (CNS), peripheral nervous system (PNS), or autonomic nervous system. When the body surveys for and attempts to eliminate tumor cells, an immune reaction is triggered against tumor antigens. This immune reaction mistakenly cross-reacts with similar proteins on neural tissues.[47] In other cases, the cause is not identified; however, a previous viral infection or a family history of autoimmune diseases may play a role. In addition, cancer treatments such as immunologic checkpoint inhibitors may also provoke autoimmune reactions leading to neurological immune-related adverse events similar in many respects to PND syndromes[48] (also see Chapter 30 for discussion of neurological syndromes associated with immune checkpoint inhibitors).

These anti-cancer immune responses often yield anti-neuronal antibodies that can be measured in the cerebrospinal fluid (CSF), as well as the serum. Antibodies facilitate the localization of an occult neoplasm associated with the PND syndrome and, in some cases, can narrow the search to a few associated organs.[48] Seronegative cases appear to be mediated by cellular immune effectors or may reflect yet to be described syndromes.[49–51] Further studies are necessary to clarify this mechanism.

Tumor prognosis is believed to be better among patients with PND syndromes as often the neoplasm is asymptomatic or undetectable at the time of presentation.[1] However, a review of large series of patients has demonstrated that the oncologic outcome of patients with PND syndromes is not different from those patients who do not have antibodies against neural tissues.[52–54]

Clinical presentation

PND syndromes may manifest in different ways such as encephalitis (inflammation of the brain), myelitis (inflammation of the spinal cord), cerebellar degeneration (ataxia, dysarthria), neuropathy (progressive numbness and weakness in lower and upper extremities), myoclonus/opsoclonus (involuntary, rapid, irregular body jerks and multidirectional eye movements), Lambert-Eaton myasthenic syndrome (LEMS; weakness of several muscle groups), and dermatomyositis (DM; proximal weakness and skin lesions). Clinical presentations may develop acutely over the course of a few days or subacutely over the course of weeks or months.

General diagnostic approach

The diagnostic evaluation for a PND syndrome should begin with a complete medical examination, including palpation of lymph nodes, breasts and testes, rectal and

Table 20.1 Paraneoplastic neurological disorder antibodies and associated cancers

Antigens	Antibody	Associated Cancers
Intracellular	anti-Tr	Hodgkin lymphoma Non-Hodgkin lymphoma[19]
	anti-PCA-2	SCLC[20]
	anti-ANNA-3	SCLC, lung, and esophageal adenocarcinoma[21]
	anti-Ma1	Breast, parotid, colon, lung, testis, and ovarian cancer[22]
	anti-Recoverin	SCLC[23]
	anti-Zic4	SCLC, Hodgkin lymphoma, ovarian cancer[24–26]
	anti-Hu (ANNA-1)	SCLC and other neuroendocrine tumors[27]
	anti-Yo (anti-PCA-1)	Breast, ovary, endometrium, and fallopian tube cancers[28]
	anti-CRMP5 (CV2)	SCLC and thymoma[29]
	anti-Ri (ANNA-2)	Breast cancer, gynecologic cancers, and SCLC[30]
	anti-Ma2	Testicular cancer[31]
	anti-amphiphysin	Breast cancer, ovarian carcinoma, SCLC[32]
Cell-surface	anti-NMDAR	Ovarian teratomas, SCLC, uterine adenocarcinoma, prostate adenocarcinoma, Hodgkin lymphoma, pineal dysgerminoma, neuroblastoma, and NETs[33–35]
	anti-LGI1	Thymoma, lung cancer, NETs, abdominal mesothelioma[36]
	anti-CASPR2	Thymomas, lung cancer, endometrial adenocarcinoma[36]
	anti-AMPAR	Hematologic malignancy, cutaneous T-cell lymphoma[37]
	anti-$GABA_A$ receptor	Prostate cancer[38]
	anti-$GABA_B$ receptor	SCLC[39]
	anti-GlyR	Hodgkin lymphoma[40]
	anti-DPPX	B-cell lymphoma[41]
	anti-mGluR1	Hodgkin lymphoma, prostate adenocarcinoma[42]
	anti-mGluR5	Hodgkin lymphoma[43]
	anti-VGCC	Brain, breast, kidney, and lung cancers[44]
	anti-Ganglionic α 3-AchR	SCLC, adenocarcinomas[45]
	anti-Muscular α 1-AchR	Thymoma, SCLC[46]

AchR, Acetylcholine receptor; *AMPAR*, α-amino-3-hydroxy-5-methyl-4-isoxazolepropionic acid receptor; *ANNA-1*, antineuronal nuclear antibody type 1; *ANNA-2*, antineuronal nuclear antibodies type 2; *ANNA-3*, antineuronal nuclear antibody type 3; *Caspr2*, contactin-associated protein 2; *CRMP5*, collapsin response mediator protein 5; *DPPX*, dipeptidyl-peptidase–like protein 6; *$GABA_A$*, gamma aminobutyric acid A; *$GABA_B$*, gamma aminobutyric acid B; *GlyR*, glycine receptor; *LGI1*, leucine-rich glioma-inactivated 1; *NETs*, neuroendocrine tumors; *NMDA*, N-methyl-D-aspartate; *PCA-2*, Purkinje cell cytoplasmic antibody type 2; *SCLC*, small-cell lung carcinoma; *VGCC*, voltage-gated calcium channel.

pelvis, and neurological examination. Diagnostic testing of the CNS includes: (1) lumbar puncture with CSF analysis (e.g., white blood cell [WBC], glucose, protein, oligoclonal bands, immunoglobulin G [IgG] index, molecular and immunologic testing, cultures, and flow cytometry), (2) MRI of the brain and/or spinal cord, and (3) electroencephalography (EEG). Paraneoplastic antibody panel testing in both serum and CSF helps to identify autoimmune markers and paraneoplastic etiologies. Electromyographic and nerve conduction studies (EMG and NCS) should be performed if neuropathy, myasthenia, or myopathy raise suspicion for PNS involvement. Serum paraneoplastic autoantibody testing alone is appropriate for evaluation of these peripheral syndromes. Serum tumor markers are also useful as part of the malignancy screen, for instance, carcinoembryonic antigen (CEA), carbohydrate antigen 19-9 (CA 19-9), cancer antigen 125 (CA-125), and prostate-specific antigen (PSA). CT of the chest, abdomen, and pelvis are helpful in evaluating for an occult malignancy, as are testicular and vaginal ultrasounds and mammography.[55] Other tests that should be included are complete blood cell count with platelets (to assess for infection and immunosuppression), prothrombin time and activated partial thromboplastin time, electrolytes and osmolarity, toxicology screen, vitamin levels, liver function tests, and infectious tests. In the event that initial tumor screening is not revealing, repeat screening 3–6 months after the initial evaluation, and every 6 months up until 4 years is advised for patients with a diagnosis of a PND syndrome.[4]

Typical findings in a PND syndrome involving the CNS include CSF pleocytosis, hyperproteinorachie (i.e., elevated spinal fluid protein), intensification of intrathecal immunoglobulin synthesis and presence of oligoclonal bands. MRI of the brain may reveal T2-weighted hyperintense signals or atrophy in different parts of the brain or spinal cord, depending of the neurological syndrome. EEG may demonstrate focal slowing, focal or diffuse paroxysmal sharp waves, or electrographic seizures.

General treatment considerations and prognosis

The first approach to a PND syndrome should be tumor treatment as appropriate for the given malignancy with hopes of removing the immune response target.[56] Studies have shown that rapid antitumor treatment is associated with a higher likelihood of neurologic improvement or stabilization as well as lower mortality rates.[57] Initial treatment includes corticosteroids (e.g., intravenous methylprednisolone or prednisone), intravenous immunoglobulin (IVIg), and plasmapheresis. Alternative immunosuppressant medications that may be considered include mycophenolate mofetil, rituximab, azathioprine, and cyclophosphamide. The latter agents are typically used for chronic immunosuppression.[58]

Some PND syndromes respond better to treatment than others. For instance, immunosuppressive therapy (e.g., corticosteroids, plasmapheresis, and IVIg) is usually effective for myasthenia gravis (MG), encephalitis, and LEMS. In contrast, syndromes such as PCD, encephalomyelitis (EM), and limbic encephalitis tend to be resistant to first-line immunotherapy and may require early use of cyclophosphamide or rituximab.[59]

The failure of a PND syndrome to respond to therapy may be related to irreversible neuronal damage. In rare cases, patients may develop a recurrent PND syndrome after recovery, revealing a cancer relapse or the development of a new primary cancer.[60]

Clinical cases: classic and common paraneoplastic neurological disorder syndromes

CASE 20.1 ENCEPHALITIS AND LIMBIC ENCEPHALITIS

Case. A 24-year-old woman without a significant past medical or family history presented to the emergency room with subacute onset of anxiety, agitation, insomnia, auditory hallucinations, and paranoid ideations with subsequent progression to mutism and catatonia, choreiform movements, seizures, and confusion. Her initial general medical examination was notable for evidence of anxiety without other neurological findings. MRI of the brain was unremarkable (Fig. 20.1). CSF assessment demonstrated a lymphocytic predominant pleocytosis (WBC: 26 cells/mm^3, 97% lymphocytes), normal glucose (72 mg/dL), low protein (14 mg/dL), normal IgG index (0.4), and no oligoclonal bands in CSF or serum. CSF venereal disease research laboratory (VDRL), Lyme, human herpesvirus 6 (HHV-6), West Nile virus (WNV), herpes simplex virus (HSV), varicella zoster virus (VZV), Epstein-Barr virus (EBV), cytomegalovirus (CMV), enterovirus polymerase chain reactions (PCRs), and serological tests were negative, as were gram stain cultures and cytology. Toxic, metabolic, and nutritional testing as well as serum tumor markers were normal. EEG demonstrated right frontotemporal seizures and episodes of lateralized body shaking without associated epileptiform changes. Anti-*N*-methyl-D-aspartate receptor (anti-NMDAR) antibodies were reported as positive at a titer of 1:160 in serum. She was treated with intravenous corticosteroids and IVIg over 5 days. CT imaging demonstrated a mass compatible with right ovarian teratoma. She underwent a laparoscopic ovarian cystectomy with the removal of the dermoid cyst on the right ovary and pathology confirmed the diagnosis of a teratoma. Three months later, she developed dysautonomia symptoms (urinary retention, hypertension, tachycardia, and hyperthermia), disorientation, inattention, confusion, agitation and aggressiveness, seizures, dysphagia, and self-injurious behaviors. A follow-up CT study demonstrated a 12-mm lesion on the left ovary contralateral to the area of prior resection, concerning for an ovarian teratoma (Fig. 20.2). She underwent resection of the left ovary, and pathology was consistent with teratoma. Following surgery, she became less violent and agitated, although she did not return to her baseline status. She received five treatments of plasmapheresis, as well as three doses of

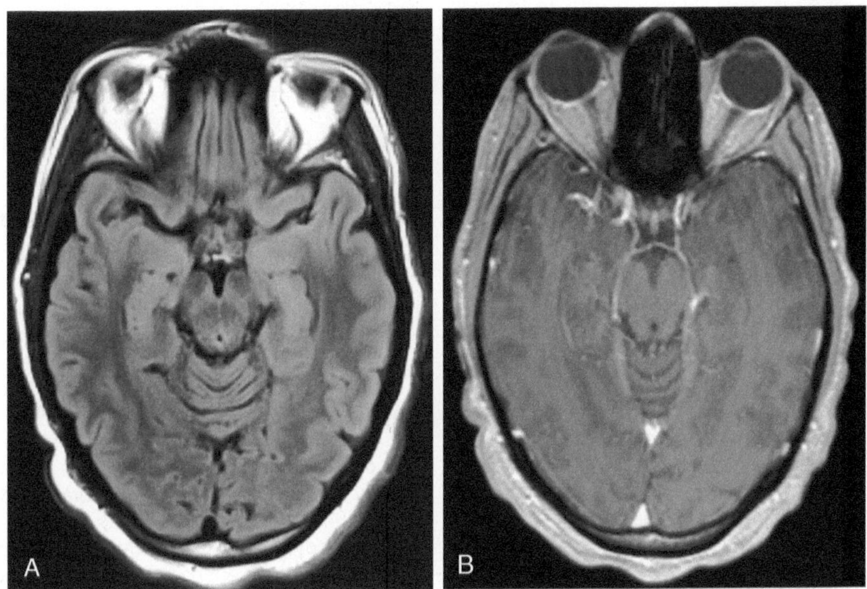

Fig. 20.1 Brain MRI of a patient with anti-NMDAR encephalitis. (A) Axial T2/fluid attenuated inversion recovery MRI and (B) T1 post-contrast sequences were unremarkable.

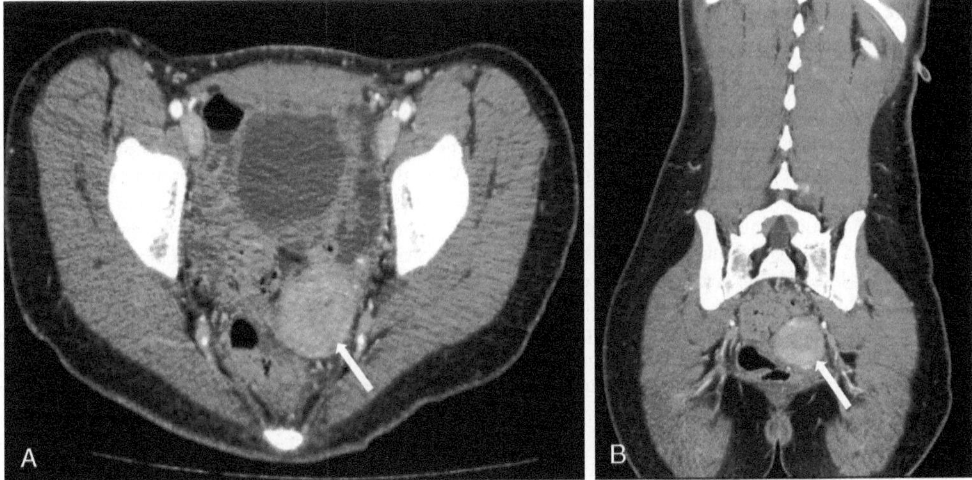

Fig. 20.2 CT scan of the abdomen and pelvis with and without contrast of a patient with anti-NMDAR encephalitis, with (A) axial image demonstrating a 2.6 × 2.4 × 2.6 cm cystic lesion concerning for tumor *(arrow)* in the posterior high left pelvis. (B) Coronal images demonstrate the mass lying along the internal iliac vessels *(arrow)*.

rituximab, with slow modest improvement. After hospital discharge, she experienced gradual improvement; however, she continued to experience episodes of movement and psychiatric disorders (bipolar mania), and cognitive impairment (inattention). This resolved in time. After nearly 5 years, she has not experienced new episodes of hallucinations, psychiatric disorders, seizures or other focal neurological symptoms. She was weaned off antipsychotic medications without issue.

Teaching Points. This case provides a typical presentation of anti-NMDAR encephalitis in the setting of ovarian teratoma and highlights several important teaching points including (1) the common neuropsychiatric features that occur at presentation in patients with encephalitis and limbic encephalitis, (2) that neuroimaging may be normal and CSF analysis may reveal subtle findings that require a high index of suspicion, and (3) source control with identification and removal of the associated neoplasm is paramount. In this case, the patient presented with prominent neuropsychiatric signs and symptoms that included hallucinations, paranoid ideations, choreiform movements, new-onset seizures, and mutism. Although primary mental illnesses can develop in the third decade, the subacute onset of symptoms required evaluation of explanatory pathology. Workup revealed only a mild lymphocytic pleocytosis and the clinician must have an appropriate index of suspicion for sending antibody testing in both the serum and CSF. In this case, control of the associated malignancy—the ovarian teratomas—was critical for managing the patient.

Paraneoplastic encephalitis

Definition and epidemiology. Encephalitis is an infectious or autoimmune condition of the brain, potentially involving the limbic system as well as other cortical and subcortical areas. Two types of autoimmune encephalitis have been described: (1) paraneoplastic encephalitis syndromes associated with cancer which typically involve antibodies to intracellular proteins, and (2) autoimmune encephalitis syndromes occurring in the absence of cancer which are more frequently observed in the setting of antibodies to cell surface proteins. Encephalitis can also occur with restricted involvement of limbic structures (e.g., hypothalamus, cingulate gyrus, insula, hippocampus, and amygdala).[61]

History. In 1968, postinflammatory changes in the mesial temporal lobes were described among patients with progressive memory loss in the setting of lung cancer.[62] Over a decade later, anti-Hu antibodies were discovered and associated with the pathogenesis of this disease. Subsequently, several antibodies have been associated with encephalitis and limbic encephalitis, including anti-Hu, anti-Ma2 (anti-TA), anti-NMDAR, anti–metabotropic glutamate receptor 5 (anti-mGluR5), anti-GABA$_B$ receptor, anti-AMPAR, anti-LGI1 and anti-CASPR2.[63–65] Not all autoimmune encephalitis and limbic encephalitis syndromes are paraneoplastic. For instance, in anti-LGI1 encephalitis, less than 10% of cases are paraneoplastic.[66–68]

Epidemiology. As paraneoplastic syndromes, encephalitis and limbic encephalitis are estimated to affect 1 per 10,000 patients with cancer, with 50% of cases occurring in the setting of SCLC, 20% with testicular tumors, and 8% with breast cancer.[69,70]

Classification. It is important to mention that not all paraneoplastic encephalitis can be categorized as limbic encephalitis. For instance, anti-NMDAR encephalitis is the most studied autoimmune encephalitis to date, and the majority do not follow the classic clinical and radiological profile for limbic encephalitis.[28,71,72] This syndrome has been identified in association with neoplasms in less than 50% of cases, mainly ovarian teratoma,[73] and in a few cases with other types of tumors such as testicular germ cell tumor,[33] Hodgkin lymphoma,[34] mediastinal teratoma,[35] and SCLC.[74]

Pathophysiology. Histopathology of patients with paraneoplastic encephalitis demonstrates T-cell infiltration, neural loss, and microglial activation in the hippocampus, amygdala, insula, orbitofrontal cortex, hippocampal gyrus, cingulate gyrus, thalamus, and hypothalamus.[75,76] Patients may have lesions in other non-limbic areas such as cerebral hemispheres, subcortical grey matter, brainstem, cerebellum, spinal cord, dorsal root, and autonomic ganglia.[77] For instance, patients with anti-CRMP5 (anti-CV2) antibodies and limbic encephalitis may have extra-limbic lesions of the cerebral cortex or basal ganglia.[78] The inflammatory changes do not necessarily correlate with the clinical presentation or neuronal loss.[79]

Whereas some paraneoplastic syndromes appear to be driven by cell-mediated inflammatory responses, others appear to be largely antibody driven. For example, anti-NMDAR encephalitis, in the presence or absence of cancer, is mediated by antibodies against the GluN1 subunit. Three immunopathogenic mechanisms have been proposed[80]:

1. Receptor internalization: antibody-mediated endocytosis of cell surface receptors that results in movement of receptors from the plasma membrane to the inside of the cell.
2. Antibody blockade of ion entry: when bound to their receptor, these antibodies obstruct enzyme function and prevent ion entry into the cell.
3. Complement-mediated cell lysis: antibody-induced activation of the complement cascade.

Molecular mimicry of the NMDA receptors appears to be the trigger of the autoimmune dysregulation.[81] The tumor cell's antigens are taken by antigen-presenting cells, activating an immune cascade, and plasma cells which produce antibodies cross-react with NMDA receptors in the brain.[82]

Clinical presentation. Encephalitis and limbic encephalitis can precede tumor diagnosis by many months or years.[83] Also, there are recent cases of patients with cancer who develop these syndromes after the initiation of immune checkpoint inhibitors (also see Chapter 30 for discussion of neurological syndromes from immune checkpoint inhibitors).[84] The clinical presentation is characterized by a subacute onset developing over days to weeks. Patients usually present with cognitive dysfunction (e.g., disorientation, altered mental status, short-term memory loss); psychiatric symptoms (e.g., change in personality, irritability, hallucinations, depression, anxiety, emotional lability, aggression, disinhibited behavior, bipolar disorder); paresis; catatonia; generalized, partial, or complex seizures; dysautonomia; and movement disorders (e.g., orofacial dyskinesia or choreoathetosis).[85] Frequently, patients initially present to medical attention when psychiatric symptoms develop, which are often first seen by a psychiatrist and misdiagnosed as an initial presentation of a psychiatric disorder in 40% of the cases.[78]

In anti-NMDAR encephalitis, adult patients typically develop memory loss and psychiatric disorders. Children, however, frequently experience seizures or movement disorders (e.g., orofacial dyskinesias, dystonic posturing, choreoathetoid movements, or general rigidity) without severe behavioral changes. Seizures commonly occur after a few weeks of onset. Patients may develop agitation or catatonia, central hypoventilation, and autonomic dysfunction.[56]

Diagnostic approach. In patients with autoimmune/paraneoplastic encephalitis or limbic encephalitis, MRI of the brain is unremarkable in more than 50% of cases, but abnormalities may become evident later.[86] Regarding autoantibody testing, both blood and CSF antibody testing should be performed given reports of increased sensitivity of CSF antibody testing over serum in anti-NMDAR encephalitis. EEG is abnormal in up to 90% of cases, commonly showing sharp and slow waves in the temporal lobes in addition to electrographic seizures.[22,87] Fluorodeoxyglucose positron emission tomography scanning (FDG-PET) scan was observed to be more sensitive than brain MRI in one retrospective study, warranting prospective evaluation.[88] In addition, occipital lobe hypometabolism appears to be a biomarker for anti-NMDAR encephalitis, suggesting the potential role of FDG-PET not only in the diagnosis of autoimmune encephalitis and limbic encephalitis but also specific antibody syndromes.[88,89] First-line screening for underlying malignancies is done with MRI, CT, and ultrasound, as appropriate for the suspected malignancy.[72] Serological tumor markers are usually negative in most patients.[90] Brain biopsy typically shows normal tissue or nonspecific inflammatory changes (e.g., neuronal loss, astrocytosis, inflammatory infiltration of perivascular and leptomeningeal tissue), and is therefore a high-risk diagnostic approach with low benefit.[22,91]

Diagnostic criteria. The diagnosis of encephalitis and limbic encephalitis is difficult and commonly involves the exclusion of other clinical syndromes, which may present similarly. Recent consensus clinical diagnostic criteria are useful in making the diagnosis of encephalitis.

Possible autoimmune or paraneoplastic encephalitis. The clinical diagnosis of possible autoimmune encephalitis can be made when three of the following criteria is present: (1) rapid progression (within 3 months) of working memory deficits, seizures, or psychiatric symptoms; (2) at least one of the following: new focal CNS findings, new onset of seizures, CSF pleocytosis, MRI suggestive of encephalitis (T2/fluid attenuated inversion recovery [FLAIR] hyperintensities in medial temporal lobes, T2/FLAIR hyperintensities in multifocal areas of grey, white matter, or both compatible with demyelination or inflammation), and (3) exclusion of other possible causes.[72,92]

Definite limbic encephalitis. The clinical diagnosis of definite limbic encephalitis requires that all four of the following criteria are met: (1) rapid progression (within 3 months) of working memory deficits, seizures or psychiatric symptoms, (2) T2-FLAIR MRI or FDG-PET scan demonstrating unilateral or bilateral abnormalities primarily in medial temporal lobes, (3) at least one of the following: CSF pleocytosis, or EEG showing epileptic or slow-wave activity involving one or both temporal lobes, (4) exclusion of other possible causes.[86]

Treatment. Encephalitis associated with cell-surface antibodies or synaptic proteins (e.g., $GABA_B$ receptor, anti-NMDAR, anti-AMPAR, anti-LGI1) is typically responsive to first-line immunosuppressive therapies. In the setting of refractory encephalitis or minimal response, rituximab or cyclophosphamide are used as second-line options.[72] Tocilizumab and bortezomib have shown additional benefits in cases of refractory anti-NMDAR encephalitis. Studies report that tocilizumab has better long-term outcomes than rituximab, whereas bortezomib therapy led to a fall in CSF antibodies levels and correlation with clinical improvement.[93] Treatment of associated seizures may require multiple anticonvulsant medications. Catatonia has been managed with benzodiazepines (e.g., lorazepam) and, in some cases, with amantadine.[94,95]

Prognosis. In general, cancer diagnosis and early treatment improve outcomes and prognosis. Patients with anti-Hu and anti-Ma/Ta antibodies have a poor prognosis given their strong associations with aggressive cancers, although seronegative cases may have a better prognosis.[96] Patients with anti-$GABA_B$ receptor encephalitis typically respond well to immunosuppressant medications.[72,97] Anti-NMDAR, anti-AMPAR, anti-$GABA_B$ receptor, anti-CASPR2, and anti-LGI1 encephalitis are also associated with excellent outcomes; however, these conditions may relapse.[97,98] For instance, among those with anti-NMDAR encephalitis, 80% achieve their clinical baseline and 12–25% experience relapse within 24 months.[99,100] The prognosis is more favorable if immunotherapy is initiated in the first 4 months of symptom onset. After discharge, a multidisciplinary group of specialists should be involved in the treatment of impairments in attention, memory, executive function, and vision. However, these sequelae could persist for many years[101–103] and impair patients' ability to return to their pre-morbid independence in daily life.[104]

CASE 20.2 ENCEPHALOMYELITIS

Case. A 42-year-old woman with a past medical history of left breast cancer treated by unilateral mastectomy, chemoradiation, and tamoxifen; migraines; and possible complex partial seizures presented to the emergency room for a subacute onset of leg weakness, fatigue, and memory loss. On examination, she had long-term memory impairment, difficulty with ambulation, and wide-based gait, with normal motor and sensory examinations. CSF findings were notable for a lymphocytic pleocytosis (WBC 120 cell/μL, 99% lymphocytes) and elevated protein (91 mg/dL), low glucose (48 mg/dL), a mildly elevated IgG index (0.9), and presence of oligoclonal bands in CSF only. CSF VDRL, Lyme, HHV-6, WNV, HSV, VZV, EBV, CMV, enterovirus PCRs, serology testing, gram stain, cultures and cytology were negative. Spinal cord and brain MRI demonstrated T2/FLAIR hyperintensities of the hypothalamus and gray matter of the spinal cord from C1 to the conus, without associated enhancement (Figs. 20.3 and 20.4). Paraneoplastic antibody testing demonstrated anti-Ri antibody in serum. In addition, erythrocyte sedimentation rate was

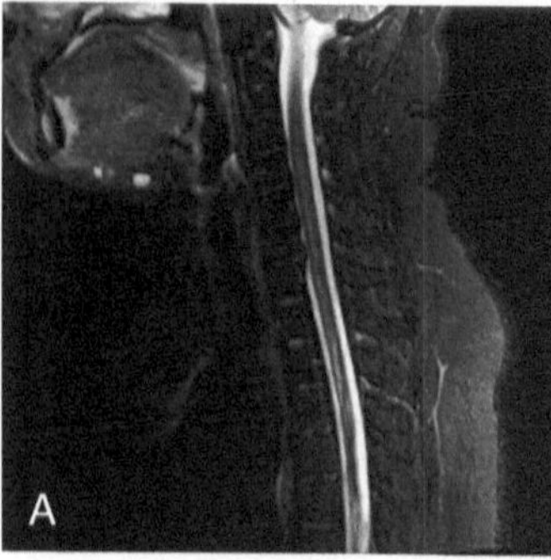

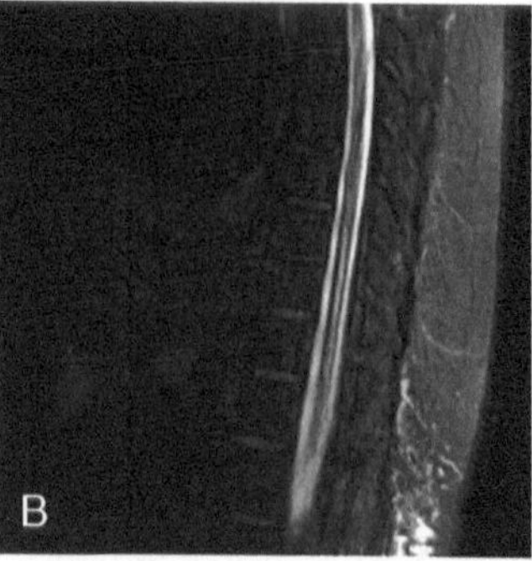

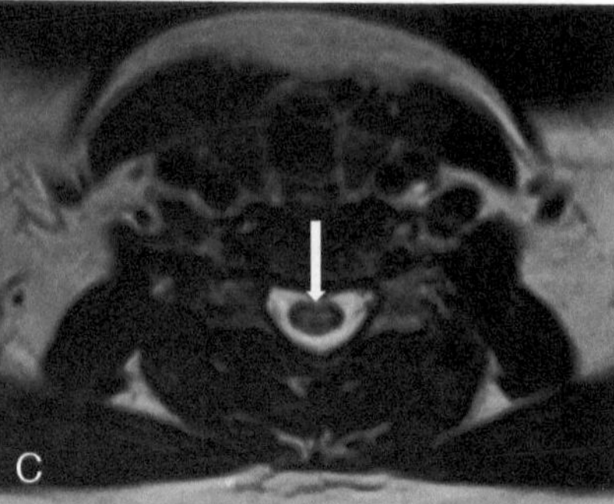

Fig. 20.3 Spinal MRI of a patient with encephalomyelitis. (A) Sagittal T2-weighted MRI of the cervical and (B) thoracic spine demonstrate a longitudinally-extensive hyperintense abnormality within the central cord, whereas (C) axial T2-weighted images demonstrate a longitudinally-extensive hyperintensity restricted to the grey matter *(arrow)*.

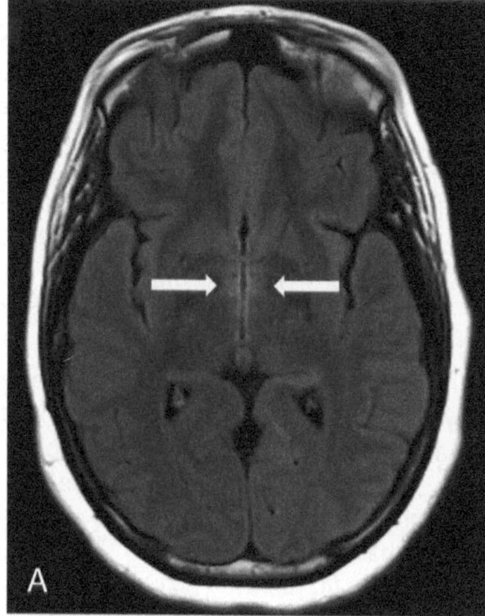

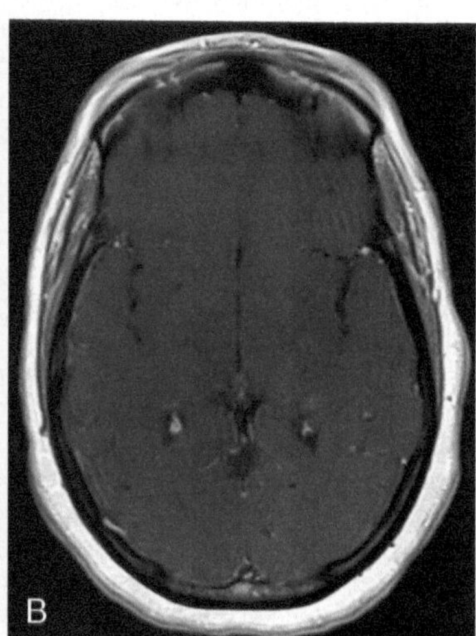

Fig. 20.4 Brain MRI of a patient with encephalomyelitis. (A) Axial T2/fluid attenuated inversion recovery images demonstrate abnormal signal hyperintensity within the hypothalamus *(arrows)* and (B) T1 post-contrast sequence does not demonstrate associated contrast enhancement.

elevated (35 mm/h) and metabolic testing including vitamin D, aldolase, copper, zinc, vitamin B_{12}, vitamin B_1, TSH, and methylmalonic acid, were all within normal limits. Serological assays for antineutrophil cytoplasmic antibodies (ANCA), double-stranded DNA, Ro/La, and syphilis were normal. Mammography and FDG-PET scan did not demonstrate evidence of breast cancer recurrence. She was treated with corticosteroids for 5 days, followed by a corticosteroid taper with improvement of her symptoms. After discharge, she slowly deteriorated despite aggressive immunotherapy, and 4 months later, she died of a cardiac arrest.

Teaching Points. This case demonstrates the spectrum of potential CNS involvement that can occur in patients with encephalomyelitis. Paraneoplastic encephalomyelitis (EM) is characterized by multifocal inflammation involving the brain, brainstem, and/or spinal cord. This case highlights the difficulty in treating patients with intracellular antigen syndromes. In contrast to the favorable outcome of the patient in Case 20.1 with a cell-surface antibody syndrome, this patient failed to respond to aggressive immunotherapy which could not rescue her progressive deterioration in neurological function, and she ultimately died.

Paraneoplastic encephalomyelitis

Definition and Epidemiology. EM is a multifocal inflammatory disorder that affects several areas of the central nervous system in association with a neoplasm, postinfectious process, or other autoimmune-related syndromes.[105] Post-infectious and post-vaccinal encephalomyelitis account for 75% of cases. Postvaccine-encephalomyelitis cases have been described with rabies, tetanus, polio, measles, mumps, rubella, Japanese B encephalitis, pertussis, and influenza vaccines.[106] In contrast, the incidence of paraneoplastic EM is unknown. Approximately 0.4% of patients with bronchial carcinoma develop this syndrome without predilection for either sex.[52] With that said, anti-Hu associated with EM is slightly more prevalent in females.[57] The most common associated malignancy is SCLC (75% of cases), although other associated cancers have been reported such as lung adenocarcinoma, multiple myeloma, lymphoma, chondrosarcoma, and neuroblastomas.[105–108] Middle-aged and older adults are typically affected.[109]

EM most frequently involves the temporal lobe limbic structures, brainstem, spinal cord, dorsal root ganglia, and autonomic nervous system.[53,110,111] Several antibodies have been associated with EM including anti-Hu, anti-CRMP5/CV2, anti-Ma2, anti-amphiphysin, anti-Yo, anti-Ta, anti-Ma1, anti-LG1, and anti-PCA-2.[25,106]

Pathophysiology. Anti-Hu antibodies are the most common antibodies detected in EM.[112] These antibodies react with RNA-binding proteins (e.g., PLE21/HuC, HuD, HuR, Hel-N1) affecting the function of the CNS.[113] Pathologic examination demonstrates perivascular and interstitial lymphocytic infiltrates, neuronophagic nodules, neuronal loss, gliosis, and plasma cell infiltration.[91,114] In addition, studies have reported the presence of HSV by PCR and 14-3-3 protein in patients with paraneoplastic EM, but the significance of these findings is still unknown.[115,116]

Clinical presentation. Generally, EM follows a subacute onset with a subsequent progression over weeks to months before achieving a clinical plateau. The typical presentation is characterized by psychiatric symptoms, cognitive impairment, seizures, cranial nerve palsies, cerebellar signs, sensory-motor neuropathy or motor neuron dysfunction, and dysautonomia.[22,53,55,57] Isolated symptoms are extremely rare, although isolated cerebellar presentations have been described.[105]

Diagnostic approach. Brain and spinal cord MRI with and without gadolinium are the image studies of choice to evaluate symptoms and signs of myelopathy. The diagnosis is supported by infratentorial and supratentorial grey and white matter lesions, and the absence of destructive hypointense white matter lesions on T1-weighted MRI in the chronic stages of the disease. However, most patients have unremarkable imaging of the brain.[117,118] In contrast, MRI abnormalities in the spinal cord are more frequent, with 60–70% of patients developing longitudinally extensive lesions often associated with contrast enhancement.[119] FDG-PET scan may show hypermetabolism of limbic structures initially, and hypometabolism during recovery. The most frequently detected antibodies include anti-Hu, anti-CRMP5/CV2, and, less frequently, anti-amphiphysin antibodies.

Treatment. Paraneoplastic EM tends to be resistant to immunosuppression, and clinical trials have not been done.[105] In this setting, the use of second-line immunotherapies such as rituximab and cyclophosphamide should be considered early. A case report described the use of rituximab and cyclophosphamide with partial improvement.[120] Prompt control of the tumor while also treating with immunosuppressive therapy may help to stabilize the course of the syndrome.[59]

Prognosis. The clinical course of paraneoplastic EM is uncertain. High titers of anti-Hu antibodies are related to worse outcomes, including death, most likely because of the strong association of this antibody with SCLC. Patients with brainstem and autonomic dysfunction, in general, develop worse outcomes and have a high mortality rate. Although resection and treatment of the associated tumor improve outcomes, neurological function rarely improves without treatment.[57,121] Paresis and paraparesis are common, and patients benefit from physical therapy and deep venous thrombosis prophylaxis. In children, the syndrome has worse outcomes and is associated with cognitive impairment and long-lasting seizures.[122] Anticonvulsants such as fosphenytoin have been used for seizure management.

CASE 20.3 PARANEOPLASTIC SUBACUTE CEREBELLAR DEGENERATION

Case. A 70-year-old woman with a past medical history of hypertension, type 2 diabetes mellitus, gallstone pancreatitis, and gastroesophageal reflux presented to the emergency room with a subacute onset of memory loss followed by progressive irritability, difficulty reading and writing, diplopia, dysarthria, and gait disturbance associated with unintentional weight loss. Her neurological examination demonstrated dysarthria, rotational nystagmus noted in all directions, dysmetria, dysdiadochokinesia, and ataxia. CSF testing revealed normal WBC (2 cell/mm^3), hyperproteinorachie (59 mg/dL), normal glucose (90 mg/dL), and presence of oligoclonal bands in CSF only. VZV, EBV, CMV, HSV PCRs and serological tests were negative, as were gram stain, cultures, and cytology. Paraneoplastic antibody testing, metabolic, and rheumatologic tests were unremarkable. Brain MRI demonstrated bilateral cerebellar atrophy and anterior temporal lobe encephalomalacia (Fig. 20.5). CT scan of the chest and abdomen demonstrated a right middle lobe nodule, multiple pulmonary nodules in the left lower lobe, and a heterogeneously enlarged left thyroid lobe with the presence of numerous hypodense nodules. Ultrasound of the thyroid demonstrated a multinodular goiter with more nodules in the left lobe as compared with the right. Thyroid biopsy did not demonstrate evidence of malignancy. FDG-PET scan revealed an active hypermetabolic right middle lobe pulmonary nodule with a prominently enlarged and hypermetabolic subcarinal lymph node (Fig. 20.6). Bronchoscopy with endobronchial ultrasound-guided biopsies confirmed a diagnosis of metastatic grade 1 neuroendocrine lung carcinoma. She underwent surgery and chemotherapy for lung cancer and received treatment with IVIg for 5 days with partial improvement. After discharge, she continued treatment with IVIg and mycophenolate as well as physical and speech therapy. Over the 2 years following diagnosis, she has experienced progressive improvement of her symptoms; however, dysphagia remains an issue.

Teaching Points. This case highlights the common and uncommon tumors associated with PND syndromes. PCD is classically associated with breast and ovarian malignancies. However, neuroendocrine tumors including small-cell carcinoma (e.g., SCLC) and hematologic malignancies such as lymphoma are not infrequently associated with PND syndromes and should be considered in patients who present with a typical clinical syndrome. Also, this patient was seronegative for a paraneoplastic autoantibody, as is observed in 50% of cases of PCD, emphasizing the importance of syndrome recognition.

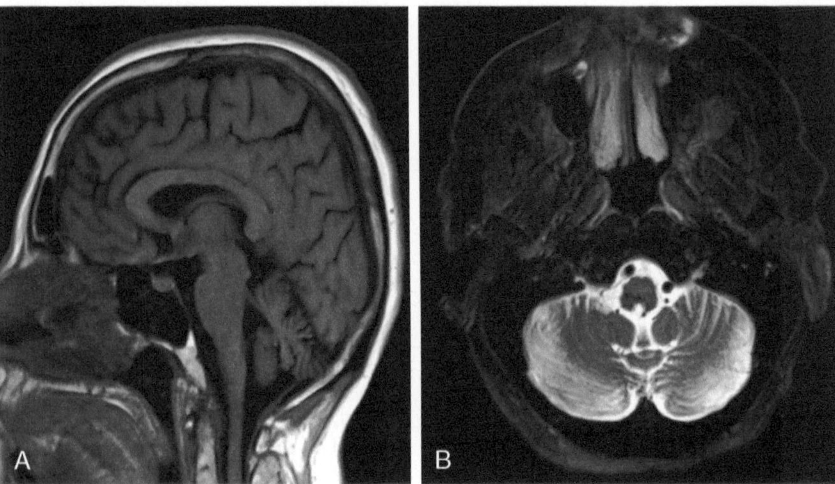

Fig. 20.5 Brain MRI of a patient with paraneoplastic subacute cerebellar degeneration. (A) Sagittal T1-weighted and (B) axial T2-weighted MRI of the brain demonstrate prominent horizontal fissures of the bilateral cerebellar hemispheres.

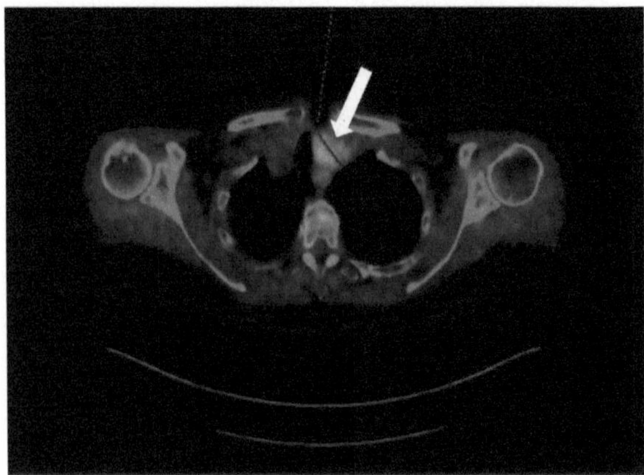

Fig. 20.6 Whole body FDG-PET scan of a patient with subacute cerebellar degeneration demonstrates a metabolically active right middle lobe pulmonary nodule with a prominently enlarged and FDG-avid subcarinal lymph node *(arrow)*. *FDG-PET*, Fluorodeoxyglucose positron emission tomography scanning.

Paraneoplastic cerebellar degeneration

Definition and epidemiology. PCD is one of the most devasting PND syndromes. This condition was first described in 1919, but its association with neoplastic tumors was established in 1951.[123] This syndrome is commonly associated with Hodgkin lymphoma, ovarian, breast, and SCLC, and rarely with prostate and gastrointestinal tumors (gastric and esophageal tumors).[13,124,125] Women are more frequently affected than men in a proportion of 7:3.[126] In the United States, PCD occurs in approximately 2 of 1,000 patients with cancer.[28] The most common and specific subtype of PCD is the syndrome related to anti-Yo (PCA-1), accounting for 50% of cases.[127] PCD manifests in different age ranges. Anti-Yo and anti-Hu associated PCD typically occurs among middle-aged patients with breast or ovarian (anti-Yo) and lung cancer (anti-Hu) whereas patients with anti-Tr associated PCD are typically young men with Hodgkin lymphoma.[128] In accordance with the rarity of this syndrome, the literature is largely limited to case series and reports.

Pathophysiology. Antibodies seem to be involved at the initial stage of the disorder; however, the T-cell immune response appears to be principally responsible for PCD (Table 20.2). The Yo antigen is a protein found in the cytoplasm that interacts with c-Myc in the Purkinje cells of the cerebellum. T cells recognize the antigen and cause severe or complete loss of Purkinje cells which is eventually seen by brain MRI.[127,129] This condition initially affects the vermis and midline cerebellum and later the cerebellar hemispheres. Approximately half of patients with PCD are seronegative for an associated antibody on commercially available testing. Thus, clinical recognition of PCD rather than reliance on antibody testing results should guide concern for malignancy.[130,131]

Clinical presentation. PCD is a condition that evolves over the course of a few weeks to months.[132] It usually starts as mild unsteadiness when walking associated with episodic vertigo, motion sickness, ataxic dysarthria, and diplopia.[13] Subsequently, it progresses to ataxia of gait and trunk, and bilateral eye abnormal movements. Limb ataxia regularly occurs after the development of gait ataxia, characterized by marked postural and intention tremor affecting activities of daily living.[129] Up to 80% of people lose the ability to ambulate or sit independently.[133]

Dysarthria can impair effective communication and contributes to social isolation, frustration, and depression.[13] Patients lose prosody and have irregular articulation, speech

Table 20.2 Antibodies and related cancers in paraneoplastic cerebellar degeneration

Antibody	Related tumor	Features
Anti-Yo	Gynecological malignancies (ovarian, pelvic related malignancies including of the fallopian tube, uterus, and cervix) Breast carcinoma	Precedes the cancer diagnosis By the time of neurological presentation, cancer is metastatic to regional lymph nodes[138]
Anti-Tr or PCA-Tr	Hodgkin lymphoma	80% of cases after diagnosis or remission Less severe Stabilize with treatment[139]
anti-Hu (ANNA-1)	SCLC (most common) Others: pancreas, prostate, cervix, and skin	Sensory or sensorimotor neuropathy (most common), cerebellar ataxia (10–20%), limbic encephalitis, or gastrointestinal dysmotility[47]
anti-Ri (ANNA-2)	Lung (SCLC and non-small cell) and breast carcinoma	50% of patients have cerebellar degeneration. A better outcome than anti-Hu or ANNA-1 Median survival >60 months PCD with opsoclonus has a better prognosis[140]
anti-CRMP5 (CV2)	SCLC Less common, thymoma	Neuropathy, dementia, chorea, cranial neuropathy, optic neuropathy Cerebellar ataxia (25%), usually in combination with the above disorders[141]

ANNA-1, Antineuronal nuclear antibodies type 1; *ANNA-2*, antineuronal nuclear antibodies type 2; *CRMP5*, collapsin response mediator protein 5; *PCA-Tr*, Purkinje cell cytoplasmic antibody Tr; *PCD*, paraneoplastic cerebellar degeneration; *SCLC*, small-cell lung carcinoma.

rate, and volume. Less commonly, patients develop dysphagia, which may require gastrostomy placement. Visual disturbances may include oscillopsia, diplopia, oculomotor palsy, and opsoclonus.[13] Other unusual associated manifestations include drowsiness, coma, dementia, and severe cognitive impairment. Mood changes are frequent, especially depression, which may be related to the damage of the cerebellar control of affect in the cerebellum.[134] However, this could also be an expected reaction to a new diagnosis of cancer and the PCD-associated disability.

Diagnostic approach. The diagnostic approach begins with clinical suspicion for PCD in the setting of subacute onset and progression of gait instability, dysarthria, vertigo, intention, and postural tremor. CSF analyses may be normal; however, inflammatory/autoimmune findings may help to differentiate PCD from other neurological disorders. Pleocytosis is present in 75% of cases (e.g., often ~20 cells, but sometimes more than 100 cells/mm^3), and hyperproteinorachie in nearly all cases.[135] High IgG index and synthesis rate suggest intrathecal antibody production. CSF oligoclonal bands are usually seen in cases of SCLC.[136] MRI of the brain is usually normal in early stages of the disease, but diffuse atrophy of the cerebellum may be seen months after symptom onset. Signal abnormalities in the brainstem and mesial temporal lobes have also been reported.[13,137]

Treatment. Therapy with corticosteroids, plasma exchange, and IVIg has not been proven to be beneficial. As such, cyclophosphamide or rituximab should be implemented early. Also, aggressive tumor therapy in association with immunosuppressive therapy appears to stabilize or improve the symptoms.[136] The impact of this therapeutic combination is still unknown.

Prognosis. Patients with PCD have a better outcome compared with neurologically healthy patients with the same associated cancers. Survival depends on the cancer type and tumor stage at the time of diagnosis. Nearly half of deaths are attributable to complications of the neurological condition and the other half due to cancer complications.[18] Survival after diagnosis of PCD varies, ranging from 10 months for SCLC and 12 months for ovarian carcinoma to 100 or more months for breast cancer and Hodgkin lymphoma.[13]

CASE 20.4 OPSOCLONUS-MYOCLONUS

Case. A 43-year-old man with a past medical history of hypertension presented to the emergency room for a subacute onset of unsteady gait, cognitive decline, generalized complex partial seizures manifesting as staring spells with facial movements, and dysphagia. The abnormal movements of his lips were increasing in frequency (6–10 times a day), lasting less than a minute, and reportedly longer during episodes of sleep. Following these episodes, he would speak in nonsensical phrases before he became reoriented. On neurological examination, he scored a 21 of a possible 30 points on the Montreal cognitive assessment

(MoCA; normal ≥26). He demonstrated disorientation, dyscalculia, hyperreflexia in his lower extremities, and Babinski's sign in the left foot. Continuous EEG demonstrated intermittent right frontotemporal sharp waves and spikes. The staring events were noted to correspond with apneic awakenings from sleep, with notable stridor during sleep. Lumbar puncture with fluoroscopic guidance demonstrated CSF pleocytosis (WBC 7 cells/mm^3), normal glucose (71 mg/dL), normal protein (35.2 mg/dL), slightly elevated IgG index (0.7), and presence of oligoclonal bands in CSF mirroring those in the serum. CSF VDRL, Lyme, HHV-6, WNV, HSV, VZV, EBV, CMV, enterovirus PCRs and serological testing, as well as gram stain, cultures, and cytology, were negative. Paraneoplastic antibody testing in the CSF and serum was negative. MRI of the brain was unremarkable. FDG-PET/CT demonstrated global hypometabolism in the brain, most notably over the right precentral gyrus, with no evidence of malignancy in the chest, abdomen, or pelvis. He was treated with high-dose IV methylprednisolone for 5 days and discharged on oral prednisone taper with close outpatient neurology follow-up. Three months later, he returned to the emergency room for a subacute onset of anxiety, panic attacks, tremulousness, worsening bilateral blurred vision complicated by feeling as though objects were "jumping around," photophobia, and short-term memory issues. A brain MRI with and without contrast demonstrated scattered periventricular and subcortical white matter T2/FLAIR hyperintensities, which likely represented chronic small vessel ischemic changes. Testicular ultrasound was normal. CT of the chest, abdomen, and pelvis revealed scattered subcentimeter hepatic hypodensities too small to characterize but likely reflecting hemangiomas or cysts. A lumbar puncture was performed and demonstrated a mild pleocytosis (WBC: 23 cells/mm^3), red blood cells 0 cells/mm^3, normal glucose (71 mg/dL), normal protein (35 mg/dL), and presence of oligoclonal bands in the CSF mirroring those in the serum. Repeated paraneoplastic antibody testing, including anti-Ri, anti-Ma1, and anti-Ta were negative. He was treated with a high dose of IV methylprednisolone with marked improvement. After discharge, he continued having episodes of anxiety and abnormal movement of his eyes, but these symptoms have been improving progressively over the subsequent 2 years of follow-up. He is currently stable without new episodes of abnormal movements or mood changes while on systemic immunosuppression with mycophenolate mofetil.

Teaching Points. Although opsoclonus-myoclonus syndrome (OMS) occurs in some children with neuroblastoma, it may also occur in adults where there is an association with SCLC and breast malignancies. Unlike this patient, anti-Hu and anti-Ri antibodies are frequently discovered in these patients. Episodes of opsoclonus may be intermittent, and, as in this case, the presentation can mimic seizures. Clinicians who recognize the subacute onset of both paroxysmal opsoclonus and myoclonus should conduct appropriate cancer screening and search for a contributory onconeuronal antibody. This case underscores the fact that, in the setting of a typical PND syndrome (e.g., OMS) and supportive neurodiagnostic evaluations suggesting CNS inflammation (e.g., lymphocytic pleocytosis), a diagnosis of possible PND syndrome can be made and treatment initiated even when a causative onconeuronal antibody or cancer are not identified.

Opsoclonus-myoclonus syndrome

Definition and epidemiology. OMS, also known as "dancing eye syndrome," is an infrequent condition. It is defined as rapid and repetitive, involuntary, irregular in amplitude and frequency ocular saccades that can occur in any direction, and is associated with ataxia, myoclonus, mood changes, and sleep disturbances. In children, its incidence is 1 in 10 million, occurring as a paraneoplastic syndrome in 2–3% of all children with neuroblastoma.[142] However, the frequency of people with OMS who develop neuroblastoma is unclear. Some case series have shown that the frequency could be between 5 and 100%. This syndrome has a median age presentation of 18 months, with a female predilection.[143,144] This condition may show a monophasic or chronic relapsing pattern. Some cases of OMS recover spontaneously in a short period of time, typically days to weeks. The majority of paraneoplastic and autoimmune cases need long-term immunosuppression treatment and have not been related to tumor recurrences.

In adults, OMS frequently occurs in association with SCLC and breast malignancies in the setting of anti-Hu and anti-Ri seropositivity. The mean age of presentation is 55 years.[145] OMS has been described in patients with other tumors (e.g., non-SCLC, ovarian teratoma, gastric adenocarcinoma, melanoma, and bladder cancer) and with other onconeural antibodies (e.g., anti-NMDAR, anti-$GABA_A$ receptor, anti-$GABA_B$ receptor, anti-DPPX, and anti-GlyR).[146,147]

Pathophysiology. Among patients with OMS, a variety of autoantibodies against various neuronal antigens found in the cerebellum and brainstem, as well as associated B- and T-cell alterations, have been described.[142,144] In children, specific antibodies have not been identified, whereas in adults this syndrome is associated with anti-Ri and anti- Hu antibodies.[143] B- and T-cell abnormalities have been reported, including an increase of the B-cell population, amplified T-cell activation, reductions in the number of helper/inducer T-cells, and augmentation of the number of suppressor/cytotoxic T cells.[148] Autopsies of adult brains demonstrate loss of Purkinje cells and dentate demyelination as well as involvement of the cerebellum and brainstem. Lesions of the dentatorubral pathway were proposed as the cause of the occurrence of OMS.[142]

Clinical presentation. In children between 1 and 3 years of age, OMS is characterized by a subacute progress of jerky unsteadiness, behavioral changes (e.g., irritability), sleep disturbance, and intermittent opsoclonus in association with abdominal or thoracic neuroblastoma.[149,150] In adults, OMS has been reported after viral gastrointestinal infections, upper respiratory illness, and in the setting of cancer. For instance, OMS was reported after febrile episodes in a series of six cases. Typical clinical presentation includes truncal ataxia that results in frequent falls, myoclonus and opsoclonus, nausea, and vomiting.[151] Less frequent symptoms include tremor, ataxia, and dysarthria. Encephalopathy, cerebellar signs, and brainstem signs may also be present.[152]

Diagnostic approach. Diagnosis of OMS is very challenging because of the rarity of the syndrome and limited clinical familiarity among physicians. Opsoclonus is frequently intermittent, and therefore close clinical observation is needed to observe an episode. In many cases, opsoclonus is misdiagnosed as another eye movement disorder or as seizures. Other symptoms, such as dysphagia, could be present and make the diagnosis more difficult.

In children, diagnosis of OMS is made if the patient has three of the following features: opsoclonus or ocular flutter, neuroblastoma, myoclonus and/or ataxia, behavioral and/or sleep disturbance in association with irritability.[8] As this paraneoplastic syndrome is associated with neuroblastoma, the current diagnostic approach for tumor detection includes a detailed MRI of abdomen and thorax, ultrasound of the neck, urinary catecholamine metabolites, and radiolabeled iodine scintigraphy scan. Antibodies related to OMS include anti-Hu, anti-Ri, and anti-PCA-1 antibodies.[26] Anti-Hu is more common in adults with OMS and frequently related to SCLC.[122,153] However, if anti-Hu is present in a child, neuroblastoma or ganglioneuroblastoma should be considered.[153] No immunological markers or brain imaging findings have been reported as specific for this disorder.[142,154]

In adults, OMS should be distinguished from other disorders (e.g., myoclonus, toxic-metabolic encephalopathy, other ataxia syndromes). CSF is typically normal but may demonstrate hyperproteinorachie or a mild lymphocytic pleocytosis.[145] Brain imaging is usually unremarkable in patients with OMS; however, it may show dorsal pontine or midbrain hyperintensities on T2-weighted images.[155] As in the presented case, paraneoplastic antibody testing is negative in the majority of adult patients.[156]

Treatment. In pediatric OMS, the evidence for the use of immunotherapy remains limited. In one study, a combination therapy of dexamethasone and cyclophosphamide at 4-week intervals was used for children with chronic relapses without evidence of recurrent neuroblastoma. Other uncontrolled studies report better outcomes with rituximab, corticotropin (ACTH), and IVIg. In addition, the treatment of neuroblastoma with chemotherapy may be useful; however, data is contradictory and unconvincing.[142]

In adults with OMS, there is no treatment consensus. Therapies such as ACTH and corticosteroids have been described, as well as cyclophosphamide and IVIg. Other medications frequently used for symptomatic treatment include baclofen, clonazepam, propranolol, thiamine, chloramphenicol, and valproic acid, which may help to reduce eye movements. Trazadone has been effective for the management of irritability and sleep problems.[142]

Prognosis. Outcomes in OMS are varied. A minority of patients achieve their baseline, but most experience a broad range of chronic neurological disabilities (e.g., motor and cognitive difficulties). In children, patients with low-grade tumors (e.g., ganglioneuroblastoma) have a markedly better oncologic outcome in comparison with patients with neuroblastoma without the neurological syndrome. In addition, prognosis in children without metastasis is excellent, with a 3-year survival of 100%.[157,158]

Many pediatric patients remain with neurological sequelae. In a retrospective study of patients with OMS, 80% developed motor, cognitive, language, and behavioral sequelae and 66% experienced intellectual disability.[159] Although, studies have demonstrated that a more aggressive treatment may help patients to reach their neurological baseline. Relapses are associated with infections and B-cell population expansion.[160]

OMS in adults tends to respond poorly to immunotherapy. Nevertheless, case reports have demonstrated good outcomes with the use of corticosteroids, cyclophosphamide, and IVIg for immunosuppression along with clonazepam and topiramate.[161,162] Relapses are frequent, and some may remain with cerebellar dysfunction (ataxic gait).[146,163] Prognosis is poor in patients with cancer or untreated tumors.

CASE 20.5 PARANEOPLASTIC SENSORY NEURONOPATHY

Case. A 71-year-old previously healthy woman presented to the emergency room for a subacute onset of vision symptoms consisting of ptosis and conjugate gaze impairment, imbalance, dysphagia, dysarthria, dysphonia, and weight loss (32 pounds) over a 2-month period. Neurological examination revealed decreased visual acuity and sluggish response in the left eye, intermittent ptosis of the left eye, hypophonic voice, dysarthria, weak elevation of the right palate, bilateral decreased light touch and vibration in distal lower extremities, and unsteady gait. A lumbar puncture yielded CSF with normal WBC (4 cells/mm^3), normal glucose (71 mg/dL), normal protein (35 mg/dL), CSF VDRL, Lyme, HHV-6, CMV, EBV, HSV, VZV, enterovirus, WNV PCRs, and serology testing were negative, as were gram stain, cultures, and cytology. Brain MRI demonstrated numerous scattered and confluent T2/FLAIR subcortical, periventricular, and deep white matter hyperintensities with an orientation perpendicular to the callososeptal interface and sparing the structures of the posterior cranial fossa. EMG/NCS showed sensory-motor axonal polyneuropathy in lower extremities as well as mild right median and ulnar neuropathy. Repetitive nerve stimulation test did not reveal electrodecremental responses suggestive of a neuromuscular junction disorder. Malignancy evaluation was undertaken, and a CT Chest revealed a nodule in the right upper lobe of the lung with a necrotic hilar and ipsilateral mediastinal adenopathy concerning for primary lung malignancy, which was biopsied (Fig. 20.7). Pathologic examination of the lymph node led to the diagnosis of SCLC in association with paraneoplastic sensory motor neuronopathy. Anti-Hu antibodies were detected in serum. She was treated with IVIg for 5 days with marked improvement. She was subsequently started on a low corticosteroid dose of 10 mg daily. Afterward, she received treatment with cisplatin and etoposide as well as whole-brain radiation.

Teaching Points. This case provides a classic presentation for a patient with anti-Hu associated paraneoplastic sensory neuronopathy or ganglionopathy. As was the case for this patient, there is a strong association with SCLC. Although studies have suggested that over 80% of SCLC patients may possess underlying anti-Hu antibodies, only a subset of these patients will develop

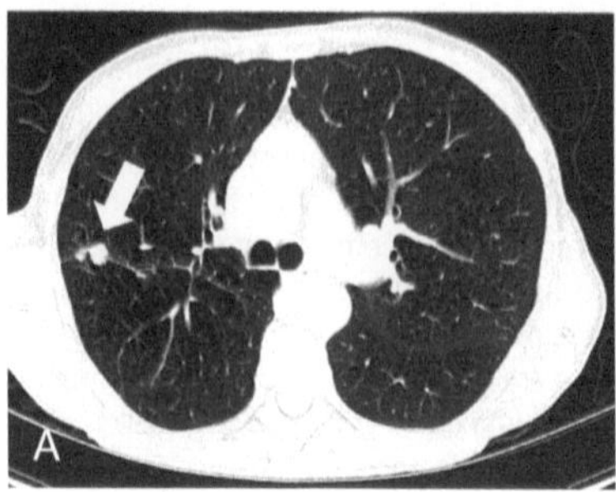

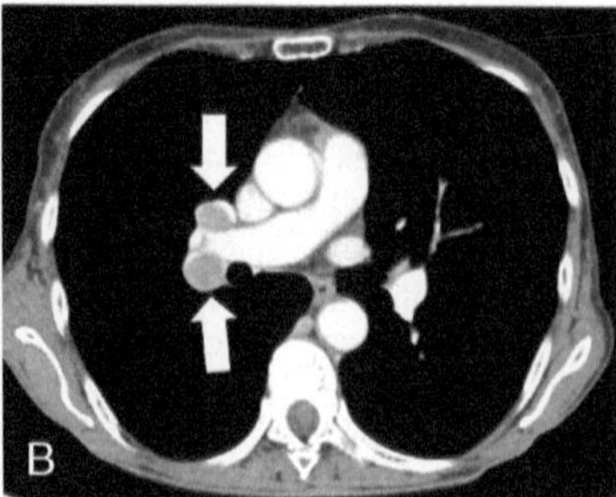

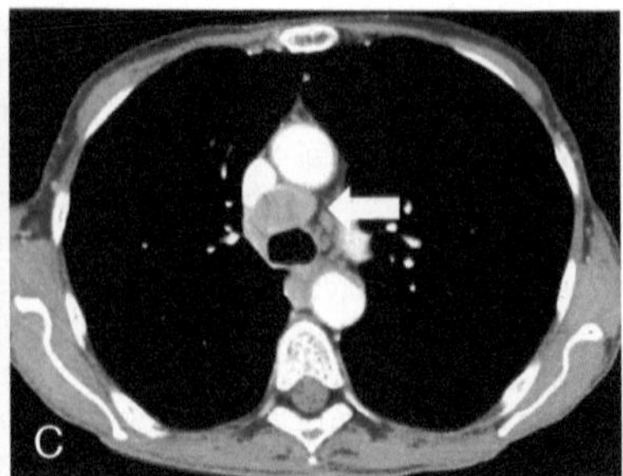

Fig. 20.7 Axial Chest CT scan of a patient with Lambert-Eaton myasthenic syndrome demonstrates (A) 1-cm nodular opacity in the posterior right upper lobe and extensive centrilobular emphysematous (arrow), (B) enlarged right hilar lymph nodes compressing the superior right pulmonary vein, as well as pulmonary arterial tree *(arrows)*, and (C) enlarged necrotic paratracheal lymph nodes *(arrow)*.

symptomatic neurological findings, underscoring the importance of establishing a clinical-serologic link in these patients. As with this patient, response to treatment can be quite favorable.

Paraneoplastic subacute sensory neuronopathy

Definition and epidemiology. The peripheral nervous system is impaired in one-third of patients with a PND syndrome.[164] Paraneoplastic subacute sensory neuronopathy (PSSN) is one of these conditions that affect the peripheral nerves in the setting of a neoplasm. It commonly affects middle-aged and older adults and follows a rapid clinical progression.[165] This disorder is associated with SCLC in 80% of cases, but also other cancers such as breast, ovarian, sarcoma, and Hodgkin lymphoma.[53] Approximately 85% of cases are associated with anti-Hu and anti-CV2/CRMP5, whereas 16% are seronegative.[166] PSSN has a broad variation in the clinical presentation and progression of neuropathy, pattern, and degree of the autonomic, sensory, and motor involvement, and we will discuss these together as PSSN.[167]

Pathophysiology. The primary neurological localization of PSSN is within the dorsal root ganglia.[168] Studies suggest that damage to the dorsal root ganglia is the result of CD8+ cytotoxic T-cell infiltration and vasculitis.[168] These changes produce a significant loss of cell bodies and axons of sensory neurons.[169] Lesions are multifocal, typically well circumscribed, and may extend to the sympathetic ganglia. In the setting of pain predominance and ataxia, biopsies have demonstrated loss of small myelinated and unmyelinated fibers. Biopsies in patients with isolated ataxia have shown exclusive loss of large myelinated fibers.

Clinical presentation. PSSN has a subacute onset and a variety of sensory impairments that manifest as a sensory ataxia.[170] Sensory disturbances are distributed asymmetrically in a polyneuropathy pattern that may affect the face, scalp, trunk, hands, arms, or proximal legs and finally feet.[165] The manifestations produce sensory ataxia due to loss of proprioceptive and kinesthetic sensation manifesting as pseudoathetosis in the fingers and hands, as well as Romberg's sign in association with absent reflexes. Cranial nerves may also be involved producing hypoacusia and loss of taste.[166] In addition to the classic presentation of a pure sensory ataxia, other manifestations may be present including allodynia, hyperalgesia to mechanical stimuli without sensory ataxia, and painful dysesthesia.[171] Motor and autonomic involvement may also be present and manifest with urinary retention, constipation, and orthostatic hypotension. Isolated motor manifestations do not rule out this disorder. For instance, a study of 20 patients with anti-Hu seropositive PSSN reported 5% of patients who developed motor symptoms exclusively.[172]

Diagnostic approach. CSF analysis commonly reveals elevated protein concentration, pleocytosis, and intrathecal oligoclonal bands.[165] MRI of the spine with gadolinium may show spinal nerve root enhancement. Electrophysiological studies show decreased or absence of sensory nerve action potentials with normal or mild decreased sensory conduction velocities and normal motor conduction velocities.[171] Isolated sensory nerve involvement is rarely demonstrated in PSSN, and motor nerve involvement may be evident despite the absence of motor function impairment. For instance, in one retrospective study, electrophysiological testing demonstrated a reduction of compound muscle action potentials in patients with pain as an isolated symptomatic manifestation.[170]

Prognosis. The recognition of PSSN is essential as this syndrome improves the chances of cancer detection and treatment. Immunosuppressive therapy before, during, and after antineoplastic therapy has shown benefits in only a few cases.[173] Also, the diagnosis and treatment of the tumor help to stabilize the sensory impairment; however, the evolution of this paraneoplastic neurological syndrome appears to be independent of cancer progression. Mortality depends on the type and stage of cancer.

CASE 20.6 LAMBERT-EATON MYASTHENIC SYNDROME

Case. A 68-year-old man with a past medical history of gastric adenocarcinoma and chronic pleural effusions was evaluated for a 1-year course of back pain and progressive weakness of the lower extremities. His initial general medical examination showed mild weakness in psoas muscles, areflexia, and steppage gait. Electrodiagnostic studies revealed reduced right median, peroneal, and tibial compound muscle action potential (CMAP) amplitudes. Right ulnar CMAP showed normal distal latency, decreased amplitude, and slowing of conduction velocity across the elbow. Repetitive nerve stimulation at 3 Hz of the right median nerve demonstrated evidence of significant decrement at baseline suggestive of a neuromuscular junctional disorder. After 10 seconds of sustained exercise, there was an increment of greater than 100% from baseline, supporting a presynaptic junctional process. P/Q type voltage-gated calcium channel antibodies (VGCC) were detected in serum, consistent with Lambert-Eaton myasthenic syndrome (LEMS). He was treated with pyridostigmine, IVIg, and 3,4 diaminopyridine with improvement. Initial neoplastic screening with chest CT scan, esophagogastroduodenoscopy (EGD), colonoscopy, and FDG-PET scan were unrevealing. He continued in regular cancer screening every 6 months for 2 years.

Two years later, EGD revealed Barret's esophagus and gastritis with biopsies demonstrating intestinal metaplasia. Colonoscopy revealed a 5 cm partially obstructing fungating mass in the ascending colon that was treated with right hemicolectomy. Pathology reported well-differentiated adenocarcinoma. Subsequently, he was treated with chemotherapy. He continues on 3-4 diaminopyradine 15 mg four times daily with marked improvement of his back pain and ambulation.

Teaching Points. This patient presented with typical findings of myasthenia and electrodiagnostic studies that suggested a presynaptic junctional disorder. The presence of P/Q-type voltage-gated calcium channel (P/Q type VGCC) antibodies further supported diagnosis of Lambert-Eaton myasthenic syndrome. This case highlights the importance of cancer screening in patients with a diagnosed PND syndrome. Appropriate cancer screening should continue for 2–5 years after the PND syndrome diagnosis as the onset of neurological symptoms can pre-date the discovery of cancer, as was the case for this patient.

Lambert-Eaton myasthenic syndrome

Definition and epidemiology. LEMS is a rare autoimmune condition that affects the neuromuscular junction.[58,174] This disorder is related to neoplasms as well as other non-paraneoplastic syndromes such as autoimmune thyroid disease, rheumatoid arthritis, and lupus.[58] The prevalence of the paraneoplastic form of LEMS is approximately 3–4 per million population, a 10 times lower annual incidence rate than other neuromuscular autoimmune diseases.[58] The median age of onset is 60 years, and patients are more commonly male (59–70% of patients). In contrast, non-tumor LEMS has two demographic peaks, one with a mean age at 35 years and a second at 60 years of age, without gender predominance.[58] LEMS most commonly presents in association with SCLC (50–60%), but other tumors have been described such as prostate carcinoma, lymphoma, leukemia, and thymoma. LEMS itself is rarely life-threatening; however, patients with LEMS have a low survival rate given its association with cancer.

Pathophysiology. P/Q-type VGCCs are large transmembrane channels present on the presynaptic membrane which when open, allow the entry of calcium into the presynaptic nerve terminal. Subsequently, acetylcholine (ACh) containing vesicles in the presynaptic neuron release ACh into the synapse to bind to receptors on the postsynaptic endplate, leading to its subsequent depolarization. In the setting of LEMS, the antibodies bind the P/Q-type VGCC, leading to their internalization and a consequent decrease in Ach released into the synapse, leading to a reduction in the action potential of the postsynaptic endplate. As a result, muscle as well as autonomic and central nervous system functions are impaired.[175]

LEMS is mediated by Ig G antibodies against presynaptic P/Q-type VGCCs in up to 90% of patients. SCLC is a tumor with neuroendocrine characteristics that expresses proteins similar to P/Q-type VGCCs on its surface. The immune system develops antibodies to the SCLC proteins that are cross-reactive with the P/Q-type VGCC on the presynaptic terminals.[58,175] Antibodies against the transcriptional factor SOX1 have also been reported in patients with paraneoplastic LEMS; however, the pathogenicity of these antibodies remains unclear.

Clinical presentation. LEMS can be easily misdiagnosed because of its variable and non-specific clinical presentation.[58] The typical presentation is characterized by a gradual progression of proximal weakness of legs and arms followed subsequently by involvement of the hands, feet, and cranial muscles. In contrast to MG, its evolution follows a caudocranial pattern, typically affecting the oculobulbar muscles last.[175,176] Physical examination may demonstrate areflexia and only minimal weakness disproportionate to a patient's symptomatic report.[58,177] A classic characteristic of this disorder is increased reflexes and muscle strength following muscle contraction (post-exercise facilitation).[58,178] Other described symptoms include fatigue, weight loss, blurred vision, diplopia, dysphagia, and neck weakness, as well as autonomic symptoms (e.g., dry eyes, dry mouth, xerostomia, erectile dysfunction, constipation, and hyperhidrosis). Less common symptoms are orthostatic hypotension, cardiac arrhythmias, gastroparesis with intestinal pseudo-obstruction, and urinary retention.[58,172]

In the setting of unexplained dyspnea, diaphragmatic muscle weakness derived from phrenic injury should be considered. SCLC is the second most common cause of diaphragmatic paralysis due to its rapid and aggressive invasion to surrounding regions including the phrenic nerves. The left phrenic nerve is more frequently affected than the right due to its proximity with the aortopulmonary window lymph nodes. This finding is usually associated with an irreversibly advanced disease.[172]

Diagnostic approach. LEMS should be suspected in the setting of proximal muscle weakness in legs and arms, diminished tendon reflexes or areflexia, and myopathic gait in the setting of electromyographic evidence of presynaptic deficits in neuromuscular transmission and seropositivity for anti-VGCC antibodies (present in 80–90% of patients).[58,179]

Electromyography and nerve conduction studies are the main diagnostic studies in the evaluation of LEMS. Repetitive nerve stimulation (RNS) demonstrates reduced amplitude of the resting CMAP and decreasing CMAP amplitudes during low rate stimulation, and this should be observed in at least two distal muscles.[58] This decremental response indicates pathology in the neuromuscular junction but does not differentiate LEMS from MG. RNS with high-frequency (20–50 Hz) stimulation or immediately after a brief maximal voluntary contraction (15–20 s) is necessary to distinguish these two and localize the pathology to the presynaptic terminus (e.g., LEMS) or postsynaptic terminus (e.g., MG). A LEMS diagnosis is established if the increase in amplitude is at least 100%, although this cut off can be decreased to 60% to increase sensitivity (97%).[58]

Single-fiber electromyography (sfEMG) has higher sensitivity but lower specificity than RNS for the diagnosis of LEMS. LEMS and MG may be differentiated through the evaluation of the neuromuscular jitter by sfEMG at different frequencies. A neuromuscular jitter is the latency from the stimulus to its response after a nerve stimulation recorded by sfEMG. In patients with LEMS, this latency is markedly increased but decreases with low stimulation rates. In contrast, MG is characterized by high latencies in the setting of low stimulation and a decrement after stimulation rates above 10 Hz.[58,174]

The presence of anti–P/Q-type VGCC antibodies is highly suggestive of LEMS; nevertheless, their absence does not exclude the disorder. Antibodies against the alpha-1A subunit of VGCC are frequently related to autoimmune LEMS in absence of tumor, whereas SOX1 antibodies have been associated with paraneoplastic LEMS in the setting of SCLC. Anti-muscarinic M1 receptor and anti-synaptotagmin antibodies also have been reported; however, the diagnostic value of these assays has not been established. Correlations between respective antibody titers and disease severity are not known.[58]

For oncologic screening, conventional chest x-rays or bronchoscopy have low sensitivity in the detection of lung tumors, and a CT of the thorax is often warranted. If it is normal, an FDG-PET scan is suggested.[58] In those without evidence of cancer at time of initial screening, tumor screening should be continued regularly at least two to three times per year for 2 years after initial symptoms. The DELTA-P score is helpful to assess the need for further screening and incorporate patient age at symptoms onset, loss of weight, bulbar dysfunction, smoking status, sexual dysfunction, and Karnofsky performance status scale.[58,179]

In cases where no cancer is identified in thus non-paraneoplastic LEMS, the additional differential diagnoses and coincident syndromes to consider and evaluate for include: Hashimoto's thyroiditis, autoimmune inflammatory myopathies, primary rheumatologic disorders, and systemic vasculitides, among others. Diseases that have similarities with LEMS should also be investigated for such as MG, Parkinson's disease, amyotrophic lateral sclerosis, myotonic dystrophy type 2, and Guillain-Barre syndrome.[58] MG typically presents with craniocaudally progression of oculobulbar and muscle weakness.[58] AChR antibodies are frequently present in concomitance with a thymoma.

Treatment. Treatment is based on symptomatic control and immunosuppressive therapy.[58] Symptomatic control is achieved with medications that extend the activity of acetylcholine or generally increase the availability of neurotransmitters within the synapse. Also, 3,4 diaminopyridine, is an effective option for the symptomatic treatment of LEMS. Side effects are rare, but seizures may occur with this medication.[58] In some cases, patients have benefited from combination therapy with pyridostigmine and 3,4 diaminopyridine.[58,174]

Promising alternative therapies include derivatives of proteasome inhibitors. Recent studies involving proteasome inhibitors have demonstrated that the medications can eliminate plasma cells effectively, produce cytotoxicity in tumor cells, and inhibit dendritic cell maturation.[58,174] Further study of these medications in the treatment of LEMS is needed.

Prognosis. The prognosis is dependent of tumor presence and degree of muscle weakness and distribution. Mortality is related to the underlying tumor, especially in the setting of an aggressive cancer such as SCLC. Studies have demonstrated better survival in this group, although this observation may be related to lead-time bias.[175]

CASE 20.7 PARANEOPLASTIC DERMATOMYOSITIS (DM)

Case. A 20-year-old man with an unremarkable past medical history developed fever, sore throat, and cough followed by diffuse proximal muscle weakness, dysphagia, and rash involving the knuckles and fingers within a period of 3 weeks. The initial neurological examination demonstrated tachycardia, areflexia, and proximal greater than distal weakness. Head CT and Brain MRI were unremarkable. Laboratory studies were notable for creatine kinase (CK) 49,680 U/L, aspartate aminotransferase 1,761 U/L, and alanine aminotransferase 513 U/L. Metabolic and rheumatologic testing were negative. An EMG/NCS was compatible with an irritative myopathy showing strikingly abnormal EMG in proximal muscles on the right and reduced CMAP amplitudes in the legs. RNS was normal. A muscle biopsy demonstrated an inflammatory myopathy with perifascicular myofiber atrophy and necrosis, as well as perimysial perivascular chronic inflammation, consistent with a diagnosis of DM. Cancer screening included CT of the chest, abdomen, and pelvis with and without contrast that demonstrated a suspicious-appearing abnormality in the distal stomach. For severe dysphagia, a percutaneous endoscopic gastrostomy was required, and a mass in the antrum was discovered during the procedure. A biopsy of the mass was negative for malignancy and instead revealed nodular pancreatic heterotopia in the antral mucosa with erosive active chronic *Helicobacter pylori* gastritis. He was treated with high-dose IV steroids and IVIg for 5 days with partial improvement. In addition, *H. pylori* was treated with lansoprazole, amoxicillin, and clarithromycin. Long-term management included methotrexate weekly, IVIg monthly, and prolonged prednisone taper.

Teaching Points. This patient presented with typical examination and paraclinical findings of DM. Characteristic histopathologic findings on muscle biopsy including demonstration of an inflammatory myopathy in the setting of perifascicular myofiber atrophy, necrosis, and perimysial perivascular chronic inflammation confirmed the diagnosis of DM. Patients with DM are at increased risk for cancer, particularly those with evidence of other connective tissue diseases.

Definition and epidemiology. DM is an uncommon inflammatory myopathy of unknown etiology, which produces erythematous eruptions in photo-exposed areas of the face, the upper eyelids, anterior neck, extensors surfaces of the forearms, and the dorsum of the hands and knuckles in association with proximal muscle weakness.[180] First described in 1975,[181] DM is associated with higher risk for cancer with an incidence of 7 to 30%.[182–184] This disorder affects adolescents, young adults, and older patients, particularly males in a ratio of 2:1.[181] Cancers frequently related to DM include testicular, bladder, prostate, ovary, pancreatic, gastric, colorectal, and non-Hodgkin lymphoma. Males usually develop nasopharyngeal carcinoma, lung, and liver cancer, whereas females develop breast, lung, or nasopharyngeal cancer. Connective tissue diseases in the setting of DM have a strong association with malignancy.[185]

Pathophysiology. The pathogenesis is not clear; however, an immune-mediated mechanism is likely involved given that tumor antigens may share similarities with proteins of muscle and skin.[186] Antibodies against Mi2, Ku, and RNP antigens have been described in association with DM.

Clinical presentation. Dermatologic manifestations frequently precede the appearance of myopathy. Pathognomonic cutaneous changes include heliotrope rash and Gottron's papules. Other common manifestations include the presence of prelingual telangiectasias, cuticular overgrowth, nailfold infarcts, poikiloderma, scaly erythema, pruritic scalp rash, and photosensitivity in the setting of myositis.[181] Paraneoplastic DM can precede, overlap, or follow the diagnosis of an underlying malignancy. Other organs that might be affected by DM include the lungs, esophagus, and heart.[181]

Diagnostic approach. The diagnostic approach to DM includes serum CK and aldolase (which are frequently elevated), EMG and nerve conduction studies, muscle biopsy (which is helpful to rule out infiltrative processes as well as demonstrate characteristic myopathic changes), as well as consideration of biopsy of the pharyngeal recess (otherwise known as the fossa of Rosenmüller).[181]

Treatment. Response to corticosteroid therapy is poor and immunosuppressive or cytotoxic therapies are usually necessary along with treatment of the underlying tumor. Skin disease is treated with photoprotection, topical corticosteroids, antimalarials, and low-dose methotrexate. In addition to immunosuppressive therapy, muscle weakness is frequently treated with rest, range of motion physical therapy, and nutritional support. The exact frequency with which this phenomenon occurs is unknown, so patients should be monitored while on long-term immunosuppressive therapy. Prognosis is, in general, poor.[186]

Paraneoplastic mononeuritis multiplex

Although not a classic paraneoplastic neurological disorder, mononeuritis multiplex (MM) is the most common form of paraneoplastic neuropathy.[187] This condition is extremely painful and asymmetric with asynchronous sensory and motor peripheral neuropathy involving two or more distant nerve areas.[187,188] As the disease progresses, the neuropathy affects multiple nerves, becoming less multifocal and more symmetrical as the syndrome progresses. The distribution is usually bilateral and patchy initially.[188] As a syndrome, MM is associated with primary and secondary vasculitides, amyloidosis, direct tumor involvement, and viral infections (e.g., HIV, hepatitis, parvovirus B19), as well as paraneoplastic processes. Tumors associated with paraneoplastic MM are prostate cancer, lymphomas, leukemias, renal cell carcinomas, lung adenocarcinoma, SCLC, and rarely non-SCLC. Paraneoplastic MM commonly manifests 2 to 10 months before the identification of the malignant tumor. Various antibodies have been reported in association with paraneoplastic MM including anti-Hu, anti-Yo, and anti-Ri; however, 10% of patients are seronegative. Other manifestations may help with the diagnosis (e.g., rapid progression, short latency between the diagnosis of cancer, and development of neuropathy and severe presentation). The diagnostic approach includes tumor screening by abdominal and thoracic CT scan, gonadal ultrasound, and consideration for FDG-PET. EMG and nerve conduction studies frequently reveal severe sensory-motor axonal neuropathy. Treatment is focused on neoplasm eradication and symptom control. Immunosuppression with plasmapheresis and cyclophosphamide has been described but their effectiveness is still uncertain.[189,190]

Future directions

There are still aspects of PND syndromes that remain unresolved. For instance, the mechanisms leading to antitumor immunity and their secondary effects in the central, peripheral, and autonomic nervous systems remain to be fully described. Studies are needed to evaluate the current effectiveness of the standard first- and second-line immunosuppressive therapies as well as new immunotherapies. A better understanding of the role of oncologic therapy is necessary to improve survival rates. Finally, studies are needed to evaluate the risk factors that predispose to PND syndromes and possibly neurological immune-related adverse events in patients treated with immune checkpoint inhibitor therapy for cancer (see Chapter 30 for discussion of neurological immune-related adverse events with immune checkpoint inhibitors).

Conclusion

PND syndromes are a diverse category of disorders thought to be the consequence of immune responses directed primarily at neoplasms. These syndromes may affect any part of the autonomic, central, and peripheral nervous system. The diagnosis of a PND syndrome is difficult and may require CSF and serum analysis, antibody testing, focused neurological imaging, and diagnostics, as well as neoplasm screening depending on the specific syndrome identified. In patients presenting with one of the common PND syndromes, presentations outlined in this chapter (Table 20.3), clinicians should have a high index of suspicion even in the absence of anti-neuronal antibodies or underlying cancer diagnosis. Outcomes and prognosis depend on tumor type and early initiation of immunosuppression and cancer therapy.

Table 20.3 Summary of clinical pearls

PND syndromes discussed in this chapter	Commonly associated tumors	Commonly associated antibodies
Encephalitis and Limbic encephalitis	Ovarian teratoma Few cases: testicular germ cell tumor, Hodgkin lymphoma, mediastinal teratoma and SCLC	anti-NMDAR[33–35]
	SCLC, NETs	anti-GAD65[191]
	SCLC, thyroid, breast, and ovarian cancer	anti-AMPAR[37]
	SCLC and other neuroendocrine tumors	anti-Hu (anti-ANNA-1)[192,193]
	Germ-cell tumors of the testis	anti-Ma2[194]
	SCLC, lung, and esophageal adenocarcinoma	anti-ANNA-3[21]
	Breast, parotid, colon, lung, testis, and ovarian cancer	anti-Ma1[22]
	Urogenital cancer	anti-ROCK2[195]
Encephalomyelitis	SCLC and other neuroendocrine tumors	anti-Hu (ANNA-1)[27]
	SCLC, breast cancer	anti-Amphiphysin[196]
	SCLC and other neuroendocrine tumors, thymoma, breast cancer, lymphomas	anti-GAD65[191]
Cerebellar degeneration	Breast, ovary, endometrium, and fallopian tube cancers	anti-Yo (anti-PCA-1)[28]
	SCLC, thymoma	anti-CV2 (anti-CRMP5)[29]
	Breast cancer, gynecologic cancers, and SCLC	anti-Ri (anti-ANNA-2)[30]
	Hodgkin lymphoma	anti-Tr (anti-PCA-Tr)[19]
	SCLC	anti-PCA-2[20]
	SCLC, lung, and esophageal adenocarcinoma	anti-ANNA-3[197]
	Breast, parotid, colon, lung, testis, and ovarian cancer	anti-Ma1[198]
	SCLC, Hodgkin lymphoma, ovarian cancer	anti-Zic4[24–26]
	SCLC, lung cancer, breast, multiple myeloma	anti-Homer3[199,200]
	Melanoma, ovarian cancer, breast cancer, lymphomas	anti-ITPR1[201]
	Non-SCLC, hepatobiliary carcinoma, colorectal cancer	anti-CARP VIII[202,203]
	Ovarian cancer	anti-Ca/ARHGAP26[204]
	SCLC	anti-TRIM46[205]
Opsoclonus-myoclonus	SCLC, non-SCLC, breast cancer, ovarian cancer, pancreatic adenocarcinoma	anti-$GABA_B$ receptor[39]
	SCLC and other neuroendocrine tumors, thymoma, breast cancer, lymphomas	anti-GAD65[206]
Sensory neuronopathy	SCLC	anti-Hu anti-CV2/CRMP5 anti-amphiphysin[166]
Lambert-Eaton myasthenic syndrome	SCLC, thymoma	anti-CV2 (anti-CRMP5)[207]
	SCLC	anti-PCA-2[20]
	SCLC	anti-VGCC[44]

Table 20.3 Summary of clinical pearls—Cont'd

PND syndromes discussed in this chapter	Commonly associated tumors	Commonly associated antibodies
Dermatomyositis	Testicular, bladder, prostate, gynecological tumors	anti-Mi2, anti-Ku, and anti-RNP[185]
Mononeuritis multiplex	SCLC, prostate, and hematologic malignancies	anti-Hu, anti-Yo, and anti-Ri[189,190]

AMPAR, α-Amino-3-hydroxy-5-methyl-4-isoxazolepropionic acid receptor; *ANNA-1*, antineuronal nuclear antibodies type 1; *ANNA-2*, antineuronal nuclear antibodies type 2; *ANNA-3*, antineuronal nuclear antibody type 3; *ARHGAP26*, Rho GTPase-activating protein 26; *CARP*, anti-carbamylated protein; *CRMP5*, Collapsin Response Mediator Protein 5; *$GABA_A$*, Gamma aminobutyric acid A receptor; *GAD65*, glutamic acid decarboxylase 65; *ITPR1*, inositol 1,4,5-trisphosphate receptor type 1; *NETs*, neuroendocrine tumors; *NMDA*, N-methyl-D-aspartate; *PCA-1*, Purkinje cell cytoplasmic antibody type 1; *PCA-2*, Purkinje cell cytoplasmic antibody type 2; *PCA-Tr*, Purkinje cell cytoplasmic antibody Tr; *PKC-g*, anti-protein kinase C; *RNP*, Sm and nuclear ribonucleoprotein; *ROCK2*, Rho-associated protein kinase 2; *SCLC*, small-cell lung carcinoma; *TRIM46*, tripartite motif-containing protein 46; *VGCC*, voltage-gated calcium channel antibody.

References

1. Kannoth S. Paraneoplastic neurologic syndrome: a practical approach. *Ann Indian Acad Neurol*. 2012;15(1):6–12.
2. Darnell RB, Posner JB. Paraneoplastic syndromes involving the nervous system. *N Engl J Med*. 2003;349(16):1543–1554.
3. Chatterjee M, Hurley LC, Tainsky MA. Paraneoplastic antigens as biomarkers for early diagnosis of ovarian cancer. *Gynecol Oncol Rep*. 2017;21:37–44.
4. Titulaer MJ, Soffietti R, Dalmau J, et al. Screening for tumours in paraneoplastic syndromes: report of an EFNS task force. *Eur J Neurol*. 2011;18(1):19–e3.
5. Gozzard P, Woodhall M, Chapman C, et al. Paraneoplastic neurologic disorders in small cell lung carcinoma: a prospective study. *Neurology*. 2015;85(3):235–239.
6. Dalmau J, Rosenfeld MR. Paraneoplastic syndromes of the CNS. *Lancet Neurol*. 2008;7(4):327–340.
7. Honnorat J, Antoine JC. Paraneoplastic neurological syndromes. *Orphanet J Rare Dis*. 2007;2:22.
8. Berzero G, Psimaras D. Neurological paraneoplastic syndromes: an update. *Curr Opin Oncol*. 2018;30(6):359–367.
9. Berger B, Bischler P, Dersch R, Hottenrott T, Rauer S, Stich O. "Non-classical" paraneoplastic neurological syndromes associated with well-characterized antineuronal antibodies as compared to "classical" syndromes—more frequent than expected. *J Neurol Sci*. 2015;352(1–2):58–61.
10. McKeon A, Pittock SJ. Paraneoplastic encephalomyelopathies: pathology and mechanisms. *Acta Neuropathol*. 2011;122(4):381–400.
11. Bien CG, Vincent A, Barnett MH, Becker AJ, Blumcke I, Graus F, et al. Immunopathology of autoantibody-associated encephalitides: clues for pathogenesis. *Brain*. 2012;135(Pt 5):1622–1638.
12. Jones AL, Flanagan EP, Pittock SJ, et al. Responses to and outcomes of treatment of autoimmune cerebellar ataxia in adults. *JAMA Neurol*. 2015;72(11):1304–1312.
13. Rojas I, Graus F, Keime-Guibert F, et al. Long-term clinical outcome of paraneoplastic cerebellar degeneration and anti-Yo antibodies. *Neurology*. 2000;55(5):713–715.
14. Berzero G, Karantoni E, Dehais C, et al. Early intravenous immunoglobulin treatment in paraneoplastic neurological syndromes with onconeural antibodies. *J Neurol Neurosurg Psychiatry*. 2018;89:789–792.
15. Joubert B, Honnorat J. Autoimmune channelopathies in paraneoplastic neurological syndromes. *Biochim Biophys Acta*. 2015;1848(10 Pt B):2665–2676.
16. Dalmau J, Graus F. Antibody-mediated encephalitis. *N Engl J Med*. 2018;378(9):840–851.
17. Hughes EG, Peng X, Gleichman AJ, et al. Cellular and synaptic mechanisms of anti-NMDA receptor encephalitis. *J Neurosci*. 2010;30(17):5866–5875.
18. Ohkawa T, Fukata Y, Yamasaki M, et al. Autoantibodies to epilepsy-related LGI1 in limbic encephalitis neutralize LGI1-ADAM22 interaction and reduce synaptic AMPA receptors. *J Neurosci*. 2013;33(46):18161–18174.
19. Peltola J, Hietaharju A, Rantala I, Lehtinen T, Haapasalo H. A reversible neuronal antibody (anti-Tr) associated paraneoplastic cerebellar degeneration in Hodgkin's disease. *Acta Neurol Scand*. 1998;98(5):360–363.
20. Vernino S, Lennon VA. New Purkinje cell antibody (PCA-2): marker of lung cancer-related neurological autoimmunity. *Ann Neurol*. 2000;47(3):297–305.
21. Sauri T, Izquierdo À, Ramió-Torrentà L, Sanchez-Montañez À, Bosch-Barrera J, Porta R. Paraneoplastic limbic encephalitis in a male with squamous cell carcinoma of the lung. *J Clin Neurol*. 2015;11(1):87–91.
22. Gultekin SH, Rosenfeld MR, Voltz R, Eichen J, Posner JB, Dalmau J. Paraneoplastic limbic encephalitis: neurological symptoms, immunological findings and tumour association in 50 patients. *Brain*. 2000;123(Pt 7):1481–1494.
23. Adamus G, Guy J, Schmied JL, Arendt A, Hargrave PA. Role of anti-recoverin autoantibodies in cancer-associated retinopathy. *Invest Ophthalmol Vis Sci*. 1993;34(9):2626–2633.
24. Kerasnoudis A, Rockhoff M, Federlein J, Gold R, Krogias C. Isolated ZIC4 antibodies in paraneoplastic cerebellar syndrome with an underlying ovarian tumor. *Arch Neurol*. 2011;68(8):1073. https://doi.org/10.1001/archneurol.2011.176.

25. Eye PG, Wang B, Keung ES, Tagg NT. Anti-ZIC4 associated paraneoplastic cerebellar degeneration in a patient with both diffuse large B-cell lymphoma and incidental smoldering multiple myeloma. *J Neurol Sci*. 2018;384:36–37. https://doi.org/10.1016/j.jns.2017.11.005.
26. Bataller L, Wade DF, Graus F, Stacey HD, Rosenfeld MR, Dalmau J. Antibodies to Zic4 in paraneoplastic neurologic disorders and small-cell lung cancer. *Neurology*. 2004;62(5):778–782.
27. Buetow MP, Eggenberger E. ANNA-1—Induced encephalitis associated with noninvasive thymoma. *Am J Roentgenol*. 2002;179(3):802–803. https://doi.org/10.2214/ajr.179.3.1790802.
28. Venkatraman A, Opal P. Paraneoplastic cerebellar degeneration with anti-Yo antibodies—a review. *Ann Clin Transl Neurol*. 2016;3(8):655–663.
29. de la Sayette V, Bertran F, Honnorat J, Schaeffer S, Iglesias S, Defer G. Paraneoplastic cerebellar syndrome and optic neuritis with anti-CV2 antibodies: clinical response to excision of the primary tumor. *Arch Neurol*. 1998;55(3):405–408.
30. Goyal MK, Bhatkar S, Modi M, et al. Anti-Ri antibody-mediated paraneoplastic cerebellar degeneration: a rare, treatable yet poorly recognized entity. *Neurol India*. 2016;64:1033–1035.
31. Hazzan MA, Neto HRS, Mendonça FGB, et al. Anti-Ma2 encephalitis: beyond testicular cancer—the association with other urogynecologic tumors (P6.092). *Neurology*. 2018;90(suppl 15):P6.092. Available at: http://n.neurology.org/content/90/15_Supplement/P6.092.abstract.
32. Qiao L, Guan HZ, Ren H, et al. Paraneoplastic neurological syndromes associated with anti-amphiphysin antibodies. 2016;49:769–774.
33. Eker A, Saka E, Dalmau J, et al. Testicular teratoma and anti-N-methyl-D-aspartate receptor-associated encephalitis. *J Neurol Neurosurg Psychiatry*. 2008;79:1082–1083.
34. Zandi MS, Irani SR, Follows G, Moody AM, Molyneux P, Vincent A. Limbic encephalitis associated with antibodies to the NMDA receptor in Hodgkin lymphoma. *Neurology*. 2009;73(23):2039–2040.
35. Stover DG, Eisenberg R, Johnson DH. Anti-N-methyl-D-aspartate receptor encephalitis in a young woman with a mature mediastinal teratoma. *J Thorac Oncol*. 2010;5(11):1872–1873.
36. Wang M, Cao X, Liu Q, Ma W, Guo X, Liu X. Clinical features of limbic encephalitis with LGI1 antibody. *Neuropsychiatr Dis Treat*. 2017;13:1589–1596.
37. Joubert B, Kerschen P, Zekeridou A, et al. Clinical spectrum of encephalitis associated with antibodies against the alpha-amino-3-hydroxy-5-methyl-4-isoxazolepropionic acid receptor: case series and review of the literature. *JAMA Neurol*. 2015;72(10):1163–1169.
38. Abdul M, Mccray SD, Hoosein NM. Expression of gamma-aminobutyric acid receptor (subtype A) in prostate cancer. *Acta Oncol*. 2008;47(8):1546–1550. https://doi.org/10.1080/02841860801961265.
39. Armangué T, Sabater L, Torres-Vega E, Martínez-Hernández E, Ariño H, Petit-Pedrol M, et al. Clinical and immunological features of opsoclonus-myoclonus syndrome in the era of neuronal cell surface antibodies. *JAMA Neurol*. 2016;73(4):417–424.
40. Borellini L, Lanfranconi S, Bonato S, et al. Progressive encephalomyelitis with rigidity and myoclonus associated with anti-GlyR antibodies and Hodgkin's Lymphoma: a case report. *Front Neurol*. 2017;8:401.
41. Hara M, Ariño H, Petit-Pedrol M, et al. DPPX antibody-associated encephalitis: main syndrome and antibody effects. *Neurology*. 2017;88(14):1340–1348.
42. Lopez-Chiriboga AS, Komorowski L, Kümpfel T, et al. Metabotropic glutamate receptor type 1 autoimmunity: clinical features and treatment outcomes. *Neurology*. 2016;86(11):1009–1013.
43. Spatola M, Sabater L, Planagumà J, et al. Encephalitis with mGluR5 antibodies: symptoms and antibody effects. *Neurology*. 2018;90(22):e1964–e1972.
44. Bekircan-Kurt CE, Derle Çiftçi E, Kurne AT, Anlar B. Voltage gated calcium channel antibody-related neurological diseases. *World J Clin Cases*. 2015;3(3):293–300.
45. Bansal P, Zutshi D, Suchdev K, Azher I, Mohamed W. Alpha 3 ganglionic acetylcholine receptor antibody associated refractory status epilepticus. *Seizure*. 2016;35:1–3. https://doi.org/10.1016/j.seizure.2015.12.008.
46. Kazarian M, Laird-Offringa IA. Small-cell lung cancer-associated autoantibodies: potential applications to cancer diagnosis, early detection, and therapy. *Mol Cancer*. 2011;10:33.
47. Pittock SJ, Kryzer TJ, Lennon VA. Paraneoplastic antibodies coexist and predict cancer, not neurological syndrome. *Ann Neurol*. 2004;56(5):715–719.
48. Hoftberger R, Rosenfeld MR, Dalmau J. Update on neurological paraneoplastic syndromes. *Curr Opin Oncol*. 2015;27(6):489–495.
49. Bernal F, Graus F, Pifarré A, Saiz A, Benyahia B, Ribalta T. Immunohistochemical analysis of anti-Hu-associated paraneoplastic encephalomyelitis. *Acta Neuropathol*. 2002;103(5):509–515.
50. Plonquet A, Gherardi RK, Créange A, et al. Oligoclonal T-cells in blood and target tissues of patients with anti-Hu syndrome. *J Neuroimmunol*. 2002;122(1–2):100–105.
51. Roberts WK, Deluca IJ, Thomas A, et al. Patients with lung cancer and paraneoplastic Hu syndrome harbor HuD-specific type 2 CD8+ T cells. *J Clin Invest*. 2009;119(7):2042–2051.
52. Graus F, Keime-Guibert F, Reñe R, et al. Anti-Hu-associated paraneoplastic encephalomyelitis: analysis of 200 patients. *Brain*. 2001;124(Pt 6):1138–1148.
53. Dalmau J, Graus F, Rosenblum MK, Posner JB. Anti-Hu--associated paraneoplastic encephalomyelitis/sensory neuronopathy. A clinical study of 71 patients. *Medicine (Baltimore)*. 1992;71(2):59–72.
54. Lucchinetti CF, Kimmel DW, Lennon VA. Paraneoplastic and oncologic profiles of patients seropositive for type 1 antineuronal nuclear autoantibodies. *Neurology*. 1998;50(3):652–657.
55. Sillevis Smitt P, Grefkens J, de Leeuw B, et al. Survival and outcome in 73 anti-Hu positive patients with paraneoplastic encephalomyelitis/sensory neuronopathy. *J Neurol*. 2002;249(6):745–753.
56. Titulaer MJ, McCracken L, Gabilondo I, et al. Treatment and prognostic factors for long-term outcome in patients with anti-NMDA receptor encephalitis: an observational cohort study. *Lancet Neurol*. 2013;12(2):157–165.
57. Foster AR, Caplan JP. Paraneoplastic limbic encephalitis. *Psychosomatics*. 2009;50(2):108–113.
58. Schoser B, Eymard B, Datt J, Mantegazza R. Lambert-Eaton myasthenic syndrome (LEMS): a rare autoimmune presynaptic disorder often associated with cancer. *J Neurol*. 2017;264(9):1854–1863.

59. Shams'ili S, de Beukelaar J, Gratama JW, et al. An uncontrolled trial of rituximab for antibody associated paraneoplastic neurological syndromes. *J Neurol*. 2006;253(1):16–20.
60. Ducray F, Graus F, Vigliani MC, et al. Delayed onset of a second paraneoplastic neurological syndrome in eight patients. *J Neurol Neurosurg Psychiatry*. 2010;81(8):937–939.
61. Altabakhi IW, Babiker HM. Paraneoplastic limbic encephalitis. In: *Treasure Island (FL)*. StatPearls Publishing; 2020.
62. Corsellis JA, Goldberg GJ, Norton AR. "Limbic encephalitis" and its association with carcinoma. *Brain*. 1968;91(3):481–496.
63. Rosenfeld MR, Titulaer MJ, Dalmau J. Paraneoplastic syndromes and autoimmune encephalitis: five new things. *Neurol Clin Pract*. 2012;2(3):215–223.
64. Kubota A, Tajima T, Narukawa S, et al. [Anti-Ma2, anti-NMDA-receptor and anti-GluRepsilon2 limbic encephalitis with testicular seminoma: short-term memory disturbance]. *Rinsho Shinkeigaku*. 2012;52(9):666–671.
65. Inoue T, Kanno R, Moriya A, et al. A case of paraneoplastic limbic encephalitis in a patient with invasive thymoma with anti-glutamate receptor antibody-positive cerebrospinal fluid: a case report. *Ann Thorac Cardiovasc Surg*. 2018;24(4):200–204.
66. Lai M, Huijbers MGM, Lancaster E, et al. Investigation of LGI1 as the antigen in limbic encephalitis previously attributed to potassium channels: a case series. *Lancet Neurol*. 2010;9(8):776–785.
67. Irani SR, Michell AW, Lang B, et al. Faciobrachial dystonic seizures precede Lgi1 antibody limbic encephalitis. *Ann Neurol*. 2011;69(5):892–900.
68. Vincent A, Bien CG, Irani SR, Waters P. Autoantibodies associated with diseases of the CNS: new developments and future challenges. *Lancet Neurol*. 2011;10(8):759–772.
69. Mauermann ML. Neurologic complications of lymphoma, leukemia, and paraproteinemias. *Continuum (Minneap Minn)*. 2017;23(3, Neurology of Systemic Disease):669–690.
70. Collao-Parra JP, Romero-Urra C, Delgado-Derio C. [Autoimmune encephalitis. A review]. *Rev Med Chil*. 2018;146(3):351–361.
71. Dalmau J, Gleichman AJ, Hughes EG, et al. Anti-NMDA-receptor encephalitis: case series and analysis of the effects of antibodies. *Lancet Neurol*. 2008;7(12):1091–1098.
72. Dalmau J, Lancaster E, Martinez-Hernandez E, Rosenfeld MR, Balice-Gordon R. Clinical experience and laboratory investigations in patients with anti-NMDAR encephalitis. *Lancet Neurol*. 2011;10(1):63–74.
73. Kumpfel T, Gerdes LA, Heck C, Pruss H. Delayed diagnosis of extraovarian teratoma in relapsing anti-NMDA receptor encephalitis. *Neurol Neuroimmunol Neuroinflamm*. 2016;3(4):e250.
74. Graus F, Saiz A, Lai M, et al. Neuronal surface antigen antibodies in limbic encephalitis: clinical-immunologic associations. *Neurology*. 2008;71(12):930–936.
75. Shen K, Xu Y, Guan H, et al. Paraneoplastic limbic encephalitis associated with lung cancer. *Sci Rep*. 2018;8(1):6792.
76. Toro J, Cuellar-Giraldo D, Duque A, Minota K, Patino J, Garcia M. Seronegative paraneoplastic limbic encephalitis associated with thymoma. *Cogn Behav Neurol*. 2017;30(3):125–128.
77. Kinirons P, Fulton A, Keoghan M, Brennan P, Farrell MA, Moroney JT. Paraneoplastic limbic encephalitis (PLE) and chorea associated with CRMP-5 neuronal antibody. *Neurology*. 2003;61(11):1623–1624.
78. Kellinghaus C, Kraus J, Blaes F, Nabavi DG, Schäbitz WR. CRMP-5-autoantibodies in testicular cancer associated with limbic encephalitis and choreiform dyskinesias. *Eur Neurol*. 2007;57:241–243.
79. Duyckaerts C, Derouesne C, Signoret JL, Gray F, Escourolle R, Castaigne P. Bilateral and limited amygdalohippocampal lesions causing a pure amnesic syndrome. *Ann Neurol*. 1985;18(3):314–319.
80. Dowben JS, Kowalski PC, Keltner NL. Biological perspectives: anti-NMDA receptor encephalitis. *Perspect Psychiatr Care*. 2015;51(4):236–240.
81. Li L, Hanahan D. Hijacking the neuronal NMDAR signaling circuit to promote tumor growth and invasion. *Cell*. 2013;153(1):86–100.
82. Martinez-Hernandez E, Horvath J, Shiloh-Malawsky Y, Sangha N, Martinez-Lage M, Dalmau J. Analysis of complement and plasma cells in the brain of patients with anti-NMDAR encephalitis. *Neurology*. 2011;77(6):589–593.
83. Kodama T, Numaguchi Y, Gellad FE, Dwyer BA, Kristt DA. Magnetic resonance imaging of limbic encephalitis. *Neuroradiology*. 1991;33(6):520–523.
84. Astaras C, de Micheli R, Moura B, Hundsberger T, Hottinger AF. Neurological adverse events associated with immune checkpoint inhibitors: diagnosis and management. *Curr Neurol Neurosci Rep*. 2018;18(1):3.
85. Graus F, Escudero D, Oleaga L, et al. Syndrome and outcome of antibody-negative limbic encephalitis. *Eur J Neurol*. 2018;25(8):1011–1016.
86. Gable MS, Sheriff H, Dalmau J, Tilley DH, Glaser CA. The frequency of autoimmune N-methyl-D-aspartate receptor encephalitis surpasses that of individual viral etiologies in young individuals enrolled in the California Encephalitis Project. *Clin Infect Dis*. 2012;54(7):899–904.
87. Lawn ND, Westmoreland BF, Kiely MJ, Lennon VA, Vernino S. Clinical, magnetic resonance imaging, and electroencephalographic findings in paraneoplastic limbic encephalitis. *Mayo Clin Proc*. 2003;78(11):1363–1368.
88. Probasco JC, Solnes L, Nalluri A, et al. Abnormal brain metabolism on FDG-PET/CT is a common early finding in autoimmune encephalitis. *Neurol Neuroimmunol Neuroinflamm*. 2017;4(4):e352.
89. Urbach H, Soeder BM, Jeub M, Klockgether T, Meyer B, Bien CG. Serial MRI of limbic encephalitis. *Neuroradiology*. 2006;48(6):380–386.
90. Lu X, Chen X, Huang L, Zhu C, Gu Y, Ye S. Anti-alpha-internexin autoantibody from neuropsychiatric lupus induce cognitive damage via inhibiting axonal elongation and promote neuron apoptosis. *PLoS One*. 2010;5(6):e11124.
91. Dalmau J, Graus F, Villarejo A, et al. Clinical analysis of anti-Ma2-associated encephalitis. *Brain*. 2004;127(Pt 8):1831–1844.
92. Schermann H, Ponomareva IV, Maltsev VG, Yakushev KB, Sherman MA. Clinical variants of limbic encephalitis. *SAGE Open Med Case Rep*. 7:2050313X19846042.
93. Scheibe F, Prüss H, Mengel AM, et al. Bortezomib for treatment of therapy-refractory anti-NMDA receptor encephalitis. *Neurology*. 2017;88(4):366–370.
94. Fink M, Taylor MA. The catatonia syndrome: forgotten but not gone. *Arch Gen Psychiatry*. 2009;66(11):1173–1177.
95. Blanpied TA, Clarke RJ, Johnson JW. Amantadine inhibits NMDA receptors by accelerating channel closure during channel block. *J Neurosci*. 2005;25(13):3312–3322.

96. Rojas-Marcos I, Graus F, Sanz G, Robledo A, Diaz-Espejo C. Hypersomnia as presenting symptom of anti-Ma2-associated encephalitis: case study. *Neuro Oncol*. 2007;9(1):75–77.
97. Lai M, Hughes EG, Peng X, et al. AMPA receptor antibodies in limbic encephalitis alter synaptic receptor location. *Ann Neurol*. 2009;65(4):424–434.
98. Boronat A, Sabater L, Saiz A, Dalmau J, Graus F. GABA(B) receptor antibodies in limbic encephalitis and anti-GAD-associated neurologic disorders. *Neurology*. 2011;76(9):795–800.
99. Platt MP, Agalliu D, Cutforth T. Hello from the other side: how autoantibodies circumvent the blood-brain barrier in autoimmune encephalitis. *Front Immunol*. 2017;8:442.
100. Iizuka T, Yoshii S, Kan S, et al. Reversible brain atrophy in anti-NMDA receptor encephalitis: a long-term observational study. *J Neurol*. 2010;257(10):1686–1691.
101. Finke C, Kopp UA, Pajkert A, et al. Structural hippocampal damage following anti-N-methyl-D-aspartate receptor encephalitis. *Biol Psychiatry*. 2016;79(9):727–734.
102. Iizuka T, Kaneko J, Tominaga N, Someko H, Nakamura M, Ishima D, et al. Association of progressive cerebellar atrophy with long-term outcome in patients with anti-N-methyl-D-aspartate receptor encephalitis. *JAMA Neurol*. 2016;73(6):706–713.
103. Brandt AU, Oberwahrenbrock T, Mikolajczak J, et al. Visual dysfunction, but not retinal thinning, following anti-NMDA receptor encephalitis. *Neurol Neuroimmunol Neuroinflamm*. 2016;3(2):e198.
104. Yeshokumar AK, Gordon-Lipkin E, Arenivas A, et al. Neurobehavioral outcomes in autoimmune encephalitis. *J Neuroimmunol*. 2017;312:8–14.
105. Wu Y-J, Lai M-L, Huang C-W. Reversible postvaccination paraneoplastic encephalomyelitis in a patient with lung adenocarcinoma. *Int J Neurosci*. 2010;120(12):792–795.
106. Ances BM, Vitaliani R, Taylor RA, et al. Treatment-responsive limbic encephalitis identified by neuropil antibodies: MRI and PET correlates. *Brain*. 2005;128(Pt 8):1764–1777.
107. Verschuuren J, Twijnstra A, De Baets M, Thunnissen F, Dalmau J, van Breda Vriesman P. Hu antigens and anti-Hu antibodies in a patient with myxoid chondrosarcoma. *Neurology*. 1994;44(8):1551–1552.
108. Dalmau J, Furneaux HM, Gralla RJ, Kris MG, Posner JB. Detection of the anti-Hu antibody in the serum of patients with small cell lung cancer—a quantitative western blot analysis. *Ann Neurol*. 1990;27(5):544–552.
109. Moyano MS, Gutierrez-Gutierrez G, Gomez-Raposo C, et al. Paraneoplastic encephalomyelitis: is it an oropharyngeal or a lung cancer complication? *Oncol Lett*. 2011;2(1):171–174.
110. Henson RA, Hoffman HL, Urich H. Encephalomyelitis with carcinoma. *Brain*. 1965;88(3):449–464.
111. Sheng B, Mak VWM, Lee HKK, Li HL, Lee IPO, Wong S. Multiple myeloma presenting with acute disseminated encephalomyelitis: causal or chance link? *Neurology*. 2006;67(10):1893–1894.
112. Hinman MN, Lou H. Diverse molecular functions of Hu proteins. *Cell Mol Life Sci*. 2008;65(20):3168–3181.
113. Jean WC, Dalmau J, Ho A, Posner JB. Analysis of the IgG subclass distribution and inflammatory infiltrates in patients with anti-Hu-associated paraneoplastic encephalomyelitis. *Neurology*. 1994;44(1):140–147.
114. Saiz A, Graus F, Dalmau J, Pifarre A, Marin C, Tolosa E. Detection of 14-3-3 brain protein in the cerebrospinal fluid of patients with paraneoplastic neurological disorders. *Ann Neurol*. 1999;46(5):774–777.
115. Sharshar T, Auriant I, Dorandeu A, et al. Association of herpes simplex virus encephalitis and paraneoplastic encephalitis—a clinico-pathological study. *Ann Pathol*. 2000;20(3):249–252.
116. Adam VN, Budinčević H, Mršić V, Stojčić EG, Matolić M, Markić A. Paraneoplastic limbic encephalitis in a patient with adenocarcinoma of the colon: a case report. *J Clin Anesth*. 2013;25(6):491–495.
117. Schwarz S, Mohr A, Knauth M, Wildemann B, Storch-Hagenlocher B. Acute disseminated encephalomyelitis: a follow-up study of 40 adult patients. *Neurology*. 2001;56(10):1313–1318.
118. Lancaster E. Paraneoplastic disorders. *Continuum (Minneap Minn)*. 2017;23(6, Neuro-oncology):1653–1679.
119. Flanagan EP, McKeon A, Lennon VA, et al. Paraneoplastic isolated myelopathy: clinical course and neuroimaging clues. *Neurology*. 2011;76(24):2089–2095.
120. Honnorat J, Didelot A, Karantoni E, et al. Autoimmune limbic encephalopathy and anti-Hu antibodies in children without cancer. *Neurology*. 2013;80(24):2226–2232.
121. Greenfield JG. Subacute spino-cerebellar degeneration occurring in elderly patients. *Brain [Internet]*. 1934;57(2):161–176. https://doi.org/10.1093/brain/57.2.161.
122. Darnell RB, DeAngelis LM. Regression of small-cell lung carcinoma in patients with paraneoplastic neuronal antibodies. *Lancet*. 1993;341(8836):21–22.
123. Greenlee JE, Brashear HR. Antibodies to cerebellar Purkinje cells in patients with paraneoplastic cerebellar degeneration and ovarian carcinoma. *Ann Neurol*. 1983;14(6):609–613.
124. Trotter JL, Hendin BA, Osterland CK. Cerebellar degeneration with Hodgkin disease. An immunological study. *Arch Neurol*. 1976;33(9):660–661.
125. Vernino S. Paraneoplastic cerebellar degeneration. *Handb Clin Neurol*. 2012;103:215–223.
126. Leypoldt F, Wandinger KP. Paraneoplastic neurological syndromes. *Clin Exp Immunol*. 2014;175(3):336–348.
127. Cui D, Xu L, Li WY, Qian WD. Anti-Yo positive and late-onset paraneoplastic cerebellar degeneration associated with ovarian carcinoma: a case report. *Medicine (Baltimore)*. 2017;96(32):e7362.
128. Afzal S, Recio M, Shamim S. Paraneoplastic cerebellar ataxia and the paraneoplastic syndromes. *Proc (Bayl Univ Med Cent)*. 2015;28:217–220.
129. Bolla L, Palmer RM. Paraneoplastic cerebellar degeneration. Case report and literature review. *Arch Intern Med*. 1997;157(11):1258–1262.
130. Ducray F, Demarquay G, Graus F, et al. Seronegative paraneoplastic cerebellar degeneration: the PNS Euronetwork experience. *Eur J Neurol*. 2014;21(5):731–735.
131. Graus F, Lang B, Pozo-Rosich P, Saiz A, Casamitjana R, Vincent A. P/Q type calcium-channel antibodies in paraneoplastic cerebellar degeneration with lung cancer. *Neurology*. 2002;59(5):764–766.
132. Durieux V, Coureau M, Meert AP, Berghmans T, Sculier JP. Autoimmune paraneoplastic syndromes associated to lung cancer: a systematic review of the literature. *Lung Cancer*. 2017;106:102–109.
133. Shams'ili S, Grefkens J, de Leeuw B, et al. Paraneoplastic cerebellar degeneration associated with antineuronal antibodies: analysis of 50 patients. *Brain*. 2003;126(Pt 6):1409–1418.
134. Vernino S, O'Neill BP, Marks RS, O'Fallon JR, Kimmel DW. Immunomodulatory treatment trial for paraneoplastic neurological disorders. *Neuro Oncol*. 2004;6(1):55–62.

135. Candler PM, Hart PE, Barnett M, Weil R, Rees JH. A follow up study of patients with paraneoplastic neurological disease in the United Kingdom. *J Neurol Neurosurg Psychiatry*. 2004;75(10):1411–1415.
136. Peterson K, Rosenblum MK, Kotanides H, Posner JB. Paraneoplastic cerebellar degeneration. I. A clinical analysis of 55 anti-Yo antibody-positive patients. *Neurology*. 1992;42(10):1931–1937.
137. Cocconi G, Ceci G, Juvarra G, et al. Successful treatment of subacute cerebellar degeneration in ovarian carcinoma with plasmapheresis. *A Case Report Cancer*. 1985;56(9):2318–2320.
138. Rojas-Marcos I, Rousseau A, Keime-Guibert F, et al. Spectrum of paraneoplastic neurologic disorders in women with breast and gynecologic cancer. *Medicine (Baltimore)*. 2003;82(3):216–223.
139. Bernal F, Shams'ili S, Rojas I, et al. Anti-Tr antibodies as markers of paraneoplastic cerebellar degeneration and Hodgkin's disease. *Neurology*. 2003;60(2):230–234. Available at: http://n.neurology.org/content/60/2/230.abstract.
140. Pittock SJ, Lucchinetti CF, Lennon VA. Anti-neuronal nuclear autoantibody type 2: paraneoplastic accompaniments. *Ann Neurol*. 2003;53(5):580–587.
141. Yu Z, Kryzer TJ, Griesmann GE, Kim K, Benarroch EE, Lennon VA. CRMP-5 neuronal autoantibody: marker of lung cancer and thymoma-related autoimmunity. *Ann Neurol*. 2001;49(2):146–154.
142. Pang KK, de Sousa C, Lang B, Pike MG. A prospective study of the presentation and management of dancing eye syndrome/opsoclonus-myoclonus syndrome in the United Kingdom. *Eur J Paediatr Neurol*. 2010;14(2):156–161.
143. Galstyan A, Wilbur C, Selby K, Hukin J. Opsoclonus-myoclonus syndrome: a new era of improved prognosis? *Pediatr Neurol*. 2017;72:65–69.
144. Luque FA, Furneaux HM, Ferziger R, Rosenblum MK, Wray SH, Schold SCJ, et al. Anti-Ri: an antibody associated with paraneoplastic opsoclonus and breast cancer. *Ann Neurol*. 1991;29(3):241–251.
145. Bataller L, Graus F, Saiz A, Vilchez JJ. Clinical outcome in adult onset idiopathic or paraneoplastic opsoclonus-myoclonus. *Brain*. 2001;124(Pt 2):437–443.
146. Armangue T, Sabater L, Torres-Vega E, et al. Clinical and immunological features of opsoclonus-myoclonus syndrome in the era of neuronal cell surface antibodies. *JAMA Neurol*. 2016;73(4):417–424.
147. Pike M. Opsoclonus-myoclonus syndrome. *Handb Clin Neurol*. 2013;112:1209–1211.
148. Pranzatelli MR, Travelstead AL, Tate ED, et al. B- and T-cell markers in opsoclonus-myoclonus syndrome: immunophenotyping of CSF lymphocytes. *Neurology*. 2004;62(9):1526–1532.
149. Matthay KK, Blaes F, Hero B, et al. Opsoclonus myoclonus syndrome in neuroblastoma a report from a workshop on the dancing eyes syndrome at the advances in neuroblastoma meeting in Genoa, Italy, 2004. *Cancer Lett*. 2005;228(1–2):275–282.
150. Klaas JP, Ahlskog JE, Pittock SJ, et al. Adult-onset opsoclonus-myoclonus syndrome. *Arch Neurol*. 2012;69(12):1598–1607.
151. Anderson NE, Budde-Steffen C, Rosenblum MK, et al. Opsoclonus, myoclonus, ataxia, and encephalopathy in adults with cancer: a distinct paraneoplastic syndrome. *Medicine (Baltimore)*. 1988;67(2):100–109.
152. Antunes NL, Khakoo Y, Matthay KK, et al. Antineuronal antibodies in patients with neuroblastoma and paraneoplastic opsoclonus-myoclonus. *J Pediatr Hematol Oncol*. 2000;22(4):315–320.
153. Aquilina A, Dingli N, Aquilina J. Postintervention acute opsoclonus myoclonus syndrome. *BMJ Case Rep*. 2017;2017.
154. Hormigo A, Dalmau J, Rosenblum MK, River ME, Posner JB. Immunological and pathological study of anti-Ri-associated encephalopathy. *Ann Neurol*. 1994;36(6):896–902.
155. Armangue T, Titulaer MJ, Sabater L, et al. A novel treatment-responsive encephalitis with frequent opsoclonus and teratoma. *Ann Neurol*. 2014;75(3):435–441.
156. Kanjanasut N, Phanthumchinda K, Bhidayasiri R. HIV-related opsoclonus-myoclonus-ataxia syndrome: report on two cases. *Clin Neurol Neurosurg*. 2010;112(7):572–574.
157. Rudnick E, Khakoo Y, Antunes NL, et al. Opsoclonus-myoclonus-ataxia syndrome in neuroblastoma: clinical outcome and antineuronal antibodies—a report from the Children's Cancer Group Study. *Med Pediatr Oncol*. 2001;36(6):612–622.
158. Mitchell WG, Brumm VL, Azen CG, Patterson KE, Aller SK, Rodriguez J. Longitudinal neurodevelopmental evaluation of children with opsoclonus-ataxia. *Pediatrics*. 2005;116(4):901–907.
159. Brunklaus A, Pohl K, Zuberi SM, de Sousa C. Outcome and prognostic features in opsoclonus-myoclonus syndrome from infancy to adult life. *Pediatrics*. 2011;128(2):e388–e394.
160. Bartos A. Effective high-dose clonazepam treatment in two patients with opsoclonus and myoclonus: GABAergic hypothesis. *Eur Neurol*. 2006;56:240–242.
161. Fernandes TD, Bazan R, Betting LE, da Rocha FCG. Topiramate effect in opsoclonus-myoclonus-ataxia syndrome. *Arch Neurol*. 2012;69(1):133.
162. Wong A. An update on opsoclonus. *Curr Opin Neurol*. 2007;20(1):25–31.
163. Pelosof LC, Gerber DE. Paraneoplastic syndromes: an approach to diagnosis and treatment. *Mayo Clin Proc*. 2010;85(9):838–854.
164. Koike H, Sobue G. Paraneoplastic neuropathy. *Handb Clin Neurol*. 2013;115:713–726.
165. Gozzard P, Maddison P. Which antibody and which cancer in which paraneoplastic syndromes? *Pract Neurol*. 2010;10(5):260–270.
166. Graus F, Dalmau J. Paraneoplastic neuropathies. *Curr Opin Neurol*. 2013;26(5):489–495.
167. Ichimura M, Yamamoto M, Kobayashi Y, et al. Tissue distribution of pathological lesions and Hu antigen expression in paraneoplastic sensory neuronopathy. *Acta Neuropathol*. 1998;95(6):641–648.
168. Antoine JC, Mosnier JF, Honnorat J, et al. Paraneoplastic demyelinating neuropathy, subacute sensory neuropathy, and anti-Hu antibodies: clinicopathological study of an autopsy case. *Muscle Nerve*. 1998;21(7):850–857.
169. McKeon A, Lennon VA, Lachance DH, Fealey RD, Pittock SJ. Ganglionic acetylcholine receptor autoantibody: oncological, neurological, and serological accompaniments. *Arch Neurol*. 2009;66(6):735–741.
170. Oki Y, Koike H, Iijima M, et al. Ataxic vs painful form of paraneoplastic neuropathy. *Neurology*. 2007;69(6):564–572.
171. Camdessanché JP, Antoine JC, Honnorat J, et al. Paraneoplastic peripheral neuropathy associated with anti-Hu antibodies. A clinical and electrophysiological study of 20 patients. *Brain*. 2002;125(Pt 1):166–175.

172. Merino-Ramirez MA, Bolton CF. Review of the diagnostic challenges of Lambert-Eaton syndrome revealed through three case reports. *Can J Neurol Sci*. 2016;43(5):635–647.
173. Giometto B, Vitaliani R, Lindeck-Pozza E, Grisold W, Vedeler C. Treatment for paraneoplastic neuropathies. *Cochrane Database Syst Rev*. 2012;12:CD007625.
174. Hulsbrink R, Hashemolhosseini S. Lambert-Eaton myasthenic syndrome—diagnosis, pathogenesis and therapy. *Clin Neurophysiol*. 2014;125(12):2328–2336.
175. Titulaer MJ, Wirtz PW, Kuks JBM, et al. The Lambert-Eaton myasthenic syndrome 1988–2008: a clinical picture in 97 patients. *J Neuroimmunol*. 2008:201–202. 153–158.
176. O'Neill JH, Murray NM, Newsom-Davis J. The Lambert-Eaton myasthenic syndrome. A review of 50 cases. *Brain*. 1988;111(Pt 3):577–596.
177. Odabasi Z, Demirci M, Kim DS, et al. Postexercise facilitation of reflexes is not common in Lambert-Eaton myasthenic syndrome. *Neurology*. 2002;59(7):1085–1087.
178. Shibayama T, Ueoka H, Nishii K, et al. Complementary roles of pro-gastrin-releasing peptide (ProGRP) and neuron specific enolase (NSE) in diagnosis and prognosis of small-cell lung cancer (SCLC). *Lung Cancer*. 2001;32(1):61–69.
179. Titulaer MJ, Maddison P, Sont JK, et al. Clinical Dutch-English Lambert-Eaton Myasthenic syndrome (LEMS) tumor association prediction score accurately predicts small-cell lung cancer in the LEMS. *J Clin Oncol*. 2011;29(7):902–908.
180. Callen JP. Dermatomyositis and malignancy. *Clin Dermatol*. 1993;11(1):61–65.
181. Tang MM, Thevarajah S. Paraneoplastic dermatomyositis: a 12-year retrospective review in the department of dermatology Hospital Kuala Lumpur. *Med J Malaysia*. 2010;65(2):138–142.
182. Symmons DP, Sills JA, Davis SM. The incidence of juvenile dermatomyositis: results from a nation-wide study. *Br J Rheumatol*. 1995;34(8):732–736.
183. Callen JP. Relation between dermatomyositis and polymyositis and cancer. *Lancet*. 2001;357(9250):85–86.
184. Buchbinder R, Hill CL. Malignancy in patients with inflammatory myopathy. *Curr Rheumatol Rep*. 2002;4(5):415–426.
185. Bientinesi R, Ragonese M, Pinto F, Bassi PF, Sacco E. Paraneoplastic dermatomyositis associated with panurothelial transitional cell carcinoma: a case report and literature review. *Clin Genitourin Cancer*. 2016;14(2):e199–e201.
186. Ekiz E, Ozkok A, Ertugrul NK. Paraneoplastic mononeuritis multiplex as a presenting feature of adenocarcinoma of the lung. *Case Rep Oncol Med*. 2013;2013:457346.
187. Sheikh AAE, Sheikh AB, Tariq U, et al. Paraneoplastic mononeuritis multiplex: a unique presentation of non-Hodgkin lymphoma. *Cureus*. 2018;10:e2885.
188. Antoine JC, Mosnier JF, Absi L, Convers P, Honnorat J, Michel D. Carcinoma associated paraneoplastic peripheral neuropathies in patients with and without anti-onconeural antibodies. *J Neurol Neurosurg Psychiatry*. 1999;67(1):7–14.
189. Liang BC, Albers JW, Sima AA, Nostrant TT. Paraneoplastic pseudo-obstruction, mononeuropathy multiplex, and sensory neuronopathy. *Muscle Nerve*. 1994;17(1):91–96.
190. Martin AC, Friedlander M, Kiernan MC. Paraneoplastic mononeuritis multiplex in non-small-cell lung carcinoma. *J Clin Neurosci*. 2006;13(5):595–598.
191. Arino H, Höftberger R, Gresa-Arribas N, et al. Paraneoplastic neurological syndromes and glutamic acid decarboxylase antibodies. *JAMA Neurol*. 2015;72(8):874–881.
192. Lalani N, Haq R. Prognostic effect of early treatment of paraneoplastic limbic encephalitis in a patient with small-cell lung cancer. *Curr Oncol*. 2012;19(5):e353–e357.
193. Alamowitch S, Graus F, Uchuya M, Reñé R, Bescansa E, Delattre JY. Limbic encephalitis and small cell lung cancer. Clinical and immunological features. *Brain*. 1997;120(Pt 6):923–928.
194. Kimura M, Onozawa M, Fujisaki A, et al. Anti-Ma2 paraneoplastic encephalitis associated with testicular germ cell tumor treated by carboplatin, etoposide and bleomycin. *Int J Urol*. 2008;15(10):942–943.
195. Popkirov S, Ayzenberg I, Hahn S, et al. Rho-associated protein kinase 2 (ROCK2): a new target of autoimmunity in paraneoplastic encephalitis. *Acta Neuropathol Commun*. 2017;5(1):40.
196. Antoine JC, Absi L, Honnorat J, et al. Antiamphiphysin antibodies are associated with various paraneoplastic neurological syndromes and tumors. *Arch Neurol*. 1999;56(2):172–177.
197. Chan KH, Vernino S, Lennon VA. ANNA-3 anti-neuronal nuclear antibody: marker of lung cancer-related autoimmunity. *Ann Neurol*. 2001;50(3):301–311.
198. Fayyaz B, Gunawan F, Obah E. "A Story Unheard": anti-Ta associated paraneoplastic cerebellar degeneration in a female. *J Comm Hosp Intern Med Perspect*. 2019;9:162–164.
199. Zuliani L, Sabater L, Saiz A, Baiges JJ, Giometto B, Graus F. Homer 3 autoimmunity in subacute idiopathic cerebellar ataxia. *Neurology*. 2007;68(3):239–240.
200. Höftberger R, Sabater L, Ortega A, Dalmau J, Graus F. Patient with homer-3 antibodies and cerebellitis. *JAMA Neurol*. 2013;70(4):506–509.
201. Berzero G, Hacohen Y, Komorowski L, et al. Paraneoplastic cerebellar degeneration associated with anti-ITPR1 antibodies. *Neurol Neuroimmunol Neuroinflamm*. 2017;4(2):e326.
202. Nishikata M, Nishimori I, Taniuchi K, et al. Carbonic anhydrase-related protein VIII promotes colon cancer cell growth. *Mol Carcinog*. 2007;46(3):208–214.
203. Akisawa Y, Nishimori I, Taniuchi K, et al. Expression of carbonic anhydrase-related protein CA-RP VIII in non-small cell lung cancer. *Virchows Arch*. 2003;442(1):66–70.
204. Jarius S, Martínez-García P, Hernandez AL, et al. Two new cases of anti-Ca (anti-ARHGAP26/GRAF) autoantibody-associated cerebellar ataxia. *J Neuroinflammation*. 2013;10:7.
205. van Coevorden-Hameete MH, van Beuningen SFB, Perrenoud M, et al. Antibodies to TRIM46 are associated with paraneoplastic neurological syndromes. *Ann Clin Transl Neurol*. 2017;4(9):680–686.
206. Armangué T, Sabater L, Torres-Vega E, et al. Clinical and immunological features of opsoclonus-myoclonus syndrome in the era of neuronal cell surface antibodies. *JAMA Neurol*. 2016;73(4):417–424. https://doi.org/10.1001/jamaneurol.2015.4607.
207. Li H, Zhang A, Hao Y, Guan H, Lv Z. Coexistence of Lambert-Eaton myasthenic syndrome and autoimmune encephalitis with anti-CRMP5/CV2 and anti-GABAB receptor antibodies in small cell lung cancer: a case report. *Medicine (Baltimore)*. 2018;97(19):e0696.

Chapter | 21 |

Perineural spread of cancer

Kutluay Uluc, Laszlo Szidonya, Joao Prola Netto, and Prakash Ambady

CHAPTER OUTLINE

Introduction

Perineural invasion (PNI) refers to a rare type of contiguous spread of neoplastic cells from their primary site along the potential space between or beneath the layers of perineurium. This entity is best described in cancers of the head and neck but is also well described in other solid tumors. Exact pathogenesis remains unclear, but proximity of the primary tumor to major nerves and plexus and the tumor cell's ability to infiltrate and proliferate within the perineural space, as well as directed molecular interactions between the tumor and its microenvironment, are thought to play an important role. The clinical presentation varies depending on the nerves involved. Developing a broad differential to include direct compression of nerves by tumors, delayed effects of prior radiation therapy, infections, and paraneoplastic syndromes as well as work-up for other common causes of neuropathies is encouraged. Contrast-enhanced magnetic resonance imaging is the imaging modality of choice, but a biopsy is frequently required for confirmation of diagnosis. Accurate detection may help predict prognosis and guide therapy. We recommend a multidisciplinary approach in selecting the curative and palliative treatment options.

Classification of perineural invasion

PNI refers to a rare type of contiguous spread of neoplastic cells from their primary site along the potential space between or beneath the layers of perineurium (Fig. 21.1). It is defined as "tumor in close proximity to nerve and involving at least 33% of its circumference or tumor cells within any of the three layers of the nerve sheath (epineurium, perineurium and endoneurium)."[1] It was first described in 1952 by Dr. Frederick Mohs and Dr. Theodore Lathrop as "silent" extensions along the nerve sheath.[2] Even though this phenomenon is frequently discussed in patients with primary head and neck malignancies, it is well defined in malignancies of the pancreas, prostate, and colorectum.[3–8] Perineural invasion can be broadly divided into two main categories based on the patient's clinical presentation:

- *Microscopic perineural invasion* (MPNI) is the asymptomatic type (60–70%) where diagnosis is made on surveillance imaging, biopsy, or autopsy.
- *Clinical perineural invasion* (CPNI) is the symptomatic type (30–40%).[9,10]

Another approach to their classification is to differentiate between the type and caliber of nerve that is involved:

- *Perineural invasion (*PNI) is used to describe involvement of small, unnamed nerves around a tumor.
- *Perineural spread* (PNS) is the term used when there is evidence of invasion and spread along a larger, named nerve or cranial nerves.[11]

Although both can result in symptoms, PNS is generally considered to be more aggressive and frequently presents with neuropathy of the affected nerve.[12,13]

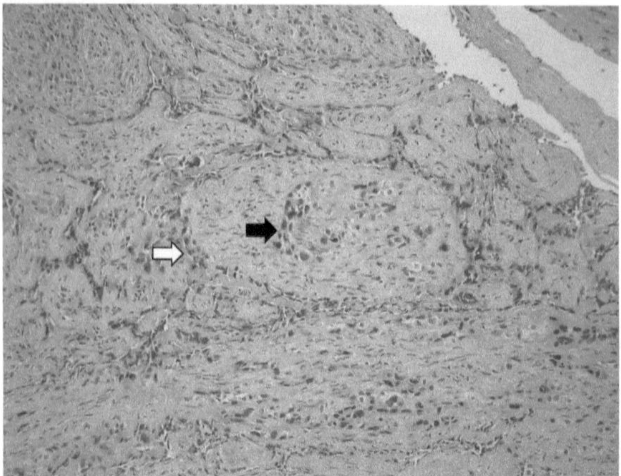

Fig. 21.1 Histopathologic stain of perineural invasion showing cancer cells (squamous cell carcinoma) invading the perineurium and endoneurium. The *white arrow* points to the perineural invasion and the *black arrow* points to endoneural invasion.

Pathogenesis

The exact pathogenesis remains unclear, but the proximity of the primary tumor to major nerves and plexus and the tumor cell's ability to infiltrate and proliferate within the perineural space, as well as directed molecular interactions between the tumor and its microenvironment, are thought to play an important role.[1] Additionally, tumor-associated macrophages, Schwann cells, and other cells in the tumor microenvironment such as fibroblasts and extracellular matrix adhesion proteins may play an important role in perineural invasion and spread. A review of the literature suggests that cells capable of producing neurotropins, including nerve growth factor, brain-derived neurotropic factor, and glial cell line–derived neurotrophic factor, are linked to PNI in multiple type of cancers.[1–16] Similarly, several studies have suggested that prostate tumor cells located adjacent to nerves have increased proliferation rates compared to those located further away, suggesting a dynamic interaction.[17,18] Evidence of PNI predisposes locoregional recurrence even after complete resection. The presence of PNI is independently associated with decreased survival.[19–21] Due to its prognostic and predictive implications, the College of American Pathologists recommends including perineural space invasion in histopathologic reports for all cutaneous and head and neck malignancies.[22] It is estimated that around 2–6% of patients with malignant head and neck tumors have evidence of PNS, whereas other tumors, such as prostate cancer, may demonstrate up to 75% PNI without significant PNS.[7,10,23–30]

Clinical presentation

In head and neck cancers, PNS frequently affects cranial nerves V (CN V) and VII (CN VII).[19–21,24,31–33] Patients with high-grade or poorly differentiated tumors, tumors involving the mid-face, male gender, and large primary tumors are at a higher risk of developing PNI.[10,23–30] Presenting symptoms are subtle, variable, and usually progress over the years. If the CN V is affected, symptoms include numbness (72%), pain (46%), or paresthesia. Patients may describe this sensation as ants crawling underneath the skin (formication) (10%). Similarly, patients may present with lower motor neuron type facial palsy if the CN VII is affected (33%).[10,34,35] The pattern of nerve involvement is closely related to the primary location of the tumor. For example, tumors of the supraorbital region tend to invade CN V1 (ophthalmic nerve), whereas tumors of the medial cheek invade CN V2 (47%) (maxillary nerve). Similarly, tumors of the temporal region invade CN V2 and CN V3 (mandibular nerve), whereas tumors of the peri-auricular region invade CN VII (26%).[34,35] The subtleness of the symptoms and slow progression over months to years may cause an incorrect diagnosis, such as Bell's palsy or trigeminal neuralgia. A high index of suspicion and good history will help broaden the differential diagnosis and aid in early detection.

Clinical cases

CASE 21.1 BRACHIAL PLEXUS INVOLVEMENT IN BREAST CANCER: PERINEURAL SPREAD VERSUS RADIATION-INDUCED PLEXOPATHY

Case. A 58-year-old woman presented with progressive radicular pain in her left arm. Pain was reported to start in the posterior neck, then radiate to the right axilla, posterior arm, and dorsal forearm into the thumb and index finger. She also reported weakness of hand grip and clawing of her left hand. Symptoms progressed very slowly after onset. On examination, atrophy but no fasciculation was noted, along with weakness in the flexors and extensors of the wrist and intrinsic muscles of the left hand. Hyporeflexia was noted in the left biceps, triceps, and brachioradialis. There was no evidence of Horner syndrome.

Her oncology history was significant for locally advanced right-sided breast cancer treated with surgical resection and local radiation therapy over 20 years prior to onset of her presenting symptoms. Due to her history of prior radiation, radiation-induced brachial plexopathy (RIBP) was considered in addition to disease progression with involvement of the brachial plexus.

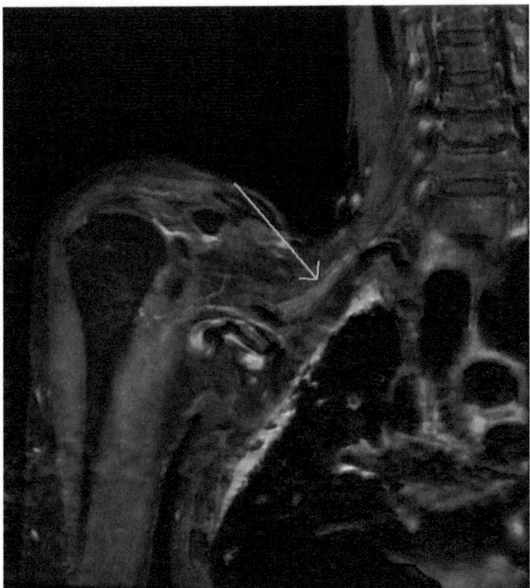

Fig. 21.2 Coronal MRI (post-contrast T1-weighted images) demonstrates abnormal enlargement of the brachial plexus *(white arrow)*. In patients with a prior history of radiation therapy, the absence of focal mass or displacement of adjacent structures may help broaden the differential to include treatment-related changes.

However, nerve conduction studies and electromyogram were unremarkable. Of note, evidence of myokymic discharges was not documented in this study. Contrast-enhanced MRI of the brachial plexus demonstrated abnormal enhancement and enlargement of the right brachial plexus along with involvement of the right pleura/lung (Fig. 21.2). PET/CT did not demonstrate evidence of tumor recurrence. Follow-up imaging did not show significant changes in the pattern of enhancement seen in the brachial plexus, and a presumptive diagnosis of RIBP rather than perineural spread was made. Biopsy was deferred but was considered upon clinical or radiographic progression.

Teaching Points: Imaging Evaluation and Diagnostic Studies for Perineural Spread. This case highlights the important role of imaging in the evaluation of patients with suspected perineural spread. Imaging may include any combination of CT, MRI, and positron emission tomography (PET). For the patient in this case, serial neuroimaging was critical in differentiating between neoplastic and non-neoplastic process as MRI findings were not definitive, and the lack of tumor recurrence on FDG-PET favored a radiation-induced brachial plexopathy but was not definitive.

Imaging evaluation and diagnostic studies

Contrast-enhanced MRI is the gold standard for establishing an imaging diagnosis of PNI.[19] Even with the best effort, imaging studies may be negative at the time of presentation.[36] Sensitivity of imaging studies is higher in symptomatic patients (CPNI), but false-negative results have been reported even in this patient population.[34,36,37] Overall, imaging studies can be negative in up to 45% of patients in PNI.[32,34,37–44] Follow-up MRI may be useful in case of negative initial imaging.[45]

Even though it is challenging, effort for early diagnosis is important, given its prognostic value. T1-weighted gadolinium-enhanced MRI is used to identify asymmetrical enlargement or abnormal enhancement around the cranial nerves.[33,36,46,47] Abnormal enhancement implies diffuse enhancement of the nerve with loss of the distinction between the nerve and the perineural vascular plexus.[33] Fat-suppression sequences are helpful, since this decreases artifacts surrounding the skull base foramina.[33,36,46,47] Furthermore, sharing relevant findings such as trophy in facial muscles or muscles of mastication denervation may prompt the radiologist to look for subtle evidence on imaging.[48,49]

In some studies, the specificity of the MRI is reported to be increased to 95–100% by using targeted MRI sequences to the suspected nerves (aka MR neurography).[50,51] However, the long procedure time and movement artifacts can limit its utility. CT also plays an important role, especially for lesions that are close to bony structures and involve the skull base. In these cases, bone destruction or enlargement and erosion of foramina may be better appreciated on CT scans.[33,36] Although lacking the spatial resolution of CT or MRI, techniques such as FDG-PET/CT scans may further aid in diagnosis by demonstrating linear or curvilinear signal changes that represent their metabolic activity.[52] A combination of CT and MRI with selected use of FDG-PET may increase the detection rate and improve the understanding of disease extent.[33,53]

Evaluation is more challenging in patients who have received prior radiotherapy where radiation-induced peripheral neuropathy (RIPN), such as radiation-induced plexitis, can present in a similar manner. In these cases, use of 3 Telsa MRI may increase sensitivity.[54] RIPN is a rare but relatively well-described complication of radiation therapy. Radiation-related changes often occur early after radiation; however, as was the case for this patient, neuronal injury can occur even decades after initial exposure to radiation.[55–57]

Metastasis to regional lymph nodes is uncommon, but some reports suggest that rates may be higher in patients with PNI.[58–60] Evaluation of these lymph nodes with MRI or CT with contrast may assist in making a diagnosis. Ultrasound-guided fine-needle aspiration and/or sentinel lymph node biopsy can be obtained if lymph nodes are identified on imaging studies.[24,33,61] Depending on the clinical presentation and clinical history, cerebrospinal fluid (CSF) studies can be considered, especially when leptomeningeal enhancement is noted by imaging. However, the yield is low and, in most cases, the only abnormality identified is high CSF protein level.[62,63]

Ultimately, biopsy of the involved nerve may be necessary to confirm the diagnosis.[64] Even after an open biopsy, diagnosis of PNI may be challenging. Peritumoral fibrosis may mimic PNI by imaging as well as on histologic sections, especially on hematoxylin and eosin stains.[21,65] Addition of p75NGFR immunostaining with or without the S-100 immunostaining may be helpful in differentiating fibrosis versus invasion.[66]

Clinical Pearls

1. Contrast-enhanced MRI is the gold standard for establishing an imaging diagnosis of PNI, but false-negative rates are high and may fail to demonstrate active disease in at least 45% of patients.
2. A combination of CT and MRI with selected use of FDG-PET may increase the detection rate and improve the understanding of disease extent.

Teaching Points: Differential Diagnosis of Perineural Spread. This case also highlights the role of imaging in guiding the clinical evaluation and informing the differential diagnosis. Imaging in this case revealed a neural lesion on contrast-enhanced MRI that did not show increased uptake on FDG-PET and showed stability on serial imaging that favored radiation-induced brachial plexitis as opposed to a direct neoplastic or perineural process.

Differential diagnosis of perineural spread

In cases where imaging studies are positive, the differential diagnosis is relatively narrowed. When imaging shows abnormal enhancement of the affected nerve with or without enlargement of the foramina or expansion of the nerve, the differential diagnosis includes neoplastic, inflammatory, and infectious causes[45,67–69]:

1. Neoplastic differential diagnoses: primary neural tumors, PNI, traumatic injury, paraneoplastic syndromes, lymphoma
2. Inflammatory differential diagnoses: granulomatous diseases (e.g., sarcoidosis)
3. Infectious differential diagnoses: histiocytosis, mucormycosis, aspergillus, viral neuritis, IgG disease, syphilis, and Lyme disease

Biopsy or a close imaging follow-up may help in differentiating between these pathologies and PNI.[69] CT-guided biopsy can be used for lesions involving V3 in the foramen ovale (Fig. 21.3). Ultrasound-guided fine-needle aspiration is usually used for peripheral nerves suspected to be involved with tumor, especially the auriculotemporal and the greater auricular nerves.[69]

When the imaging studies are negative, differential diagnosis varies depending on the nerve being affected. If CN V is affected, the differential diagnosis includes imaging-negative diagnoses like cluster headaches, dental pain, giant cell arteritis, glossopharyngeal neuralgia, vascular or direct compression of the trigeminal nerve, migraine, multiple sclerosis, otitis media, postherpetic neuralgia, paroxysmal hemicranias, sinusitis, and temporomandibular joint syndrome.[70] If CN VII is affected, the differential diagnosis will include Bell's palsy, Lyme disease, stroke, multiple sclerosis, Guillain-Barre syndrome, sarcoidosis, direct compression from tumors (parotid, acoustic schwannoma, etc.), or Ramsay Hunt/Zoster syndrome.[71] Although PNI is a feature of local invasiveness, sometimes it can be seen in certain benign breast lesions such as sclerosing adenosis, complex sclerosing lesion/radial scar, and ductal carcinoma in situ.[72,73] Some authors have suggested this is epithelial glands that are displaced into the perineural space which may mimic PNI. This may be a potential source of misdiagnosis and may not represent true invasion and thus may have minimal clinical impact on outcomes.[72,74,75]

At times it may be challenging to differentiate between the possible etiologies of abnormal imaging given the complex clinical history of these patients. Abnormal enhancement of neural structures may be due to prior radiation to the field or perineural invasion (Fig. 21.2).

Clinical Pearls

1. The differential diagnosis of a new-onset brachial plexopathy in a cancer patient includes perineural spread and radiation-induced brachial plexopathy.
2. For these patients, the presence of pain should favor perineural spread or locoregional cancer recurrence, whereas the absence of pain should favor radiation-induced brachial plexopathy.

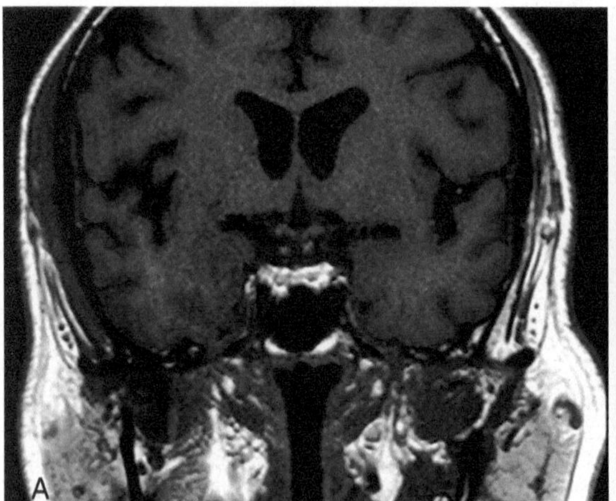

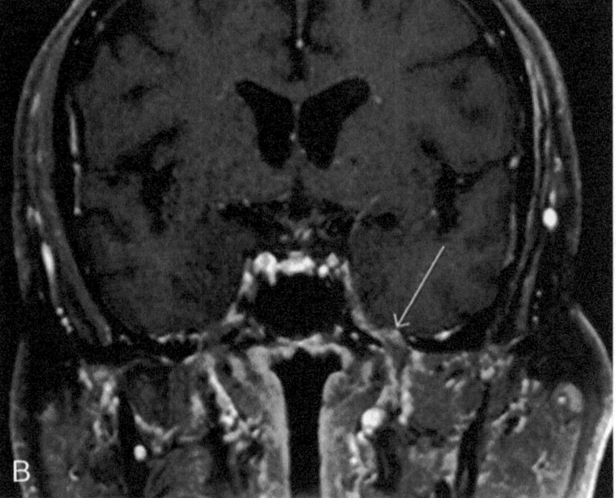

Fig. 21.3 T1-weighted MRI pre- (A) and post-contrast (B) images demonstrating abnormal enhancement of the CN V3 in the foramen ovale on the left side *(white arrow)*.

CASE 21.2 TRIGEMINAL NEURALGIA PAIN IN PATIENT WITH HEAD AND NECK CANCER

Case. A 67-year-old man presented with intermittent facial pain in the left lower face. Pain was exacerbated by chewing and exposure to cold. His oncologic history was significant for stage I squamous cell carcinoma (SCC) of the tongue treated with partial glossectomy 9 years prior to presentation, followed by radical left-sided neck dissection (levels 1b, 2a, 3, and 4), left segmental mandibulectomy, left partial glossectomy, left partial pharyngectomy, and left first molar dental extraction 7 years later (2 years prior to the current presentation). Pathology demonstrated well-differentiated SCC with no perineural or angiolymphatic invasion. No adjuvant therapy was initiated at that time because a clear surgical margin was achieved and there was no evidence of draining lymph nodes involvement.

At presentation, CT did not demonstrate any abnormal cranial foramina dilatation; however, contrast-enhanced MRI demonstrated asymmetrical enhancement of the left mandibular nerve within the foramen ovale without overt mass concerning for early perineural spread of tumor (Fig. 21.4). Facial pain was refractory to medical management and he subsequently underwent CT-guided trigeminal tractotomy for symptom control with transient improvement in pain for 16 months. A second left-sided CT-guided trigeminal tractotomy was performed with significant improvement in his pain. No addition antitumor therapies were initiated, and the lesion was monitored with serial imaging. A routine PET/CT performed approximately 1 year later demonstrated a focus of intense uptake in the left oral cavity highly concerning for malignancy. Biopsy of this lesion confirmed well-differentiated SCC.

Teaching Points: Symptomatic and Cancer-Directed Management of Perineural Invasion. This case highlights the clinical presentation and treatment options available to patients with perineural invasion. Clinicians need a high index of suspicion for this diagnosis. New facial pain or cranial neuropathy in a patient with a history of head and neck cancer should prompt an evaluation for PNI. Unfortunately, symptomatic treatments are often poorly effective and early diagnosis with appropriate cancer-directed therapies are the best approach.

Symptomatic treatment of perineural invasion

Symptomatic treatment of perineural invasion poses a significant problem and, in general, symptomatic patients tend to have a worse overall prognosis compared to asymptomatic patients.[43] Conservative medical management is recommended initially with local therapies such as nerve blocks. Tractotomy is reserved for refractory symptoms. Symptoms are generally progressive, and improvement reported only in 7% to 23 % of patients.[32,35]

Definitive treatment options for perineural invasion

Treatment starts with diagnosis. Early diagnosis of PNI improves prognosis.[76] Treatment options are surgical resection with or without removal of involved nerves, radiotherapy to region of the primary tumor with or without including the involved nerves, chemotherapy, or a combination of these therapies depending on the clinical situation.[28,34,77–81]

Surgery. Surgical resection with clear margins may improve survival rates compared to other treatment modalities.[79,82] Mohs micrographic surgery has been proposed as the surgical approach with highest chance of obtaining negative margins.[83] But this may not be possible due to anatomical limitations and extent of disease.[79] Williams et al. described zonal classification to aid decision making in selecting the patients for surgical resection.[48,50] In general, the extension of PNI beyond the gasserian and geniculate ganglion is usually deemed unresectable.[50]

Postoperative recurrence risks. Recurrence may occur after surgery even after negative margins are obtained, possibly due to a phenomenon called "skip" lesions. This is a histologic finding seen in PNI.[32,84] Thus the decision to pursue

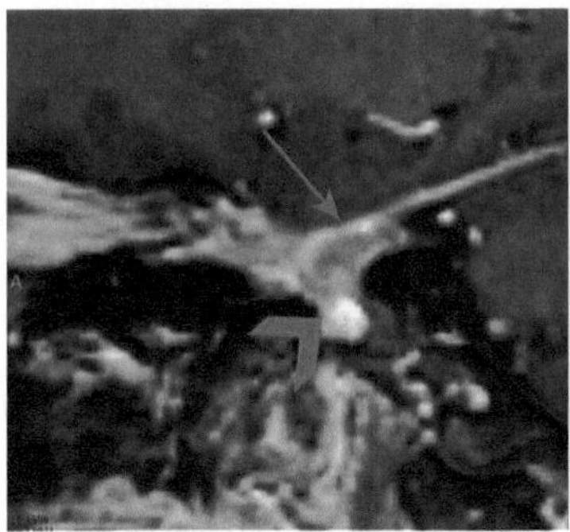
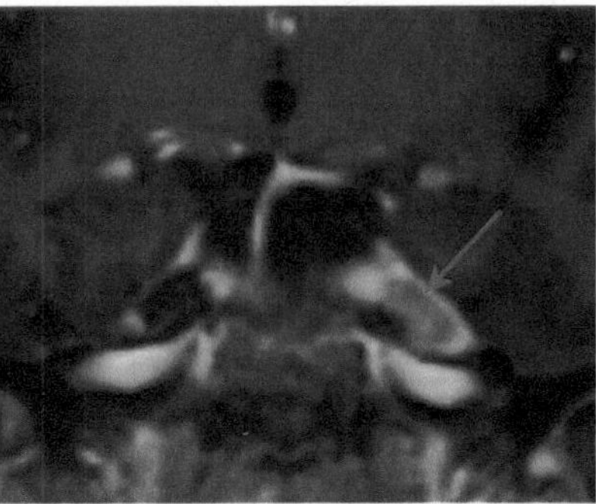
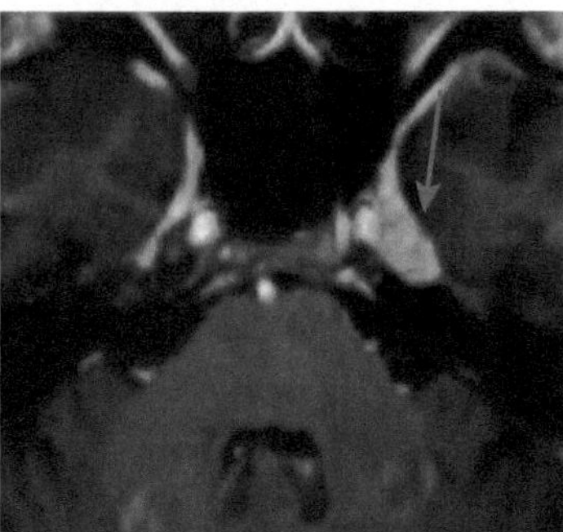

Fig. 21.4 A 67-year-old male with squamous cell cancer presents with intermittent progressive pain in the left mandible region. Sagittal, coronal, and axial post-contrast T1 demonstrates nodular thickening and enhancement of the left trigeminal nerve (*arrow*) with extension along the V3 segment through the foramen ovale (*arrowhead*).

a *"negative margin"* surgery is complex and must weigh the morbidity of surgery against the higher radiation doses and larger radiation fields used to treat residual postoperative disease.[79,85] Planning of the dose and the field of radiotherapy depends on the margin positivity after surgery.[21] Higher doses and larger fields, including incorporation of the skull base and regional lymph nodes, are necessary to improve local control rates.[21] Intensity modulated radiotherapy and proton beam therapy are other novel radiotherapy options proposed to treat this challenging problem (see Chapter 3 for further discussion of types of radiotherapy in neuro-oncology).[21]

Postoperative survival rates. Overall median progression free-survival with radiotherapy for CPNI was 5 months; median overall survival was 60 months.[34] Locoregional control rate is 69% at 5 years in cases with PNI compared to 78% in cases without PNI after postoperative radiotherapy.[86] There is a significant difference in local control rates in patients with MPNI and CPNI, ranging between 78% and 87% for MPNI compared to 45% and 55% for CPNI.[24,32,76] Extension to skull base significantly decreases local control to 25%.[76] Five-year overall absolute survival in patients treated with surgical resection and adjuvant radiotherapy is 55% for MPNI and 50% for CPNI.[24,32] Despite the therapeutic benefit of adjuvant radiotherapy, this is not without risk of complications and can be expensive and time consuming.[21] Up to 10% of patients will experience soft tissue necrosis, bone exposure, and osteoradionecrosis with adjuvant radiation therapy. Moreover, definitive radiotherapy can cause transient central nervous system syndrome, fistula, or wound infection in one-third of patients.[76]

Chemotherapy options. In addition to surgery and radiotherapy, many chemotherapeutic agents have been suggested for treatment of PNI. Cisplatin, doxorubicin, bleomycin, peplomycin, methotrexate, 5-fluorouracil, and cetuximab are some of the proposed agents.[87–90] Erlotinib and intrathecal chemotherapy has been also suggested for successful treatment of a patient with SCC with PNI.[91] Data on postoperative radiotherapy and concurrent chemotherapy is limited.[92] Their efficacy may be low due to blood-nerve barrier causing limits the delivery of these agents.

Clinical Pearls

1. Early diagnosis of PNI is critical for prompt initiation of treatment, as neurological deficits are poorly rescued once significant dysfunction has developed.
2. Surgical resection with the goal of clear margins must be balanced against the risk of postoperative morbidity from neurological insult.
3. Five-year survival in patients treated with surgical resection and adjuvant radiotherapy is 55% for patients with microscopic PNI and 50% for symptomatic patients.

Conclusion

PNI is a sign of poor prognosis in patients with head and neck cancers. For this reason, an effort for early diagnosis should be made. After the diagnosis, aggressive surgical, radiation, and chemotherapy may improve the outcome. There is no consensus in management of PNI, especially amongst surgeons and radiation oncologists.[19] We recommend a multidisciplinary approach in selecting the curative and palliative treatment options.

References

1. Liebig C, Ayala G, Wilks JA, Berger DH, Albo D. Perineural invasion in cancer: a review of the literature. *Cancer.* 2009;115(15):3379–3391.
2. Mohs FE, Lathrop TG. Modes of spread of cancer of skin. *AMA Arch Derm Syphilol.* 1952;66(4):427–439.
3. Liu B, Lu KY. Neural invasion in pancreatic carcinoma. *Hepatobiliary Pancreat Dis Int.* 2002;1(3):469–476.
4. Harnden P, Shelley MD, Clements H, et al. The prognostic significance of perineural invasion in prostatic cancer biopsies: a systematic review. *Cancer.* 2007;109(1):13–24.
5. Liebig C, Ayala G, Wilks J, et al. Perineural invasion is an independent predictor of outcome in colorectal cancer. *J Clin Oncol.* 2009;27(31):5131–5137.
6. Johnston M, Yu E, Kim J. Perineural invasion and spread in head and neck cancer. *Expert Rev Anticancer Ther.* 2012;12(3):359–371.
7. Zareba P, Flavin R, Isikbay M, et al. Perineural invasion and risk of lethal prostate cancer. *Cancer Epidemiol Biomarkers Prev.* 2017;26(5):719–726.
8. Capek S, Howe BM, Amrami KK, Spinner RJ. Perineural spread of pelvic malignancies to the lumbosacral plexus and beyond: clinical and imaging patterns. *Neurosurg Focus.* 2015;39(3):E14.
9. Veness MJ. Perineural spread in head and neck skin cancer. *Australas J Dermatol.* 2000;41(2):117–119.
10. Mendenhall WM, Parsons JT, Mendenhall NP, et al. Carcinoma of the skin of the head and neck with perineural invasion. *Head Neck.* 1989;11(4):301–308.
11. Brown IS. Pathology of perineural spread. *J Neurol Surg B Skull Base.* 2016;77(2):124–130.
12. Panizza B, Warren T. Perineural invasion of head and neck skin cancer: diagnostic and therapeutic implications. *Curr Oncol Rep.* 2013;15(2):128–133.
13. Roh J, Muelleman T, Tawfik O, Thomas SM. Perineural growth in head and neck squamous cell carcinoma: a review. *Oral Oncol.* 2015;51(1):16–23.
14. Kolokythas A, Cox DP, Dekker N, Schmidt BL. Nerve growth factor and tyrosine kinase A receptor in oral squamous cell carcinoma: is there an association with perineural invasion? *J Oral Maxillofac Surg.* 2010;68(6):1290–1295.
15. He S, Chen CH, Chernichenko N, et al. GFRalpha1 released by nerves enhances cancer cell perineural invasion through GDNF-RET signaling. *Proc Natl Acad Sci U S A.* 2014;111(19):E2008–E2017.

16. Gao L, Bo H, Wang Y, Zhang J, Zhu M. Neurotrophic factor artemin promotes invasiveness and neurotrophic function of pancreatic adenocarcinoma in vivo and in vitro. *Pancreas.* 2015;44(1):134–143.
17. Ayala GE, Wheeler TM, Shine HD, et al. In vitro dorsal root ganglia and human prostate cell line interaction: redefining perineural invasion in prostate cancer. *Prostate.* 2001;49(3):213–223.
18. Ayala GE, Dai H, Ittmann M, et al. Growth and survival mechanisms associated with perineural invasion in prostate cancer. *Cancer Res.* 2004;64(17):6082–6090.
19. Parker GD, Harnsberger HR. Clinical-radiologic issues in perineural tumor spread of malignant diseases of the extracranial head and neck. *Radiographics.* 1991;11(3):383–399.
20. Feasel AM, Brown TJ, Bogle MA, Tschen JA, Nelson BR. Perineural invasion of cutaneous malignancies. *Dermatol Surg.* 2001;27(6):531–542.
21. Mendenhall WM, Amdur RJ, Hinerman RQ, et al. Skin cancer of the head and neck with perineural invasion. *Am J Clin Oncol.* 2007;30(1):93–96.
22. Pathologists College of American. *Cancer Protocol Templates.* Accessed: February, 2019. Available at: https://www.cap.org/protocols-and-guidelines/cancer-reporting-tools/cancer-protocol-templates.
23. Ojiri H. Perineural spread in head and neck malignancies. *Radiat Med.* 2006;24(1):1–8.
24. Mendenhall WM, Ferlito A, Takes RP, et al. Cutaneous head and neck basal and squamous cell carcinomas with perineural invasion. *Oral Oncol.* 2012;48(10):918–922.
25. Buda-Okreglak EM, Walden MJ, Brissette MD. Perineural CNS invasion in primary cutaneous follicular center lymphoma. *J Clin Oncol.* 2007;25(29):4684–4686.
26. Leibovitch I, Huilgol SC, Selva D, Hill D, Richards S, Paver R. Cutaneous squamous cell carcinoma treated with Mohs micrographic surgery in Australia II. perineural invasion. *J Am Acad Dermatol.* 2005;53(2):261–266.
27. Leibovitch I, Huilgol SC, Selva D, Richards S, Paver R. Basal cell carcinoma treated with Mohs surgery in Australia III. perineural invasion. *J Am Acad Dermatol.* 2005;53(3):458–463.
28. Goepfert H, Dichtel WJ, Medina JE, Lindberg RD, Luna MD. Perineural invasion in squamous cell skin carcinoma of the head and neck. *Am J Surg.* 1984;148(4):542–547.
29. Mendenhall WM, Amdur RJ, Williams LS, Mancuso AA, Stringer SP, Price Mendenhall N. Carcinoma of the skin of the head and neck with perineural invasion. *Head Neck.* 2002;24(1):78–83.
30. Rowe DE, Carroll RJ, Day Jr CL. Prognostic factors for local recurrence, metastasis, and survival rates in squamous cell carcinoma of the skin, ear, and lip. Implications for treatment modality selection. *J Am Acad Dermatol.* 1992;26(6):976–990.
31. Ibrahim M, Parmar H, Gandhi D, Mukherji SK. Imaging nuances of perineural spread of head and neck malignancies. *J Neuro Ophthalmol.* 2007;27(2):129–137.
32. Garcia-Serra A, Hinerman RW, Mendenhall WM, et al. Carcinoma of the skin with perineural invasion. *Head Neck.* 2003;25(12):1027–1033.
33. Galloway TJ, Morris CG, Mancuso AA, Amdur RJ, Mendenhall WM. Impact of radiographic findings on prognosis for skin carcinoma with clinical perineural invasion. *Cancer.* 2005;103(6):1254–1257.
34. Gluck I, Ibrahim M, Popovtzer A, et al. Skin cancer of the head and neck with perineural invasion: defining the clinical target volumes based on the pattern of failure. *Int J Radiat Oncol Biol Phys.* 2009;74(1):38–46.
35. Balamucki CJ, Mancuso AA, Amdur RJ, et al. Skin carcinoma of the head and neck with perineural invasion. *Am J Otolaryngol.* 2012;33(4):447–454.
36. Su CY, Lui CC. Perineural invasion of the trigeminal nerve in patients with nasopharyngeal carcinoma. Imaging and clinical correlations. *Cancer.* 1996;78(10):2063–2069.
37. Williams LS, Mancuso AA, Mendenhall WM. Perineural spread of cutaneous squamous and basal cell carcinoma: CT and MR detection and its impact on patient management and prognosis. *Int J Radiat Oncol Biol Phys.* 2001;49(4):1061–1069.
38. Zhu JJ, Padillo O, Duff J, Hsi BL, Fletcher JA, Querfurth H. Cavernous sinus and leptomeningeal metastases arising from a squamous cell carcinoma of the face: case report. *Neurosurgery.* 2004;54(2):492–498; discussion 498–499.
39. Farasat S, Yu SS, Neel VA, et al. A new american joint committee on cancer staging system for cutaneous squamous cell carcinoma: creation and rationale for inclusion of tumor (T) characteristics. *J Am Acad Dermatol.* 2011;64(6):1051–1059.
40. Takubo K, Takai A, Yamashita K, et al. Light and electron microscopic studies of perineural invasion by esophageal carcinoma. *J Natl Cancer Inst.* 1985;74(5):987–993.
41. Anderson C, Krutchkoff D, Ludwig M. Carcinoma of the lower lip with perineural extension to the middle cranial fossa. *Oral Surg Oral Med Oral Pathol.* 1990;69(5):614–618.
42. Osguthorpe JD, Abel CG, Lang P, Hochman M. Neurotropic cutaneous tumors of the head and neck. *Arch Otolaryngol Head Neck Surg.* 1997;123(8):871–876.
43. Dodd GD, Dolan PA, Ballantyne AJ, Ibanez ML, Chau P. The dissemination of tumors of the head and neck via the cranial nerves. *Radiol Clin North Am.* 1970;8(3):445–461.
44. Nemzek WR, Hecht S, Gandour-Edwards R, Donald P, McKennan K. Perineural spread of head and neck tumors: how accurate is MR imaging? *AJNR Am J Neuroradiol.* 1998;19(4):701–706.
45. Neuroradiology AJO. *Perineural Spread on FDG-PET/CT.* Accessed: August 18, 2016. http://www.ajnr.org/ajnr-case-collections-diagnosis/perineural-spread-fdg-petct.
46. Weber AL. Computed tomography and magnetic resonance imaging of the nasopharynx. *Isr J Med Sci.* 1992;28(3–4):161–168.
47. Caldemeyer KS, Mathews VP, Righi PD, Smith RR. Imaging features and clinical significance of perineural spread or extension of head and neck tumors. *Radiographics.* 1998;18(1):97–110, quiz 147.
48. Ginsberg LE. MR imaging of perineural tumor spread. *Magn Reson Imaging Clin N Am.* 2002;10(3):511–525,vi.
49. Russo CP, Smoker WR, Weissman JL. MR appearance of trigeminal and hypoglossal motor denervation. *AJNR Am J Neuroradiol.* 1997;18(7):1375–1383.
50. Gandhi MR, Panizza B, Kennedy D. Detecting and defining the anatomic extent of large nerve perineural spread of malignancy: comparing "targeted" MRI with the histologic findings following surgery. *Head Neck.* 2011;33(4):469–475.
51. Baulch J, Gandhi M, Sommerville J, Panizza B. 3T MRI evaluation of large nerve perineural spread of head and neck cancers. *J Med Imaging Radiat Oncol.* 2015;59(5):578–585.
52. Paes FM, Singer AD, Checkver AN, Palmquist RA, De La Vega G, Sidani C. Perineural spread in head and neck malignancies: clinical significance and evaluation with 18F-FDG PET/CT. *Radiographics.* 2013;33(6):1717–1736.

53. Arcas A, Bescos S, Raspall G, Capellades J. Perineural spread of epidermoid carcinoma in the infraorbital nerve: case report. *J Oral Maxillofac Surg*. 1996;54(4):520–522.
54. Penn R, Abemayor E, Nabili V, Bhuta S, Kirsch C. Perineural invasion detected by high-field 3.0-T magnetic resonance imaging. *Am J Otolaryngol*. 2010;31(6):482–484.
55. Khan M, Ambady P, Kimbrough D, et al. Radiation-induced myelitis: initial and follow-up MRI and clinical features in patients at a single tertiary care institution during 20 years. *AJNR Am J Neuroradiol*. 2018;39(8):1576–1581.
56. Bowen BC, Verma A, Brandon AH, Fiedler JA. Radiation-induced brachial plexopathy: MR and clinical findings. *AJNR Am J Neuroradiol*. 1996;17(10):1932–1936.
57. Kori SH, Foley KM, Posner JB. Brachial plexus lesions in patients with cancer: 100 cases. *Neurology*. 1981;31(1):45–50.
58. Moore BA, Weber RS, Prieto V, et al. Lymph node metastases from cutaneous squamous cell carcinoma of the head and neck. *Laryngoscope*. 2005;115(9):1561–1567.
59. Cherpelis BS, Marcusen C, Lang PG. Prognostic factors for metastasis in squamous cell carcinoma of the skin. *Dermatol Surg*. 2002;28(3):268–273.
60. Fagan JJ, Collins B, Barnes L, D'Amico F, Myers EN, Johnson JT. Perineural invasion in squamous cell carcinoma of the head and neck. *Arch Otolaryngol Head Neck Surg*. 1998;124(6):637–640.
61. Wagner JD, Evdokimow DZ, Weisberger E, et al. Sentinel node biopsy for high-risk nonmelanoma cutaneous malignancy. *Arch Dermatol*. 2004;140(1):75–79.
62. Maroldi R, Ambrosi C, Farina D. Metastatic disease of the brain: extra-axial metastases (skull, dura, leptomeningeal) and tumour spread. *Eur Radiol*. 2005;15(3):617–626.
63. Kesari S, Batchelor TT. Leptomeningeal metastases. *Neurol Clin*. 2003;21(1):25–66.
64. Esmaeli B, Ahmadi MA, Gillenwater AM, Faustina MM, Amato M. The role of supraorbital nerve biopsy in cutaneous malignancies of the periocular region. *Ophthalmic Plast Reconstr Surg*. 2003;19(4):282–286.
65. Hassanein AM, Proper SA, Depcik-Smith ND, Flowers FP. Peritumoral fibrosis in basal cell and squamous cell carcinoma mimicking perineural invasion: potential pitfall in Mohs micrographic surgery. *Dermatol Surg*. 2005;31(9 Pt 1):1101–1106.
66. Lewis Kelso R, Colome-Grimmer MI, Uchida T, Wang HQ, Wagner Jr RF. p75(NGFR) immunostaining for the detection of perineural invasion by cutaneous squamous cell carcinoma. *Dermatol Surg*. 2006;32(2):177–183.
67. Marsot-Dupuch K, Matozza F, Firat MM, Iyriboz AT, Chabolle F, Tubiana JM. Mandibular nerve: MR versus CT about 10 proved unusual tumors. *Neuroradiology*. 1990;32(6):492–496.
68. Ong CK, Chong VF. Imaging of perineural spread in head and neck tumours. *Canc Imag*. 2010;10(Spec no A):S92–S98.
69. Gandhi M, Sommerville J. The imaging of large nerve perineural spread. *J Neurol Surg B Skull Base*. 2016;77(2):113–123.
70. Zakrzewska JM. Diagnosis and differential diagnosis of trigeminal neuralgia. *Clin J Pain*. 2002;18(1):14–21.
71. Tiemstra JD, Khatkhate N. Bell's palsy: diagnosis and management. *Am Fam Physician*. 2007;76(7):997–1002.
72. Gobbi H, Jensen RA, Simpson JF, Olson SJ, Page DL. Atypical ductal hyperplasia and ductal carcinoma in situ of the breast associated with perineural invasion. *Hum Pathol*. 2001;32(8):785–790.
73. Tsang WY, Chan JK. Neural invasion in intraductal carcinoma of the breast. *Hum Pathol*. 1992;23(2):202–204.
74. Mate TP, Carter D, Fischer DB, et al. A clinical and histopathologic analysis of the results of conservation surgery and radiation therapy in stage I and II breast carcinoma. *Cancer*. 1986;58(9):1995–2002.
75. Roses DF, Bell DA, Flotte TJ, Taylor R, Ratech H, Dubin N. Pathologic predictors of recurrence in stage 1 (TINOMO) breast cancer. *Am J Clin Pathol*. 1982;78(6):817–820.
76. Han A, Ratner D. What is the role of adjuvant radiotherapy in the treatment of cutaneous squamous cell carcinoma with perineural invasion? *Cancer*. 2007;109(6):1053–1059.
77. Frunza A, Slavescu D, Lascar I. Perineural invasion in head and neck cancers - a review. *J Med Life*. 2014;7(2):121–123.
78. Huyett P, Gilbert M, Liu L, Ferris RL, Kim S. A model for perineural invasion in head and neck squamous cell carcinoma. *J Vis Exp*. 2017;(119):55043.
79. Dean NR, White HN, Carter DS, et al. Outcomes following temporal bone resection. *Laryngoscope*. 2010;120(8):1516–1522.
80. Byers RM, O'Brien J, Waxler J. The therapeutic and prognostic implications of nerve invasion in cancer of the lower lip. *Int J Radiat Oncol Biol Phys*. 1978;4(3–4):215–217.
81. Terashi H, Kurata S, Tadokoro T, et al. Perineural and neural involvement in skin cancers. *Dermatol Surg*. 1997;23(4):259–264, discussion 264–265.
82. Lawrence N, Cottel WI. Squamous cell carcinoma of skin with perineural invasion. *J Am Acad Dermatol*. 1994;31(1):30–33.
83. Cottel WI. Perineural invasion by squamous-cell carcinoma. *J Dermatol Surg Oncol*. 1982;8(7):589–600.
84. Matorin PA, Wagner Jr RF. Mohs micrographic surgery: technical difficulties posed by perineural invasion. *Int J Dermatol*. 1992;31(2):83–86.
85. Dunn M, Morgan MB, Beer TW. Perineural invasion: identification, significance, and a standardized definition. *Dermatol Surg*. 2009;35(2):214–221.
86. Langendijk JA, Slotman BJ, van der Waal I, Doornaert P, Berkof J, Leemans CR. Risk-group definition by recursive partitioning analysis of patients with squamous cell head and neck carcinoma treated with surgery and postoperative radiotherapy. *Cancer*. 2005;104(7):1408–1417.
87. Padhya TA, Cornelius RS, Athavale SM, Gluckman JL. Perineural extension to the skull base from early cutaneous malignancies of the midface. *Otolaryngol Head Neck Surg*. 2007;137(5):742–746.
88. Suen JK, Bressler L, Shord SS, Warso M, Villano JL. Cutaneous squamous cell carcinoma responding serially to single-agent cetuximab. *Anti Canc Drugs*. 2007;18(7):827–829.
89. Bernier J, Domenge C, Ozsahin M, et al. Postoperative irradiation with or without concomitant chemotherapy for locally advanced head and neck cancer. *N Engl J Med*. 2004;350(19):1945–1952.
90. Bauman JE, Eaton KD, Martins RG. Treatment of recurrent squamous cell carcinoma of the skin with cetuximab. *Arch Dermatol*. 2007;143(7):889–892.
91. van Vugt VA, Saria MG, Javier A, Kesari N, Turpin T, Kesari S. Neurological improvement of perineural and leptomeningeal spread of squamous cell carcinoma treated with intrathecal chemotherapy and systemic EGFR inhibition. *CNS Oncol*. 2017;6(4):269–274.
92. Gorayski P, Foote M, Porceddu S, Poulsen M. The role of postoperative radiotherapy for large nerve perineural spread of cancer of the head and neck. *J Neurol Surg B Skull Base*. 2016;77(2):173–181.

Chapter | 22 |

Cancer-associated plexopathy

Mary Jane Lim-Fat, Patrick Y. Wen, and Ugonma N. Chukwueke

CHAPTER OUTLINE

Introduction

Despite the development of new therapies and related neurological complications, the two main considerations in patients with a history of cancer presenting with a brachial or lumbar plexopathy is neoplastic plexopathy or radiation-induced plexopathy. A focused cancer history and neurological examination can aid in localization and in narrowing down the differential diagnosis. Cancer-related plexopathies are more common, tend to be painful, and have a more rapid onset than radiation-induced plexopathies, which present in a more indolent fashion over the course of months to years following radiation therapy. Although imaging is helpful to visualize the degree of plexus involvement and to assess for locoregional disease, it is difficult to distinguish the two on the basis of imaging alone. Nerve conduction studies (NCS) and electromyography (EMG) can be useful if myokymic changes are present, as these are associated with radiation-induced plexopathies. Unfortunately, both types of plexopathies are treated with supportive measures, and survival and quality of life may be limited in many of the affected patients.

Approach to plexopathies

Cancer and cancer-associated treatments can have direct and indirect effects on all parts of the nervous system including the brachial and lumbar plexus. In a patient with a known history of cancer, plexopathies can be caused by trauma from surgery or anesthesia, metastatic tumor spread, radiation therapy, chemotherapy, immunotherapy, and radiation-induced tumors. Cancer patients are also susceptible to acute plexopathies that are unrelated to their malignancy or its treatment. A thorough understanding of neuroanatomy is essential, as the clinical examination and diagnostic studies can help with localization and point to a specific etiology. Cancer history with particular attention to pathology, prior treatments for cancer including any surgeries, radiation therapy (including type, field, and dose delivered), conventional chemotherapies, targeted molecular therapies, and immunotherapies, as well as any clinical trial protocol should be noted. In patients without a known history of cancer, a family history of cancer and risk factors for malignancies should be investigated (e.g., smoking history, HIV or immunosuppression, prior history of radiation, and tumor predisposition syndromes among others). Relevant history for non–cancer-related causes of plexopathies including diabetes, recent vaccinations, and intercurrent illnesses should also be determined. Imaging modalities, including magnetic resonance imaging (MRI) or computed tomography (CT) scans, and electrophysiologic testing with NCS and EMG are useful adjuncts to aid the diagnosis of plexopathies.

Brachial plexopathy

Anatomy

The brachial plexus consists of the ventral rami of the C5–C8 nerve roots (Fig. 22.1). These later form three distinct trunks: superior (C5, C6), medial (C7), and inferior (C8–T1), which are then further subdivided into dorsal and ventral divisions. The dorsal divisions converge to form the posterior cord from which emerge the thoracodorsal nerve (to the latissimus dorsi), the subscapular nerve (to the subscapularis), the axillary nerve (to the deltoid), and the radial nerve (motor innervation to the triceps, brachioradialis, biceps, wrist extensor, finger extensors, and sensory innervation to the posterior aspect of the arm and forearm). The ventral divisions give off the lateral and the medial cords. The lateral cord branches into the musculocutaneous nerve (motor innervation to the biceps, brachialis, coracobrachialis, and sensation to the radial aspect of the forearm). The lateral cord also converges later on with the medial cord to form the median nerve (with motor innervation to the forearm flexors, pronator teres and pronator quadratus, thumb flexors and lumbricals, and sensation to the medial palm and first three and a half fingers). The medial cord also supplies the ulnar nerve, which in turn supplies the intrinsic muscles of the hand and some of the flexors of the hand and digits (flexor carpi ulnaris, flexor digitorum profundus II and IV, abductor, opponens and flexor of the fifth digit, and sensation to the ulnar aspect of the palm).

The sympathetic chain connects to the brachial plexus through the gray rami communicantes, and involvement of the brachial plexus, especially of the C8 and T1 nerve roots, can present with Horner syndrome consisting of ptosis, miosis, and anhidrosis through the disruption of second order sympathetic fibers.

Lumbosacral plexopathy

Anatomy

The lumbosacral plexus consists of the ventral rami of L1–S2 nerve roots and is subdivided into the lumbar and sacral plexus (Fig. 22.2). The lumbar plexus has anterior and posterior divisions, with the anterior division giving rise to the iliohypogastric, ilioinguinal, and genitofemoral nerves (supplied by L1 and L2), which provide sensory innervation to the lower abdomen, upper thigh, and lateral perineum; and the obturator nerve (supplied

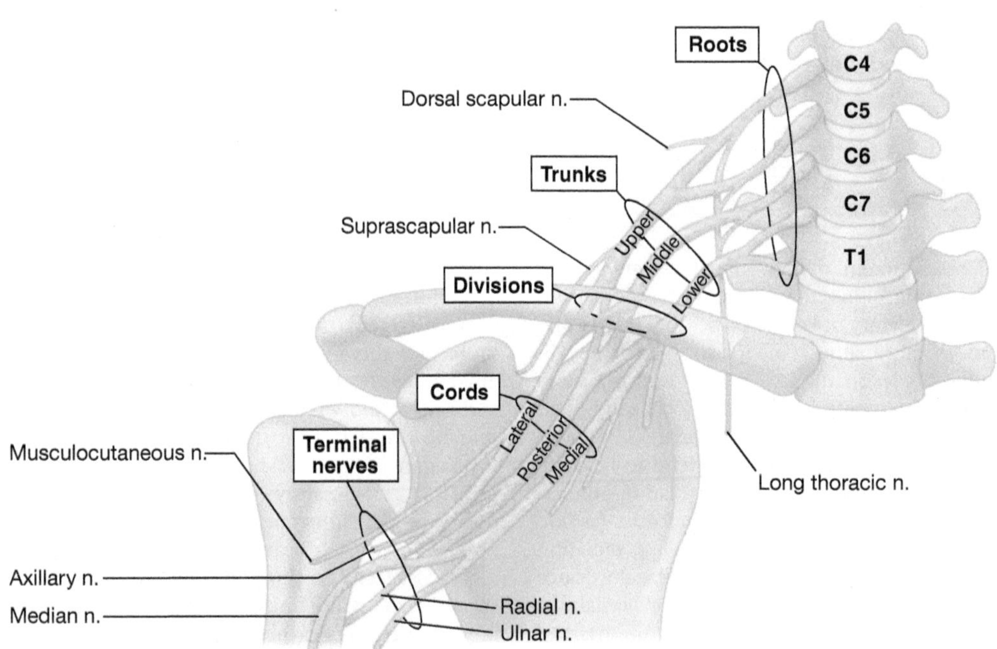

Fig. 22.1 Diagrammatic illustration of the brachial plexus. *n*, nerve. (Reprinted with permission from Ferrante MA. Brachial plexopathies: classification, causes, and consequences. *Muscle Nerve*. 2004;30(5);547–568.)

by L2–L4), which provides motor innervation to the adductors and gracilis muscles. The posterior division of the lumbar plexus is made up of the iliohypogastric and lateral femoral cutaneous nerves (L2–L3) with sensory afferents from the lateral hip and thigh; and the femoral nerve (L2–L3), which provides motor fibers to the psoas, iliacus, sartorius, and quadriceps. It also receives sensory afferents from the anterior thigh and medial upper leg. The sacral plexus consists of the ventral rami of S1–S4, as well as a branch of the lower lumbar plexus (L4–L5). The sacral plexus is further subdivided into the anterior division, which provides motor fibers to the quadratus femoris and hamstrings; and the tibial nerve (L4–S3), which provides motor fibers for the foot dorsiflexors and intrinsic foot muscles. The posterior division branches into the common peroneal nerve (supplied by L2–S2) to the peroneal muscles, tibialis anterior, extensor digitorum, and extensor hallucis and has sensory afferents from the lateral leg, dorsal foot, and toes. It also gives off the superior (L4–S1) and inferior (L5–S2) gluteal nerves supplying the gluteus muscles. The posterior division is the origin of the sciatic nerve, which divides into the common peroneal and tibial nerves, and the posterior femoral cutaneous nerve (S1–S3), which carries sensory information from the posterior thigh. The perineum is innervated by another branch of the sacral plexus, the pudendal nerve (S2–S4).

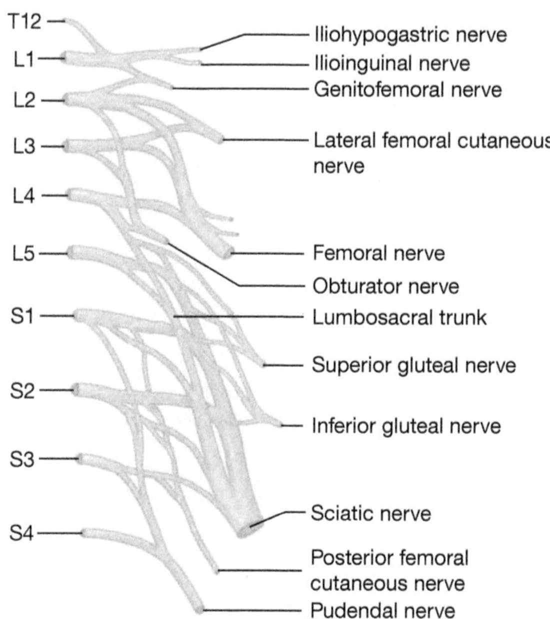

Fig. 22.2 Diagrammatic illustration of the lumbosacral plexus. (Reprinted with permission from Brazis P, Masdeu J, Biller J. *Localization in Clinical Neurology.* 5th ed. Philadelphia: Lippincott Williams & Wilkins; 2007.)

Clinical cases

CASE 22.1 NEOPLASTIC BRACHIAL PLEXOPATHY

Case. A 60-year-old right-handed female with history of epidermal growth factor receptor (EGFR)-wildtype non–small-cell lung cancer (NSCLC) was referred for worsening right arm pain. Her oncologic history begins 9 years ago when she was diagnosed with locally advanced (stage 3B unresectable) right lung adenocarcinoma. She was treated with concurrent cisplatin and etoposide chemotherapy and right lung and mediastinal radiation. She thereafter received two adjuvant cycles of cisplatin and pemetrexed and her systemic disease remained well controlled until she presented with right posterior shoulder pain radiating down her arm into her fourth and fifth digits. She had noted some difficulty with fine finger movements with the right hand, although no focal weakness had been observed. A few weeks following the onset of her pain, she also started noticing numbness and tingling in her right hand.

Neurological examination revealed normal mental status, right-sided ptosis, and miosis but no other cranial nerve deficit. Muscle bulk was normal except for right thenar and first dorsal interosseous (FDI) atrophy. The remainder of the neurological examination, including sensory examination and reflexes, was within normal limits.

NCS and EMG showed electrophysiologic evidence of denervation to axons supplied by the right C8 and T1 nerve roots and lower trunk of the brachial plexus. MRI of the cervical spine and brachial plexus showed a nodular heterogeneously enhancing soft tissue lesion extending from the right lung apex and pleural surface into the supraclavicular fossa, surrounding the right brachial plexus (Fig. 22.3). This finding was felt to be consistent with involvement of the brachial plexus by pulmonary and pleural metastasis. Interval enlargement of several mediastinal and axillary lymph nodes was also observed.

Her clinical presentation and electrodiagnostic studies were indicative of a neoplastic brachial plexopathy, predominantly involving the lower trunk. Given her locoregional progression, she was started on ramucirumab and docetaxel. Palliative radiation to the brachial plexus was discussed but deferred for the time being. She was started on gabapentin and lidocaine transdermal patch for pain relief. She was also referred to a palliative care specialist and started physical therapy with some improvement of her symptoms.

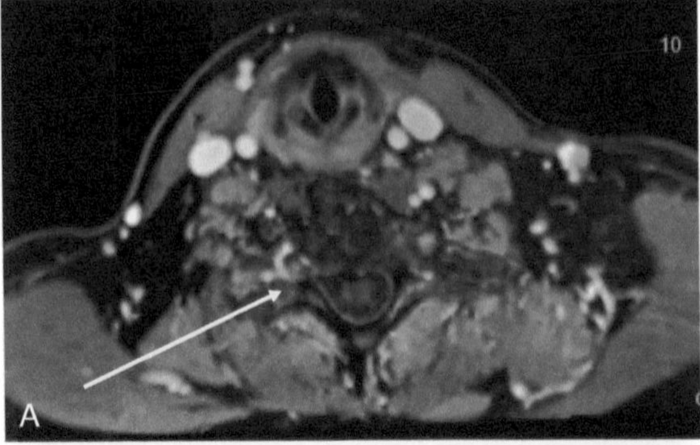

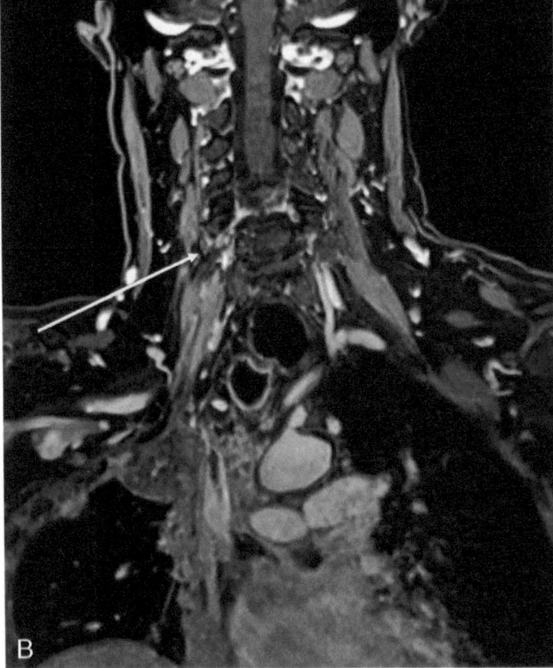

Fig. 22.3 MRI of the brachial plexus with axial (A) and coronal (B) post-contrast T1 sequences showing enhancement around the right brachial plexus *(arrow),* but also right apical, pleural, and mediastinal metastasis, consistent with neoplastic brachial plexopathy.

Clinical Pearls

1. The presentation of a neoplastic brachial plexopathy is frequently in the form of worsening pain in the neck, shoulder, or arm over the span of weeks to months.
2. In such cases, Horner syndrome may be present, especially with the involvement of the lower trunk.
3. The lower plexus is most often involved in cancer-related brachial plexopathies, and electrodiagnostic studies can be helpful to confirm localization.
4. MRI images of the cervical spine and plexus are required to assess for bulky locoregional disease that may be amenable to treatment with surgery or radiation therapy.

Teaching Points: Approach to Neoplastic Brachial Plexopathy

Pathophysiology of neoplastic brachial plexopathies

Although primary tumors arising from the brachial plexus can cause neurological symptoms, the vast majority of cancer-related brachial plexopathies are due to local extension of an adjacent tumor or metastasis of a more distant neoplasm. These plexopathies can occur due to the direct pressure of a local mass but more frequently are caused by the invasion of cancer cells along nerves or connective tissue surrounding the brachial plexus. The brachial plexus is in close proximity to the lung, breast, and lymphatic system and is therefore at higher risk of involvement from metastases compared to other parts of the peripheral nervous system (Fig. 22.4). Although some tumors may directly extend from adjacent tissue and organs into the nervous plexus, secondary invasion from metastases through regional lymph nodes or through tracking along the epineurium can also occur. A large retrospective review at a single institution in the 1980s identified about 2% of patients with cancer being referred for neurological evaluation as having a brachial plexopathy. Of these, up to 75% were due to direct metastasis from lung, breast cancer, or systemic lymphoma.[1] Non-Hodgkin lymphoma in particular has been associated with 90% of neurolymphomatosis, which can involve the brachial plexus in a variable presentation of neuropathy, radiculopathy, or plexopathy.[2]

Primary tumors of the brachial plexus include schwannomas or neurofibromas (see Chapter 9, Case 9.1 for imaging features of brachial plexus peripheral nerve sheath tumors), which are both rare when occurring sporadically. In the context of neurofibromatosis type 1 (NF1), neurofibromas are the most common benign tumor to occur in this familial tumor predisposition syndrome (see Chapter 16 for further discussion of NF1). In NF1, a mutation of the tumor suppressor gene neurofibromin leads to overactivity of the p21 *ras,* which in turn causes cell growth, differentiation, and benign tumor formation. Although these neurofibromas can occur in a plexiform distribution (e.g., involving fascicles of a nerve or branches of a large nerve), the term plexiform neurofibroma does not indicate involvement of a nerve plexus and their location can be varied across the peripheral nervous system. Malignant transformation of a neurofibroma can lead to development of malignant peripheral nerve sheath tumors (MPNST) in which early diagnosis and surgical management can improve survival outcomes (also see Chapter 16 for discussion of NF1 and Chapter 9, Case 9.3 for imaging of MPNST).[3]

Clinical Presentation

Brachial plexopathy from direct invasion of a primary or metastatic tumor typically presents with signs and symptoms related to the anatomic location of involvement. The most common symptom described is pain, which is present in about 75% of patients, followed by sensory changes in up to 25%.[1] The distribution of pain may vary from patient to patient. It is typically described as arising in the shoulder or axilla when the upper plexus is involved from metastases originating from

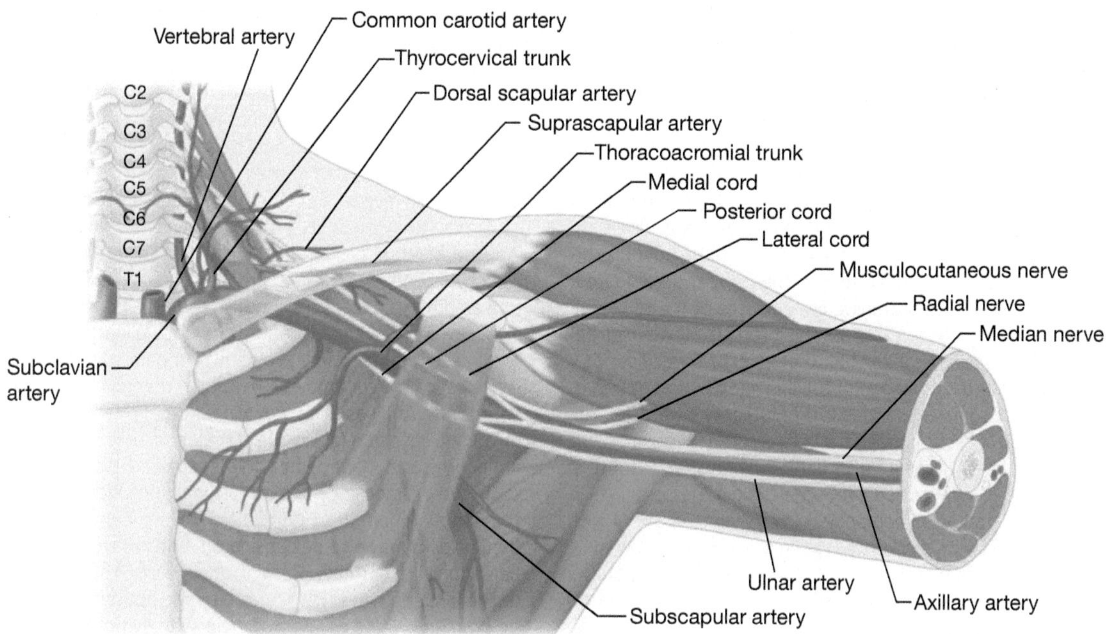

Fig. 22.4 The brachial plexus and its relationship to adjacent structures reflects its vulnerability to compression or infiltration from tumors of the head and neck, lung, breast, and lymph nodes. (Reprinted with permission from Ferrante MA. Brachial plexopathies: classification, causes, and consequences. *Muscle Nerve*. 2004;30(5);547–568.)

cervical lymph nodes or other head and neck tumors. Pain arising from the elbow and radiating to the medial arm and hands, however, is felt to be more common and is often the presenting symptom if the lower plexus is involved, as is the case in some Pancoast tumors that arise from the region around the superior sulcus of the lung. Up to 75% of patients affected by a painful neoplastic plexopathy present with involvement of either the lower or upper brachial plexus, with the remaining 25% of patients with global involvement of the entire plexus involving C5–T1.

Progressive weakness, atrophy, and sensory changes of the upper extremity may also evolve over time. In primary tumors of the brachial plexus, sensory changes may be more gradual and present in the form of progressive paresthesia without significant pain. A unilateral Horner syndrome may also be present in about 25% of patients, when the sympathetic trunk or sympathetic ganglia are affected, especially when the upper thoracic or lower cervical roots are involved. About 30% of cases with a unilateral Horner syndrome will also have concurrent epidural involvement and MRI of the cervical and thoracic spine is therefore recommended for such presentations.

Diagnostic Imaging

Imaging of the brachial plexus has evolved with the advent of higher resolution MRI and new applications of ultrasound methods. MRI of the brachial plexus can provide high spatial resolution and contrast delineation, allowing for determination of location and degree of involvement of brachial plexus pathologies.

Benign peripheral nerve sheath tumors. Benign primary neoplasms of the brachial plexus such as peripheral nerve sheath tumors can have specific features on MRI. These tumors are usually well-circumscribed, avidly enhancing ovoid lesions along the parent nerve. Characteristic appearance of peripheral nerve sheath tumors include the target sign, split fat sign, fascicular sign, and string sign.[4] Although these radiologic signs apply both to schwannomas and neurofibromas, schwannomas tend to be eccentric to the parent nerve without infiltrating within the fascicles, whereas neurofibromas are not encapsulated and typically infiltrate the nerve fascicles. Plexiform neurofibromas are usually readily identifiable on MRI due to the diffuse enlargement of several nerve branches, often referred to as a "bag of worms." Enhancement of plexiform neurofibromas can be heterogeneous and appear much larger in size than solitary neurofibromas. MPNSTs can have a similar imaging profile as other soft tissue sarcomas, but can be distinguished from benign peripheral nerve sheath tumors due to their size (typically larger than 7 cm), perilesional edema, peripheral enhancement, and intratumoral cystic change.[5]

Brachial plexus metastasis or neoplastic invasion. In the setting of involvement of the brachial plexus from direct adjacent mass effect from a locally occurring secondary tumor, or secondary metastasis, lesions of the brachial plexus may be focal or diffusely infiltrating. There can be solid enhancement of bulky or nodular metastasis, and thickening of nerve roots on neuroimaging. In the case of neurolymphomatosis, diffuse enhancement along the perineural space may be visible. Nerve enlargement, isointensity to muscle on T1, hyperintensity on T2, and focal or diffuse enhancement may also be present.[2]

Peripheral nerve ultrasound. Although ultrasound techniques have allowed for a fairly reliable and rapid bedside assessment of the brachial plexus, it has not been routinely integrated in the workup of neoplastic plexopathies. It is the most helpful to visualize elements of the brachial plexus when an MRI is contraindicated, not tolerated due to claustrophobia, or not readily available.[6] Visualization of the nerve roots is limited by the shadowing of the transverse processes of the vertebral bodies, but all other fascicles of the brachial plexus can be mapped by ultrasound, in the hands of an experienced sonographer with good knowledge of brachial plexus anatomy. It is particularly helpful in visualizing loss of integrity in the brachial plexus or adjacent structures caused by trauma, neoplasms, or radiation fibrosis. Ultrasound of benign nerve sheath tumors reveal typically well-defined hypoechoic ovoid masses.

Positron emission tomography. Most patients with brachial plexus metastases have advanced systemic malignancy. Systemic staging with PET-CT of the body, CT chest, and mammogram, among others, is therefore an essential part of the workup of neoplastic plexopathies. In addition, MRI of the cervical or thoracic spine may also be required if proximal root involvement with extension into the spinal cord or epidural space is suspected.

Electrophysiologic testing. Electrodiagnostic studies with NCS and EMG can be helpful in assessing for localization and degree of involvement in neoplastic brachial plexopathies. Sensory or motor involvement may be present, and may specifically point to specific radicular, branch, division, or nerve involvement.[7] NCS may reveal axonal loss with low or absent sensory potentials from the ulnar, medial, or antebrachial nerves. Needle examination can show spontaneous activity and motor units consistent with a denervating process. However, there is no specific feature on nerve conduction or needle EMG that may delineate a neoplastic cause from some other etiologies of brachial plexopathy. Myokymia, which can be seen in radiation-induced brachial plexopathies, is absent in neoplastic brachial plexopathy. Comparing nerve conductions on the affected side to the normal side can provide an estimate for the degree of injury and potential for recovery.

Occasionally, surgical exploration and biopsy may be required to confirm pathologic diagnosis, specifically if no clear primary neoplasm is identified; however, it is usually preferable to biopsy a more accessible lesion if present, as nerve biopsy can result in permanent neurological damage.

Management

Management of neoplastic brachial plexopathies can vary greatly depending on symptom burden and systemic involvement. It is typically focused on treatment of the primary malignancy with systemic agents or with radiation to sites of bulky locoregional metastasis. Surgical debulking is seldom used due to the intricate anatomy of the region involved. Targeted therapies (e.g., with tyrosine kinase inhibitors), in lung cancer, such as the anaplastic lymphoma kinase rearranged (ALK) inhibitors and the EGFR tyrosine kinase inhibitors, have been increasingly used in subtypes of non–small-cell lung cancer. Endocrine therapy and HER2-targeted therapy are also part of the treatment armamentarium for certain types of breast cancer. Radiation therapy is used for locoregional disease for palliative purposes, or after first-line systemic therapy has failed, with some improvement or reversal of pain or neurological deficits.[8]

Survival may be limited for many patients with neoplastic-induced brachial plexopathy due to advanced stage cancer. Symptom control and improvement of quality of life are therefore a primary concern. Pain from neoplastic brachial plexopathies can be challenging, and a multidisciplinary approach is often recommended. Involvement of a pain specialist or palliative care physician may be helpful in managing progressive symptoms. Analgesia for neuropathic pain can be targeted through transcutaneous nerve stimulators, duloxetine, tricyclic antidepressants, gabapentin, or pregabalin. Opiate analgesics, transdermal lidocaine, and occasionally infusion pumps are sometimes required. In particularly severe cases, local anesthetic blocks may also be considered, and in severe intractable pain, dorsal rhizotomy, dorsal root entry zone surgery, plexus dissection, and neurolysis remain salvage options. Physical and occupational therapy can also help with symptom relief and prevention of loss of function and contractures.

CASE 22.2 RADIATION-INDUCED BRACHIAL PLEXOPATHY

Case. A 75-year-old female presented to the neurology clinic with over a year history of progressive paraesthesias in the left upper extremity. She had a remote 20-year history of breast cancer (presumed triple negative, treated at an outside facility), for which she underwent a left lumpectomy and external beam radiation therapy to the whole breast, followed by adjuvant chemotherapy with doxorubicin, cyclophosphamide first, then paclitaxel. She was under surveillance with no evidence of systemic recurrence since then. She first noted tingling in her hand, which interfered with her ability to play the violin. Although initially intermittent, this gradually became more persistent, to the point where her entire arm would feel numb when lying supine at night. She also eventually developed a painful sensation in the form of shooting pain around the left scapula.

On examination, she had normal mental status and cranial nerve examinations. Bulk and tone were normal in the upper and lower extremities. She was noted to have weakness of the left shoulder abduction (4/5), abductor pollicis brevis (4+/5), and extensor indicis (4+/5). Sensation was subjectively reduced over the left lateral arm into the thumb.

A nerve conduction study and EMG showed:

- Normal left median and ulnar compound muscle action potentials with normal f wave latencies
- Moderately reduced left median D2, 3, ulnar D5, superficial radial, and musculocutaneous sensory nerve action

potentials are all moderately reduced in amplitude, with preserved conduction velocity
- Mild to moderate chronic reinnervation in muscles on the left on needle study (particularly in the left deltoid, biceps, and extensor indicis proprius)
- No myokymia on needle study

Overall this study was felt to be abnormal, with electrophysiologic evidence of a chronic brachial plexopathy of moderate severity affecting the left arm, with muscles and nerves from the upper and lower trunks affected equally.

An MRI of the C-spine did not show any significant degenerative disease or visible metastasis to account for any structural impingement of nerve roots or plexus. MRI of the brachial plexus revealed abnormal T1 and T2 dark, soft tissue around the trunks of the brachial plexus, and this was felt to be most consistent with fibrosis with loss of most of the surrounding adipose tissue (Fig. 22.5). This abnormality also corresponded with the distribution of chronic left apical lung scarring, an asymmetrically small left clavicle, and atrophic left shoulder girdle musculature, all likely related to prior radiation therapy. At the level of the radiation port, the nerves of the brachial plexus were found to be matted together with the adjacent subclavian vasculature. There were no imaging findings to suggest the presence of residual or recurrent tumor.

Teaching Points: Risk Factors for Radiation-Induced Brachial Plexopathy. Treatment-related complications, in particular radiation injury to the plexus, is an important differential diagnosis and can be difficult to elucidate in patients with a known cancer diagnosis. Radiation-induced brachial plexopathy (RIBP) can develop in patients undergoing radiation for tumors located in the neck, axilla, or chest wall (most commonly breast, lung, cervical, or nasopharyngeal cancers) or their metastases. The highest incidence is in patients with a history of radiotherapy for breast cancer, in particular if the tolerance dose for the brachial plexus is exceeded. In patients with breast cancer, a total axillary dose >50 Gy has been associated with a higher risk of RIBP.[9] Individual fraction doses of 2.5 to 6.0 Gy in particular have been associated with higher risk of neurological impairment.[10] In addition, higher cumulative dose over the entire treatment course, shortened overall treatment time, and larger than standard fraction doses (>2 Gy/fraction), concurrent or sequential cytotoxic treatment, and extent of axillary dissection have all been found to confer a higher risk of RIBP.[11] Modern radiotherapeutic regimens have led to lower rates and milder cases of RIBP due to more precise and reduced dose delivery to the brachial plexus.

Clinical Pearls

1. Radiation-induced brachial plexopathy (RIBP) can occur years following the initial course of radiation therapy.
2. The progression of symptoms may occur in an indolent fashion over months and even years and is typically in the form of sensory symptoms, pain, and worsening weakness and atrophy.
3. Although classically thought to involve the upper plexus, RIBP can also involve the lower plexus or entire plexus, as is the case in this scenario.
4. Imaging of the brachial plexus may reveal radiotherapy-related changes in other adjacent anatomical structures such as the lung, bones, and connective tissue.

Approach to Radiation-Induced Brachial Plexopathy

Pathophysiology. The exact biologic mechanism underlying RIBP is still poorly understood. Autopsy studies and pathologic evaluation of surgical biopsies have revealed fibrosis around the brachial plexus, leading to entrapment of nerve fibers and subsequent endoneurium thickening. Demyelination can subsequently occur and obliteration of small blood vessels in the epineural plexus is also frequent. This supports the "double crush" phenomenon in which the first insult caused by irradiation and related changes in the nerves leads to decreased ability for nerve repair in the face of fibrosis, entrapment, and chronic ischemia. The long latency to the development of symptoms (few months up to 30 years after radiation treatment) may be in support of this theory.[9] It remains unclear, however, as to why 60–90% of patients have progressive

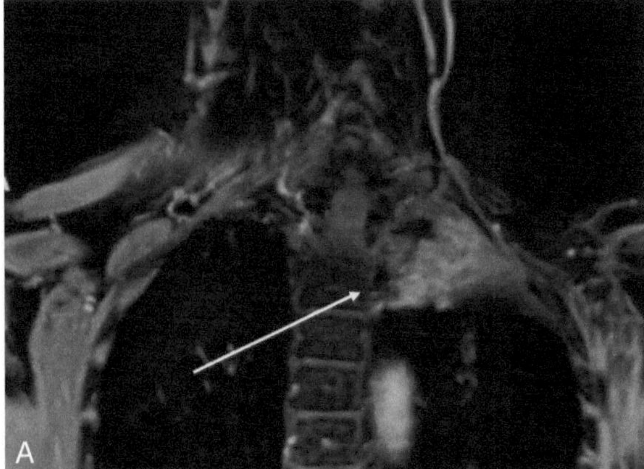

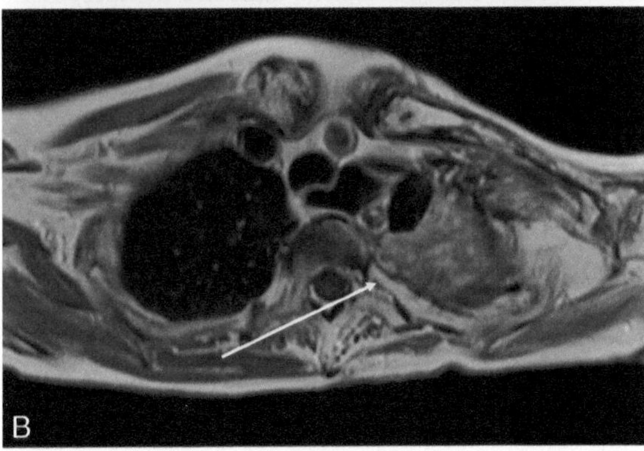

Fig. 22.5 MRI of the brachial plexus with coronal (A) and axial fluid attenuated inversion recovery (B) sequences showing fibrosis of the left lung apex and matting of the brachial plexus with surrounding structures, consistent with radiation-induced brachial plexopathy.

severe neurological deficits, whereas in the remainder of patients, progression plateaus and spontaneously ceases after 1–3 years.[12]

Clinical presentation. RIBP can present with progressive sensory changes including numbness, pain, and paresthesias as well as motor deficits in the form of worsening weakness or atrophy. While the presentation makes it difficult to clinically distinguish radiation-induced plexopathy from neoplastic brachial plexopathy, certain characteristics are unique to each form of plexopathy. In general, RIBP is less painful, and the upper plexus has been classically thought to be more commonly involved (due to the higher prevalence in breast cancer and the radiation field involved), although patients may also experience involvement of the lower plexus and the entire plexus.[1] Pain or paresthesia occurring less than 6 months following radiation, and rapid progression of symptoms would also favor neoplastic involvement over radiation injury which can progress over years in an indolent fashion. Horner syndrome is less likely to occur in patients with RIBP, and occasionally cutaneous signs of radiation effects can be seen (poikiloderma, telangiectasias, atrophy, hyperpigmentation, and lymphedema). The presence of a focal mass or known adjacent neoplasm would also favor direct plexus invasion from cancer or its metastasis as opposed to radiation injury.

Diagnostic studies. Neuroimaging studies with MRI can show diffuse thickening of nerve roots and fibrosis around the plexus in RIBP. Fibrosis of other adjacent structures, such as the lung apex and pericardium, may also be present. However, frequently, in the absence of visualized metastatic disease, it may be difficult to distinguish RIBP from cancer-related plexopathy using imaging alone. PET imaging usually shows hypometabolism, which may be helpful in distinguishing RIBP from neoplastic plexopathies. Although electrophysiologic studies in RIBP can show abnormal motor units and sensory NCS in the affected plexus segments, the most helpful feature, when present, is myokymic discharges on EMG. Myokymia is present in 63% of patients and not typically associated with neoplasm-related plexopathies.[13] Although not sensitive, this is felt to be a specific feature for RIBP. Clinically, myokymia is defined as a spontaneous, involuntary, and undulating worm-like localized movement in a specific muscle but is rarely reported by patients. Rather, myokymic discharges that can be seen spontaneously on needle study are the corresponding spontaneous single motor unit firing that occur either at regular or irregular intervals. Myokymia is thought to be associated with the demyelinating process underlying some cases of RIBP.

Management. There is no established treatment to reverse or improve nerve injury from radiation therapy. A phase II study of hyperbaric oxygen for the treatment of RIBP did not provide evidence of improvement in functional outcome.[14] One case report describes resolution of conduction block on NCS in a patient with RIBP in which anticoagulation was started,[15] suggesting that revascularization could help in radiation injury repair in some cases. Whereas bevacizumab is used to treat radiation necrosis in the central nervous system,[16] there is currently no evidence for the use of bevacizumab in RIBP. Antioxidant therapy with vitamin B_1-B_6 is routinely used, although the evidence is currently lacking. As fibrosis and atrophy are felt to contribute to nerve injury, the combined use of clodronate and pentoxifylline-tocopherol (PENTOCLO) has also been investigated due to the combined biologic effects, with some reported neurological benefit for RIBP.[17,18] Similar to neoplastic brachial neuropathies, a multidisciplinary approach aimed at symptom control and functional preservation with physical and occupational therapy can be helpful for patients with RIBP. Given the lack of effective treatment strategies, continued efforts are being made to improve delineation and delivery of radiation therapy to head and neck, breast, or lung cancers with avoidance of the brachial plexus.[19]

CASE 22.3 LUMBOSACRAL PLEXOPATHY

Case. A 50-year-old male with a past history of atypical fibrous sarcoma of the pelvic floor (measuring 12.3 × 9.7 × 8.8 cm at diagnosis), treated with surgical debulking followed by radiation therapy and another debulking surgery for local recurrence 4 years later, presented with worsening left lower extremity pain and weakness over the course of a few weeks. There were no new bowel or bladder changes, but he had been known to have hydronephrosis in the context of his bulky disease. He noted frequent tripping over his left foot. Examination revealed normal mental status and cranial nerves. Bulk and tone were normal in the upper and lower extremities. He had weakness of left dorsiflexion (4–/5), great toe extension (4–/5), ankle plantar flexion (3/5), and knee flexion (4–/5). The ankle jerk was depressed on the left, but otherwise reflexes were preserved in the upper and lower extremities. Sensation was reduced to pinprick over the bottom of his left foot and the lateral side of his calf. This was clinically felt to represent involvement of the lower lumbar and sacral nerve roots (L5, S1) or lumbosacral plexus. Imaging was performed with an MRI of the lumbosacral spine and plexus. This revealed the presence of extensive metastatic disease in the epidural space around L5–S3 but also encasing the left lumbosacral plexus (Fig. 22.6). There was increased focal enhancement within the left L5–S1 neural foramen adjacent to the exiting left L5 nerve root, concerning for recurrent/residual tumor. He therefore underwent laminectomy of L5 through S3 with epidural tumor resection. His subsequent course was complicated with local tumor recurrence requiring proton radiation, as well as systemic metastasis to his lung, for which he was started on pazopanib. Several months later and with intensive physical therapy, he slowly regained some of the power in his left lower extremity but unfortunately his locoregional disease continued to progress.

Clinical Pearls

1. A prior history of a pelvic floor tumor and new lower extremity symptoms should raise the concern for a lumbosacral plexopathy related to local disease recurrence or metastasis.

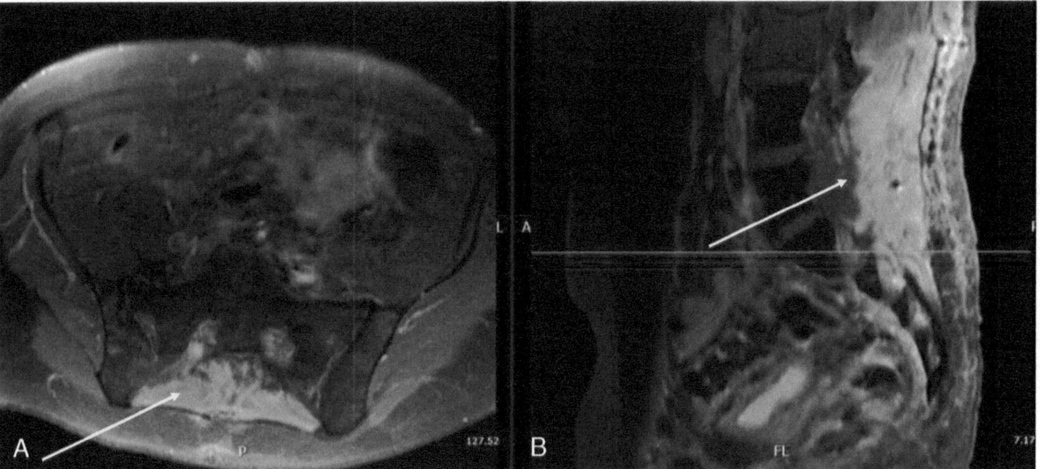

Fig. 22.6 MRI of the lumbar sacral spine with axial (A) and sagittal (B) T1 post-contrast sequences showing extensive locoregional recurrence of the pelvic floor fibrous tumor, involving the epidural space at L5–S3.

2. Electrodiagnostic studies are not required to confirm localization if the imaging findings can account for the localization suggested by the clinical examination.

Teaching Points: Approach to Cancer-Associated Lumbosacral Plexopathy

Pathophysiology. Neoplastic lumbosacral plexopathies are typically associated with tumors of the abdominal or pelvic cavity through direct invasion. Colorectal or gynecological cancers, retroperitoneal sarcomas, lymphomas, or sacral chordomas account for over 75% of cases of plexopathies, whereas primary neoplasms outside the abdominal cavity (breast or lung cancer) are involved in about 25% of cases.[20] This is typically due to bulky disease extension into the lumbosacral plexus, but can also be caused by direct invasion of the plexus through connective tissue or the epineurium. Rarely, involvement of the lumbosacral plexus occurs due to compression from lymph node or bony metastases.

Clinical presentation. Signs and symptoms associated with neoplastic invasion of the lumbosacral plexus depend on the level of anatomic involvement. A review of 85 patients with lumbosacral plexopathy showed involvement of lower plexus in about 50%, the upper plexus in 30%, and the entire plexus in 20%.[20] Progressive and severe pain is almost always the presenting complaint (up to 98%),[20] and may have radicular or referred features. It is often worse in the supine position or with certain movements or weight bearing. Other progressive neurological symptoms such as weakness and sensory complaints can evolve over time in about 60% of patients.[20] Bowel and bladder changes and sexual dysfunction are not typically present unless bilateral lumbosacral plexopathies are present. A palpable abdominal or pelvic mass can be present on examination. Leg swelling or hydronephrosis in the presence of neurological symptoms involving the perineum or lower extremities should raise the suspicion for a neoplastic plexopathy.

Diagnostic studies. MRI of the plexus, and MRI of the abdomen and pelvis can be helpful in identifying structural lesions and locoregional disease or metastasis. Typically, increased T2/fluid attenuated inversion recovery signal in the plexus, with or without enhancement, can be present. A local mass compressing the plexus or thickening and/or nodular enhancement of the plexus can also indicate the presence of neoplastic plexopathy. A PET-CT may be helpful in detecting active cancer in the area adjacent to the plexus and can occasionally show increased avidity in the area of the plexus itself. NCS and EMG may be helpful for localization and prognostication as described above.

Management. The same principles of management apply to lumbosacral plexopathies, with regards to pain management and allied health involvement. In addition, consultation from urological specialists may be required in the case of bladder dysfunction.

Radiation-Induced Lumbosacral Plexopathy

Radiation to cancers of the pelvic floor or abdomen can lead to radiation-induced lumbosacral plexopathies, with doses as low as 1700 cGy. As is the case with brachial plexopathies, it can be difficult to distinguish radiation-induced from neoplastic lumbosacral plexopathies. Pain is a prominent feature in almost all cases of neoplastic lumbosacral plexopathies (98%), whereas it is only present in about 10% of radiation-induced plexopathies. Bilateral plexus involvement can also be more common in radiation-induced lumbosacral plexopathy. The time of onset of radiation-induced lumbosacral plexopathy varies between 1–5 years (range of 1 month to 31 years).[20]

Table 22.1 Features of neoplastic vs. radiation-induced plexopathies

Features	Neoplastic plexopathy	Radiation-induced plexopathy
Onset of symptoms	Rapid evolution of symptoms, usually corresponding to increased burden of systemic disease	Months to years from last treatment to onset of symptoms
Location of involvement	Lower brachial plexus in the case of lung neoplasms, although entire plexus may be involved	Upper brachial plexus when related to radiation in context of breast neoplasm, although entire plexus may be involved
Pain	Tends to be more severe and progressive, uniformly present in neoplastic lumbar plexopathies	Slowly progressive when present, indolent in nature
Other associated clinical features	Horner syndrome (lower brachial plexus), lymphedema	Dermatitis, telangiectasias, atrophy, hyperpigmentation, and lymphedema
Imaging findings	MRI or CT may reveal large burden of locoregional disease MRI of the plexus may show thickening of nerve roots PET imaging may reveal increased avidity in the plexus	MRI of the plexus may show fibrosis of surrounding structures and organs as well as matting of nerve roots
EMG/NCS findings	No pathognomonic features	Myokymia present in about 60% of cases

EMG, Electromyography; *NCS*, nerve conduction study.

Other cancer-related plexopathies

Although these will be covered separately in other chapters, direct invasion of malignancy (Chapter 21), paraneoplastic plexopathies (Chapter 20), and immune-checkpoint blockade associated plexopathy (Chapter 29) are other causes of brachial and lumbar plexopathies. In particular, an inflammatory demyelinating neuropathy has been described in immune-checkpoint blockade using cytotoxic T-lymphocyte associated protein 4 (CTLA-4) or programmed death 1 (PD-1)/ programmed death ligand 1 (PDL-1) inhibitors. Patients with cancer can also be at higher risk of infections due to an immunocompromised state while under chemotherapy, and infectious and postinfectious plexopathies remain a consideration. Other considerations are malnutrition and cachexia, which may in turn cause metabolic or nutritional neuropathies and plexopathies.

Conclusion

Brachial and lumbosacral plexopathies can occur in cancer patients as a result of the malignancy itself or of cancer-targeted therapy. Careful history taking and examination skills can aid in localization. Cancer-related plexopathies are more common and tend to be painful and more rapid in onset than radiation-induced plexopathies, which present in a more indolent fashion (Table 22.1). EMG/NCS can be useful if myokymic changes are present and imaging can show locoregional or systemic progression suggestive of a neoplastic plexopathy. Supportive measures and a multidisciplinary approach with palliative care, pain, and rehabilitation specialists are essential, as survival and quality of life may be limited in many of the affected patients.

References

1. Kori SH, Foley KM, Posner JB. Brachial plexus lesions in patients with cancer: 100 cases. *Neurology*. 1981;31(1): 45–50.
2. Bourque PR, Warman Chardon J, Bryanton M, Toupin M, Burns BF, Torres C. Neurolymphomatosis of the brachial plexus and its branches: case series and literature review. *Can J Neurol Sci*. 2018;45(2):137–143.
3. Pacelli J, Whitaker CH. Case of the month brachial plexopathy due to malignant peripheral nerve sheath tumor in neurofibromatosis type 1: case report and subject review. *Muscle Nerve*. 2006;33:697–700.
4. Stilwill SE, Mills MK, Hansford BG, et al. Practical approach and review of brachial plexus pathology with operative correlation: what the radiologist needs to know. *Semin Roentgenol*. 2019;54:92–112.
5. Wasa J, Nishida Y, Tsukushi S, et al. MRI features in the differentiation of malignant peripheral nerve sheath tumors and neurofibromas. *AJR Am J Roentgenol*. 2010;194(6):1568–1574.

6. Griffith JF. Ultrasound of the brachial plexus. *Semin Musculoskelet Radiol.* 2018;22(3):323–333.
7. Seror P. Brachial plexus neoplastic lesions assessed by conduction study of medial antebrachial cutaneous nerve. *Muscle Nerve.* 2001;24(8):1068–1070.
8. Kamenova B, Braverman AS, Schwartz M, et al. Effective treatment of the brachial plexus syndrome in breast cancer patients by early detection and control of loco-regional metastases with radiation or systemic therapy. *Int J Clin Oncol.* 2009;14(3):219–224.
9. Schierle C, Winograd JM. Radiation-induced brachial plexopathy: review. Complication without a cure. *J Reconstr Microsurg.* 2004;20(2):149–152.
10. Friberg S, Rudn BI. Hypofractionation in radiotherapy. An investigation of injured Swedish women, treated for cancer of the breast. *Acta Oncol (Madr).* 2009;48(6):822–831.
11. Lindberg K, Grozman V, Lindberg S, et al. Radiation-induced brachial plexus toxicity after SBRT of apically located lung lesions. *Acta Oncol.* 2019;58:1178–1186.
12. Killer HE, Hess K. Natural history of radiation-induced brachial plexopathy compared with surgically treated patients. *J Neurol.* 1990;237(4):247–250.
13. Harper CM, Thomas JE, Cascino TL, Litchy WJ. Distinction between neoplastic and radiation-induced brachial plexopathy, with emphasis on the role of EMG. *Neurology.* 1989;39(4): 502–502.
14. Pritchard J, Anand P, Broome J, et al. Double-blind randomized phase II study of hyperbaric oxygen in patients with radiation-induced brachial plexopathy. *Radiother Oncol.* 2001;58(3):279–286.
15. Soto O. Case of the month radiation-induced conduction block: resolution following anticoagulant therapy. *Muscle Nerve.* 2005;31:642–645.
16. Levin VA, Bidaut L, Hou P, et al. Randomized double-blind placebo-controlled trial of bevacizumab therapy for radiation necrosis of the central nervous system. *Int J Radiat Oncol Biol Phys.* 2011;79(5):1487–1495.
17. Delanian S, Lefaix JL, Pradat PF. Radiation-induced neuropathy in cancer survivors. *Radiother Oncol.* 2012;105(3):273–282.
18. Delanian S, Lefaix J-L, Maisonobe T, Salachas F, Pradat P-F. Significant clinical improvement in radiation-induced lumbosacral polyradiculopathy by a treatment combining pentoxifylline, tocopherol, and clodronate (pentoclo). *J Neurol Sci.* 2008;275(1–2):164–166.
19. Hall WH, Guiou M, Lee NY, et al. Development and validation of a standardized method for contouring the brachial plexus: preliminary dosimetric analysis among patients treated with IMRT for head-and-neck cancer. *Int J Radiat Oncol Biol Phys.* 2008;72(5):1362–1367.
20. Jaeckle KA. Neurologic manifestations of neoplastic and radiation-induced plexopathies. *Semin Neurol.* 2010;30(3):254–262.

Chapter | 23 |

Cancer complications in patients with hematologic malignancies

Cristina Valencia-Sanchez, Molly Knox, and Maciej M. Mrugala

CHAPTER OUTLINE

Introduction

Malignant cells of both B-cell and T-cell origin have a predilection for infiltrating into the cerebrospinal fluid (CSF) and the meningeal membranes surrounding the brain and the spinal cord. Central nervous system (CNS) involvement can occur at presentation, with systemic progression, and at relapse. In patients with lymphoma, neoplastic involvement may be leptomeningeal (see Chapter 15, Case 15.2), intraparenchymal, intramedullary, and/or epidural. Unique syndromes include lymphomatosis cerebri and neurolymphomatosis. Neurological complications are more frequent with non-Hodgkin lymphoma (NHL) than with Hodgkin lymphoma (HL). CNS involvement by leukemia includes leptomeningeal or intracranial metastases and extramedullary myeloid tumors. Intracranial hemorrhage is also a common complication of leukemia.[1]

The incidence of CNS involvement is highest in aggressive lymphomas such as Burkitt lymphoma and acute lymphoblastic leukemia (ALL), ranging from 30% to 50%, and CNS prophylaxis is routinely used in the treatment protocols. In patients with diffuse large B-cell lymphoma (DLBCL), the overall CNS relapse risk is 2–5%, and CNS prophylaxis is reserved for high-risk patients.[2] Neurological involvement with acute myelogenous leukemia (AML) is rare, less than 5%, and even rarer in chronic lymphocytic leukemia (CLL), occurring in less than 1% of patients.[1]

CNS involvement can be difficult to diagnose. The clinical presentation varies widely depending on the site of involvement. Brain and spine MRI, CSF analysis with cytology, and flow cytometry may assist in diagnosis.

Rarely, NHL and HL may be associated with paraneoplastic syndromes. Limbic encephalitis, paraneoplastic cerebellar degeneration, and granulomatous angiitis of the CNS are the typical paraneoplastic syndromes associated with HL.[3]

This chapter reviews the spectrum of neurologic complications associated with lymphoma and leukemia through six representative cases.

Clinical cases

CASE 23.1 LEPTOMENINGEAL RECURRENCE

Case. A 71-year-old male presented with altered mental status. He had a history of B-cell NHL diagnosed 5 months prior to presentation. He initially presented with abdominal and back pain and was found to have a mesenteric and paraspinal mass extending from T6 to T10, with spinal and epidural involvement. Biopsy of the mesenteric mass was consistent with high-grade, CD10+ B-cell lymphoma with MYC and BCL-2 rearrangements (double-hit). Bone marrow biopsy and CSF were negative for disease. He received radiation treatment for the paraspinal mass and chemotherapy with rituximab plus bendamustine for three cycles, the last cycle being completed 1 month prior to current presentation. Recent PET scan had shown partial response with residual mesenteric and paraspinal masses.

The patient then developed visual disturbances and incoordination 6 weeks prior to current presentation. He was eventually found in his car confused with incoherent speech. On examination, he was lethargic with eyelid opening apraxia, dysarthria, and increased tone in bilateral upper extremities and right lower extremity.

The differential diagnosis for suspected subacute encephalopathy included toxic, metabolic, infectious, inflammatory, and neoplastic conditions, which are summarized in Table 23.1.

Brain MRI showed increased T2 signal in the dorsal midbrain, medial thalami, hypothalamus, optic tracts, anterior fornix, and periventricular white matter. There was aqueductal effacement and enlargement of the lateral ventricles suggestive of obstructive hydrocephalus (Fig. 23.1A). Post-gadolinium images showed abnormal enhancement of the leptomeninges and septum pellucidum (Fig. 23.1B). Electroencephalogram (EEG) showed generalized slowing. CSF analysis revealed elevated protein (57 mg/dL) with normal white blood cell (WBC) count and glucose level. Cytology was negative. Flow cytometry was not performed due to paucity of cells present in the CSF. Due to finding of hydrocephalus, ventriculoperitoneal shunt was placed and the patient experienced significant improvement of mental status. Flow cytometry of ventricular fluid showed an atypical B-cell population, positive for CD19, CD20, and CD10. Diagnosis of leptomeningeal recurrence of NHL was made and treatment with high-dose intravenous (IV) methotrexate and rituximab was initiated.

Teaching Points: Diagnosis and Management of Lymphomatous Meningitis. Leptomeningeal involvement by NHL results from the multifocal seeding of the leptomeninges by cancer cells (also see Chapter 15, Case 15.2). Many patients have concurrent leptomeningeal and parenchymal involvement.[4] Leptomeningeal disease may be seen in 4–15% of patients with NHL.[5] It is very rare in patients with HL.[6]

The clinical presentation of leptomeningeal involvement is typically characterized by multifocal neurological signs including cranial neuropathies (diplopia, facial weakness, hearing loss, imbalance, vertigo, dysphagia, hoarseness), extremity weakness or sensory changes, occasionally spinal cord symptoms (incontinence), headache, and communicating hydrocephalus.[5] Testing should include MRI of the entire neuroaxis and CSF analysis including cytology and flow cytometry. In hematologic malignancies, flow cytometry is significantly more sensitive in detecting abnormal cells in CSF than conventional cytology and should be routinely used when lymphomatous involvement is suspected.[7] Consideration should be given for radionuclide CSF flow study to evaluate for obstruction if bulky disease or hydrocephalus occurs, as impaired CSF flow is a relative contraindication for intrathecal (IT) chemotherapy.[5]

MRI demonstrates focal or diffuse leptomeningeal contrast enhancement, subarachnoid nodules, or intradural root enlargement with enhancement. CSF may reveal lymphocytosis, increased protein, and low glucose. A unique CSF feature in leptomeningeal HL is eosinophilic pleocytosis, and identification of Reed-Sternberg cells in the CSF gives the definitive diagnosis.[6]

First-line treatment of NHL leptomeningeal metastases is typically high-dose intravenous (IV) methotrexate. Other com-

Table 23.1 Differential diagnosis for subacute encephalopathy in Case 23.1

Differential diagnoses	Test results
Infectious encephalitis Virus: HSV1/2, VZV, EBV, HHV-6, CMV, arbovirus, JC virus, HIV Bacterial: Lyme, TB, listeria, syphilis Fungal/Parasitic	Negative serum and CSF studies
Neoplastic: CNS lymphoma, primary CNS malignancy, brain metastases	CSF cytology from the ventricular fluid showed atypical B-cells
Autoimmune or paraneoplastic encephalitis by a neural antibody	Negative neural antibodies in serum and CSF
Inflammatory: CNS vasculitis	MRI not typical, negative ANA, ENA, ANCA
Metabolic/endocrine encephalopathy: uremic, hepatic, hyponatremia, hypo/hyperthyroid, hypoglycemia, vitamin B_{12} deficiency	Complete metabolic panel, TSH, vitamin B_{12} within normal limits
Toxic encephalopathy: alcohol, chemotherapy, CO	No history of exposure to alcohol or CO
Creutzfeldt-Jakob disease	No other associated signs (ataxia, myoclonus) MRI and EEG not typical

ANA, Antinuclear antibody; *ANCA*, antineutrophil cytoplasmic antibody; *CMV*, cytomegalovirus; *CNS*, central nervous system; *CSF*, cerebrospinal fluid; *CO*, carbon monoxide; *EBV*, Epstein–Barr virus; *ENA*, extractable nuclear antigens; *HHV-6*, human herpes virus 6; *HIV*, human immunodeficiency virus; *HSV*, herpes simplex virus; *JC* virus, John Cunningham virus; *TB*, tuberculosis; *TSH*, thyroid stimulating hormone; *VZV*, varicella-zoster virus.

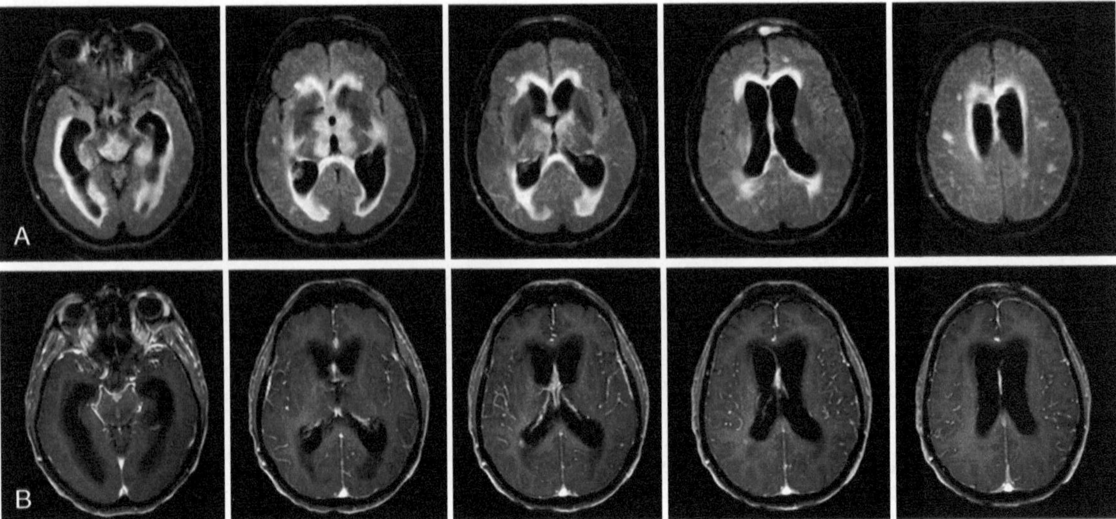

Fig. 23.1 (A) Axial MRI fluid-attenuated inversion recovery images showing increased T2 signal intensity in the dorsal midbrain, medial thalami, hypothalamus, optic tracts, anterior fornix, and periventricular white matter. Enlargement of the lateral ventricles is suggestive of obstructive hydrocephalus. (B) Axial T1 post-gadolinium MRI showing abnormal enhancement of the leptomeninges and septum pellucidum.

monly used drugs are cytarabine and thiotepa. If no CSF flow obstruction is detected, IT chemotherapy can also be considered.[5] Clinical trials of new IT agents such as rituximab are underway.[4] Focal radiotherapy might be needed to treat bulky disease obstructing CSF pathways,[5] but because of its significant toxicity, it is rarely used.

For NHL patients with leptomeningeal metastases, prolonged overall survival was associated with being near the median age, with an early diagnosis, a low International Prognosis Index score, higher Karnofsky Performance Scores, and concurrent parenchymal involvement.[4]

In leukemia, leptomeningeal involvement is most common in ALL. It is identified in less than 10% of adults at diagnosis, but occurs in 30% to 50% of patients at leukemic relapse. Due to the high incidence of CNS involvement, CNS prophylaxis is recommended in all patients with ALL.[2]

Clinical Pearls

1. Lymphomatous infiltration of the leptomeninges is the most common neurologic complication of NHL.
2. The clinical presentation of leptomeningeal metastases is characterized by multifocal neurological signs and symptoms affecting the brain, cranial nerves, spinal cord, and exiting nerve roots. It may also cause obstructive hydrocephalus.
3. MRI demonstrating leptomeningeal enhancement and CSF analysis including cytology and flow cytometry are typically needed for diagnosis of leptomeningeal involvement.
4. Treatment strategies for leptomeningeal disease typically include a combination of IT and systemic chemotherapy.

CASE 23.2 INTRACRANIAL METASTASES

Case. A 64-year-old female presented with a breast mass and axillary lymphadenopathy. Biopsy of the breast mass demonstrated DLBCL, whereas the axillary lymph node biopsy revealed small lymphocytic lymphoma with evidence of clonal B-cells. It was unclear if the two cancers were clonally related. She had no neurological symptoms at the time of diagnosis and brain MRI was normal. She underwent six cycles of rituximab, cyclophosphamide, doxorubicin, vincristine, and prednisone (R-CHOP), as well as two doses of IT methotrexate (e.g., CNS prophylaxis for high-risk disease). Following R-CHOP, she received consolidative radiation to her breast and had no evidence of recurrent lymphoma for 2 years. She then presented with confusion and brain MRI showed an enhancing mass in the splenium of the corpus callosum that was hypermetabolic on CT-PET. CSF flow cytometry revealed a clonal B-cell population, and the diagnosis of secondary CNS lymphoma was made. She underwent treatment with nine cycles of methotrexate, rituximab, and temozolomide (MRT) followed by consolidation with etoposide and cytarabine, with resolution of her brain lesion. One year later, her family noted progressive cognitive difficulties, and a repeat brain MRI showed new enhancing lesions in the left cerebellum, brainstem, and left basal ganglia (Fig. 23.2). CSF analysis revealed a small lambda monotypic B-cell population confirming CNS relapse. She was reinitiated on MRT for six cycles with resolution of the brain lesions, and then placed on monthly maintenance high-dose IV methotrexate for 12 months, in addition to 6 months of maintenance temozolomide.

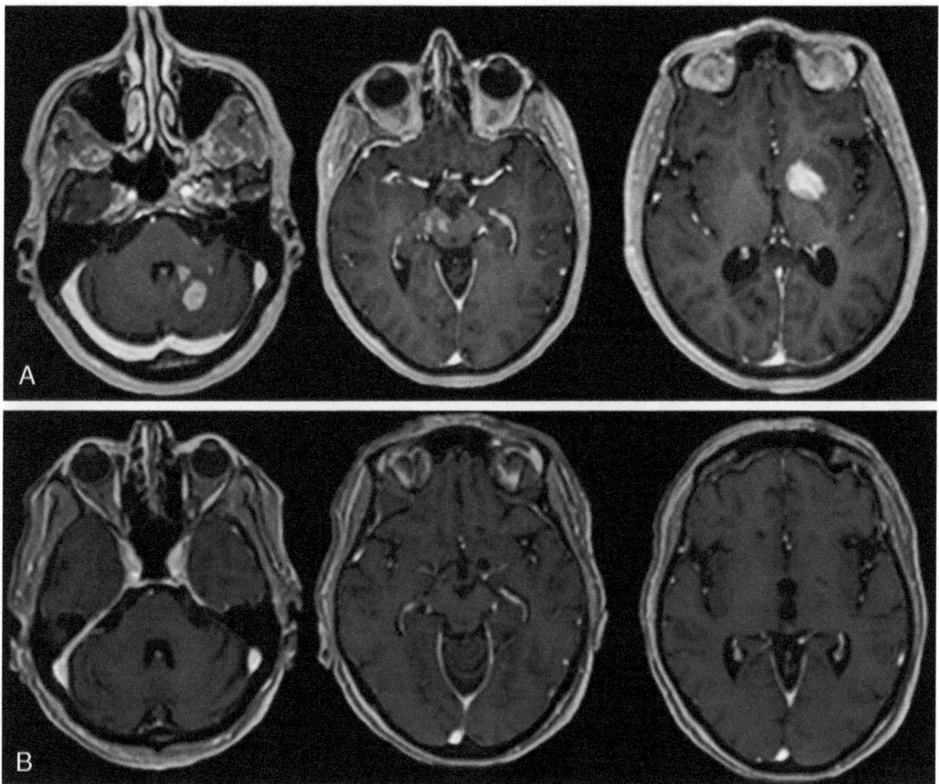

Fig. 23.2 Axial T1 post-gadolinium brain MRI from the patient's second central nervous system (CNS) recurrence, pre- and posttreatment. (A) CNS relapse with enhancing lesions of the left cerebellum, brainstem, and left basal ganglia. (B) Images obtained 6 months after treatment initiation showing resolution of the enhancing lesions.

Teaching Points: CNS Recurrence May Occur in High-Risk Systemic Lymphoma. Routine CNS prophylaxis in DLBCL is only recommended in patients with high-risk of CNS involvement. Initial involvement of the breast indicates a more aggressive form, with a 9–27% risk of developing secondary CNS lymphoma.[8] This patient was therefore considered high-risk and treated with two doses of IT methotrexate. National Comprehensive Cancer Network (NCCN) guidelines currently recommend four to eight doses of IT chemotherapy, although treatment practices vary greatly due to lack of clear evidence.[9] CNS recurrence often presents in isolation soon after diagnosis or after completion of chemotherapy (4.7–9 months).[9] Parenchymal metastases occur in 1% to 2% of NHL and in 0.2% to 5% of HL.[1] Compared with other lymphomas, DLBCL is more likely to manifest with a parenchymal lesion than leptomeningeal disease. Common clinical presentations of a new parenchymal mass include new-onset headaches, focal deficits, and changes in mental status, coma, or seizures. Workup of suspected CNS relapse should include MRI of the brain with and without contrast, CSF cytology and flow cytometry, and evaluation for systemic recurrence. Parenchymal lesions on brain MRI are typically multiple, homogeneously enhancing, and periventricular, sometimes accompanied by leptomeningeal or subependymal enhancement. Treatment of secondary CNS lymphoma includes systemic high-dose methotrexate and rituximab, frequently R-CHOP, with recent evidence supporting the use of temozolomide.[10] Newer agents are currently being explored, such as ibrutinib[11] and lenalidomide.[12] Surgery is reserved for lesions causing mass effect and treatment with radiation has failed to show improvement in survival.[8]

Clinical Pearls

1. Parenchymal metastases are less common than leptomeningeal disease in secondary CNS lymphoma, with the exception of DLBCL.
2. Treatment of secondary CNS lymphoma with parenchymal disease is similar to that of primary CNS lymphoma (see Chapter 13 for discussion of treatment for primary CNS lymphoma), including systemic high-dose methotrexate, rituximab, and temozolomide as primary treatment options. Emerging treatment agents include lenalidomide, ibrutinib, and immune therapies.

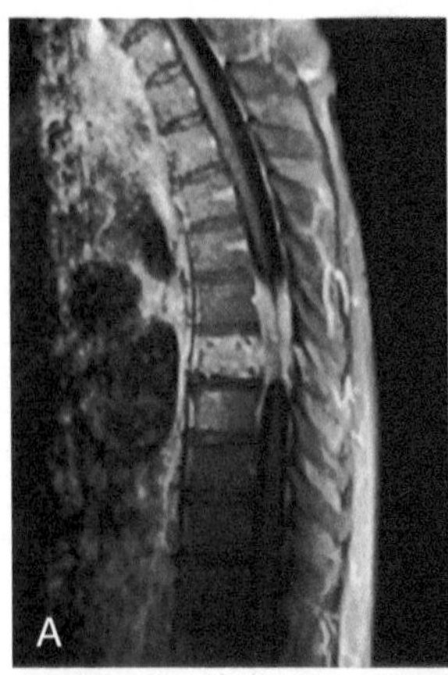

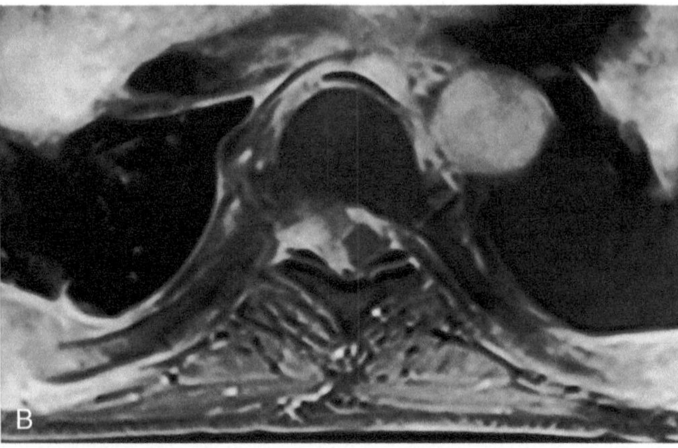

Fig. 23.3 (A) Sagittal and (B) axial MRI of the thoracic spine with contrast. Thoracic spine MRI reveals lymphoma replacing bodies of T7 and T8. There is a large rind of epidural tumor extending from T5–6 to T7–8 interspace with cord compression and deformity throughout these segments, without obvious spinal cord signal abnormality.

CASE 23.3 EPIDURAL METASTASES

Case. A 55-year-old male on chronic immunosuppression for orthotopic deceased-donor liver transplantation with concomitant renal transplantation 10 years prior presented with shortness of breath. Laboratory studies were pertinent for anemia, hypercalcemia, and elevated uric acid. CT Chest revealed a large left pleural effusion, lytic bone lesions to the chest wall, and mediastinal lymphadenopathy. Skeletal survey showed additional lesions to the T7 vertebrae and the left ilium. He underwent bone biopsy of the chest wall lesion and pathology showed a monomorphic post-transplant lymphoproliferative disorder, CD20-positive large B-cell lymphoma type, Epstein–Barr virus (EBV) negative. The day he was scheduled to begin treatment with R-CHOP, he developed sudden lower extremity weakness while walking and described a tingling sensation in his hands and feet. Two hours later he could no longer support his weight and had urinary retention. Neurological examination revealed 4/5 strength to his right lower extremity, left hip flexor 2/5, left knee flexor 4/5, and left dorsiflexion and plantar flexion 4/5. Sensation was intact and he had brisk patellar reflexes bilaterally. Urgent spine MRI revealed spinal cord compression due to epidural tumor at the T5–6 interspace extending down to the T7–8 interspace. Osseous involvement with lymphoma was noted at C4, T7, T8, L3, and L5 (Fig. 23.3). He was given 10 mg of IV dexamethasone, and a foley catheter was placed. Neurosurgery and radiation oncology were consulted and chose to proceed with urgent radiation given the radiosensitive nature of his tumor. He was placed on a dexamethasone taper and completed 30 Gy of radiotherapy in 10 fractions targeting T5–9 spine with complete resolution of his weakness and urinary retention.

Teaching Points: Epidural Spinal Cord Compression—a Neuro-Oncologic Emergency. Primary and secondary spinal involvement from hematologic malignancy is rare. Epidural disease occurs in 2% to 5% of patients with NHL and 0.2% of patients with HL.[13] In leukemia, spinal involvement presents as extramedullary myeloid tumors, also known as chloromas or granulocytic sarcomas, and has incidence of 3% in acute and chronic myelogenous leukemia.[14] Multiple myeloma is better known for causing epidural spinal cord compression, affecting up to 6% of patients throughout the course of disease.[15] The mechanism of epidural disease includes spread from the vertebrae to the epidural space, which allows the tumor to encircle the thecal sac and cause obstruction of the venous plexus, which ultimately results in vasogenic edema of the spinal cord. This can lead to spinal cord infarction and permanent loss of strength if untreated. The most common site of involvement is the thoracic spine. Signs and symptoms that would necessitate urgent spinal imaging in a patient with hematologic malignancy includes severe back pain, worse with movement or level specific, radicular pain, loss of gait function, ataxia, hyperreflexia, Lhermitte's phenomenon, and bowel, bladder, or erectile dysfunction. MR imaging is the gold standard and will typically reveal a homogeneous enhancing mass. Emergent treatment includes high-dose steroids and radiation. Surgical decompression or spinal column stabilization may be considered in specific cases. In our case, surgical intervention was not ideal given the rapid presentation and radiosensitive nature of the tumor. Surgery could have further delayed treatment with radiation due to the risk of delayed skin healing.

Clinical Pearls

1. Red flag symptoms of spinal cord compression in a patient with known cancer such as back pain, lower extremity weakness, incontinence, and gait instability should prompt urgent neurologic evaluation and spinal MR imaging.
2. Initial treatment includes intravenous dexamethasone 10 mg IV followed by 4 mg every 6 hours to reduce vasogenic edema with close monitoring of patient's symptoms and neurological examination.
3. Hematologic malignancies are radiosensitive and urgent treatment should be provided to reduce the risk of permanent neurological injury.

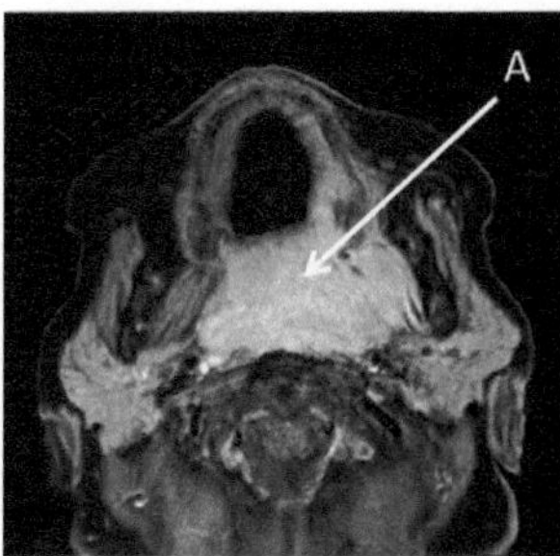

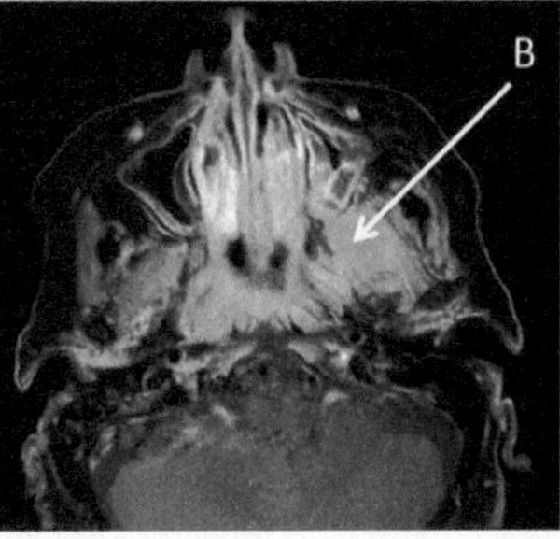

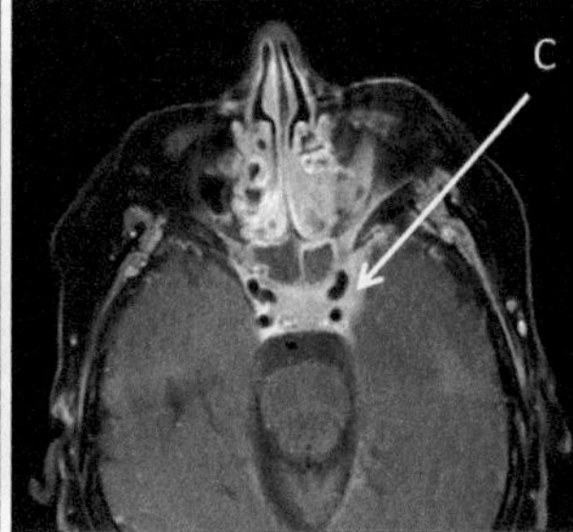

Fig. 23.4 Axial T1 post-gadolinium brain MRI showing a large homogeneously enhancing mass (*arrows* A and B) centered on the nasopharynx with extension to the left pterygoid musculature, left palate, and superiorly to involve left cavernous sinus and Meckel's cave. There is also slight abnormal enhancement and thickening of the anterior dura within the left middle cranial fossa (*arrow* C).

CASE 23.4 NEUROLYMPHOMATOSIS

Case. A 71-year-old female with rheumatoid arthritis on immunosuppression presented with 2 months of headaches, left ear fullness, sinus drainage, and night sweats. CT of the head and sinuses revealed a massive sinonasal and nasopharyngeal tumor measuring 6.4 cm × 7 cm × 5.1 cm. MRI Brain revealed intracranial extension with involvement of the left cavernous sinus and Meckel's cave with slight involvement of the dura of the left middle cranial fossa, but no abnormal parenchymal enhancement (Fig. 23.4). She underwent biopsy of the mass, with flow cytometric study and morphologic evaluation showing DLBCL, EBV positive. CSF analysis and bone marrow biopsy were negative for involvement. She was treated with three cycles of R-CHOP and received one round of IT methotrexate. Consolidative radiation therapy was performed with post-treatment PET/CT showing excellent response. One year later she complained of numbness to her left cheek and pain with chewing. Neurological examination was pertinent for diminished sensation of left V2 to pinprick, causing concern for secondary CNS involvement. Repeat MRI Brain revealed non–mass-like enhancement of the left pterygopalatine fossa extending into the foramen rotundum. Repeat CSF analysis with flow cytometry and cytology was negative for disease. She was treated with four cycles of high-dose intravenous methotrexate for neurolymphomatosis affecting the left trigeminal nerve in V2 distribution, and experienced improvement in facial symptoms. Unfortunately, after treatment concluded, her symptoms returned, with additional complaints of intermittent electrical pain across her left cheek and eye. She was placed on lenalidomide for 1 month but failed to improve. Treatment was then changed to ibrutinib with good response.

Teaching Points: Neurolymphomatosis Is a Rare Complication of Lymphoma Requiring High Index of Suspicion. Neurolymphomatosis (NL) is neoplastic lymphocytic invasion of cranial nerves (CN), peripheral nerve roots, or plexus by non-Hodgkin lymphoma. It is a rare neurologic manifestation occurring in an estimated 3% of cases, and is more common with aggressive subtypes such as DLBCL.[16] It may present in patients with active or remitted systemic lymphoma, primary leptomeningeal disease, or as the only site of involvement.

There are four clinical presentations of NL:

1. Painful polyneuropathy or polyradiculopathy
2. Cranial neuropathy
3. Painless polyneuropathy
4. Peripheral mononeuropathy

The cauda equina is commonly affected in the painful polyneuropathy/polyradiculopathy subtype and the sciatic nerve is the most common mononeuropathy. Cranial neuropathy often presents as a Bell's palsy (CN VII), recurrent or bilateral, CN VI and CN III palsy, or as seen in our case, trigeminal (CN V) neuropathy with or without tic douloureux.

MRI is the most sensitive and specific noninvasive diagnostic tool, and may reveal enlargement and enhancement of nerves, roots, or plexus. Fluorodeoxyglucose (FDG)-PET may be a useful tool to identify sites of potential biopsy, as biopsy is the gold standard for diagnosis of NL.[16] Pathology reveals tumor cell infiltration of the endoneurium and perineurium. Treatment with corticosteroids should be avoided prior to biopsy, as it may result in a non-diagnostic sample. CSF should also be evaluated, as meningeal dissemination will occur in 20–40% of patients.[16] Treatment of NL is similar to that of primary CNS lymphoma, involving high-dose IV methotrexate as first line. In cases associated with systemic lymphoma, combination chemotherapy regimens such as CHOP or MCHOD (methotrexate, cyclophosphamide, vincristine, Adriamycin, and dexamethasone) may be used. IT chemotherapy should be initiated if there is evidence of coleptomeningeal involvement. Radiation therapy is of benefit in chemotherapy refractory cases or in systemic lymphoma with bulky disease.

In our case, long-term high-dose IV methotrexate was not feasible due to a high risk of kidney injury. Ibrutinib was ultimately chosen for its favorable CNS penetration after the patient was placed on and could not tolerate lenalidomide. Both ibrutinib and lenalidomide are being explored for use in cases of refractory or recurrent lymphoma involving the CNS.[11,12] Treatment response exceeds 50%; however, overall prognosis is poor, with median survival of 10 months following diagnosis.[16]

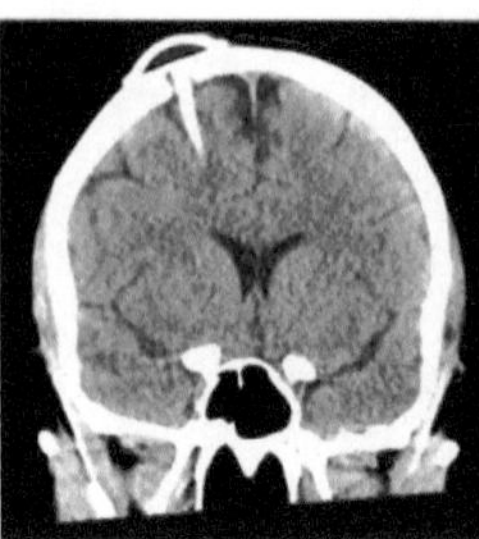
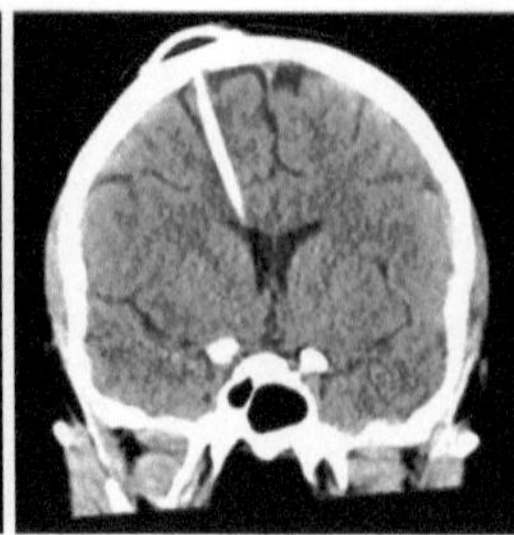
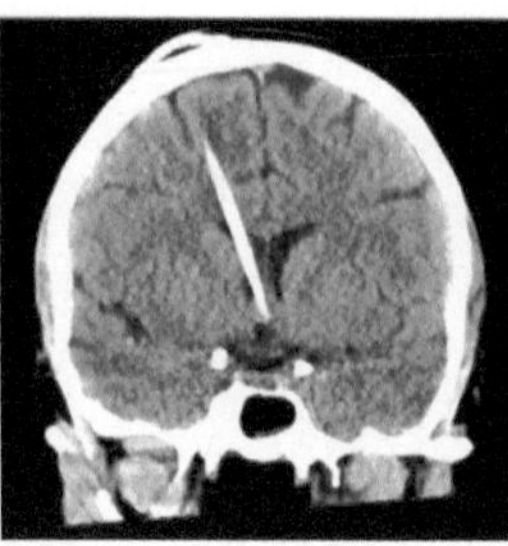
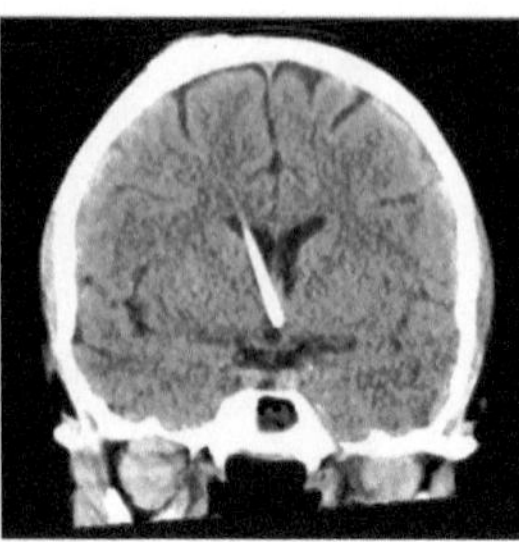

Fig. 23.5 Coronal CT showing trajectory of Ommaya reservoir.

Clinical Pearls

1. Neurolymphomatosis is a rare manifestation of lymphoma, and may manifest as a painful radiculopathy, cranial neuropathy, painless polyneuropathy, or mononeuropathy.
2. MR imaging is useful for diagnosis; however, nerve biopsy is the gold standard of diagnosis and will show lymphomatous cell infiltration in the perineurium and endoneurium.
3. Treatment of neurolymphomatosis involves high-dose IV methotrexate with ibrutinib and lenalidomide as possible options for refractory cases.

CASE 23.5 CENTRAL NERVOUS SYSTEM PROPHYLAXIS IN HEMATOLOGIC MALIGNANCY

Case. A 28-year-old female presented with intermittent chest pain. Workup revealed a WBC count of 83.2 × 10^9/L, with 26% blasts in peripheral smear. Bone marrow biopsy was consistent with B lymphoblastic leukemia, with t (9:22), BCR/ABL fusion, monosomy 7, and MYC+. She initiated induction chemotherapy with rituximab followed by IV dexamethasone, cyclophosphamide, vincristine and doxorubicin, and oral dasatinib (Hyper-CVAD regimen).

The patient reported no neurological symptoms and her neurological examination was normal. She had a history of Arnold–Chiari malformation. Due to the requirement of multiple lumbar punctures for administration of IT chemotherapy, an Ommaya reservoir was placed (Fig. 23.5). Cytology and flow cytometry of the CSF sample from the ventricle were negative for disease. She received prophylactic IT chemotherapy, with methotrexate on day 2 plus IT cytarabine on day 8 of each treatment cycle.

After cycle three of induction treatment, bone marrow biopsy showed morphologic remission but persistent minimal residual disease (MRD), so she was treated with blinatumomab and achieved MRD negative status. The patient then received allogenic stem cell transplant, after conditioning with cyclophosphamide and total body irradiation.

Teaching Points: Approach to Prophylaxis of Brain and Leptomeningeal Recurrence in High-Risk Lymphoma. Burkitt lymphoma and ALL have a high CNS relapse risk, about 30–50%. The risk of CNS recurrence for patients with DLBCL, with the current standard of R-CHOP chemotherapy, is much lower, about 2–5%.[2] The prevalence of CNS involvement in ALL is sufficiently high that all patients routinely receive prophylactic treatment to eradicate occult disease that would otherwise lead to a relapse. Lumbar puncture should be performed in all newly diagnosed patients and it is recommended to administer the first dose of IT chemotherapy at that time.[17]

Because oral and IV chemotherapy drugs penetrate poorly from the blood into the CNS, ALL cells can escape the full cytotoxic effects of systemic chemotherapy. IT methotrexate or cytarabine are often given in combination with high-dose IV methotrexate and/or cytarabine. Therapeutic levels of methotrexate and cytarabine can be achieved in the CSF when administered IV in high doses. The frequency of IT therapy treatments is greater during induction and consolidation courses and then becomes less frequent during prolonged maintenance therapy.[17]

In patients with DLBCL, the overall CNS relapse risk is 2–5%. CNS prophylaxis, in addition to the standard R-CHOP chemotherapy, is reserved for high-risk patients.[2] Factors known to be associated with a high risk of CNS relapse include elevated lactate dehydrogenase, >1 extra-nodal site of involvement, Eastern Cooperative Oncology Group (ECOG) performance score >1, advanced stage (III/IV) disease, extra-nodal involvement of testes, kidneys, adrenal gland, uterine, breast, and bone marrow, dual MYC/BCL2 expression, and activated B-cell subtype.[2]

DLBCL CNS relapses often occur within the brain parenchyma, either in isolation or concurrently with leptomeningeal disease. As such, CNS prophylaxis should have adequate penetrance to the CNS parenchyma. IT chemotherapy alone, with methotrexate and/or cytarabine, is insufficient to prevent parenchymal CNS recurrences because it does not adequately penetrate the brain parenchyma. IT chemotherapy is typically used in combination with systemic CNS penetrants such as high-dose methotrexate.[2]

Clinical Pearls

1. The prevalence of CNS involvement in ALL is sufficiently high that all patients should routinely receive CNS prophylaxis.

2. CNS prophylaxis in DLCBL is reserved for high-risk patients.
3. The best prophylactic strategy is yet to be determined, but regimens typically include IT chemotherapy in combination with systemic chemotherapy. Ommaya reservoir placement for IT therapy may be desirable in some patients due to the need of frequent injections and superior distribution of the drug after intraventricular administration.

CASE 23.6 PARANEOPLASTIC NEUROLOGICAL SYNDROMES

Case. A 45-year-old female presented with a subacute cerebellar syndrome. Ten years prior to presentation, she was diagnosed with mucosa-associated lymphoid tissue (MALT) lymphoma of the parotid gland and nasopharynx that required surgical resection and four infusions of rituximab. One year later, she had recurrent disease presenting with an axillary adenopathy. She received chemotherapy with R-CHOP for six cycles. She was in remission for the following 8 years.

The patient then presented for new complaints of back pain and fever, followed by 8 weeks of progressive neurological symptoms including headache, vertigo, dysarthria, diplopia, left-sided tremor, and gait difficulties.

Neurological examination was significant for mild ataxic dysarthria, nystagmus on right and left gaze, large amplitude postural and action tremor in the left upper extremity, bilateral upper and lower extremity dysmetria, and marked truncal and gait ataxia, requiring assistance to walk. She had palpable lymphadenopathy in the left groin.

Her laboratory studies were significant for anemia and leukopenia with normal platelet count. Sedimentation rate was elevated at 75 and aspartate transaminase/alanine aminotransferase were elevated at 425 and 447 mg/dL, respectively. MRI Brain showed a vascular anomaly of the left cerebellar hemisphere (which did not explain the patient's clinical presentation) but was otherwise unremarkable (Fig. 23.6). CSF studies revealed 8 WBC, mildly elevated protein (47 mg/dL), and elevated IgG synthesis rate, with no evidence of lymphoma cells. Paraneoplastic evaluation in serum and CSF were negative. PET/CT revealed widely disseminated lymphadenopathy and cutaneous lesions suggestive of lymphoma recurrence. Biopsy of the lymphadenopathy showed low-grade B-cell lymphoma with plasmacytic differentiation consistent with marginal zone lymphoma.

The patient initiated a trial with IV methylprednisolone 1000 mg daily for 3 days and then weekly for 3 weeks. She did not notice any improvement of her neurological symptoms. A decision was made to treat lymphoma with a combination of rituximab and bendamustine. After six cycles of treatment, lymphoma was in remission and PET-CT was consistent with complete response. Unfortunately, she had no improvement of her neurological symptoms and her dysarthria had worsened. She received treatment with IV immunoglobulins (IVIG) for 3 days followed by weekly for 8 weeks, followed by monthly treatments for 9 months. She initially experienced mild improvement of nystagmus and tremor but no significant improvement in functional status, with persistent severe ataxia and inability to ambulate. IVIG was tapered off and eventually discontinued without significant change in her symptoms.

Teaching Points: Clinical Spectrum of Paraneoplastic Neurological Disorders With Hematologic Malignancies. Paraneoplastic neurological syndromes are rarely associated with HL and NHL, with occurrence in less than 1% of patients (also see Chapter 20 for paraneoplastic neurological syndromes). Unlike solid tumors, patients with lymphoma who develop a paraneoplastic syndrome do not usually have limited extension at the time of diagnosis. Most patients do not have an associated onconeural antibody that is detected.[3]

The most common syndromes are limbic encephalitis and paraneoplastic cerebellar degeneration (PCD) in patients with HL, and sensorimotor neuropathies and dermatomyositis in NHL. Other reported paraneoplastic syndromes include opsoclonus-myoclonus, paraneoplastic chorea, stiff-person

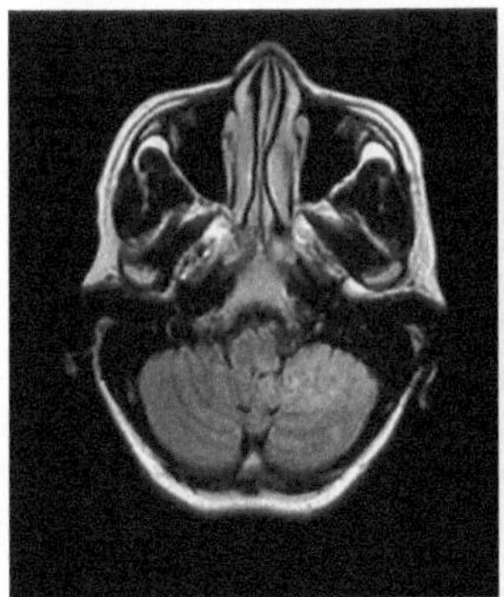
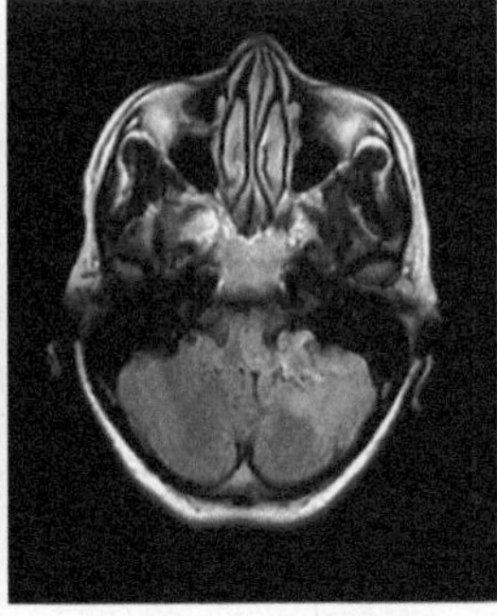
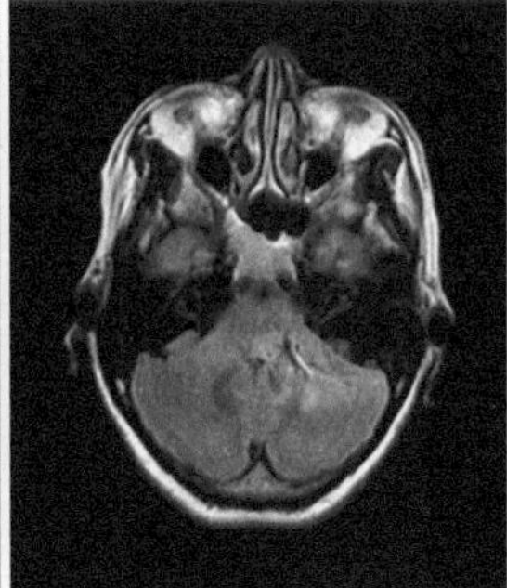
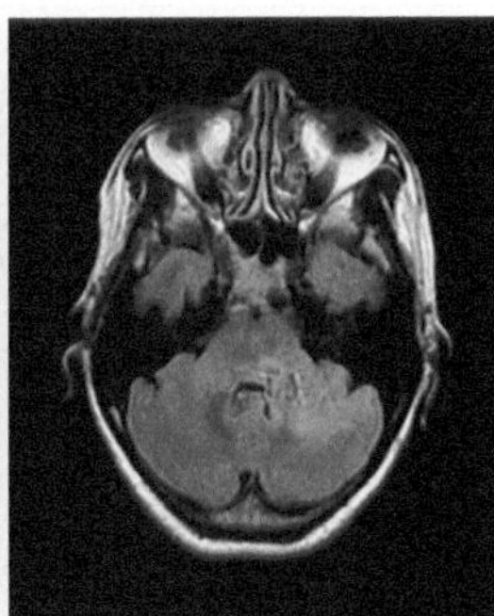

Fig. 23.6 Axial fluid-attenuated inversion recovery brain MRI showed signal abnormality involving the left cerebellar hemisphere, left cerebellar peduncles, and dorsal left pons with prominent vessels and enhancement in these regions. Findings were consistent with proliferative angiopathy of the left cerebellum with drainage into a developmental venous anomaly. (Clinical case courtesy of Dr. Andrew McKeon.)

syndrome, and myelopathy. Granulomatous angiitis is a unique paraneoplastic syndrome associated with HL.[3]

Limbic encephalitis associated with lymphoma is also known as Ophelia syndrome, and is typically associated with metabotropic glutamate receptor type 5 (mGluR5). Patients present with subacute memory loss, disorientation, confusion, depression/anxiety or psychosis with visual/auditory hallucinations, or paranoid ideation. Seizures can occur in one-half of patients. MRI demonstrates increased T2 signal in the hippocampi. Treatment of the tumor usually results in full neurologic recovery.[18]

PCD is typically associated with anti-Tr antibodies. Patients present with dizziness and vertigo that rapidly progress to severe truncal and limb ataxia, dysarthria, diplopia, and nystagmus. CSF examination usually shows pleocytosis, and the MRI studies are initially normal and later show cerebellar atrophy. PCD precedes the diagnosis of HL in 80% of the patients. The prognosis is better than that of PCD associated with solid tumors.[19] Paraneoplastic cerebellar ataxia in patients with lymphoma has also been associated with mGluR1 antibodies.[20]

Granulomatous angiitis of the CNS is a necrotizing vasculitis involving small arteries and veins along with noninfectious granulomas composed of lymphocytes, monocytes, and plasma cells. The disorder may precede or occur shortly after the diagnosis of HL. Patients present with headache, encephalopathy, and focal neurological deficits. Stroke and seizures may occur. CSF analysis is usually abnormal, with lymphocytic pleocytosis and elevated protein. Brain MRI may demonstrate small infarcts in multiple vascular territories, T2 white matter changes, gadolinium-enhancing lesions that follow a perivascular pattern, or, less frequently, hemorrhagic lesions. Cerebral angiography may show small vessel beading, suggestive of vasculitis, but it has low sensitivity. Biopsy may be needed for confirmation. Treatment is with cyclophosphamide and steroids. Patients usually recover completely after this treatment and treatment for the underlying HL.[21]

Clinical Pearls

1. Paraneoplastic syndromes are rarely associated with HL and NHL, and most cases have negative onconeural antibodies.
2. Patients with low-grade lymphomas may have accompanying devastating paraneoplastic neurological disorders. Some of these patients respond to immunotherapy.
3. PCA-Tr, mGluR1, and mGluR5 are well-recognized biomarkers of paraneoplastic neurological syndromes associated with HL.
4. Granulomatous angiitis is a unique paraneoplastic syndrome associated with HL.

Conclusion

Neurological complications associated with hematologic malignancies may occur via direct invasion of the CNS or via indirect mechanisms such as paraneoplastic syndromes. They occur more frequently in patients with NHL. Early recognition and treatment of these complications are essential to improve patient outcomes.

Acknowledgments

We thank Dr. Andrew McKeon (Departments of Laboratory Medicine and Pathology and Neurology, Mayo Clinic, Rochester, Minnesota) for providing Case 23.6: Paraneoplastic neurological syndrome.

References

1. Mauermann ML. Neurologic complications of lymphoma, leukemia, and paraproteinemias. *Continuum*. 2017;23(3):669–690.
2. Kansara R. Central nervous system prophylaxis strategies in diffuse large B cell lymphoma. *Curr Treat Options Oncol*. 2018;19(11):52.
3. Graus F, Ariño H, Dalmau J. Paraneoplastic neurological syndromes in Hodgkin and non-Hodgkin lymphomas. *Blood*. 2014;123(21):3230–3238.
4. Meng X, Yu J, Fan Q, et al. Characteristics and outcomes of non-Hodgkin's lymphoma patients with leptomeningeal metastases. *Int J Clin Oncol*. 2018;23(4):783–789.
5. Grier J, Batchelor T. Metastatic neurologic complications of non-Hodgkin's lymphoma. *Curr Oncol Rep*. 2005;7(1):55–60.
6. Grimm S, Chamberlain M. Hodgkin's lymphoma: a review of neurologic complications. *Adv Hematol*. 2011;2011:1–7.
7. Ahluwalia MS, Wallace PK, Peereboom DM. Flow cytometry as a diagnostic tool in lymphomatous or leukemic meningitis. *Cancer*. 2012;118(7):1747–1753.
8. Colocci N, Glantz M, Recht L. Prevention and treatment of central nervous system involvement by non-Hodgkin's lymphoma: a review of the literature. *Semin Neurol*. 2004;24(4):395–404.
9. Kridel R, Dietrich PY. Prevention of CNS relapse in diffuse large B-cell lymphoma. *Lancet Oncol*. 2011;12(13):1258–1266.
10. Nagle SJ, Shah NN, Ganetsky A, et al. Long-term outcomes of rituximab, temozolomide and high-dose methotrexate without consolidation therapy for lymphoma involving the CNS. *Int J Hematol Oncol*. 2017;6(4):113–121.
11. Soussain C, Choquet S, Blonski M, et al. Ibrutinib monotherapy for relapse or refractory primary CNS lymphoma and primary vitreoretinal lymphoma: final analysis of the phase II "proof-of-concept" iLOC study by the lymphoma study

association (LYSA) and the french oculo-cerebral lymphoma (LOC) network. *Eur J Cancer*. 2019;117:121–130.
12. Goldfinger M, Xu M, Bertino JR, Cooper DL. Checking in on lenalidomide in diffuse large B cell lymphoma. *Clin Lymphoma Myeloma Leuk*. 2019;19(6):e307–e311.
13. Higgins SA, Peschel RE. Hodgkin's disease with spinal cord compression. A case report and a review of the literature. *Cancer*. 1995;75(1):94–98.
14. Muss HB, Moloney WC. Chloroma and other myeloblastic tumors. *Blood*. 1973;42(5):721–728.
15. Svien HJ, Price RD, Bayrd ED. Neurosurgical treatment of compression of the spinal cord caused by myeloma. *J Am Med Assoc*. 1953;153(9):784–786.
16. Baehring JM, Batchelor TT. Diagnosis and management of neurolymphomatosis. *Cancer J*. 2012;18(5):463–468.
17. Larson RA. Managing CNS disease in adults with acute lymphoblastic leukemia. *Leuk Lymphoma*. 2018;59(1):3–13.
18. Lancaster E, Martinez-Hernandez E, Titulaer MJ, et al. Antibodies to metabotropic glutamate receptor 5 in the Ophelia syndrome. *Neurology*. 2011;77(18):1698–1701.
19. Bernal F, Shams'ili S, Rojas I, et al. Anti-Tr antibodies as markers of paraneoplastic cerebellar degeneration and Hodgkin's disease. *Neurology*. 2003;60(2):230–234.
20. Lopez-Chiriboga AS, Komorowski L, Kümpfel T, et al. Metabotropic glutamate receptor type 1 autoimmunity: clinical features and treatment outcomes. *Neurology*. 2016;86(11):1009–1013.
21. Lopez-Chiriboga AS, Sebastian Lopez-Chiriboga A, Yoon JW, et al. Granulomatous angiitis of the central nervous system associated with Hodgkin's lymphoma: case report and literature review. *J Stroke Cerebrovasc Dis*. 2018;27(1):e5–e8.

Chapter 24

Approach to the patient with radiation necrosis

Jiayi Huang, Lauren E. Henke, and Jian L. Campian

CHAPTER OUTLINE

Introduction

Cerebral radiation necrosis is a challenging and potentially devastating complication of cranial irradiation. Based on the temporal relationship to radiation therapy (RT), it can be classified as pseudoprogression (a form of early subacute injury) or radiation necrosis (a form of delayed injury). Pseudoprogression typically occurs within 3 months of fractionated RT and usually reverses spontaneously after a few weeks. Delayed radiation necrosis typically develops months or years after RT and is considered more irreversible. Radiation necrosis can have a waxing and waning clinical course but may also be relentlessly progressive.[1,2] The pathophysiology is attributed to a combination of vascular endothelial cell damage, glial cell injury, and immune-mediated reactions. These cascading events lead to increased permeability of the blood-brain barrier, followed by coagulative necrosis and demyelination.[3] Vascular endothelial growth factor (VEGF) and hypoxia-inducible factor 1α appear to be increased in the tumor micro-environment and may play important roles in the development of radiation necrosis.[4,5]

Diagnosis

Both early pseudoprogression and delayed radiation necrosis are typically characterized by increased contrast-enhancement or the appearance of ring-enhancing lesions on T1-weighed magnetic resonance imaging (MRI) sequences as well as increased vasogenic edema on T2-weighed MRI sequences. These changes may be accompanied by neurological symptoms such as headache, seizure, speech difficulty, cognitive dysfunction, or vision deficits. The clinical and imaging characteristics are indistinguishable from tumor progression or recurrence. However, they typically regress over time, and surgical resection of enhancing lesions reveals extensive necrotic tissues that may also contain minimal viable tumor cells that exhibit significant treatment-related changes.[1,2]

The diagnosis of radiation necrosis can be very challenging and can pose significant dilemma for treating physicians. Prolonged follow-up of the clinical course with imaging is often preferred; surgery with histopathologic confirmation is the gold standard for confirming the diagnosis.[2,6] However, surgery is not always possible or preferable, and observation may risk delaying salvage treatment for recurrent tumor. Advanced imaging techniques, such as MR perfusion, MR spectroscopy, and positron emission tomography (PET), have been reported by different institutional studies as effective at distinguishing radiation necrosis from tumor recurrence with mixed results.[1,6,7]

MR perfusion. In one of the largest studies on MR perfusion, Barajas et al. retrospectively analyzed 57 glioblastoma (GBM) patients who developed progressively enlarging lesions within the RT fields after chemoradiotherapy and were evaluated using MR perfusion. Their study cohort consisted of 40 patients who had histologic confirmation of recurrent tumor, 15 with histologically confirmed radiation necrosis, and 2 with clinically diagnosed radiation necrosis. Although relative cerebral blood volume (rCBV), the common parameter used to analyze MR perfusion, was statistically higher among the recurrent tumor cohort than the radiation necrosis cohort, there was significant overlap between the two groups. Overall, rCBV did not reliably distinguish recurrent GBM from radiation necrosis (sensitivity: 79%; specificity: 72%). This study showed that relative peak height (rPH), a less common parameter to analyze MR perfusion, was more accurate (sensitivity: 89%; specificity: 81%).[8] However, these findings have not been consistently replicated in other retrospective studies.[6]

MR spectroscopy. MR spectroscopy measures metabolic composition of tissue such as lipid and choline to distinguish tumor and necrosis. However, it suffers from poor spatial resolution and low reproducibility, and its accuracy has been mixed in the literature.[6,9,10]

Positron emission tomography (PET). Fluorodeoxyglucose (FDG)-based PET has generally shown modest predictive accuracy for distinguishing radiation necrosis from recurrent tumor in small retrospective studies, with sensitivity ranging from 65–81% and specificity ranging from 40–94%. Normal brain unfortunately exhibits variable FDG update and can obscure the uptake of a tumor. Radiation necrosis can also trigger repair mechanisms to increase glucose uptake, leading to a false-positive interpretation.[7] Novel amino acid tracers, such as 3,4-dihydroxy-6-(18F)-fluoro-phenylalanine (FDOPA) or (18F)-fluciclovine, may be superior to FDG for PET evaluation of suspected radiation necrosis but are not widely available in most clinics.[11] To date, none of these advanced imaging techniques have been validated in large prospective studies to reliably diagnose radiation necrosis from recurrent tumor. Thus, findings should be interpreted with caution and evaluated as part of the larger context of the patient's clinical course and other risk factors for radiation necrosis or recurrent tumor. Suspected radiation necrosis cases should ideally be managed by an experienced multidisciplinary team of neurosurgeons, radiation oncologists, and neuro-oncologists.

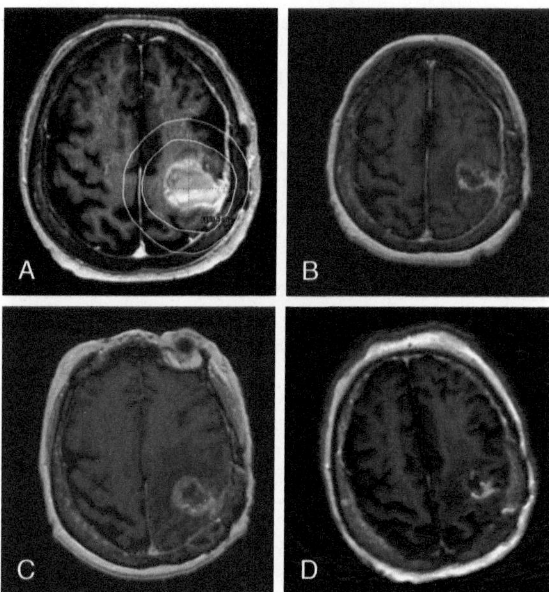

Fig. 24.1 A case of pseudoprogression of glioblastoma with *MGMT* methylation after radiation therapy (RT) and concurrent temozolomide chemotherapy. (A) T1 post-contrast axial sequence of the simulation MRI before RT (*yellow line* represents 60 Gy isodose line; *blue line* represents 46 Gy isodose line). (B) T1 post-contrast axial sequence of the MRI 1 month after RT. (C) T1 post-contrast axial sequence of the MRI 3 months after RT while receiving adjuvant temozolomide. (D) T1 post-contrast axial sequence of the MRI 5 months after RT without change of treatment, showing improvement of enhancement.

Clinical cases

CASE 24.1 PSEUDOPROGRESSION IN GLIOMA

Case. A 69-year-old female with a newly diagnosed, *IDH*-wildtype, *MGMT* promoter methylated GBM underwent a gross total resection and then received standard fractionated RT of 60 Gy in 30 fractions (Fig. 24.1A) with concurrent temozolomide. One month after completion of chemoradiotherapy, her MRI was stable (Fig. 24.1B). However, 3 months after RT, there was increased enhancement around the resection cavity (Fig. 24.1C), with the radiology report stating "increased thick rim of enhancement around the resection cavity with associated elevated cerebral blood volume and markedly increased surrounding T2 hyperintensity, concerning for tumor progression." She was continued on adjuvant temozolomide, and her MRI subsequently improved without changing her treatment (Fig. 24.1D).

Teaching Points. Approximately 20–30% of glioma patients can develop early pseudoprogression in the weeks after standard fractionated RT. As was the case for the patient presented in this case, imaging reveals findings that mimic those of tumor progression; however, in the case of pseudoprogression, serial imaging subsequently shows improvement or resolution of contrast enhancement and perilesional vasogenic edema.

The Response Assessment in Neuro-Oncology (RANO) criteria recommend that when there is worsening enhancement on MRI within 3 months of RT, progression should only be defined if the new enhancement is outside of the high-dose region (80% isodose line) of RT or if surgery confirms recurrent tumor.[12] Recognition of this phenomenon is important to accurately counsel patients and to prevent premature discontinuation of effective adjuvant therapy. Concurrent chemotherapy, immunotherapy, and tumor-specific factors such as methylation of *MGMT* gene promoter appear to increase the risk of pseudoprogression.[13–15] Interestingly, pseudoprogression has recently been reported to be less common in oligodendrogliomas with 1p/19q codeletion than *IDH*-mutant or *IDH*-wildtype astrocytomas.[16,17]

Clinical Pearls

1. Pseudoprogression is an earlier and reversible form of radiation necrosis that typically occurs within 3 months of chemoradiotherapy for glioma and resolves spontaneously.
2. Although there is no imaging modality proven to provide accurate diagnosis of radiation necrosis, MR perfusion, MR spectroscopy, or PET may be considered to help supplement the diagnostic workup.

CASE 24.2 DELAYED RADIATION NECROSIS IN GLIOMA

Case. A 56-year-old male with a grade 3 anaplastic oligodendroglioma with 1p/19q co-deletion, *IDH* mutation, and *MGMT* methylation underwent a subtotal resection. He subsequently received adjuvant chemotherapy of procarbazine/lomustine/vincristine, followed by RT using proton beam therapy to 59.4 Gy (Gray) relative biological equivalents (RBE, Fig. 24.2A). Restaging MRI after RT demonstrated stable postsurgical changes (Fig. 24.2B). Approximately 1 year after RT, MRI showed an enhancing lesion abutting the left lateral ventricle and increased enhancement around the resection cavity (Fig. 24.2C). MRI perfusion and PET were concerning for progression. Multiple core biopsies showed necrosis only, and laser interstitial thermal therapy (LITT) of the enhancing region was performed. Enhancement subsequently recurred with worsening symptoms of confusion and headache. LITT was performed again, and the patient was treated with 6 months of bevacizumab with significant improvement of the enhancement and his symptoms (Fig. 24.2D).

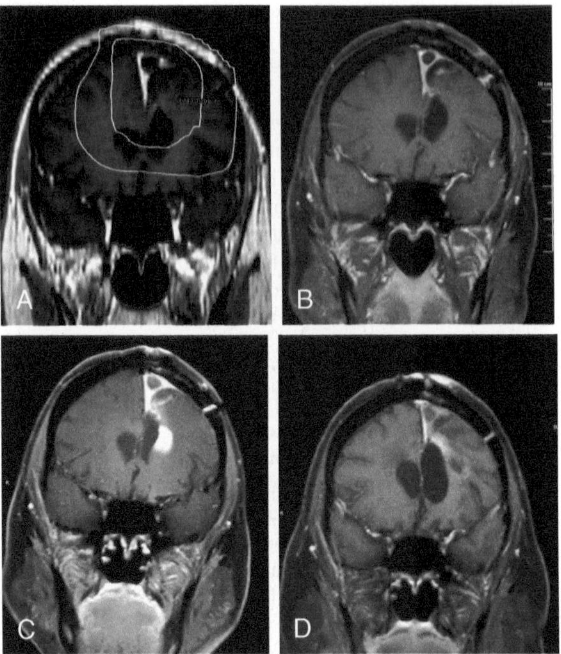

Fig. 24.2 A case of delayed radiation necrosis of 1p/19q co-deleted oligodendroglioma after proton beam therapy (PBT) and sequential procarbazine/lomustine/vincristine chemotherapy. (A) T1 post-contrast coronal sequence of the simulation MRI before PBT (*yellow line* represents 59.4 Gy (RBE) isodose line; *blue line* represents 45 Gy (RBE) isodose line). (B) T1 post-contrast coronal sequence of the MRI 1 month after PBT. (C) T1 post-contrast coronal sequence of the MRI 1 year after PBT demonstrating new enhancement. (D) T1 post-contrast coronal sequence of the MRI after laser ablation and 6 months of bevacizumab showing improved enhancement.

Teaching Points. Delayed radiation necrosis occurs in approximately 5–10% of glioma patients treated with standard fractionated RT. The median latency time of developing symptomatic radiation necrosis is approximately 1 year after RT, with the vast majority occurring within 2 years of RT. As with the patient presented in this case, radiation necrosis may follow a progressive course with recurrence of imaging findings even after initial surgical treatment.

The risk of radiation necrosis appears to be related to radiation dose, radiation fraction size, and chemotherapy use.[18] There are emerging data that 1p/19q co-deleted oligodendrogliomas may have increased risk of developing radiation necrosis than non–co-deleted astrocytomas, exhibiting relative steep dose-volume response when increasing volumes of brain are irradiated to 60 Gy. For example, a 5% increase of the percent of brain volume receiving 60 Gy is associated with approximately a 10% increase of radiation necrosis incidence for oligodendrogliomas.[19]

Clinical Pearls

1. Delayed radiation necrosis can occur months or years after fractionated RT and can continue to wax and wane even after surgical resection.
2. Surgical resection or prolonged follow up of clinical course remains the best way to establish the diagnosis of radiation necrosis at the current time.

CASE 24.3 RADIATION NECROSIS AFTER RADIOSURGERY

Case. A 72-year-old female with metastatic mesothelioma and a right temporal lobe brain metastasis was treated with a single-fraction stereotactic radiosurgery (SRS) of 21 Gy prescribed to 50% isodose line (Fig. 24.3A). She also received pemetrexed chemotherapy 3 weeks before SRS and 1 day after SRS. Three months after SRS, she developed confusion requiring hospitalization, and her MRI showed significant increase of the right temporal enhancing lesion with surrounding vasogenic edema (Fig. 24.3B). MR spectroscopy was suggestive of tumor progression. However, biopsy showed only necrosis. She was then treated with steroid with gradual resolution of the increased enhancement and edema on subsequent serial MRIs (Fig. 24.3C, D).

Teaching Points. Brain metastases are increasingly treated with SRS, typically consisting of a single fraction of high-dose RT delivered with stereotactic guidance.[20,21] The incidence of symptomatic radiation necrosis for brain metastases after single-fraction SRS is approximately 18% at 1 year.[22,23] For single-fraction SRS, the volume of brain receiving 12 Gy and tumor location appears to be the most predictive factors for radiation necrosis.[24,25] In particular, the peri-ventricular white matter is a common site of radiation necrosis, potentially owing to its relatively poor blood supply.[25a] There have been mixed reports whether concurrent administration of chemotherapy, immunotherapy, or targeted therapy with SRS may increase the risk of radiation necrosis.[26–29]

Clinical Pearls

1. In cases of suspected radiation necrosis, early involvement of a multidisciplinary team that includes neurosurgeons, radiation oncologists, and neuro-oncologists is recommended.
2. Asymptomatic cases should be initially observed with close monitoring.
3. For symptomatic cases, corticosteroids are the initial mainstay of treatment.
4. Additional treatment options for mild cases include Vitamin E and pentoxifylline; for more severe cases, surgery, interstitial laser ablation, bevacizumab, or hyperbaric oxygen may be considered.

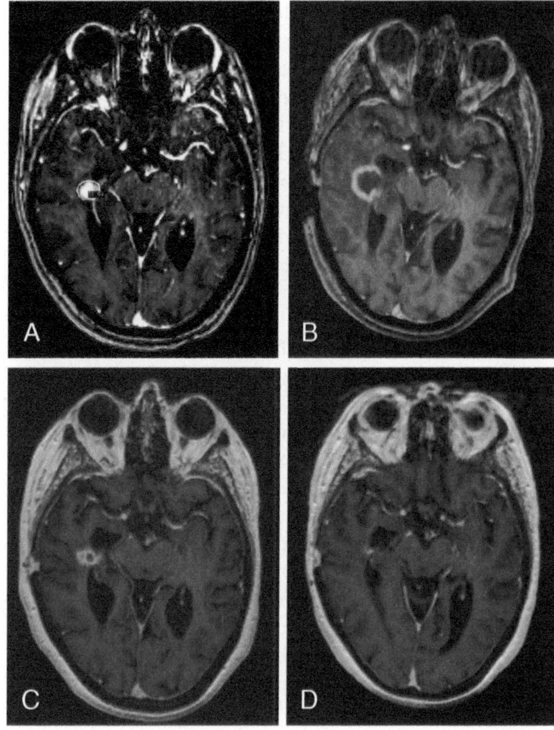

Fig. 24.3 A case of radiation necrosis of brain metastasis after stereotactic radiosurgery. (A) T1 post-contrast axial sequence on the planning MRI for radiosurgery (*yellow line* represents 21 Gy isodose line). (B) T1 post-contrast axial sequence of the MRI 3 months after radiosurgery showing increased enhancement. (C) T1 post-contrast axial sequence of the MRI 6 months after radiosurgery showing decreased size of the enhancing lesion. (D) T1 post-contrast axial sequence of the MRI 12 months after radiosurgery showing near complete resolution of enhancement.

Treatment of radiation necrosis

For suspected radiation necrosis in asymptomatic patients or with relatively small lesions, observation with shorter-interval MRI should be the first step, as many may stabilize or regress on follow-up MRI. Asymptomatic patients should be followed closely, as they may also deteriorate suddenly, and patients should contact their physicians if developing neurological symptoms. In patients with clinical symptoms or significant vasogenic edema, corticosteroids are considered first-line treatment.

Vitamin E and pentoxifylline. A small pilot study of 11 suspected patients with radiation necrosis evaluated the benefit of oral pentoxifylline 400 mg and vitamin E 400 IU twice a day and reported improvement of edema in all except one patient who subsequently was found to have recurrent tumor.[30] Given the overall tolerability and inexpensive cost of pentoxifylline and vitamin E, it is our practice to use them either alone or in conjunction with corticosteroids in mild or moderate cases and have observed anecdotal improvement in our practice. We typically continue pentoxifylline and vitamin E for 1 to 2 years as long as the patient is tolerating them and if there is observed improvement.

Surgery. For more severe cases or for corticosteroid-refractory cases, surgical resection should be entertained, which can be not only diagnostic but also therapeutic. Laser interstitial thermal therapy (LITT) is a new, minimally invasive laser ablation technique that has also shown promising results to treat radiation necrosis (see Chapter 2, Case 2.3 for further discussion of LITT as a surgical treatment).[31–33] Biopsy can be performed before laser ablation to help aid in the diagnosis. Although the exact mechanism is unclear, LITT may ablate the reactive astrocytes in the radiation necrosis region to decrease VEGF production.[32] In a recent multicenter prospective study, 44 brain metastasis patients with progressive lesions after SRS were treated with LITT. Biopsy at the time of LITT showed recurrent tumor in 20 cases (48%), radiation necrosis in 19 cases (45%), and non-diagnostic in 3 cases (7%). At the 3-month follow-up, 31% of patients stopped or reduced corticosteroid use. Among the confirmed radiation necrosis cases, the local progression-free survival rate was 91%. LITT was fairly well tolerated, with 12% of cases incurring immediate treatment-related neurological complication.[31]

Bevacizumab. If surgery or LITT is not possible, bevacizumab may be considered as the second-line medical therapy for steroid-refractory cases, which is supported by both retrospective and prospective studies.[34–37] In a small double-blinded, placebo-controlled study, 14 patients were randomized to receive either placebo or intravenous bevacizumab at a dose of 7.5 mg/kg every 3-week cycle for two cycles. The responding patients would receive two additional cycles, and non-responding patients would cross over to the other arm. None of the seven placebo patients had clinical or radiologic improvement, but all seven bevacizumab patients and the crossed-over placebo patients responded clinically and radiologically.[36] A larger, single-arm prospective study subsequently treated 38 inoperable and corticosteroid-refractory radiation necrosis patients with bevacizumab. In additional to prior corticosteroids, 53% of patients also had been treated with vitamin E, 47% anticoagulant, 11% had prior surgery, and 8% had received hyperbaric oxygen. Among this heavily treated refractory population they observed 79% radiologic response (≥30% reduction of perilesional edema continuing for ≥1 month) at 3 months, 42% improvement of performance status, and 76% with steroid reduction. Grade 3 adverse events occurred in 24% of patients, including hypertension, elevated liver enzymes, seizure, and anemia. Grade 2 intracranial hemorrhage and venous thromboembolic event occurred in 3% and 2% of patients, respectively.[38] Patients with cerebral hemorrhage or pulmonary embolism may not be able to receive bevacizumab. Bevacizumab may also cause vascular insufficiency and worsening hypoxia, which can lead to worsening radiation necrosis.[39] Since bevacizumab also has anti-neoplastic effects and is a second-line agent for recurrent glioma, initial response to bevacizumab may not confirm the diagnosis of radiation necrosis, so close follow-up is warranted. Alternatively, it has also been our clinical experience that we have had patients who initially received bevacizumab for presumed recurrent glioma and subsequently had clinical and radiologic resolution that remained stable off bevacizumab for many years. In hindsight, these cases were likely radiation necrosis.

Hyperbaric oxygen therapy. For severe radiation necrosis cases that do not respond to bevacizumab or where bevacizumab is contraindicated, hyperbaric oxygen may be considered and is supported by multiple small retrospective studies.[40–43] Hyperbaric oxygen treatment consists of a chamber with 100% oxygen with 2–2.5 times normal atmospheric pressure. The treatment is delivered 5 days a week for 20–60 sessions. The primary contraindication is uncontrolled seizure.[44] Given its more extensive time commitment, limited available facilities, and lack of prospective data, the authors would typically consider bevacizumab first before hyperbaric oxygen. However, in our practice, we have also anecdotally observed improvement of selected bevacizumab-refractory radiation necrosis cases using hyperbaric oxygen.

Conclusion

Radiation necrosis is a challenging complication after RT and can resemble recurrent tumor. Pseudoprogression is an earlier and reversible form of radiation necrosis that typically occurs within 3 months of chemoradiotherapy for glioma and resolves spontaneously. Delayed radiation necrosis can occur months or years after fractionated RT or SRS and can be more waxing and waning. Although there is no single imaging modality proven to provide accurate diagnosis of radiation necrosis, MR perfusion, MR spectroscopy, or PET may be considered to supplement the diagnostic workup. Surgical resection or prolonged follow-up of clinical course remains the best way to establish the diagnosis of radiation necrosis at the current time. As the diagnosis and management of radiation necrosis can be complex, early involvement of a multidisciplinary team consisting of neurosurgeons, radiation oncologists, and neuro-oncologists is recommended. Asymptomatic cases should be initially observed with close monitoring. For symptomatic cases, corticosteroids and/or pentoxifylline plus vitamin E should be considered. For more severe cases, surgery, interstitial laser ablation, bevacizumab, or hyperbaric oxygen may be considered depending on the clinical situation.

References

1. Chao ST, Ahluwalia MS, Barnett GH, et al. Challenges with the diagnosis and treatment of cerebral radiation necrosis. *Int J Radiat Oncol Biol Phys*. 2013;87(3):449–457.
2. Giglio P, Gilbert MR. Cerebral radiation necrosis. *Neurologist*. 2003;9(4):180–188.

3. Rahmathulla G, Marko NF, Weil RJ. Cerebral radiation necrosis: a review of the pathobiology, diagnosis and management considerations. *J Clin Neurosci*. 2013;20(4):485–502.
4. Nonoguchi N, Miyatake S, Fukumoto M, et al. The distribution of vascular endothelial growth factor-producing cells in clinical radiation necrosis of the brain: pathological consideration of their potential roles. *J Neurooncol*. 2011;105(2):423–431.
5. Nordal RA, Nagy A, Pintilie M, Wong CS. Hypoxia and hypoxia-inducible factor-1 target genes in central nervous system radiation injury: a role for vascular endothelial growth factor. *Clin Cancer Res*. 2004;10(10):3342–3353.
6. Huang J, Wang AM, Shetty A, et al. Differentiation between intra-axial metastatic tumor progression and radiation injury following fractionated radiation therapy or stereotactic radiosurgery using MR spectroscopy, perfusion MR imaging or volume progression modeling. *Magn Reson Imaging*. 2011;29(7):993–1001.
7. Verma N, Cowperthwaite MC, Burnett MG, Markey MK. Differentiating tumor recurrence from treatment necrosis: a review of neuro-oncologic imaging strategies. *Neuro Oncol*. 2013;15(5):515–534.
8. Barajas Jr RF, Chang JS, Segal MR, et al. Differentiation of recurrent glioblastoma multiforme from radiation necrosis after external beam radiation therapy with dynamic susceptibility-weighted contrast-enhanced perfusion MR imaging. *Radiology*. 2009;253(2):486–496.
9. Schlemmer HP, Bachert P, Herfarth KK, Zuna I, Debus J, van Kaick G. Proton MR spectroscopic evaluation of suspicious brain lesions after stereotactic radiotherapy. *AJNR Am J Neuroradiol*. 2001;22(7):1316–1324.
10. Zeng QS, Li CF, Zhang K, Liu H, Kang XS, Zhen JH. Multivoxel 3D proton MR spectroscopy in the distinction of recurrent glioma from radiation injury. *J Neurooncol*. 2007;84(1):63–69.
11. Chen W, Silverman DH, Delaloye S, et al. 18F-FDOPA PET imaging of brain tumors: comparison study with 18F-FDG PET and evaluation of diagnostic accuracy. *J Nucl Med*. 2006;47(6):904–911.
12. Wen PY, Macdonald DR, Reardon DA, et al. Updated response assessment criteria for high-grade gliomas: response assessment in neuro-oncology working group. *J Clin Oncol*. 2010;28(11):1963–1972.
13. Brandes AA, Franceschi E, Tosoni A, et al. MGMT promoter methylation status can predict the incidence and outcome of pseudoprogression after concomitant radiochemotherapy in newly diagnosed glioblastoma patients. *J Clin Oncol*. 2008;26(13):2192–2197.
14. Brandsma D, Stalpers L, Taal W, Sminia P, van den Bent MJ. Clinical features, mechanisms, and management of pseudoprogression in malignant gliomas. *Lancet Oncol*. 2008;9(5):453–461.
15. Roth P, Valavanis A, Weller M. Long-term control and partial remission after initial pseudoprogression of glioblastoma by anti-PD-1 treatment with nivolumab. *Neuro Oncol*. 2017;19(3):454–456.
16. Lin AL, Liu J, Evans J, et al. Codeletions at 1p and 19q predict a lower risk of pseudoprogression in oligodendrogliomas and mixed oligoastrocytomas. *Neuro Oncol*. 2014;16(1):123–130.
17. Lin AL, White M, Miller-Thomas MM, et al. Molecular and histologic characteristics of pseudoprogression in diffuse gliomas. *J Neurooncol*. 2016;130(3):529–533.
18. Ruben JD, Dally M, Bailey M, Smith R, McLean CA, Fedele P. Cerebral radiation necrosis: incidence, outcomes, and risk factors with emphasis on radiation parameters and chemotherapy. *Int J Radiat Oncol Biol Phys*. 2006;65(2):499–508.
19. Acharya S, Robinson CG, Michalski JM, et al. Association of 1p/19q codeletion and radiation necrosis in adult cranial gliomas after proton or photon therapy. *Int J Radiat Oncol Biol Phys*. 2018;101(2):334–343.
20. Brown PD, Jaeckle K, Ballman KV, et al. Effect of radiosurgery alone vs radiosurgery with whole brain radiation therapy on cognitive function in patients with 1 to 3 brain metastases: a randomized clinical trial. *JAMA*. 2016;316(4):401–409.
21. Yamamoto M, Serizawa T, Shuto T, et al. Stereotactic radiosurgery for patients with multiple brain metastases (JLGK0901): a multi-institutional prospective observational study. *Lancet Oncol*. 2014;15(4):387–395.
22. Kohutek ZA, Yamada Y, Chan TA, et al. Long-term risk of radionecrosis and imaging changes after stereotactic radiosurgery for brain metastases. *J Neurooncol*. 2015;125(1):149–156.
23. Minniti G, Scaringi C, Paolini S, et al. Single-fraction versus multifraction (3 × 9 Gy) stereotactic radiosurgery for large (>2 cm) brain metastases: a comparative analysis of local control and risk of radiation-induced brain necrosis. *Int J Radiat Oncol Biol Phys*. 2016;95(4):1142–1148.
24. Flickinger JC, Kondziolka D, Maitz AH, Lunsford LD. Analysis of neurological sequelae from radiosurgery of arteriovenous malformations: how location affects outcome. *Int J Radiat Oncol Biol Phys*. 1998;40(2):273–278.
25. Minniti G, Clarke E, Lanzetta G, et al. Stereotactic radiosurgery for brain metastases: analysis of outcome and risk of brain radionecrosis. *Radiat Oncol*. 2011;6:48.
25a. Shah R, Vattoth S, Jacob R, et al. Radiation necrosis in the brain: imaging features and differentiation from tumor recurrence. *Radiographics*. 2012;32(5):1343–1359.
26. Colaco RJ, Martin P, Kluger HM, Yu JB, Chiang VL. Does immunotherapy increase the rate of radiation necrosis after radiosurgical treatment of brain metastases? *J Neurosurg*. 2016;125(1):17–23.
27. Fang P, Jiang W, Allen P, et al. Radiation necrosis with stereotactic radiosurgery combined with CTLA-4 blockade and PD-1 inhibition for treatment of intracranial disease in metastatic melanoma. *J Neurooncol*. 2017;133(3):595–602.
28. Kim JM, Miller JA, Kotecha R, et al. The risk of radiation necrosis following stereotactic radiosurgery with concurrent systemic therapies. *J Neurooncol*. 2017;133(2):357–368.
29. Tallet AV, Dhermain F, Le Rhun E, Noël G, Kirova YM. Combined irradiation and targeted therapy or immune checkpoint blockade in brain metastases: toxicities and efficacy. *Ann Oncol*. 2017;28(12):2962–2976.
30. Williamson R, Kondziolka D, Kanaan H, Lunsford LD, Flickinger JC. Adverse radiation effects after radiosurgery may benefit from oral vitamin E and pentoxifylline therapy: a pilot study. *Stereotact Funct Neurosurg*. 2008;86(6):359–366.
31. Ahluwalia M, Barnett GH, Deng D, et al. Laser ablation after stereotactic radiosurgery: a multicenter prospective study in patients with metastatic brain tumors and radiation necrosis. *J Neurosurg*. 2018;130(3):804–811.
32. Rahmathulla G, Recinos PF, Valerio JE, Chao S, Barnett GH. Laser interstitial thermal therapy for focal cerebral radiation necrosis: a case report and literature review. *Stereotact Funct Neurosurg*. 2012;90(3):192–200.
33. Rammo R, Asmaro K, Schultz L, et al. The safety of magnetic resonance imaging-guided laser interstitial thermal therapy for cerebral radiation necrosis. *J Neurooncol*. 2018;138(3):609–617.

34. Boothe D, Young R, Yamada Y, Prager A, Chan T, Beal K. Bevacizumab as a treatment for radiation necrosis of brain metastases post stereotactic radiosurgery. *Neuro Oncol.* 2013;15(9):1257–1263.
35. Gonzalez J, Kumar AJ, Conrad CA, Levin VA. Effect of bevacizumab on radiation necrosis of the brain. *Int J Radiat Oncol Biol Phys.* 2007;67(2):323–326.
36. Levin VA, Bidaut L, Hou P, et al. Randomized double-blind placebo-controlled trial of bevacizumab therapy for radiation necrosis of the central nervous system. *Int J Radiat Oncol Biol Phys.* 2011;79(5):1487–1495.
37. Sadraei NH, Dahiya S, Chao ST, et al. Treatment of cerebral radiation necrosis with bevacizumab: the Cleveland Clinic experience. *Am J Clin Oncol.* 2015;38(3):304–310.
38. Furuse M, Nonoguchi N, Kuroiwa T, et al. A prospective, multicentre, single-arm clinical trial of bevacizumab for patients with surgically untreatable, symptomatic brain radiation necrosis. *Neurooncol Pract.* 2016;3(4):272–280.
39. Jeyaretna DS, Curry Jr WT, Batchelor TT, Stemmer-Rachamimov A, Plotkin SR. Exacerbation of cerebral radiation necrosis by bevacizumab. *J Clin Oncol.* 2011;29(7):e159–e162.
40. Aghajan Y, Grover I, Gorsi H, Tumblin M, Crawford JR. Use of hyperbaric oxygen therapy in pediatric neuro-oncology: a single institutional experience. *J Neurooncol.* 2019;141(1):151–158.
41. Chuba PJ, Aronin P, Bhambhani K, et al. Hyperbaric oxygen therapy for radiation-induced brain injury in children. *Cancer.* 1997;80(10):2005–2012.
42. Leber KA, Eder HG, Kovac H, Anegg U, Pendl G. Treatment of cerebral radionecrosis by hyperbaric oxygen therapy. *Stereotact Funct Neurosurg.* 1998;70(suppl 1):229–236.
43. Valadao J, Pearl J, Verma S, Helms A, Whelan H. Hyperbaric oxygen treatment for post-radiation central nervous system injury: a retrospective case series. *Undersea Hyperb Med.* 2014;41(2):87–96.
44. Feldmeier JJ, Hampson NB. A systematic review of the literature reporting the application of hyperbaric oxygen prevention and treatment of delayed radiation injuries: an evidence based approach. *Undersea Hyperb Med.* 2002;29(1):4–30.

Chapter 25

Neurological complications of radiation

Christina K. Cramer and Tiffany L. Cummings

CHAPTER OUTLINE

Introduction

Cognitive abilities in glioma patients are influenced by a myriad of factors: the tumor itself, depression and anxiety, fatigue, sleep dysfunction, pre–brain tumor cognitive baseline (e.g., premorbid functioning), pain, and brain tumor treatments themselves (e.g., surgery, chemotherapy, and radiation). Most often, attention, working memory, and information processing speed are affected in brain tumor patients but a wide array of cognitive symptoms can be seen.[1] Roughly 30% or more of patients alive at 4 months after chemoradiation have deficits in cognitive functioning[2] and the proportion of patients with impairment continues to rise as a function of time after treatment. The Radiation Therapy Oncology Group (RTOG) 0525 and RTOG 0825 arguably provide the best prospectively collected neurocognitive data of high-grade glioma patients.

RTOG 0825 was a prospective, randomized phase III trial in newly diagnosed patients with glioblastoma comparing standard radiation and temozolomide (TMZ) therapy with and without bevacizumab. RTOG 0825 also prospectively collected extensive neurocognitive data on all enrolled patients. In RTOG 0525, 27% of patients were classified as "declined" using the reliable change index on Hopkins verbal learning test (HVLT)-R scores at 4 months post-radiation.

Patients often experience cognitive dysfunction at baseline and following treatment that can range from mildly to severely affecting functional independence, return to work, and quality of life. Tucha et al. found cognitive impairment in over 90% of patients with supratentorial brain tumors prior to treatment.[3] The domains affected can vary but mainly include difficulties in attention/executive functioning, learning and retrieval, and motor speed. The rate of tumor growth is a predictor of cognitive impairment. In general, rapidly growing tumors like high-grade gliomas present with greater dysfunction and more widespread cognitive deficits than slow-growing, low-grade gliomas. However, the specific tumor type and tumor volume have not been shown to predict cognitive performance.[4] After chemoradiation, risk factors for the development of radiotherapy (RT)-related cognitive dysfunction include greater volume of irradiated tissue, a higher dose of RT (>2 Gy per fraction), adjuvant chemotherapy, and older age.[5,6]

Corticosteroids and antiseizure medications can also impact cognitive functioning. Although corticosteroids can improve cognitive deficits due to cerebral edema, they can also be associated with transient emotional/behavioral disturbance and attention/concentration difficulties.[7,8] Some studies show poor working memory in patients treated with antiepileptic drugs (AEDs). Others show no difference in performance when evaluating patients on newer versus older AEDs versus no AED medications.

Clinical cases

CASE 25.1 MANAGEMENT OF NEUROCOGNITIVE DYSFUNCTION IN A PATIENT WITH DIFFUSE GLIOMA AND ASSOCIATED DEPRESSION AND ANXIETY

Case. A 48-year-old, right-hand dominant Caucasian female with a master's degree presented with headache and imaging revealed a right parietal lesion measuring 2.2 × 2.3 cm on T2 fluid attenuated inversion recovery (FLAIR) imaging without enhancement or mass effect. She underwent gross total resection. Pathology revealed a WHO grade III anaplastic astrocytoma. She underwent concurrent chemotherapy (TMZ) and radiation (59.4 Gy). Preradiation neuropsychologic testing was performed after surgery and before chemoradiation. At baseline, she had high-average functioning and demonstrated difficulties with attention, concentration, executive functioning, verbal memory, and verbal fluency (Table 25.1). In addition, she had symptomatic anxiety, mild depression, and fatigue. At 3 months posttreatment, her attention and verbal memory performance had improved. However, other cognitive impairments remained stable and she continued to have symptoms of depression and anxiety. Unfortunately, she lost her job during treatment and was required to find alternative employment, exacerbating her perceived stress. Neuropsychology recommended pharmacologic intervention for treatment of her mood, referral to cancer support services for psychosocial support, and discussion of employment options. At 6 months posttreatment, impairment was noted in all areas, but her symptoms of depression and anxiety were much improved (due to pharmacologic intervention).

Teaching Points. This case highlights the multifactorial nature of neurocognitive dysfunction in patients with brain tumors. Cognition may be influenced not only by the tumor and its treatment but also by associated mood symptoms, treatment-induced fatigue, psychosocial stressors, and other factors, all of which likely contributed to the deficits in this patient. She reported significant anxiety and depressive symptoms following her diagnosis. Treatment of her mood symptoms with selective serotonin reuptake inhibitor (SSRI) therapy resulted in considerable benefit on her neurocognitive performance.

Clinical Pearls

1. The neuropsychologic evaluation should include an assessment of fatigue and depression as both occur at high rates within the brain tumor patient population and can impact cognitive functioning.
2. Neuropsychologic evaluation should be performed by a board-certified neuropsychologist who is experienced in working with brain tumor patients.
3. Neurologists and neuro-oncologists should use the neuropsychology report to guide treatment interventions which can include pharmacologic and nonpharmacologic interventions.

Table 25.1 Cognitive performance of patient in Case 25.1

	Pretreatment	Three months posttreatment	Six months posttreatment
Premorbid	86th percentile	86th percentile	86th percentile
Attention	1st percentile	4th percentile	9th percentile
Learning	21st percentile	10th percentile	2nd percentile
Memory	2nd percentile	14th percentile	1st percentile
Lexical fluency	1st percentile	3rd percentile	3rd percentile
Semantic fluency	4th percentile	1st percentile	1st percentile
Set-shifting	1st percentile	1st percentile	1st percentile
BDI-2	16/63	32/63	23/63
BAI	33/63	19/63	4/63
Fatigue	6.4/7	5.8/7	7.0/7

Lower percentiles indicate worse cognitive functioning; higher percentiles indicate better cognitive performance.
BAI, Beck Anxiety Inventory; *BDI*, Beck Depression Inventory.

CASE 25.2 MANAGEMENT OF NEUROCOGNITIVE DYSFUNCTION IN A PATIENT WITH GLIOBLASTOMA AND SLEEP DYSFUNCTION

Case. A 62-year-old, right-hand dominant Caucasian male presented after a fall and was found on imaging to have an enhancing 6.5 × 5.5 × 4.8 cm mass in the right frontal lobe. He underwent a right frontal craniotomy and pathology revealed glioblastoma. He subsequently underwent standard Stupp-style chemoradiation. Postsurgical, preradiation cognitive testing showed difficulties with effortful encoding and retrieval of novel verbal information as well as impaired visual abstract reasoning, and impaired lexical verbal fluency (Table 25.2). He had average consolidation, attention and set-shifting, and semantic verbal fluency. During his treatment course, he required prolonged corticosteroid use for management of cerebral edema and complained of severe treatment-associated fatigue and excessive daytime sleepiness. His weight increased by approximately 20 pounds during the 6 months of adjuvant chemotherapy and he developed steroid-induced myopathy and steroid-induced diabetes mellitus requiring initiation of metformin. He was found to have elevated thyroid stimulating hormone (TSH) at 10.5 IU/mL and low free thyroxine (free T4) of 2.1 ng/dL and was started on levothyroxine 50 mcg/day with improvement in thyroid studies. He was also sent for a polysomnogram which revealed obstructive sleep apnea and he was recommended to initiate home continuous positive airway pressure treatment.

At his 6-month examination, his encoding skills improved, as did his retrieval for novel verbal information though his attention and verbal fluency skills declined. He did not have any emotional/behavioral disturbance at either visit and his self-reported fatigue levels were low. Currently, he is not bothered enough by the deficits in attention or verbal fluency so no empiric treatment has been pursued.

Teaching Points. This case highlights many of the factors and their management that can be considered in high-grade glioma patients with neurocognitive dysfunction. The patient in this case developed endocrinopathy, corticosteroid-associated side effects, and was found to have newly diagnosed obstructive sleep apnea. These comorbid conditions, in combination with his underlying glioma and prior treatment, presumably contributed to the findings on neurocognitive assessment. Despite this, he was managed with minimal decline or changes in overall neurocognitive status after treatment and was able to continue to live and work independently.

Clinical Pearls

1. Cognitive impairment can indicate disease recurrence or progression so imaging should be obtained if a patient has a significant and sudden decline in cognitive performance.
2. However, cognitive impairment often increases over time after treatment for brain tumors in the absence of disease progression as a result of treatment-related damage to neural circuitry.
3. Shortened neuropsychologic examinations may be appropriate for brain tumor patients who are older or have poorer performance status as they may not have the stamina to complete a full evaluation.
4. Patients with severe cognitive impairment may not be capable of living independently. Consideration should be given in these cases to home safety evaluations, or assisted living should be discussed with the patient's family.
5. Preventive strategies are an area of very active research and include radioprotective agents, use of radiosurgery, and hippocampal-avoidance.

Table 25.2 Cognitive performance by patient in Case 25.2

	Pretreatment	Six months posttreatment
Premorbid	34th percentile	34th percentile
Attention	37th percentile	21st percentile
Learning	13th percentile	61st percentile
Memory	16th percentile	55th percentile
Lexical fluency	2nd percentile	4th percentile
Semantic fluency	93rd percentile	42nd percentile
Set-shifting	34th percentile	68th percentile
BDI-2	6/63	5/63
BAI	0/63	0/63
Fatigue	4.11/7	2.11/7

BAI, Beck Anxiety Inventory; *BDI*, Beck Depression Inventory.

Common presentations and timing of neurocognitive dysfunction after treatment

There are three phases of neurocognitive dysfunction after treatment that are classified based on the time between the administration of RT and the development of symptoms (acute, early delayed, and late delayed).[9]

- *Acute phase.* The acute phase develops shortly after the initiation of RT and may persist throughout treatment; symptoms include headache, fatigue, nausea, depression, worsening neurological signs, and problematic attention and memory skills.

- *Early delayed phase.* The early delayed phase occurs approximately a few weeks following the completion of RT to 6 months following treatment; symptoms include a transient decline in cognitive functioning (memory mainly), somnolence, fatigue, and potentially reemerging neurologic signs. The cognitive decline noted at this stage is reversible in most cases and is not predictive of deficits at later stages.[10] These effects tend to reverse by 1 year if there is no disease progression.
- *Late delayed phase.* The late delayed phase encompasses the years following treatment completion and can be identified as early as 2 years after completion, with some studies showing onset as late as 8 years posttreatment and a median of 5 years.[11] This phase is again characterized primarily by memory related deficits and is generally considered irreversible.

Serial cognitive follow-up of patients with primary brain tumors is imperative as cognitive decline can precede radiographic evidence of tumor progression by several weeks in patients with gliomas.[9,12,13]

Neurocognitive symptom cluster: neurocognitive dysfunction, fatigue, and sleep disturbance

There are multiple sources of cognitive impairment for patients with glioma; however, fatigue and sleep disturbance exacerbate subjective and objective levels of cognitive impairment in this group. Fatigue is one of the most frequently reported symptoms in patients undergoing radiation therapy and dysfunction in sleep is very closely related. Together, these symptoms produce slowing of thought and attention problems that can lead to impairments in other domains such as learning, memory, and executive functioning. These symptoms tend to be cyclical and exacerbate one another while both impact thinking at the same time.

Diagnostic evaluation and workup for neurocognitive dysfunction

When brain tumor patients or their caregivers mention cognitive impairment as a daily problem, the next step should be gathering more information. Workup generally includes an assessment of disease status to rule out progressive tumor growth and then an assessment of potential factors that may contribute to neurocognitive dysfunction (Table 25.3). Additional history should be obtained to determine the timeline of onset of the cognitive dysfunction and differentiate between rapid-onset cognitive decline versus slow, progressive cognitive deficits.

Sudden decline in cognition over days. If the decline was sudden, then a workup for delirium is undertaken. Repeat neuroimaging is often indicated in this case to rule out ischemic stroke, hemorrhage, tumor progression, or treatment-related edema. Underlying infection or pharmacologic causes should also be considered, with special attention to new medications. For patients with acute cognitive changes, inpatient hospitalization is often warranted to expedite the workup.

Slow, progressive decline in cognition over weeks. For patients with subacute or slow, progressive cognitive decline, physicians should rule out progressive disease with neuroimaging and then inquire about possible depression, review medications, and consider evaluating for endocrinopathy or metabolic abnormalities including vitamin B_{12}, folate levels, TSH, free T4, morning cortisol (in patients not taking corticosteroids), and testosterone levels (in men). Workup of cognitive dysfunction that has slowly progressed over weeks can usually be done in the outpatient setting. After brain imaging and laboratory tests, the next step is usually neuropsychologic testing (if it has not already been obtained). If there were family concerns for dementia or mild cognitive impairment prior to brain tumor diagnosis (or a strong family history of dementia), then it is also reasonable to consider the workup you would do for a patient with possible Alzheimer disease or frontotemporal dementia (which might include a lumbar puncture and brain PET scan).

In appropriate patients, excessive daytime sleepiness or other sleep dysfunction may be further evaluated to rule out comorbid obstructive sleep apnea which can contribute to

Table 25.3 **Guidelines for the diagnostic evaluation of neurocognitive dysfunction in a patient with a brain tumor**

Workup Checklist
Rule out the following: • Progressive disease with imaging • Treatment-related cerebral edema (particularly during chemoradiation) • Ischemic or hemorrhagic stroke • Infection • Medication-induced cognitive changes (e.g., especially opioids, anticholinergics, or antiepileptic medications) • Electrolyte dysfunction, kidney injury, or hepatotoxicity • Vitamin B_{12} or folate deficiency • Hormonal deficiency (e.g., thyroid, cortisol, and testosterone) • Assessment for depression • Assessment of sleep impairment/fatigue • Evaluation of obstructive sleep apnea • Neuropsychologic evaluation
• Obtain neurocognitive testing
• Treat empirically for depression and fatigue first and then memory and/or attention

neurocognitive deficits. In patients who are receiving active chemotherapy and/or radiation therapy, electrolyte disturbance and infection (e.g., urinary tract infection, pneumonia) should also be evaluated. At times, patients may develop kidney injury or uremia, hepatic toxicity, or systemic metabolic derangement that may also require laboratory investigation.

Goal of neuropsychologic testing. As imaging studies have already identified a structural lesion, the neuropsychologic evaluation in this population is not used to diagnose or localize, rather to clarify the nature and severity of cognitive impact.[13] In addition, these evaluations can assist in identifying complex emotional/behavioral and psychosocial interventions and understand concerns that, when addressed, can improve quality of life and potentially impact morbidity. Core neuropsychologic protocols include standardized instruments that have demonstrated sensitivity to the neurotoxic effects of cancer and related treatment and are typically short due to the high prevalence of fatigue in this population.

Neuropsychologic tests. The most commonly included tests are those that measure attention, executive functioning, learning and retrieval, and graphomotor speed (Table 25.4).[13–15] Assessment of emotional/behavioral functioning, fatigue, and activities of daily living is also included. Recommendations from these evaluations include psychoeducation regarding brain-behavior relationships, compensatory strategies (internal and external aids), and environmental modifications.[16,17] They can also include psychotherapy, caregiver support and education, and pharmacologic interventions.[13] Sleep hygiene and energy conservation techniques can also be offered given the treatment of sleep-related dysfunction can also contribute to cognitive and quality-of-life improvement.[18]

Treatment of neurocognitive dysfunction

Cognition directed treatment options can be partitioned into pharmacologic or nonpharmacologic treatments. Pharmacologic treatment options generally include agents used in treating dementias such as donepezil, stimulants such as methylphenidate, and wakefulness-promoting agents such as modafinil or armodafinil. Some clinicians consider off label use of other alternative agents for selected patient populations. Amantadine has been used in other disease states as a pharmacologic brain "activator" and may be attempted by some clinicians to manage bifrontal abulia. Nonpharmacologic treatments include cognitive rehabilitation and exercise programs (Table 25.5). In addition to these, treatment of associated mood, depression, anxiety, fatigue, sleep, endocrinopathy, and other associated symptoms is paramount.

Table 25.4 Common neuropsychologic tests

Test name	Skills measured	General brain ROI
Test of Premorbid Functioning (TOPF)	Pre-illness estimates of intellectual functioning from reading and demographic factors	NA
Montreal Cognitive Assessment (MoCA)	Global screening of cognitive functioning	All
Trail Making Test Part A (TMT-A) Digit Span (WAIS-IV DS)	Attention, concentration, and speed of thought	Frontal, subcortical, parietal, and cerebellar
Trail Making Test Part B (TMT-B)	Speeded cognitive set-shifting	Frontal, subcortical, and cerebellar
Hopkins Verbal Learning Test (HVLT-R)	Learning and memory	Frontal and temporal
Boston Naming Test (BNT)	Visual object naming	Temporal and parietal
Boston Diagnostic Aphasia Exam (BDAE) Complex Ideational Material	Auditory comprehension	Temporal and parietal
Controlled Oral Word Association Test (COWAT)	Verbal fluency	Frontal and temporal
Rey Complex Figure Test (RCFT)	Visual planning and organization	Frontal and parietal
Matrix Reasoning (WAIS-IV MR)	Visual abstract reasoning	Frontal
BDI-II and BAI	Emotional/behavioral status	NA
Fatigue Severity Scale	Fatigue	NA
Barthel ADL	Activities of daily living (ADL)	NA

BAI, Beck Anxiety Inventory; *BDI,* Beck Depression Inventory; *ROI,* region-of-interest; *WAIS,* Wechsler Adult Intelligence Scale.

Table 25.5 Treatment options

Symptom	Treatment	Evidence	Caution
Poor working memory	Donepezil	Secondary analysis of a randomized phase III trial[19] in brain tumor survivors showed improvement on HVLT-IR and HVLT-DR with treatment. Most effective in patients who are the most impaired.	Caution in patients with bradycardia, prolonged QT interval, or COPD.
Impaired attention or fatigue	Methylphenidate	Shown to improve attention in pediatric brain tumor survivors. Randomized phase III trial in adults[20] was negative but the study was underpowered due to patient drop-out. Can be used off-label for adults.	Cannot be used with concurrent MAOI. Cannot be used for patients with glaucoma or a history of stroke, myocardial infarction, or tachycardia.
Excessive fatigue	Armodafinil or modafinil	Randomized phase II[21] showed that armodafinil improves fatigue scores and QOL when given during and 1 month after RT for patients who have greater baseline fatigue.	Caution in patients with cardiac disease, hepatic impairment, or Tourette's syndrome.
Multiple impairments	Cognitive rehabilitation	Randomized trial[22,23] showed that a 7-week rehabilitation program improved self-reported cognitive function immediately after completion of the program and improved performance on cognitive testing 6 months after rehabilitation.	

COPD, Chronic obstructive pulmonary disease; *DR,* delayed recall; *HVLT,* Hopkins verbal learning test; *IR,* immediate recall; *MAOI,* monoamine oxidase inhibitor; *QOL,* quality of life; *RT,* radiotherapy.

Treatment of associated symptoms

Treatment of depression in brain tumor patients is analogous to treatment in non–brain tumor patients except that special attention needs to be paid to potential interactions with their other medications and to whether they have been having uncontrolled seizures. Most often, starting with SSRIs or serotonin–norepinephrine reuptake inhibitors is reasonable and makes sense. For treating sleep dysfunction, melatonin is often an initial step. Sedative-hypnotic medications such as zolpidem, eszopiclone, and others risk worsening of neurocognition, even those that are non-benzodiazepine classes of agents. Medical complications of treatment such as endocrinopathy must be recognized and interventions considered according to laboratory results (see Chapter 19 for discussion of the approach to posttreatment endocrinopathy).

Conclusion

A high proportion of patients with primary or metastatic brain tumors have cognitive impairment, which can range from mild to severe. Cognitive impairment can indicate disease recurrence or progression, so imaging should be obtained if a patient has a significant and sudden decline in cognitive performance. However, cognitive impairment often increases over time after treatment for brain tumors in the absence of disease progression as a result of treatment-related damage to neural circuitry. Neuropsychologic evaluation should be performed by a board-certified neuropsychologist who is experienced in working with brain tumor patients. The neuropsychologic evaluation should include an assessment of fatigue and depression, as both occur at high rates within the brain tumor patient population and can impact cognitive functioning. Patients with severe cognitive impairment may not be capable of living independently. Consideration should be given in these cases to home safety evaluations, or assisted living should be discussed with the patient's family. Pharmacologic treatments are available and are often combined with nonpharmacologic interventions. Preventive strategies are an area of very active research and include radioprotective agents, use of radiosurgery, and hippocampal avoidance.

References

1. Johnson DR, Sawyer AM, Meyers CA, O'Neill BP, Wefel JS. Early measures of cognitive function predict survival in patients with newly diagnosed glioblastoma. *Neuro Oncol.* 2012;14:808–816. https://doi.org/10.1093/neuonc/nos082.
2. Greene-Schloesser D, Robbins ME, Peiffer AM, Shaw EG, Wheeler KT, Chan MD. Radiation-induced brain injury: a review. *Front Oncol.* 2012;2:73. https://doi.org/10.3389/fonc.2012.00073.
3. Tucha O, Smely C, Preier M, Lange KW. Cognitive deficits before treatment among patients with brain tumors. *Neurosurgery.* 2000;47:324–333; discussion 333. https://doi.org/10.1097/00006123-200008000-00011.
4. Kayl AE, Meyers CA. Does brain tumor histology influence cognitive function? *Neuro Oncol.* 2003;5(4):255–260. https://doi.org/10.1215/S1152851703000012.
5. Behin A, Delattre JY. Neurologic sequelae of radiotherapy on the nervous system. In: Schiff D, Wen PY, eds. *Cancer Neurology in Clinical Practice.* Totowa, NJ: Humana Press; 2003:173–191.
6. DeAngelis LM, Posner JB. Side effects of radiation therapy. In: DeAngelis LM, Posner JB, eds. *Neurologic Complications of Cancer.* 2nd ed. New York: Oxford University Press; 2009:551–555.
7. Klein M, Taphoorn MJ, Heimans JJ, et al. Neurobehavioral status and health-related quality of life in newly diagnosed high-grade glioma patients. *J Clin Oncol.* 2001;19(20):4037–4047.
8. Boosma I, Vos MJ, Heimans JJ, et al. The course of neurocognitive functioning in high-grade glioma patients. *Neuro Oncol.* 2007;9(1):53–62. https://doi.org/10.1215/15228517-2016-012.
9. Armstrong CL, Goldstein B, Shera D, Ledakis GE, Tallent EM. The predictive value of longitudinal neuropsychological assessment in the early detection of brain tumor recurrence. *Cancer.* 2003;97(3):649–656. https://doi.org/10.1002/cncr.11099.
10. Armstrong CL, Hunter JV, Ledakis GE, et al. Late cognitive and radiographic changes related to radiotherapy: initial prospective findings. *Neurology.* 2002;59(1):40–48.
11. Brown PD, Jensen AW, Felten SJ, et al. Detrimental effects of tumor progression on cognitive function of patients with high-grade glioma. *J Clin Oncol.* 2006;24(34):5427–5433. https://doi.org/10.1200/JCO.2006.08.5605.
12. Meyers CA, Hess KR. Multifaceted end points in brain tumor clinical trials: cognitive deterioration precedes MRI progression. *Neuro Oncol.* 2003;5:89–95.
13. Noll KR, Bradshaw ME, Rexer J, Wefel JS. Neuropsychological practice in the oncology setting. *Arch Clin Neuropsychol.* 2018;33(3):344–353.
14. Correa DD, Ahles TA. Neurocognitive changes in cancer survivors. *Cancer J.* 2008;14(6):396–400.
15. Wefel JS, Kayl AE, Meyers CA. Neuropsychological dysfunction associated with cancer and cancer therapies: a conceptual review of an emerging target. *Br J Cancer.* 2004;90(9):1691–1696.
16. Ferguson RJ, Ahles TA, Saykin AJ, et al. Cognitive-behavioral management of chemotherapy-related cognitive change. *Psycho Oncol.* 2007;16(8):772–777.
17. Gehring K, Sitskoorn MM, Gundy CM, et al. Cognitive rehabilitation in patients with gliomas: a randomized, controlled trial. *J Clin Oncol.* 2009;27(22):3712–3722.
18. Ferreri AJ, Zucca E, Armitage J, Cavalli F, Batchelor TT. Ten years of international primary CNS lymphoma collaborative group studies. *J Clin Oncol.* 2013;31(27):3444–3445.
19. Rapp SR, Case LD, Peiffer A, et al. Donepezil for irradiated brain tumor survivors: a phase III randomized placebo-controlled clinical trial. *J Clin Oncol.* 2015;33:1653–1659. https://doi.org/10.1200/JCO.2014.58.4508.
20. Butler Jr JM, Case LD, Atkins J, et al. A phase III, double-blind, placebo-controlled prospective randomized clinical trial of d-threo-methylphenidate HCl in brain tumor patients receiving radiation therapy. *Int J Radiat Oncol Biol Phys.* 2007;69:1496–1501. https://doi.org/10.1016/j.ijrobp.2007.05.076.
21. Page BR, Shaw EG, Lu L, et al. Phase II double-blind placebo-controlled randomized study of armodafinil for brain radiation-induced fatigue. *Neuro Oncol.* 2015;17:1393–1401. https://doi.org/10.1093/neuonc/nov084.
22. Gehring K, Sitskoorn MM, Gundy CM, et al. Cognitive rehabilitation in patients with gliomas: a randomized, controlled trial. *J Clin Oncol.* 2009;27:3712–3722. https://doi.org/10.1200/JCO.2008.20.5765.
23. van der Linden SD, Sitskoorn MM, Rutten GM, Gehring K. Feasibility of the evidence-based cognitive telerehabilitation program Remind for patients with primary brain tumors. *J Neuro Oncol.* 2018;137:523–532. https://doi.org/10.1007/s11060-017-2738-8.

Chapter 26

Uncommon radiation-induced neurological syndromes

Shivani Sud, Courtney M. Vaughn, and Colette Shen

CHAPTER OUTLINE

Introduction

Cranial irradiation is used in settings ranging from definitive treatment of primary brain and head and neck cancers to palliation of metastatic disease and prophylaxis, as a single modality or in combination with surgery or systemic therapy. Common side-effect considerations include neurocognitive and inflammatory effects as well as damage to critical brain structures, which are discussed elsewhere in this text (see Chapter 24 for a discussion of radiation necrosis and Chapter 25 for neurocognitive dysfunction). Here, we provided a case-based review of rare complications of cranial irradiation. A comprehensive understanding of potential complications of radiation therapy is necessary for optimal multidisciplinary management of oncology patients. Generally, complications are related to the disease site, radiation field, radiation dose, age at time of treatment, receipt of combination therapies, and time since treatment completion.

Clinical cases

CASE 26.1 RADIATION MYELITIS

Case. A 67-year-old man with a 25 pack-year smoking history and squamous cell carcinoma of the right base of the tongue treated with a cumulative dose of 70 Gy using conventional fractionation with concurrent carboplatin. One-year post-treatment, he presented with numbness and tingling sensations in the lower extremities, elicited with neck movements, and dull, intermittent cervical neck pain exacerbated by palpation. Review of systems was otherwise negative. Neurological examination was otherwise unremarkable, and cranial nerves II–XII were intact. Imaging showed no evidence of local disease recurrence. Magnetic resonance imaging (MRI) of the spine showed mildly T2 hyperintense signal within a prominent cord at the C3–C7 levels (Fig. 26.1). The patient's symptoms and imaging are consistent with radiation myelopathy with intermittent Lhermitte syndrome. On review of radiation treatment records, the maximum dose to the spinal cord was 37 Gy. Treatment with hyperbaric oxygen was initiated and improved radiation-related xerostomia; however, radiation myelitis did not improve. Treatment with steroids decreased severity of the lower extremity nerve pain after 2 weeks. The patient now continues on long-term pentoxifylline and vitamin E.

Teaching Points. Radiation myelitis is the most common of the rare complications of spinal cord irradiation and can present as a transient early or irreversible late reaction. Other rare complications include paralysis secondary to ischemia, hemorrhage, and lower motor neuron syndrome.

Early radiation-induced myelopathy. Early radiation-induced myelopathy typically develops within 2–6 months

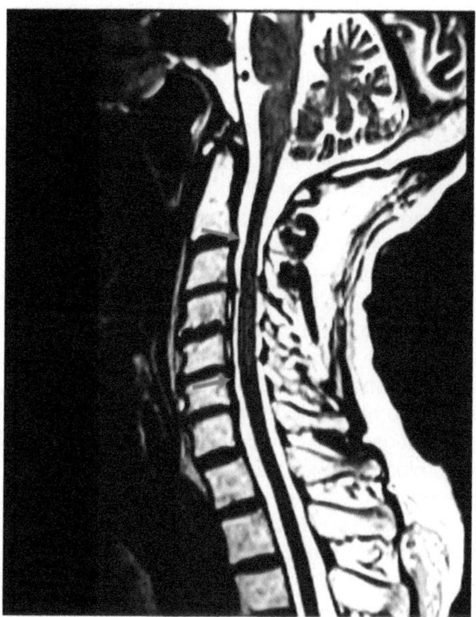

Fig. 26.1 Radiation myelitis. Sagittal plane of T2-weighted MRI demonstrating mildly T2 hyperintense signal (blue arrows) within a prominent cord at the C3–C7 levels in a patient with radiation myelitis.

following spinal irradiation and usually spontaneously resolves over 3–6 months without intervention.[1] The characteristic clinical presentation is a positive Lhermitte's sign, an electric shock-like sensation radiating to the extremities or trunk upon flexion of the neck. The incidence is estimated to be between 3–15% among patients receiving radiation to the head, neck, and upper respiratory tract.[2–4] Diagnosis is based on history, physical examination, and evaluation for alternative causes of myelopathy. The differential includes compressive disease (metastatic tumor, cervical spondylosis), demyelinating disease (multiple sclerosis), chemotherapy toxicity (platinum agents and taxanes), vitamin B_6 or B_{12} deficiency, rheumatoid disease, and trauma, among other causes of transverse myelitis.[5] Positron emission tomography demonstrating increased spinal cord metabolic uptake in the setting of Lhermitte's sign has also been described but is not necessary for diagnosis.[6] The mechanism of injury is attributed to transient damage to myelin-producing oligodendroglial cells in the irradiated field resulting in demyelination of the posterior columns of the spinal cord leading to hyperexcitability. Early radiation-induced myelopathy is a self-limited condition that does not require treatment. Neuropathy and muscle spasm can be symptomatically managed with medications such as gabapentin or carbamazepine.

Late radiation-induced myelopathy. Late radiation-induced myelopathy is chronic and typically, but not always, progressive and irreversible.[7] Onset ranges between 6–30 months posttreatment, with one series reporting a mean latency of 18.5 months following a single course of irradiation and 11.4 months following re-irradiation.[8] Symptoms are variable, ranging from minor to major sensorimotor deficits or paraplegia. Late radiation-induced myelopathy is a diagnosis of exclusion based on history, physical examination, and imaging. The differential is similar to that of early radiation-induced myelopathy with special attention to the evaluation of new metastases and disease progression. On MRI, radiation-induced myelopathy is typically characterized by intramedullary T1 hypointensity, possible focal contrast enhancement, and T2 hyperintensity (Fig. 26.1).[7,9] Pathogenesis is multifactorial and predominantly attributed to white matter injury of the spinal cord as well as vascular changes.[10–12] White matter injury includes myelin breakdown, nerve fiber degeneration and necrosis in the setting of damage to neurons and supporting cells including oligodendrocytes, astrocytes, and immune microglia cells. Vasculature-related changes include altered vascularity, telangiectasias, hyaline degeneration, edema, fibrosis, inflammation, degeneration, impaired blood flow, and hemorrhage. Treatment with radiosensitizing agents may increase risk of radiation toxicity by potentiating these mechanisms.

Risk of damage to the spinal cord can be mitigated with consideration of radiation dose, volume, and fractionation. One radiobiologic indicator of tissue sensitivity to radiation dose per fraction is the alpha/beta ratio. The spinal cord has a low alpha/beta ratio indicating high sensitivity to dose per fraction. Based on the Quantitative Analysis of Normal Tissue Effects in the Clinic (QUANTEC), a benchmark set of reviews on normal tissue toxicity secondary to radiation, the risk of radiation-induced myelopathy is less than 1% and less than 10% for total doses of 54 Gy and 61 Gy, respectively, using conventional radiotherapy fractionation of 1.8–2 Gy/fraction to the full-thickness cord.[13]

More recently, where clinically appropriate, alternative fractionation schemes have been adopted including hypofractionation, delivery of radiation over a shorter period of days or weeks compared with standard radiation therapy, and stereotactic body radiation therapy, which is the use of high doses of radiation given in a highly precise and conformal manner to a target volume over a small number of fractions.[14] QUANTEC analysis shows that when the maximum spinal cord dose is limited to the equivalent of 13 Gy in one fraction or 20 Gy in three fractions, the risk of myelopathy is <1%.[13]

Re-irradiation is considered for both palliation and definitive management of local disease progression or new disease sites. Treatment may encompass the entirety of the previously treated spinal cord or only a portion of this volume. Given the complexity of these cases, careful consideration is given to the prior radiation plan including spinal cord volume treated, dose and fractionation received, and time interval since treatment completion.[15] Per QUANTEC, when the cumulative dose from both initial and repeat irradiation to the cord is less than 60 Gy in 2 Gy equivalents, no cases of myelopathy were reported. Preclinical and metaanalysis data further suggest partial recovery of subclinical damage to the cord beginning at 6 months and increasing over 2 years posttreatment,[13] and thus a minimum time interval of 6 months from initial to repeat irradiation is recommended.[13,15]

Treatment of radiation myelitis focuses on addressing the suspected mechanisms of injury and supportive care as clinical data are limited. High-dose glucocorticoids are often empirically prescribed to reduce inflammation and edema.[12] In a 14-patient, double-blind, placebo-controlled, randomized clinical trial of symptomatic radiation necrosis of the brain, the monoclonal antibody against vascular endothelial growth factor, bevacizumab, led to radiographic and neurologic symptom improvement for all patients in the intervention arm, and case reports have suggested some improvement in radiation myelopathy with bevacizumab.[16,17] Hyperbaric oxygen is considered based on application to treating soft tissue and osteoradionecrosis; however, evidence for treating radiation myelitis is limited to case reports and preclinical data.[18,19] Anticoagulation with heparin and warfarin was evaluated in a small study of 11 patients with late radiation-induced nervous system injuries including cerebral radionecrosis and myelopathy unresponsive to glucocorticoids, which showed some recovery of function in over half of the patients, presumably due to impact on small vessel endothelial injury.[20] The combination of vitamin E and pentoxifylline, a phosphodiesterase inhibitor that reduces inflammation and also decreases erythrocyte resistance to deformation and blood viscosity, have been used in management of radiation-induced fibrosis and could be considered for radiation myelitis.[21,22]

Lower motor neuron syndrome is a delayed radiation complication with time to onset over a period of years following radiation to the lower spinal cord and cauda equina, characterized by progressive lower extremity weakness with minimal impairment of sensory, bowel, and bladder function. The etiology is controversial given the lack of radiation dose–effect relationship. Proposed mechanisms include preceding viral infection and radiculopathy secondary to vasculopathy of proximal spinal roots without significant damage to the lower motor neurons in the cord.[23,24]

Spinal cord hemorrhage, telangiectasia, and cavernous malformations can develop following radiation, though reports are exceedingly rare. Potential complications include symptomatic infarct or compression and subsequent effects.[25,26]

CASE 26.2 SMART SYNDROME: STROKE-LIKE MIGRAINE ATTACKS AFTER RADIATION THERAPY

Case. A 31-year-old woman with history of medulloblastoma at age 4 was treated with combination chemotherapy and radiation to a cumulative dose of 54 Gy using conventional fractionation and remains in remission. Twenty-six years post-treatment, she presented with 2 weeks of recurrent migraines and loss of her right visual field. With the exception of visual field cut, neurologic examination was nonfocal. On MRI, post-contrast T1-weighted images showed enhancement of the cerebral gyri sparing the white matter in the occipital lobe. On review of prior records, the region of enhancement corresponded with the prior radiation field. Given symptoms and MRI findings consistent with stroke-like migraine attacks after radiation therapy (SMART) syndrome, no further diagnostics such as biopsy were indicated. Symptoms were managed conservatively with avoidance of headache triggers, a brief course of steroids, and verapamil for migraine prophylaxis. Migraines resolved 2 weeks later, and visual field was restored. The patient has now been 1 year without recurrent episodes.

Teaching Points. SMART syndrome is a delayed complication of brain irradiation characterized by recurrent episodes of complicated migraines. This is a rare entity with approximately 40 reported cases, although it is likely underdiagnosed.[27,28] Time to onset in these cases ranges from 1–35 years, with a median of 14 years post-irradiation. Common symptoms include headache, seizure, hemianopsia, hemiparesis, and aphasia. Symptoms are often recurrent over a period of hours to weeks but generally considered reversible, although incomplete neurologic recovery has been reported.[27,29]

Differential diagnosis. The differential includes tumor recurrence, infarct, vasculitis, mitochondrial encephalomyelopathy with lactic acidosis and stroke (MELAS), posterior reversible encephalopathy (PRES), meningoencephalitis, status epilepticus, familial/sporadic hemiplegic migraine, radiation vasculopathy, cerebral autosomal dominant arteriopathy with subcortical infarcts and leukoencephalopathy (CADASIL), and toxic-metabolic derangements. Proposed diagnostic criteria by Black et al. include (1) a remote history of cranial irradiation with absence of residual or recurrent tumor; (2) prolonged characteristic symptoms of complex migraine, seizures, and/or stroke-like symptoms referable to a unilateral cortical region; (3) characteristic brain MRI findings; and (4) exclusion of alternative etiologies.[29–31]

Imaging findings. Post-contrast T1-weighted MRI may show unilateral cortical gadolinium enhancement of the cerebral gyri sparing the white matter within the prior radiation field, usually in the temporal, parietal, or occipital lobes. Transient T2 and fluid attenuated inversion recovery (FLAIR) hyperintensity, as well as susceptibility-weighted imaging (SWI) with numerous hypointensities within the periventricular white matter attributed to radiation-induced cavernous hemangiomas, have been described. These characteristic MRI findings appear 2–7 days following symptom onset.[27,30,32] In addition to symptom management, recognition of this entity is critical for preventing unnecessary invasive diagnostics such as brain biopsy.

Pathogenesis. The pathogenesis is poorly understood. Most cases are associated with a radiation dose of 50 Gy or higher, but reported doses have ranged from 15–64 Gy with highly variable treatment volumes and concurrent systemic therapies.[27,28] It has been hypothesized that SMART could result from radiation-induced injury to the vasculature or trigeminovascular system, lowered threshold for cortical-spreading depression and endothelial dysfunction resulting in characteristic migraines, cortical enhancement, and seizures.[30] Notably, surgically-induced SMART syndrome has also been reported.[33]

Treatment. Treatment for SMART is limited to conservative medical management given the dearth of clinical cases and data. Similar to management of complex migraines, avoidance of headache triggers is encouraged, and antiepileptics or a brief course of steroids may be considered. Limited case reports suggest aspirin and verapamil, a calcium channel blocker used for migraine and cluster headache prophylaxis and thought to prevent vasospasm, may reduce the frequency and severity of SMART syndrome episodes.[28,34]

CASE 26.3 HYPOTHALAMIC DYSFUNCTION

Case. A 30-year-old woman with history of right sinus and orbit rhabdomyosarcoma diagnosed at age 3 was treated with chemotherapy and radiation therapy to 59.8 Gy using conventional fractionation. At age 7, she presented with growth failure and precocious puberty. At age 9, she developed temperature dysregulation, difficulty sleeping, and excessive daytime somnolence. Examination was notable for poor dentition and impaired growth of facial bones. Imaging for chronic rhinosinusitis showed bilateral sphenoid sinus stenosis. The patient was jointly followed by pediatrics, radiation oncology, endocrinology, and neurology. She was diagnosed with panhypopituitarism and dysfunctional circadian drive but did not have adrenal insufficiency. Collectively, her conditions indicated hypothalamic and pituitary dysfunction. She was treated with growth hormone replacement and started on leuprolide followed by oral contraceptives for precocious puberty and menstrual regulation. The patient also takes levothyroxine for hypothyroidism. She was counseled on sleep hygiene and takes melatonin as needed.

Teaching Points. Dysfunction of the hypothalamus most often involves the hypothalamic-pituitary axis but can also be limited to the hypothalamus alone. The hypothalamus is located in the ventral brain above the pituitary gland and may fall within the radiation field during cranial irradiation for numerous indications including prophylactic irradiation (≤30 Gy), total-body irradiation (10–14 Gy) and treatment of primary brain, nasopharyngeal, sinonasal, skull base, and metastatic lesions (≤60 Gy). The hypothalamus releases hormones that act on the pituitary gland, forming the hypothalamic-pituitary axis to regulate multiple endocrine systems and is also involved in nonendocrine functions of temperature, appetite, and autonomic nervous system regulation. Disruptions of either the hypothalamic or pituitary component of the axis can lead to endocrine dysfunction, both of which require care coordination with endocrinology, with a focus on managing hormonal derangements.

Neuroendocrine dysfunction as a result of hypothalamic-pituitary irradiation is common among both children and adults. Hormones released by the hypothalamus include growth hormone–releasing hormone (GHRH), gonadotropin-releasing hormone (GnRH), thyrotropin-releasing hormone (TRH), corticotropin-releasing hormone (CRH), somatostatin, and dopamine. Each of the corresponding hormone axes have variable sensitivity to radiation dose, with the growth hormone (GH) axis being the most radiosensitive, followed by the thyroid hormone, adrenocorticotropic hormone (ACTH), and gonadotropin axes (Table 26.1).[35–37]

Growth hormone–releasing hormone (GHRH). GHRH stimulates the anterior pituitary gland to secrete GH. Time to onset among children is influenced by dose and estimated to be 60 months, 36 months, and 12 months for radiation doses of 15–20 Gy, 25–36 Gy and >60 Gy, respectively.[38,39] A longitudinal study of adults receiving radiation for primary nonpituitary brain tumors reported dose-dependent GH deficiency among 32% of patients.[40] Similarly, a meta-analysis showed that among adults receiving radiation for nonpituitary lesions, the median prevalence of GH deficiency was 45%.[41] GH deficiency in children causes growth impairment, and, in adults, severe deficiency has been associated with cognitive, cardiovascular, neuromuscular, metabolic, and bony abnormalities. Diagnosis is based on low GH levels following one of various GH secretion-stimulating tests, of which the insulin tolerance test remains the gold standard for radiation-induced GH deficiency.[42] Children treated with cranial irradiation are recommended to undergo routine physical examinations every 6 months until growth is complete and, if poorly growing, undergo evaluation with assessment of nutritional status, thyroid studies, and radiographs for bone age.[43] Referral to pediatric endocrinology is indicated for further evaluation and GH replacement. Due to the theoretical risk of GH replacement stimulating cancer recurrence, therapy is typically avoided for 2 years following treatment completion. Adults with severe symptomatic GH deficiency may be selectively considered for GH replacement by endocrinology.

Gonadotropin-releasing hormone (GnRH). GnRH regulates release of follicle-stimulating hormone (FSH) and luteinizing hormone (LH) from the anterior pituitary, thereby controlling sex-specific hormone secretion and onset of puberty. Central gonadotropin deficiency and hypogonadism are late onset and can occur following doses >30 Gy at a cumulative incidence of 20–60% among children and adults, with risk of dysfunction increasing with dose.[44,45] In children, doses causing severe GnRH deficiency lead to concomitant GH deficiency. This combined deficiency can lead to delayed puberty and delayed linear growth in children.[46] Conversely, radiation doses ≥18 Gy can cause central precocious puberty, with higher risk in girls and children receiving radiation treatment at a younger age.[47] In children, there is an active inhibition of GnRH secretion prepuberty. Puberty is initiated with a sustained increase in pulsatile release of GnRH from the hypothalamus. It is hypothesized that doses of 15–50 Gy injure inhibitory neurons, leading to increased GnRH secretion. Children must be carefully followed, as precocious puberty can mask GH deficiency and lead to decreased height potential due to accelerated epiphyseal closure. In adults, hypogonadism can present as fatigue, decreased sexual function and drive, and infertility. Gonadotropin deficiency is diagnosed based on history and serum levels of estrogen/testosterone, FSH, or LH. Primary pituitary versus hypothalamic hypogonadism are differentiated

Table 26.1 Pituitary-hypothalamic axis dysfunction following radiation

Condition	Dose	Presentation	Diagnostics
GH deficiency	≥18 Gy	Children: Growth delay Adults: Variable cognitive, cardiovascular, metabolic abnormalities	IGF-I, ITT, glucagon, clonidine
Central precocious puberty	≥18 Gy	Early onset of puberty	FSH, LH, estradiol (female), testosterone (male)
FSH/LH deficiency	≥30 Gy	Delayed puberty and linear growth in children	FSH, LH, estradiol (female), testosterone (male), GnRH
TSH deficiency	≥30 Gy	Fatigue, weight gain, cold intolerance, brittle hair and constipation	TSH, FT4, TRH
ACTH deficiency	≥30 Gy	Weight loss, anorexia, nausea, vomiting	Cortisol, ITT, Synacthen
Hyperprolactinemia	≥40–50 Gy	Pubertal delay in children, impotence in men, galactorrhea in women	Prolactin level

ACTH, Adrenocorticotropic hormone; *FSH,* follicle-stimulating hormone; *FT4,* free thyroxine; *GH,* growth hormone; *GnRH,* gonadotropin-releasing hormone; *IGF-1,* insulin-like growth factor 1; *ITT,* insulin tolerance test; *LH,* luteinizing hormone; *TRH,* thyrotropin-releasing hormone; *TSH,* thyroid-stimulating hormone.

based on response to GnRH stimulation. Hypogonadism may be treated with hormone replacement therapy consisting of GnRH for hypothalamic hypogonadism and with replacement of appropriate sex-specific hormones for pituitary etiology.

Thyrotropin-releasing hormone (TRH). TRH stimulates the release of thyroid-stimulating hormone (TSH) and prolactin from the anterior pituitary gland. Thyroid hormone deficiency from hypothalamic-pituitary irradiation is dose dependent, with 5-year hormone deficiency rates of 4%, 25%, and 43% from median hypothalamic and pituitary doses of ≤20 Gy, 20–40 Gy, and ≥40 Gy, respectively.[37] In addition, the thyroid itself is highly radiation-sensitive, and children undergoing craniospinal irradiation or adults receiving head and neck irradiation are at high risk of primary hypothyroidism.[48,49] Patients may present with fatigue, weight gain, cold intolerance, brittle hair, and constipation. Testing for annual free T4 and TSH is recommended. Deficiency can be corrected with administration of levothyroxine.

Corticotropin-releasing hormone (CRH). CRH stimulates the release of ACTH from the anterior pituitary. This axis is relatively radioresistant, as ACTH deficiency occurs in less than 5% of patients receiving cranial irradiation with hypothalamic-pituitary doses of <40 Gy.[37,45,48] ACTH deficiency is a late onset side-effect that is typically subclinical but may present with weight loss, anorexia, nausea, and vomiting; hypoglycemia and dilutional hyponatremia are unlikely. The insulin tolerance test, blood cortisol level measurement, and the cortisol stimulation test are commonly employed for diagnosis. Deficiency is treated with cortisol hormone replacement therapy.

Prolactin. Prolactin is released from the pituitary gland and primarily promotes lactation. Dopamine output from the hypothalamus inhibits release of prolactin. Although up to 72% of patients may have an elevated prolactin level following radiation to the hypothalamic-pituitary axis, hyperprolactinemia manifesting as pubertal delay in children, impotence in men, or galactorrhea in women is rare.[44,50] Symptomatic hyperprolactinemia may be managed with the dopamine agonists cabergoline or bromocriptine.

Data are limited on radiation-induced nonendocrine hypothalamic dysfunction. However, similar to the case presented here, it is likely that hypothalamic irradiation can lead to disruptions in thermal homeostasis, autonomic system regulation and maintenance of circadian rhythm.[51–53] In addition, hypothalamic obesity is known to result from hypothalamic tumors or injury to the hypothalamic region (e.g., surgery or radiotherapy) and is seen in 30–75% of patients treated for craniopharyngioma.[54] This form of obesity results from impaired leptin signaling, thus simulating a state of starvation where energy expenditure is reduced and adipogenesis and insulin secretion are increased. As lifestyle and pharmacologic interventions are minimally effective, the best strategy is to limit hypothalamic damage upfront, for example, by treating craniopharyngiomas with more conservative surgery followed by conformal radiotherapy as opposed to gross total resection.[55,56]

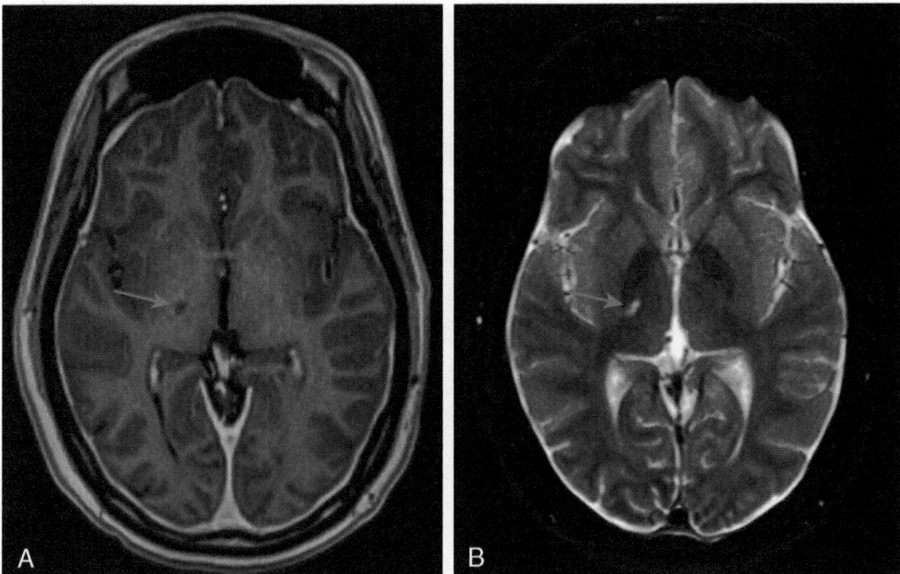

Fig. 26.2 Post-radiation stroke. (A) Axial plane of T1-weighted MRI showing subacute right capsular lacunar infarct (blue arrow). Diffuse scattered foci of microhemorrhage compatible with sequelae of radiation treatment. (B) Axial plane of T2-weighted MRI showing hyperintense lesion (blue arrow) in the right posterior limb internal capsule consistent with capsular lacunar infarct.

CASE 26.4 POST-RADIATION VASCULOPATHY AND STROKE

Case. A 21-year-old man with history of suprasellar immature teratoma with drop metastases in the lumbar spine was treated with neoadjuvant chemotherapy, resection, and adjuvant craniospinal irradiation with cranial boost to a cumulative dose of 54 Gy (with conventional fractionation) at age 14. He continued on adjuvant azacitidine. Treatment was complicated by secondary panhypopituitarism within 1 year. Seven years following treatment, he presented with new left lower extremity weakness requiring the use of a wheelchair. Physical examination was notable for abnormal left-sided muscle tone and gait ataxia. MRI Brain showed a new subacute right capsular lacunar infarct (Fig. 26.2). The patient was started on aspirin 81 mg daily. He is currently being monitored by pediatric oncology for craniospinal recurrence.

Teaching Points. Post-radiation vasculopathy is a late-onset complication potentially manifesting as ischemic or hemorrhagic cerebrovascular accidents (CVA), vascular occlusive disease, vascular malformations, or intracranial hemorrhage. Incidence is higher among those who received radiation as children compared with adults. The pathophysiology of radiation-induced vascular injury is complex and attributed to multiple changes including progressive endothelial loss, disruption of the blood-brain barrier, inflammation, vasogenic edema, and thrombosis followed by long-term effects on vascular remodeling including atheroma formation, endothelial proliferation, adventitial fibrosis, basement membrane thickening, and eventual vessel dilation.[57]

Among adults, incidence of post-radiation CVA using fractionated radiation is estimated between 12–21% at 20 years based on retrospective review; however, a comparison of patients receiving radiation versus surgery found no difference in CVA risk.[58–60] In a Dutch study identifying patients with pituitary adenoma as being at greater risk of CVA mortality relative to the general population, the primary stroke risk factors were preexisting coronary or peripheral artery disease.[59] The Childhood Cancer Survival Study estimates cumulative incidence of stroke of 0.73% and 5.6% at 25 years among children with leukemia and brain tumors, respectively. Risk of stroke increased in a dose-dependent manner above 30 Gy with the highest risk after doses of ≥50 Gy.[61] Additional risk factors in children include relative location of the tumor to the circle of Willis, administration of chemotherapy, neurofibromatosis type 1 (NF1) status, and age <5 years at the time of radiation.[57]

The Children's Oncology Group recommends annual evaluation including neurologic examination for children exposed to cranial irradiation ≥18 Gy and brain MRI, neurology/neurosurgery involvement, and revascularization procedures as indicated.[62] Stroke prevention strategies including aggressive management of comorbid conditions such as diabetes, heart disease, hypercholesterolemia, and hyperlipidemia should be employed. Management of stroke is the same as in the general population, including urgent CT scan, consultation of neurosurgery for hemorrhagic stroke, and initiation of tissue plasminogen activator if applicable or alternative anti-coagulant agents depending on clinical circumstances. Patients with a history of stroke should be followed by neurology and initiated on secondary prevention including antihypertensive

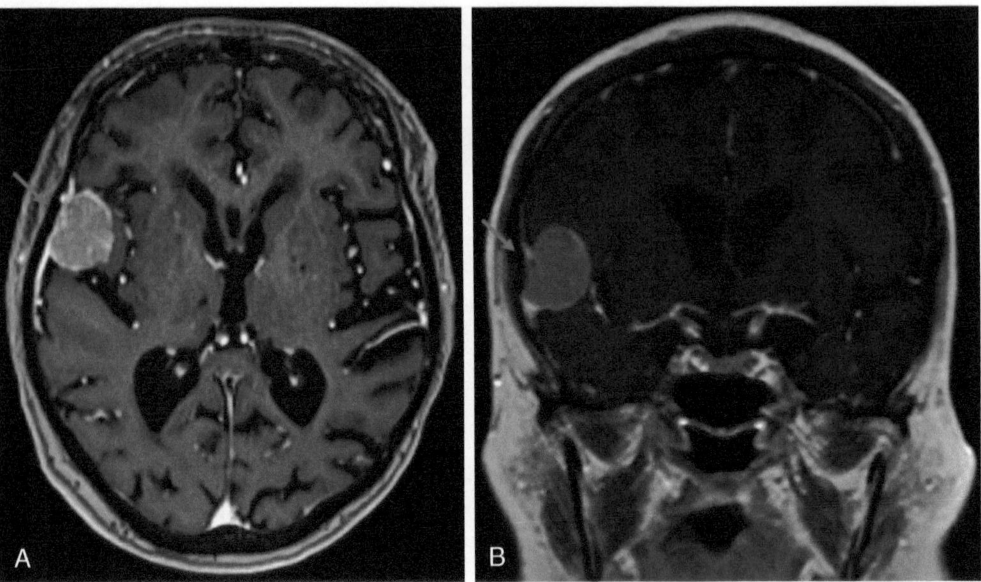

Fig. 26.3 Radiation-induced meningioma. (A) Axial plane and (B) coronal plane of T1-weighted post-gadolinium MRI showing dural-based 3 × 2 cm solid lesion (blue arrows) with mild mass effect consistent with characteristic meningioma appearance on MRI.

therapy, statin therapy, antithrombotic therapy, and lifestyle modification.[63]

Moyamoya disease is characterized by progressive stenosis and occlusion of the intracranial internal carotid arteries and their proximal branches, with subsequent development of smaller collateral vessels ("moyamoya" means "puff of smoke" in Japanese and describes the appearance of clusters of small collateral vessels). Associated symptoms and conditions are broadly related to brain ischemia (stroke, transient ischemic attacks, headaches, seizures) and dysfunction of collateral vasculature (hemorrhage, headache). Moyamoya disease primarily affects children but can also be seen in adults. The estimated incidence of Moyamoya in children with acute lymphoblastic leukemia receiving 18–24 Gy prophylactic cranial irradiation was 0.46% at 8 years and in those with primary brain tumors was 3.5%, with a median time to diagnosis of 46 months.[64,65] Radiation dose above 50 Gy, tumor location, and NF1 were associated with more rapid onset of Moyamoya.[65]

Interventions for radiation-induced vaso-occlusive disease are limited. A prospective nonrandomized study of carotid angioplasty and stenting for high-grade (≥70%) radiation-induced carotid stenosis using atherosclerotic stenosis as a control showed a higher rate of in-stent restenosis among patients with radiation-induced disease.[66]

Vascular malformations including cavernous malformation, telangiectasia, and aneurysm are potential delayed side effects of radiation that are typically asymptomatic but can hemorrhage. The incidence of cavernous malformations is estimated to be 6.7% at 20 years among children undergoing cranial irradiation for a variety of neoplasms; however, in a study of medulloblastoma patients, an incidence of 43% at 10 years was observed.[67,68] Risk of hemorrhage is estimated to be about 1% per year for previously unruptured lesions,[69,70] and thus serial follow up with MRI and consideration of resection is advised for enlarging lesions.[67]

Lacunar infarcts are small noncortical infarcts in the deep parenchyma of the brain that appear on MRI as foci of white matter loss. A study of children with brain tumors found that 6% of patients treated with either combination or single modality radiation or chemotherapy developed lacunes at a median interval of 2.0 years. Age less than 5 at time of radiation was the most significant predictor. All lacunar lesions were clinically silent without associated change in intelligence quotient scores.[71]

CASE 26.5 RADIATION-INDUCED MENINGIOMA

Case. A 75-year-old woman with history of posterior fossa ependymoma 32 years prior was treated with resection and adjuvant radiation to a cumulative dose to the resection bed of 45 Gy. At age 68, she was diagnosed with a temporal meningioma following incidental identification of a 2.8 × 2.1 × 2.7 cm right temporal mass on surveillance MRI (Fig. 26.3). Her meningioma is located within a region that received low radiation dose at the time of treatment for her ependymoma. Given growth over time, the meningioma was managed with radiation using stereotactic radiosurgery to a dose of 13 Gy in one fraction.

Teaching Points. Meningiomas are tumors arising from the meninges surrounding the brain and spinal cord and are the most common primary central nervous system (CNS) tumors, accounting for approximately one-third of cases (also see Chapter 10 for the general approach to the meningioma patient). Whereas the vast majority of meningiomas arise spontaneously, prior exposure to ionizing radiation is an established acquired risk factor for development of meningioma, and meningiomas are in fact the most common secondary CNS tumors following cranial radiotherapy.[72,73] Other predisposing conditions include neurofibromatosis type 2 (Chapter 16), schwannomatosis, and, potentially, prior history of breast cancer and obesity.[74] The incidence of spontaneous meningiomas increases with age, peaking in the fifth and sixth decades.[75] The vast majority of spontaneous meningiomas are nonmalignant and are characterized at the time of presentation as World Health Organization (WHO) grade I, II, or III in 80.6%, 17.4%, and 2.1% of cases, respectively.[75]

With regard to radiation-induced meningioma (RIM), data from the "Tinea capitis cohort," 11,000 children treated with low dose irradiation (<15 Gy) for scalp fungal infection and two matched control groups who did not receive radiotherapy, show that treated children received a brain dose of 1–2 Gy and had a relative risk of 9.5 for development of meningioma.[76] The mean latency period from radiation exposure to development of RIM was 36 years. In a report from the Childhood Cancer Survivor Study evaluating new CNS neoplasms in over 14,000 long-term survivors of pediatric malignancy, radiation exposure was associated with an increased risk of developing meningioma, with an odds ratio of 9.9 compared with matched controls, at a median interval of 17 years after original cancer diagnosis.[72] A systematic review of 251 reported cases of RIM showed an average age of primary lesion diagnosis of 13.0 ± 13.5 years, average radiation dose delivered to the primary lesion of 38.8 ± 16.8 Gy, and a latency period to development of meningioma of 22.9 ± 11.4 years. The latency period was shorter for patients who developed higher-grade meningiomas and those receiving radiation doses greater than 15 Gy. Higher radiation dose was associated with higher meningioma grade and development of multiple meningiomas. Similar to prior studies, recurrence of RIM occurred in 18% of patients.[77,78] The 5-year and 10-year survival rates for all patients with RIM in this study were 77.7% and 66.1%, respectively.[78]

Criteria for RIM are inferred from Cahan's criteria for radiation-induced sarcoma as follows: (1) the tumor must arise within the irradiated field; (2) a sufficient latency period must have elapsed between irradiation and induced malignancy; (3) the radiation-induced tumor must be a different histology than the primary tumor; and (4) the tissue from which the secondary malignancy arose must have been normal, for example, without genetic predisposition to tumor development such as Li-Fraumeni disease, tuberous sclerosis, neurofibromatosis, etc.[79]

The question arises are there significant differences between spontaneous meningiomas and RIM? Studies of patients with RIM suggest younger age at diagnosis, more calvarial tumors, increased recurrence rate, greater proportion of multiple meningiomas and tumors with higher histopathologic grade, and more complex cytogenetic aberrations compared with spontaneous meningiomas.[77,78,80] For example, although approximately 20% of spontaneous meningiomas are atypical or malignant (grade II or III), these studies suggest that higher-grade meningiomas comprise 30–38% of RIM. In addition, whereas spontaneous meningiomas have a female predominance with a female:male ratio of approximately 1.7:1, this difference is no longer seen in RIM.

Similar to spontaneous meningioma, RIM is managed with surgery and/or radiation therapy, although radiotherapy is considered more cautiously in the setting of re-irradiation depending on time interval from prior radiation and tumor/patient factors. Patients with small (<2 cm), asymptomatic lesions may consider active surveillance with annual MRI. When treatment is necessary, surgical resection is preferred when feasible, as this can be curative and provides tissue for pathology, especially given prior radiotherapy. If the lesion is inaccessible or the patient is not a surgical candidate, re-irradiation can be used. Adjuvant radiation is favored in the treatment of malignant meningioma and some subtotally resected nonmalignant lesions to improve local control. The role of systemic therapy in the management of meningioma is limited.[81]

CASE 26.6 RADIATION-INDUCED GLIOMA/GLIOBLASTOMA

Case. A 40-year-old man with history of acute lymphoblastic leukemia treated with chemotherapy and prophylactic cranial irradiation to a dose of 18 Gy at age 16. He developed progressive leg weakness and gait instability 6 months ago and now presents due to 2 weeks of severe headaches. MRI with contrast showed heterogeneously enhancing masses in the right frontal lobe with central necrosis, thick rim enhancement, and surrounding vasogenic edema on T1- and T2-weighted images (Fig. 26.4). Biopsy showed glioblastoma, MGMT unmethylated, IDH wildtype, TERT promotor mutated. The mass was not resectable. He was treated with primary re-irradiation to a dose of 50 Gy with concurrent and adjuvant temozolomide.

Teaching Points. Gliomas are brain and spinal cord tumors that arise from glial cells including astrocytes, oligodendrocytes, and ependymal cells. This broad classification includes heterogeneous tumor types that vary with regard to biologic aggressiveness but are often referred to as low grade and high grade for WHO grade I–II and III–IV gliomas, respectively. Gliomas are further characterized by histopathology and molecular diagnostic tests including IDH1/IDH2 mutations, 1p/19q co-deletion, ATRX mutation, TP53 mutation, H3 K27M mutation, BRAF alterations and RELA fusion (see Chapter 1 for molecular review of neuropathology).[82] Glioblastomas are highly aggressive and are the most common malignant CNS tumor.

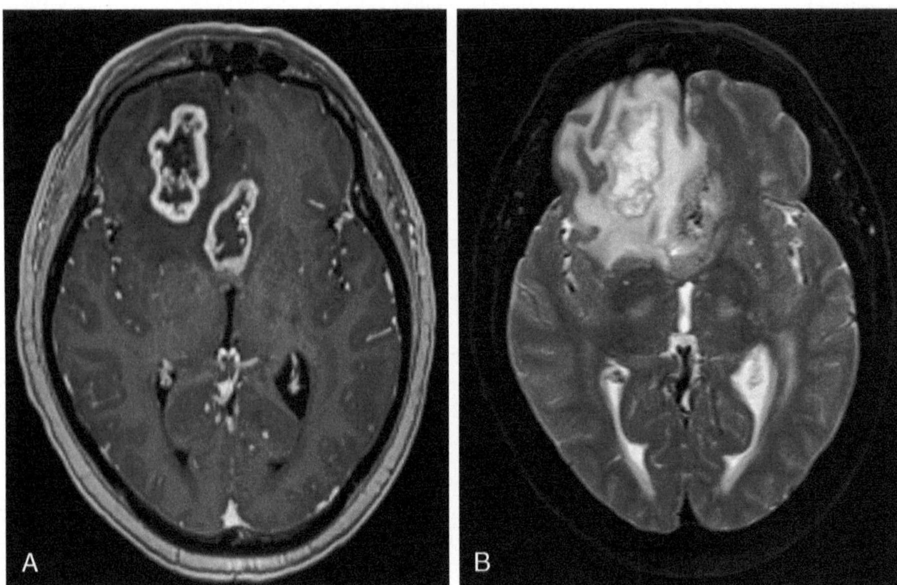

Fig. 26.4 Radiation-induced glioblastoma. (A) Axial plane of T1-weighted post-gadolinium MRI and (B) axial plane of T2-weighted MRI show heterogeneously enhancing masses in the right frontal lobe with central necrosis, thick rim enhancement, and surrounding vasogenic edema, consistent with characteristic glioblastoma appearance on MRI.

Radiation-induced gliomas (RIG) are a rare but known entity following cranial irradiation, second to radiation-induced meningiomas.[72] Criteria for RIG are similar to those for other secondary neoplasms per modified Cahan criteria, including occurrence within the irradiated field, sufficient latency between radiation and new neoplasm development, distinct tumor histology compared with the primary lesion, and absence of genetic predisposition to tumor development.[79]

A systematic review of 296 reported cases of RIG showed average age of primary lesion diagnosis of 16.0 ± 15.8 years, average radiation dose delivered to the primary lesion of 37.6 ± 20.0 Gy, and a latency period to development of glioma of 9 years. Secondary gliomas were categorized as grade I, II, III, or IV in approximately 0.3%, 11%, 30%, and 59% of reported cases, respectively. The median overall survival was 11 months, with a 2-year survival rate of 20.2%. On subset analysis, receipt of combination surgery, chemotherapy, and radiation for RIG was associated with an improved 2-year survival rate of 28.5%.[83] In a report from the Childhood Cancer Survivor Study evaluating new CNS neoplasms in over 14,000 long-term survivors of pediatric malignancy, the standardized incidence ratio for glioma was 8.7, and the excess relative risk of glioma development was a linear 0.33/Gy compared with matched controls.[72] Data from the Tinea capitis cohort showed similar findings, with excess relative risk of malignant brain tumors decreasing with increasing age at the time of radiation.[84] In a more recent retrospective French study of 4581 pediatric cancer patients treated with modern, more conformal radiotherapy, 50% of secondary CNS tumors developed in regions that received a dose <2.5 Gy.[85] Thus, future directions to reduce the risk of secondary neoplasm include minimizing low-dose radiation to the brain through use of highly conformal techniques and evaluation of active scanning proton beam therapy for children.[86]

When comparing RIG with spontaneously occurring gliomas, several clinical features differ, but molecular-genetic characteristics have thus far been found to be similar. A study of nine patients with RIG indicated younger age at diagnosis, higher tumor histologic grade, and atypical tumor location compared with spontaneous gliomas, but molecular-genetic alterations appeared to be similar to de novo high grade gliomas.[87] However, a more recent study of pediatric RIG using gene expression microarray profiling suggested greater homogeneity of gene expression in RIG compared with de novo pediatric glioblastomas, with high overlap in gene expression patterns between RIG and pilocytic astrocytomas.[88]

Patients should be referred to a multidisciplinary neuro-oncology team for management of RIG. Biopsy of the lesion is recommended for histology and molecular testing to determine the diagnosis. Management of gliomas in general consists of surgical resection or biopsy followed by adjuvant systemic and/or radiation therapy depending on extent of surgery and histologic and molecular features. Although use of radiotherapy in the management of RIG may be more conservative, a retrospective study showed significantly worse survival outcomes in patients who were not treated with re-irradiation for RIG. Patients who received re-irradiation to a mean dose of 50 Gy had a 1-, 2-, and 5-year overall survival rates of 58.9%, 20.5%, and 6.8%, compared with 15.1%, 3%, and 0%, respectively, for those who did not receive re-irradiation.[89]

Table 26.2 Summary of rare complications of cranial irradiation

Complication	Symptoms	Onset post-radiation	Diagnostics	Treatment	Multidisciplinary teams
Late radiation myelitis	Insidious variable isolated or combination sensory, motor deficits	6–30 months	H&P MRI	Glucocorticoids Bevacizumab Hyperbaric oxygen Vitamin E Pentoxifylline	Radiation Oncology Neurology
SMART syndrome	Headache, seizure, hemianopsia, hemiparesis, aphasia	Late complication, 1 year–indefinite	H&P MRI	Steroids Antiepileptics Verapamil Aspirin	Radiation Oncology Neurology
Hypothalamic dysfunction	Variable based on axes impacted. Growth delay, precocious puberty, pubertal delay fatigue, weight gain, cold intolerance, weight loss, galactorrhea, thermal dysregulation, loss of circadian rhythm, obesity	1–5 years	H&P Diagnostic testing specific to hormone deficiency	Hormone replacement	Radiation Oncology Neurology Endocrinology Pediatrics depending on age
Post-RT vasculopathy/ stroke	Ischemic, hemorrhagic stroke symptoms, vaso-occlusive disease	Late complication, 1 year–indefinite	H&P MRI	Acute stroke management Aggressive secondary prevention	Radiation Oncology Neurology Primary care and specialists managing cardiovascular risk
RT-induced meningioma	Incidental on imaging, headaches, seizures, focal neurologic deficits	Late complication, 5 year–indefinite	H&P MRI Consider biopsy	Resection Primary radiation therapy	Radiation Oncology Neurosurgery
RT-induced glioma/ glioblastoma	Headaches, seizures, focal neurologic deficits	5 year–indefinite	H&P MRI Biopsy	Surgical resection, systemic therapy including temozolomide, radiation therapy	Radiation Oncology Neurosurgery Medical Oncology

H&P, History and physical examination; *RT,* radiation therapy; *SMART,* stroke-like migraine attacks after radiation therapy.

Conclusion

Cranial radiotherapy is an integral component in the treatment of CNS and head and neck primary cancers, metastatic cancers, and hematologic malignancies for prophylaxis. Although cranial irradiation is generally well tolerated, common and rare adverse events do occur. Rare complications and clinical pearls are summarized in Table 26.2. Future directions in optimizing radiation safety include further study of the radiation parameters related to complications such as dose, treatment fields, fractionation schedule, and method of radiation delivery. The interaction between radiation and new systemic therapies including targeted agents and immunotherapy is an active area of investigation. Modern radiation therapy techniques including intensity modulated radiation therapy and stereotactic radiosurgery allow for highly conformal dose distributions and sparing of critical structures. Proton beam therapy may variably reduce normal tissue toxicity and further improve dose conformity, thereby reducing risk of complications, and has generally been adopted in the treatment of many pediatric CNS malignancies where available. In the rapidly evolving oncology landscape, multidisciplinary management of patients is necessary for cancer treatment and management of complications.

References

1. Esik O, Csere T, Stefanits K, et al. A review on radiogenic Lhermitte's sign. *Pathol Oncol Res*. 2003;9:115–120.
2. Fein DA, Marcus RB, Parsons JT, Mendenhall WM, Million RR. Lhermitte's sign: incidence and treatment variables influencing risk after irradiation of the cervical spinal cord. *Int J Radiat Oncol Biol Phys*. 1993;27:1029–1033.
3. Leung WM, Tsang NM, Chang FT, Lo CJ. Lhermitte's sign among nasopharyngeal cancer patients after radiotherapy. *Head Neck*. 2005;27:187–194.
4. Ko HC, Power AR, Sheu RD, et al. Lhermitte's Sign following VMAT-based head and neck radiation-insights into mechanism. *PloS One*. 2015;10:e0139448.
5. Khare S, Seth D. Lhermitte's Sign: the current status. *Ann Indian Acad Neurol*. 2015;18:154.
6. Esik O, Csere T, Stefanits K, et al. Increased metabolic activity in the spinal cord of patients with long-standing Lhermitte's sign. *Strahlenther Onkol*. 2003;179:690–693.
7. Khan M, Ambady P, Kimbrough D, et al. Radiation-induced myelitis: initial and follow-up MRI and clinical features in patients at a single tertiary care institution during 20 years. *AJNR Am J Neuroradiol*. 2018;39:1576–1581.
8. Wong CS, Van Dyk J, Milosevic M, Laperriere NJ. Radiation myelopathy following single courses of radiotherapy and retreatment. *Int J Radiat Oncol Biol Phys*. 1994;30:575–581.
9. Wang PY, Shen WC, Jan JS. Serial MRI changes in radiation myelopathy. *Neuroradiology*. 1995;37:374–377.
10. Okada S, Okeda R. Pathology of radiation myelopathy. *Neuropathology*. 2001;21:247–265.
11. Schultheiss TE, Kun LE, Ang KK, Stephens LC. Radiation response of the central nervous system. *Int J Radiat Oncol Biol Phys*. 1995;31:1093–1112.
12. Wong CS, Fehlings MG, Sahgal A. Pathobiology of radiation myelopathy and strategies to mitigate injury. *Spinal Cord*. 2015;53:574–580.
13. Kirkpatrick JP, van der Kogel AJ, Schultheiss TE. Radiation dose-volume effects in the spinal cord. *Int J Radiat Oncol Biol Phys*. 2010;76:S42–S49.
14. Potters L, Kavanagh B, Galvin JM, et al. American Society for Therapeutic Radiology and Oncology (ASTRO) and American College of Radiology (ACR) practice guideline for the performance of stereotactic body radiation therapy. *Int J Radiat Oncol Biol Phys*. 2010;76:326–332.
15. Nieder C, Grosu AL, Andratschke NH, Molls M. Update of human spinal cord reirradiation tolerance based on additional data from 38 patients. *Int J Radiat Oncol Biol Phys*. 2006;66:1446–1449.
16. Chamberlain MC, Eaton KD, Fink J. Radiation-induced myelopathy: treatment with bevacizumab. *Arch Neurol*. 2011;68:1608–1609.
17. Psimaras D, Tafani C, Ducray F, et al. Bevacizumab in late-onset radiation-induced myelopathy. *Neurology*. 2016;86:454–457.
18. Calabrò F, Jinkins JR. MRI of radiation myelitis: a report of a case treated with hyperbaric oxygen. *Eur Radiol*. 2000;10:1079–1084.
19. Sminia P, van der Kleij AJ, Carl UM, Feldmeier JJ, Hartmann KA. Prophylactic hyperbaric oxygen treatment and rat spinal cord re-irradiation. *Cancer Lett*. 2003;191:59–65.
20. Glantz MJ, Burger PC, Friedman AH, Radtke RA, Massey EW, Schold Jr SC. Treatment of radiation-induced nervous system injury with heparin and warfarin. *Neurology*. 1994;44:2020–2027.
21. Gothard L, Cornes P, Earl J, et al. Double-blind placebo-controlled randomised trial of vitamin E and pentoxifylline in patients with chronic arm lymphoedema and fibrosis after surgery and radiotherapy for breast cancer. *Radiother Oncol*. 2004;73:133–139.
22. Magnusson M, Höglund P, Johansson K, et al. Pentoxifylline and vitamin E treatment for prevention of radiation-induced side-effects in women with breast cancer: a phase two, double-blind, placebo-controlled randomised clinical trial (Ptx-5). *Eur J Cancer*. 2009;45:2488–2495.
23. Bowen J, Gregory R, Squier M, Donaghy M. The post-irradiation lower motor neuron syndrome neuronopathy or radiculopathy? *Brain J Neurol*. 1996;119(Pt 5):1429–1439.
24. Esik O, Vönöczky K, Lengyel Z, Sáfrány G, Trón L. Characteristics of radiogenic lower motor neurone disease, a possible link with a preceding viral infection. *Spinal Cord*. 2004;42:99–105.
25. Jabbour P, Gault J, Murk SE, Awad IA. Multiple spinal cavernous malformations with atypical phenotype after prior irradiation: case report. *Neurosurgery*. 2004;55:1431.
26. Allen JC, Miller DC, Budzilovich GN, Epstein FJ. Brain and spinal cord hemorrhage in long-term survivors of malignant pediatric brain tumors: a possible late effect of therapy. *Neurology*. 1991;41:148–150.
27. Rigamonti A, Lauria G, Mantero V, Filizzolo M, Salmaggi A. SMART (stroke-like migraine attack after radiation therapy) syndrome: a case report with review of the literature. *Neurol Sci*. 2016;37:157–161.
28. Zheng Q, Yang L, Tan LM, Qin LX, Wang CY, Zhang HN. Stroke-like migraine attacks after radiation therapy syndrome. *Chin Med J (Engl.)*. 2015;128:2097–2101.
29. Black DF, Morris JM, Lindell EP, et al. Stroke-like migraine attacks after radiation therapy (SMART) syndrome is not always completely reversible: a case series. *AJNR Am J Neuroradiol*. 2013;34:2298–2303.
30. Black D, Bartleson J, Bell M, Lachance D. SMART: stroke-like migraine attacks after radiation therapy. *Cephalalgia*. 2006;26:1137–1142.
31. Singh AK, Tantiwongkosi B, Moise AM, Altmeyer WB. Stroke-like migraine attacks after radiation therapy syndrome: case report and review of the literature. *NeuroRadiol J*. 2017;30:568–573.

32. Khanipour Roshan S, Salmela MB, McKinney AM. Susceptibility-weighted imaging in stroke-like migraine attacks after radiation therapy syndrome. *Neuroradiology*. 2015;57:1103–1109.
33. Maloney PR, Rabinstein AA, Daniels DJ, Link MJ. Surgically induced SMART syndrome: case report and review of the literature. *World Neurosurg*. 2014;82:240.e7–240, e12.
34. Solomon GD. Verapamil prophylaxis of migraine: a double-blind, placebo-controlled study. *J Am Med Assoc*. 1983;250:2500.
35. Littley MD, Shalet SM, Beardwell CG, Robinson EL, Sutton ML. Radiation-induced hypopituitarism is dose-dependent. *Clin Endocrinol*. 1989;31:363–373.
36. Rose SR, Horne VE, Howell J, et al. Late endocrine effects of childhood cancer. *Nat Rev Endocrinol*. 2016;12:319–336.
37. Vatner RE, Niemierko A, Misra M, et al. Endocrine deficiency as a function of radiation dose to the hypothalamus and pituitary in pediatric and young adult patients with brain tumors. *J Clin Oncol*. 2018;36:2854–2862.
38. Clayton PE, Shalet SM. Dose dependency of time of onset of radiation-induced growth hormone deficiency. *J Pediatr*. 1991;118:226–228.
39. Crowne E, Gleeson H, Benghiat H, Sanghera P, Toogood A. Effect of cancer treatment on hypothalamic–pituitary function. *Lancet Diabetes Endocrinol*. 2015;3:568–576.
40. Agha A, Sherlock M, Brennan S, et al. Hypothalamic-pituitary dysfunction after irradiation of nonpituitary brain tumors in adults. J Clin Endocrinol Metab. 90:6355–6360.
41. Appelman-Dijkstra NM, Kokshoorn NE, Dekkers OM, et al. Pituitary dysfunction in adult patients after cranial radiotherapy: systematic review and meta-analysis. *J Clin Endocrinol Metab*. 2011;96:2330–2340.
42. Darzy KH, Aimaretti G, Wieringa G, Gattamaneni HR, Ghigo E, Shalet SM. The usefulness of the combined growth hormone (GH)-releasing hormone and arginine stimulation test in the diagnosis of radiation-induced GH deficiency is dependent on the post-irradiation time interval. *J Clin Endocrinol Metab*. 2003;88:95–102.
43. Nandagopal R, Laverdière C, Mulrooney D, Hudson MM, Meacham L. Endocrine late effects of childhood cancer therapy: a report from the children's oncology group. *Horm Res*. 2008;69:65–74.
44. Pai HH, Thornton A, Katznelson L, et al. Hypothalamic/pituitary function following high-dose conformal radiotherapy to the base of skull: demonstration of a dose–effect relationship using dose–volume histogram analysis. *Int J Radiat Oncol*. 2001;49:1079–1092.
45. Constine LS, Woolf PD, Cann D, et al. Hypothalamic-pituitary dysfunction after radiation for brain tumors. *N Engl J Med*. 1993;328:87–94.
46. Rappaport R, Brauner R, Czernichow P, et al. Effect of hypothalamic and pituitary irradiation on pubertal development in children with cranial tumors. *J Clin Endocrinol Metab*. 1982;54:1164–1168.
47. Ogilvy-Stuart AL, Clayton PE, Shalet SM. Cranial irradiation and early puberty. *J Clin Endocrinol Metab*. 1994;78:1282–1286.
48. Livesey EA, Hindmarsh PC, Brook CG, et al. Endocrine disorders following treatment of childhood brain tumours. *Br J Cancer*. 1990;61:622–625.
49. Ling S, Bhatt AD, Brown NV, et al. Correlative study of dose to thyroid and incidence of subsequent dysfunction after head and neck radiation. *Head Neck*. 2017;39:548–554.
50. Samaan NA, Vieto R, Schultz PN, et al. Hypothalamic, pituitary and thyroid dysfunction after radiotherapy to the head and neck. *Int J Radiat Oncol Biol Phys*. 1982;8:1857–1867.
51. Saper CB, Scammell TE, Lu J. Hypothalamic regulation of sleep and circadian rhythms. *Nature*. 2005;437:1257–1263.
52. Rosen GM, Bendel AE, Neglia JP, Moertel CL, Mahowald M. Sleep in children with neoplasms of the central nervous system: case review of 14 children. *Pediatrics*. 2003;112:e46–e54.
53. Khan RB, Merchant TE, Sadighi ZS, et al. Prevalence, risk factors, and response to treatment for hypersomnia of central origin in survivors of childhood brain tumors. *J Neuro Oncol*. 2018;136:379–384.
54. Lustig RH. Hypothalamic obesity after craniopharyngioma: mechanisms, diagnosis, and treatment. *Front Endocrinol*. 2011;2:60.
55. Merchant TE, Kiehna EN, Sanford RA, et al. Craniopharyngioma: the St. Jude Children's Research Hospital experience 1984–2001. *Int J Radiat Oncol Biol Phys*. 2002;53:533–542.
56. Cohen M, Bartels U, Branson H, Kulkarni AV, Hamilton J. Trends in treatment and outcomes of pediatric craniopharyngioma, 1975–2011. *Neuro Oncol*. 2013;15:767–774.
57. Murphy ES, Xie H, Merchant TE, Yu JS, Chao ST, Suh JH. Review of cranial radiotherapy-induced vasculopathy. *J Neuro Oncol*. 2015;122:421–429.
58. Flickinger JC, Nelson PB, Taylor FH, Robinson A. Incidence of cerebral infarction after radiotherapy for pituitary adenoma. *Cancer*. 1989;63:2404–2408.
59. Sattler MG, Vroomen PC, Sluiter WJ, et al. Incidence, causative mechanisms, and anatomic localization of stroke in pituitary adenoma patients treated with postoperative radiation therapy versus surgery alone. *Int J Radiat Oncol Biol Phys*. 2013;87:53–59.
60. Brada M, Burchell L, Ashley S, Traish D. The incidence of cerebrovascular accidents in patients with pituitary adenoma. *Int J Radiat Oncol Biol Phys*. 1999;45:693–698.
61. Bowers DC, Liu Y, Leisenring W, et al. Late-occurring stroke among long-term survivors of childhood leukemia and brain tumors: a report from the Childhood Cancer Survivor Study. *J Clin Oncol*. 2006;24:5277–5282.
62. Morris B, Partap S, Yeom K, Gibbs IC, Fisher PG, King AA. Cerebrovascular disease in childhood cancer survivors: a children's Oncology Group Report. *Neurology*. 2009;73:1906–1913.
63. Kernan WN, Ovbiagele B, Black HR, et al. Guidelines for the prevention of stroke in patients with stroke and transient ischemic attack: a guideline for healthcare professionals from the American Heart Association/American Stroke Association. *Stroke*. 2014;45:2160–2236.
64. Kikuchi A, Maeda M, Hanada R, et al. Moyamoya syndrome following childhood acute lymphoblastic leukemia. *Pediatr Blood Cancer*. 2007;48:268–272.
65. Ullrich NJ, Robertson R, Kinnamon DD, et al. Moyamoya following cranial irradiation for primary brain tumors in children. *Neurology*. 2007;68:932–938.
66. Yu SC, Zou WX, Soo YO, et al. Evaluation of carotid angioplasty and stenting for radiation-induced carotid stenosis. *Stroke*. 2014;45:1402–1407.
67. Strenger V, Sovinz P, Lackner H, et al. Intracerebral cavernous hemangioma after cranial irradiation in childhood. Incidence and risk factors. *Strahlenther Onkol*. 2008;184:276–280.
68. Lew S, Morgan JN, Psaty E, Lefton DR, Allen JC, Abbott R. Cumulative incidence of radiation-induced cavernomas in long-term survivors of medulloblastoma. *J Neurosurg*. 2006;104:103–107.

69. Kondziolka D, Monaco EA, Lunsford LD. Cavernous malformations and hemorrhage risk. *Prog Neurol Surg*. 2013;27:141–146.
70. Al-Holou WN, O'Lynnger TM, Pandey AS, et al. Natural history and imaging prevalence of cavernous malformations in children and young adults. *J Neurosurg Pediatr*. 2012;9:198–205.
71. Fouladi M, Langston J, Mulhern R, et al. Silent lacunar lesions detected by magnetic resonance imaging of children with brain tumors: a late sequela of therapy. *J Clin Oncol*. 2000;18(4):824–831.
72. Neglia JP, Robinson LL, Stovall M, et al. New primary neoplasms of the central nervous system in survivors of childhood cancer: a report from the Childhood Cancer Survivor Study. *J Natl Cancer Inst*. 2006;98:1528–1537.
73. Yonehara S, Brenner AV, Kishikawa M, et al. Clinical and epidemiologic characteristics of first primary tumors of the central nervous system and related organs among atomic bomb survivors in Hiroshima and Nagasaki, 1958–1995. *Cancer*. 2004;101:1644–1654.
74. Wiemels J, Wrensch M, Claus EB. Epidemiology and etiology of meningioma. *J Neuro Oncol*. 2010;99:307–314.
75. Ostrom QT, Gittleman H, Truitt G, Boscia A, Kruchko C, Barnholtz-Sloan JS. CBTRUS Statistical Report: primary brain and other central nervous system tumors diagnosed in the United States in 2011–2015. *Neuro Oncol*. 2018;20:iv1–iv86.
76. Ron E, Modan B, Boice Jr JD, et al. Tumors of the brain and nervous system after radiotherapy in childhood. *N Engl J Med*. 1988;319:1033–1039.
77. Sadetzki S, Flint-Richter P, Ben-Tal T, Nass D. Radiation-induced meningioma: a descriptive study of 253 cases. *J Neurosurg*. 2002;97:1078–1082.
78. Yamanaka R, Hayano A, Kanayama T. Radiation-induced meningiomas: an exhaustive review of the literature. *World Neurosurg*. 2017;97:635–644. e8.
79. Cahan WG, Woodard HQ, Higinbotham NL, Stewart FW, Coley BL. Sarcoma arising in irradiated bone: report of eleven cases. 1948. *Cancer*. 1998;82:8–34.
80. Al-Mefty O, Topsakal C, Pravdenkova S, Sawyer JR, Harrison MJ. Radiation-induced meningiomas: clinical, pathological, cytokinetic, and cytogenetic characteristics. *J Neurosurg*. 2004;100:1002–1013.
81. Goldbrunner R, Minniti G, Preusser M, et al. EANO guidelines for the diagnosis and treatment of meningiomas. *Lancet Oncol*. 2016;17:e383–e391.
82. Louis DN, Perr A, Reifenberger G, et al. The 2016 World Health Organization classification of tumors of the central nervous system: a summary. *Acta Neuropathol*. 2016;131:803–820.
83. Yamanaka R, Hayano A, Kanayama T. Radiation-induced gliomas: a comprehensive review and meta-analysis. *Neurosurg Rev*. 2018;41:719–731.
84. Sadetzki S, Chetrit A, Freedman L, Stovall M, Modan B, Novikov I. Long-term follow-up for brain tumor development after childhood exposure to ionizing radiation for tinea capitis. *Radiat Res*. 2005;163:424–432.
85. Diallo I, Haddy N, Adjadj E, et al. Frequency distribution of second solid cancer locations in relation to the irradiated volume among 115 patients treated for childhood cancer. *Int J Radiat Oncol*. 2009;74:876–883.
86. Prasad G, Haas-Kogan DA. Radiation-induced gliomas. *Expert Rev Neurother*. 2009;9:1511–1517.
87. Brat DJ, James CD, Jedlicka AE, et al. Molecular genetic alterations in radiation-induced astrocytomas. *Am J Pathol*. 1999;154:1431–1438.
88. Donson AM, Erwin NS, Kleinschmidt-DeMasters BK, Madden JR, Addo-Yobo SO, Foreman NK. Unique molecular characteristics of radiation-induced glioblastoma. *J Neuropathol Exp Neurol*. 2007;66:740–749.
89. Paulino AC, Mai WY, Chintagumpala M, Taher A, Teh BS. Radiation-induced malignant gliomas: is there a role for reirradiation? *Int J Radiat Oncol Biol Phys*. 2008;71:1381–1387.

Chapter | 27 |

Approach to the patient with a delayed posttreatment CNS neurotoxicity

Amy Pruitt

CHAPTER OUTLINE

Introduction

With significant advances in cancer treatment, both the number of long-term cancer survivors and the complications to which these patients are vulnerable have grown. These complications can involve the peripheral and/or central nervous systems, significantly impairing quality of life (QOL) and not infrequently affecting overall survival. This chapter complements other chapters' discussion of treatment-related complications, concentrating on those that occur after the acute phase of chemotherapy or combined modality regimens. The chapter begins with a brief discussion of some of the peripheral nervous system complications that can occur following chemotherapy and targeted treatments for cancer—and some of these are discussed in further detail in subsequent chapters (see Chapter 28 for discussion of chemotherapy induced peripheral neuropathy). This is followed by a case-based review of central nervous system complications of systemic therapies. Complications unique to immunotherapies and chimeric antigen receptor (CAR) T-cell interventions are covered in Chapters 29 and 30, respectively.

Overview of chemotherapy

Table 27.1 summarizes the common complications of cytotoxic and targeted therapies based on the syndrome, etiology, and acuity of the neurological problem.[1] Table 27.2 emphasizes the special adverse effects and drug interactions of corticosteroids, one of the most ubiquitous agents used in oncology. Corticosteroid complications are both dose and duration dependent.[2]

Both nervous and extra-nervous complications may occur following systemic treatments for cancer. Within the neuroaxis, both central nervous system (CNS) and peripheral nervous system (PNS) complications can occur. In the PNS, chemotherapy-induced peripheral neuropathy (CIPN) is the most common late complication of chemotherapy,

Table 27.1 Complications of chemotherapy and immunotherapy

Central nervous system toxicities	Conventional chemotherapy	Biologic and immunologic therapies
Acute encephalopathy (within hours to 24 hours after therapy delivered)	Ifosfamide, methotrexate, cytarabine, cisplatin[a], 5-fluorouracil, vinca alkaloids[b]	Vascular endothelial growth factor (VEGF) inhibitors (posterior reversible encephalopathy syndrome [PRES]), interferon alfa, interleukin-2, corticosteroids
Subacute encephalopathy	Procarbazine[c], methotrexate, nelarabine	
Multifocal leukoencephalopathy	Capecitabine	
Delayed encephalopathy	Methotrexate, high-dose multidrug regimens (anthracyclines)[d]	Tacrolimus, sirolimus, cyclosporine
Headache[e]	Ixabepilone, nelarabine, tamoxifen, etoposide, fludarabine	
PRES	Cytarabine, gemcitabine, cyclophosphamide, methotrexate, cisplatin, carboplatin	Cyclosporine/tacrolimus/sirolimus, rituximab, nivolumab, pembrolizumab, bevacizumab, other VEGF inhibitors
Seizures	Methotrexate, busulfan, cytarabine, cisplatin, etoposide, dacarbazine, carmustine, paclitaxel	Chimeric antigen receptor T-cell therapy, interferon alfa, VEGF inhibitors
Acute focal deficit (demyelinating, arterial/venous ischemia)	L-asparaginase, methotrexate, fludarabine	Pembrolizumab[f], nivolumab[f]
Cerebellar syndrome	5-Fluorouracil, nelarabine, cytarabine, capecitabine	
Lymphocytic meningitis	Methotrexate, cytarabine[g]	Trastuzumab, intravenous immunoglobulin (IVIG)
Myelopathy	Methotrexate, cytarabine (intrathecal), cisplatin (transient demyelination with Lhermitte sign)	Ipilimumab
Hearing loss	Cisplatin, vincristine, oxaliplatin	Tacrolimus
Optic neuropathy	Fludarabine, tamoxifen	Bevacizumab (with radiation therapy), tacrolimus, crizotinib
Peripheral nervous system toxicities	**Conventional cytotoxic chemotherapy**	**Biologic and immunologic therapies**
Chronic, mostly sensory polyneuropathy	Docetaxel, paclitaxel, cisplatin, vincristine (also motor, cranial nerves, autonomic), bortezomib, ixabepilone, thalidomide (sensory and autonomic)	Brentuximab
Acute inflammatory demyelinating polyradiculoneuropathy (AIDP)/chronic inflammatory demyelinating polyradiculoneuropathy (CIDP)		Ipilimumab, nivolumab, pembrolizumab, tacrolimus
Myasthenia	Cisplatin	Ipilimumab, interferon alfa, interleukin-2, nivolumab, pembrolizumab[h]

Continued

Table 27.1 Complications of chemotherapy and immunotherapy—cont'd

Myopathy	Gemcitabine	Aromatase inhibitors, ipilimumab, corticosteroids, selumetinib, nivolumab, pembrolizumab[h]
Infections		
Viral		
Cytomegalovirus, human herpesvirus 6	High-dose induction therapy with various chemotherapy agents 0–1 month post transplantation	
Varicella-zoster virus, herpes simplex virus	Corticosteroids, mycophenolate 1–6 months post transplantation	Tacrolimus, cyclosporine, sirolimus
Progressive multifocal leukoencephalopathy (JC virus)	Leflunomide, azathioprine	Rituximab, alemtuzumab, brentuximab, mycophenolate, ibrutinib, tacrolimus, multiple combination regimens that deplete CD4+ counts
Fungal		
Aspergillus, Candida	Prolonged neutropenia from chemotherapy or posttransplant regimen	Ibrutinib

[a]Hypomagnesemia, seizures, syndrome of inappropriate secretion of antidiuretic hormone [SIADH].
[b]Syndrome of SIADH, also seen with cisplatin and cyclophosphamide.
[c]Procarbazine: weak monoamine oxidase inhibitor can produce hypertensive encephalopathy, headache, or delirium after administration with sympathomimetic agents or after consumption of tyramine-containing foods.
[d]Particularly anthracycline-based regimens producing chemo brain.
[e]Headache soon after administration as a prominent feature absent PRES or encephalopathy.
[f]Pseudoprogression.
[g]Any intrathecal agent can produce lymphocytic meningitis
[h]Combinations of myopathy and myasthenia gravis have been reported with various PD1 and PDL1 inhibitors.
Data modified from Pruitt AA. Epidemiology, treatment and complications of central nervous system metastases. *Continuum (Minneap Minn).* 2017;23(6):1580–1600.

whereas in the CNS, neurocognitive dysfunction is the most common. Systemically, a number of late effects predispose patients to infectious, toxic, metabolic, and immune-mediated complications of cancer treatment including long-term hematologic toxicities, endocrinopathies, and infections.

Hematologic toxicities

High-grade cytopenias are less common in standard adult brain tumor therapy than in regimens for other malignancies. Nitrosoureas are more likely than temozolomide to produce significant cytopenias, but chronic high-grade lymphopenia with the latter can predispose to *Pneumocystis jirovecii* (PJP) and other infections. It is recommended that PJP prophylaxis be given to patients being treated with chemoradiation on the Stupp regimen (see Chapter 4 for background on evidence-based chemotherapies for brain tumors). PJP has been reported in other brain tumor patients treated with chemotherapy and radiation such as primary CNS lymphoma (PCNSL). It is appropriate to follow serial lymphocyte counts and consider prophylaxis when lymphocyte counts are <500 cells/mL, but no clear guidelines have been prospectively validated.

The American Society of Clinical Oncology (ASCO) recommends a threshold of 10,000 platelets for prophylactic transfusion in solid tumors, but clinicians may consider a threshold of 20,000 for patients with necrotic tumors at increased risk of intracranial hemorrhage: there is an absence of firm data. For neurosurgery, platelet counts of >100,000 are preferable and should be at least >75,000 cells/mL.[3]

Endocrine and fertility issues

Alkylating agents are among the most gonadotoxic chemotherapy drugs, resulting in follicular depletion, destruction of oocytes, and premature ovarian failure. In some men,

Table 27.2 Adverse effects and drug interactions of corticosteroids[a]

Common	Uncommon
Myopathy	Psychosis
Weight gain	Hiccups
Peripheral edema	Epidural lipomatosis
Behavioral changes	Avascular necrosis
Insomnia	Allergy suppression
Glucose intolerance	Gastric irritation/ hemorrhage
Tremor	Infections (PJP, PML, VZV)[b]
Reduced taste	Steroid dependence
Osteopenia/osteoporosis	
Oral candidiasis (thrush)	
Cerebral atrophy	
Enhanced steroid potency	**Diminished steroid potency (CYP 3A4 inducers)**
Cirrhosis	Barbiturates
Hypothyroidism	Phenytoin
Macrolide antibiotics	Carbamazepine
Ketoconazole	Rifampin
Thalidomide	
Enhanced coagulation effect	
Warfarin	

[a]Most adverse effects are dose and duration dependent and largely independent of specific corticosteroid preparation chosen.
[b]See Table 27.1 for other infections associated with chemotherapy regimens that can include corticosteroids.

drugs such as temozolomide may have deleterious effects on sperm counts, sperm motility, and sperm density that appear to be transient in most but may be permanent.

Treatment-induced infectious complications

Immune-suppressive agents such as cyclophosphamide, azathioprine, mycophenolate mofetil, cyclosporine, tacrolimus, mitoxantrone, and methotrexate predispose patients to a wide range of bacterial, fungal, and viral pathogens, whereas immunomodulatory drugs confer a generally lower risk of infection, as they target only one or a few immune system components. Table 27.1 summarizes reported CNS infections associated with commonly used antineoplastic agents. Common among these infections is reactivation of herpesviruses with disseminated varicella zoster (VZV) or cytomegalovirus (CMV). Rituximab-related infections include progressive multifocal leukoencephalopathy (PML), CMV, enterovirus meningoencephalitis, increased severity of West Nile, Babesiosis, and PJP. Reactivation of hepatitis B can occur and re-vaccination may be necessary.

Clinicians should consider the patient's underlying cancer diagnosis and treatment regimen when evaluating infectious complications. For patients on active treatment, timing of prophylactic and vaccination strategies should be considered to avoid blood count nadir. Clinicians should be aware of transfusion safety, travel and zoonotic exposures, community and nosocomial epidemiologic trends, and remember that presentation and course of any pathogen in a cancer patient may be different from those of patients without immune-compromising conditions. Radiation and chemotherapy complications may mimic infection with novel syndromes.[4]

Chemotherapy-induced peripheral neuropathy

CIPN (also see Chapter 28 for further case-based discussion of CIPN) is among the most common long-term adverse effect of many antineoplastic agents, and decreases QOL in cancer survivors with symptoms that include pain in the hands and feet with associated inability to complete basic activities of daily living (ADLs) and risk of falling.[5] It has been estimated that injuries are three times as common in patients with CIPN as in those without neuropathy. CIPN is likely underdiagnosed by clinicians, especially in younger age groups.[6] CIPN may require dose modifications and treatment interruptions, thereby negatively influencing patient survival as well. The most common offending drugs include docetaxel and paclitaxel (e.g., taxanes), platinum compounds, vinca alkaloids, and the proteasome inhibitor bortezomib. For these drugs, neuropathy may be the dose-limiting toxicity. A metaanalysis of over 4,000 patients estimated CIPN prevalence to be about 68% at the end of the first month and 30% at 6 months.[7] In a study of 121 childhood cancer survivors who received chemotherapy before age 17 with a median of 8.5 years of follow-up, over half treated with vinca alkaloids and platinum compounds continued to have lower limb sensory axonal neuropathy and deficits in manual dexterity, distal sensation, and balance consistent with CIPN. Often these symptoms (which may be greater in the presence of comorbidities such as diabetes mellitus and patients' age) are not specifically addressed in follow-up of childhood cancer survivors, and multimodal testing with objective neurophysiologic measures and subjective patient-reported outcome measures is important.[8]

Treatment-related peripheral neuropathies must be distinguished from those similarly appearing immune-mediated neuropathies associated with a limited number of cancers such as multiple myeloma (e.g., POEMS), thymoma (e.g., anti-CV2 sensorimotor), lymphoplasmacytic lymphoma (previously known as Waldenstrom's), and small-cell lung cancer (e.g., paraneoplastic anti-Hu antibody dorsal root ganglionopathy) (see Chapter 20 for further discussion of paraneoplastic neurological syndromes). Sensory neurons in the dorsal root ganglia lack a blood-brain barrier (BBB) and therefore can be more vulnerable to systemically administered chemotherapy toxins than are motor neurons. Large myelinated fibers are affected by platinum drugs and small fibers are preferentially affected by taxanes and microtubule poisons such as vincristine.[9] Toxicity is dose dependent and may continue to worsen after cessation of chemotherapy, a phenomenon called coasting. The neuropathy from oxaliplatin and bortezomib improves slowly, though up to a third of patients may have persistent discomfort with burning dysesthesias, proprioceptive problems, and/or allodynia that impair QOL.

Unfortunately, no therapy for CIPN has been approved by the Food and Drug Administration (FDA), and duloxetine is the only drug with modest demonstrated benefit in a prospective randomized clinical trial (RCT).[10] Neurologic consultants offer helpful input by ruling out alternative explanations, including immune-mediated demyelinating neuropathies or spinal cord pathology that require investigation with imaging or spinal fluid sampling for leptomeningeal involvement. Neurologists can define the severity of neuropathy to guide decisions about whether symptoms will be worsened by additional neurotoxic regimens.[11]

Clinical cases

The following cases illustrate the often-multifactorial dilemmas that result from successful cancer therapy.

CASE 27.1 ONGOING INFECTIOUS RISKS MANY YEARS AFTER SUCCESSFUL CHEMOTHERAPY

Case. A 68-year-old man presented with a 3-month history of clumsiness of the left hand, balance difficulties, and dysarthria. Forty-one years earlier he had been treated for stage 1A nodular sclerosing Hodgkin's disease with mechlorethamine hydrochloride, vincristine, procarbazine, and prednisone (MOPP), splenectomy, and extended field radiation of 2000 cGY to the mantle field (e.g., all lymph node areas in the neck, chest, and arms). Coronary artery disease presented at age 50 years (he had stopped smoking at age 35 years), and he underwent triple coronary artery bypass grafting. MRI showed a non-enhancing lesion of the left cerebellum (Fig. 27.1). The differential diagnosis was thought to be PML versus a low-grade radiation–induced glial neoplasm. He was HIV negative with a CD4+ count of 170 cells/mL (duration unknown, as it had not been regularly measured in the many decades since his original treatment). He had acellular cerebrospinal fluid (CSF) that was negative for John Cunningham virus (JCV). However, brain biopsy revealed PML, and he received pembrolizumab as part of an investigational trial. Subsequently, he was found to have a second, probably radiation-induced tumor, a mesothelioma subsequently found on PET/CT.

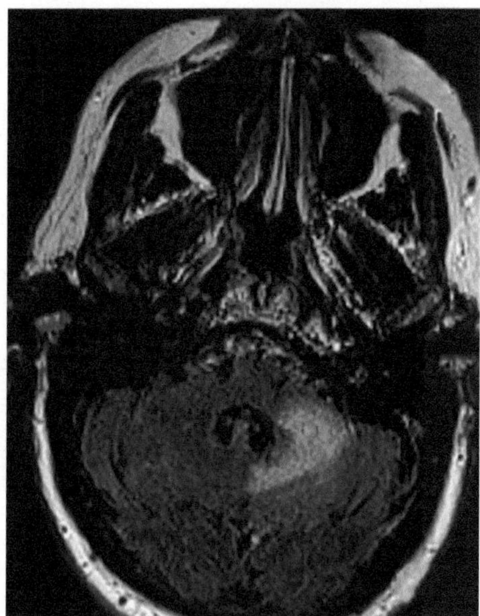

Fig. 27.1 This MRI fluid-attenuated inversion recovery sequence shows an area of hyperintensity in the left cerebellum that does not produce significant mass effect and that did not show enhancement on gadolinium-enhanced MRI sequences (not shown). The radiographic differential diagnosis was low-grade glial neoplasm or progressive multifocal leukoencephalopathy.

Teaching Points. This case demonstrates the long-term risk of infection that extends well beyond the initial active treatment period. A high index of suspicion was needed, as commercially available testing for JCV was initially negative and a brain biopsy was required to establish the diagnosis and open up options for clinical trial therapy.

Clinical Pearls

1. The risk for infection continues well beyond the active treatment period.

2. CSF can be negative for JC virus when tested by commercially available methods.
3. CSF formulas in immunocompromised patients can fail to reflect inflammation in the presence of cytopenias or impaired immune response.
4. PML can have variable appearances with or without contrast enhancement.
5. Immunocompromised patients should have screening CT/MRI before lumbar puncture.
6. There is no established therapy for PML, but pembrolizumab is being investigated.[12]

CASE 27.2 IS THE PROBLEM CAUSED BY THE DISEASE ITSELF OR SOME OTHER COMPLICATION?

Case. A 57-year-old woman initially treated for stage IIIA Hodgkin's lymphoma with ABVD (i.e., first-line treatment regimen consisting of Adriamycin, bleomycin, vinblastine, and dacarbazine) at age 44 years. At age 55 years, she had a recurrence treated with gemcitabine, docetaxel, and brentuximab. While still on chemotherapy treatment, she presented with 6 weeks of progressive leg pain and weakness with bladder dysfunction (a cauda equina syndrome). MRI showed enhancement of the cauda equine roots. CSF protein was 192 mg/dL, glucose 59 mg/dL, and white blood cells (WBC) 38 lymphocytes/mL with negative cytology on two successive lumbar punctures.

Teaching Point #1: Is this syndrome likely to be due to recurrent Hodgkin lymphoma? The clinician should first recognize that this neurological syndrome is unlikely to be explained by recurrent Hodgkin disease. CNS involvement in Hodgkin disease is extremely rare. However, clinicians must consider non-Hodgkin lymphoma, a second hematologic malignancy that is more likely to spread to the CNS.

Case 27.2 – Continued

The patient then developed sudden bilateral vision loss. An inflammatory process such as neuromyelitis optica (NMO) was considered, and IV methylprednisolone 1000 mg daily was administered for 5 days. Her physicians were considering adding rituximab when she developed multiple cranial nerve palsies including left cranial nerve (CN) III, bilateral CN V, and right CN VIII palsies.

Teaching Point #2: What other tests should be done on the CSF? At this point, the patient had evidence of disease involving the cauda equine, cranial nerves, and vision which localized to the CSF. Neoplastic workup was negative and a strong consideration was for an infectious source including herpesvirus infection. Table 27.1 indicates the herpesvirus-associated syndromes and cancer treatment regimens that confer the highest risk. In this patient, subsequent CSF sampling showed protein 299 mg/dL, glucose 56 mg/dL, and 47 WBC cells/mL. VZV polymerase chain reaction (PCR) was negative but VZV IgG was >4000 and IgM >3.67, confirming varicella-zoster infection.

Posttreatment VZV meningoencephalitis. VZV IgM in serum or CSF is indicative of acute infection with VZV. PCR is less likely to be helpful more than 1 week after symptom onset. As this patient was more than 1 week out from symptom onset, the appropriate test is an antibody radio of VZV-specific IgG/total IgG in CSF test to VZV-specific IgG/total IgG in the serum. She was treated with acyclovir with no recovery of vision.

Clinical Pearls

1. Up to 15% of leukemia and lymphoma patients will have symptomatic dermatomal VZV infection. Post-herpetic neuralgia is more than three times as frequent in cancer patients as in those without cancer who develop shingles.
2. Systemic neurologic syndromes from zoster include: the well-known dermatomal or disseminated skin lesions, focal segmental weakness, acute encephalitis or myelitis, vasculopathy with large and small vessel arteritis—40% of whom have no history of rash and up to one-third who have no CSF pleocytosis.[13]
3. Ocular manifestations of VZV include Ramsay-Hunt syndrome, pontine myelitis infarction of one or more cranial nerves, acute monocular visual loss with temporal arteritis-like presentation, and acute outer retinal necrosis (this patient).
4. The new VZV subunit vaccine (Shingrix) is appropriate for immunocompromised patients.

CASE 27.3 TREATMENT-INDUCED NEUROCOGNITIVE DYSFUNCTION (CHEMO BRAIN AND CAVERNOMA)

Case. At age 11, a now 69-year old man, who has four cousins and a sister with brain tumors, had a grade II cerebellar astrocytoma resected and treated with an unknown dose of radiation therapy. He did well through childhood, but high-frequency hearing loss necessitated a hearing aid by age 34 years. Dysarthria developed in his mid-40s, and by age 50 years he had balance problems and loss of smell and taste. At age 60 years, he had a wide-based gait and frequent falls. Since age 68 years he has had progressive short-term memory problems. An MRI scan from 23 years earlier reportedly showed cerebellar atrophy and superficial siderosis. A cochlear implant was required at age 68 years.

Laboratory evaluation showed chronic cytopenias with leukopenia 3.1–3.8 cells/mL, platelet count of 121,000–136,000 cells/mL. Physical examination showed that he was hypertensive with dysarthria, scanning speech, wide-based gait, and ataxia of his arms and legs; handwriting was illegible. MRI scan at age 69 is shown in Fig. 27.2.

Teaching Points. This progressive speech and gait disorder (e.g., cerebellar ataxia) coupled with hearing loss and with the characteristic MRI findings is consistent with **superficial siderosis**. Some patients also have myelopathy, the

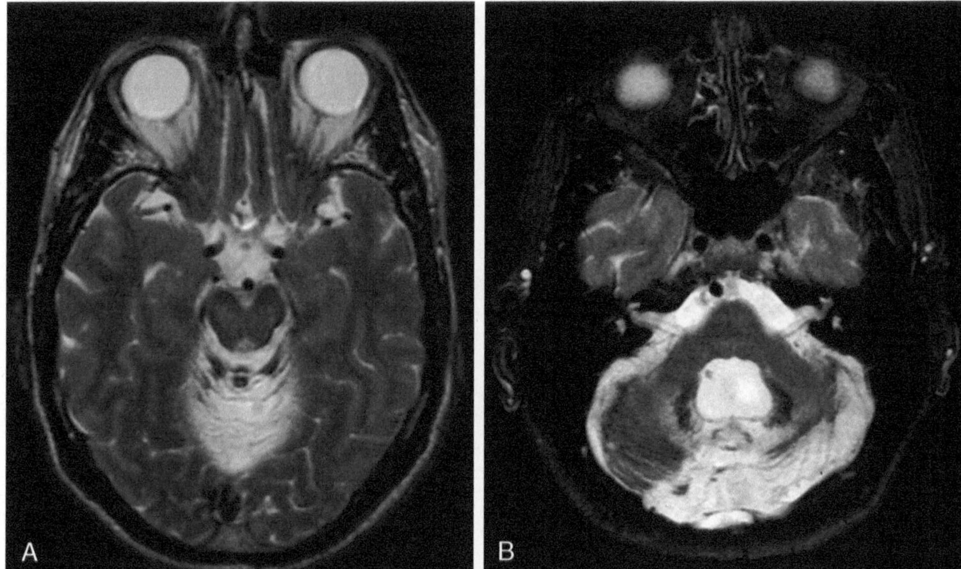

Fig. 27.2 (A) There is a rim of hypointense signal around the brainstem on T2-weighted MRI sequence and (B) marked cerebellar atrophy with compensatory IVth ventricle enlargement along with similar hypointense signal consistent with superficial siderosis in the cerebellar folia.

third component of the triad—cerebellar ataxia, myelopathy, and hearing loss. Superficial siderosis is a neurodegenerative condition caused by deposition of hemosiderin on the surface of the brain, spinal cord, and cranial nerves. Importantly, MRI scan did not show communicating hydrocephalus, which can also present with a gait disorder and cognitive dysfunction.

Clinical Pearls

1. Radiation in childhood leads to many long-term sequelae including endocrinopathies, vasculopathy, neurocognitive dysfunction, and risk of second malignancy among others. The patient did not have cavernous angiomata or communicating hydrocephalus and had no evidence of a secondary neoplasm, both differential considerations in this situation.
2. Superficial siderosis is a syndrome usually appearing many years after cranial surgery or traumatic brain injury, particularly in the posterior fossa. The pathophysiology is deposition of hemosiderin around the brainstem and cerebellar folia; the MRI signature is a rim of hypointensity around the basal cisterns and in the cerebellum.
3. Differential diagnosis of late-onset cognitive change after cancer treatment, as in this patient, should include interrogation of endocrine status (see Chapter 25 for further discussion of evaluating patients with treatment-induced neurocognitive dysfunction).
4. Chronic cytopenias raise the risk of a myelodysplastic syndrome, and such patients require lifelong surveillance.

CASE 27.4 CHEMO BRAIN

Case. A 43-year-old woman completed systemic chemotherapy for HER2+ breast cancer, completing treatment 3 years before neurologic evaluation. She has complained that her memory has never been the same since treatment; she cannot multitask, is always tired, and yet sleeps poorly. She now has to limit her work hours. Complete metabolic panel, blood count, and thyroid functions were normal. She was given a trial of duloxetine and then of nortriptyline, neither of which improved her symptoms.

Teaching Points. This patient suffers from what has been loosely called "chemo brain," first characterized in women after breast cancer chemotherapy. Studies have been conflicting. In one study of 206 participants (166 patients and 60 control subjects), patients demonstrated overall cognitive decline and scored consistently worse on Go/No-Go trials. Only chemotherapy patients showed decline in reaction time on a computerized alertness test. Overall cognitive performance correlated with self-reported cognitive problems at 1-year posttreatment.

PET scans have shown decreased activity in the left dorsolateral prefrontal cortex correlating with decreased processing speed. MRI scans are often normal but, in some studies of cancer survivors, with long intervals after cancer treatment, a higher prevalence of deep and infratentorial cerebral micro-hemorrhages has been reported (Fig. 27.3). In these patients, white matter lesion volume was similar to non-cancer controls.

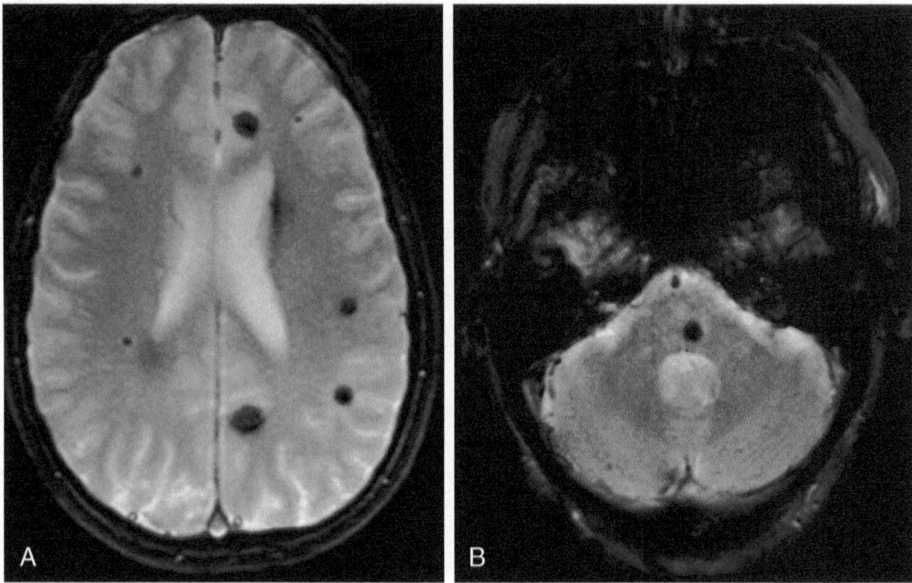

Fig. 27.3 Numerous radiation-induced cavernous angiomas are seen on the susceptibility weighted or gradient echo sequences both (A) supra- and (B) infratentorially.

Theories to explain chemo brain include recognition that chemotherapy can affect the coagulation profile of an individual, as seen by an increase in the rate of prothrombotic sequelae in patients on chemotherapy compared with those who did not receive chemotherapy. Additionally, it is thought that chemotherapy compounds may cause endothelial dysfunction with resultant arterial stiffening leading to chronic hypertension. Abnormal blood pressure fluctuation correlates with deep brain micro-bleeds (hypertensive arteriopathy). The elucidation of chemo brain potentially emerging from micro-hemorrhages and resultant white matter damage on imaging is an important issue that warrants future studies in cancer patients of all ages.[14–16]

Other cognitive changes may have more specific etiologies. For example, a patient who develops delirium after receiving capecitabine or 5-fluorouracil, drugs that inhibit pyrimidine biosynthesis and thereby decrease ammonia utilization, should be checked for hyperammonemia. If this is present, search for mutations among urea cycle–related genes should be undertaken.[17]

Clinical Pearls

1. Chemo brain is not explained exclusively by affective disorder or posttraumatic stress disorder.
2. Early detection of cerebral micro-hemorrhages requires attention to specific susceptibility-weighted imaging MRI sequences and may represent an opportunity to adjust therapeutic strategies before cognitive impairment becomes clinically detectable.
3. Specific attention to rigorous hypertension and other vascular risk factor treatment is indicated.

CASE 27.5 POSTTREATMENT LEUKOENCEPHALOPATHY

Case. A 47-year-old woman presented with a pathologic fracture of T10 and was diagnosed with metastatic estrogen receptor–positive, progesterone receptor–negative, and HER2-negative breast cancer. She was treated with anastrozole, denosumab, and palbociclib. Focal radiation therapy centered at T10 was completed in 10 sessions. Carcinomatous meningitis was suspected based on posterior fossa areas of leptomeningeal enhancement. She received seven intrathecal methotrexate treatments. Subsequent brain MRI showed diffuse white matter changes correlating with complaints of short-term memory impairment and imbalance (Fig. 27.4).

Teaching Points. While the combination of methotrexate and radiation therapy is particularly prone to cause progressive white matter changes, methotrexate alone, intrathecally or systemically, has produced similar complications. Work from the Monje laboratory has helped to elucidate the mechanism for methotrexate-induced chemotherapy toxicity, namely depletion of oligodendrocyte lineage cells that affect myelination and impair cognition in mice. There appears to be chronic microglial activation. Notably, microglial depletion can rescue glial cell dysregulation and cognitive deficits in mice but has yet to be translated into clinical treatments.[18]

Clinical Pearls

1. Delayed leukoencephalopathy has been seen in transplant recipients receiving cyclosporine or tacrolimus. The diffuse leukoencephalopathy resembles that of Case 27.5.

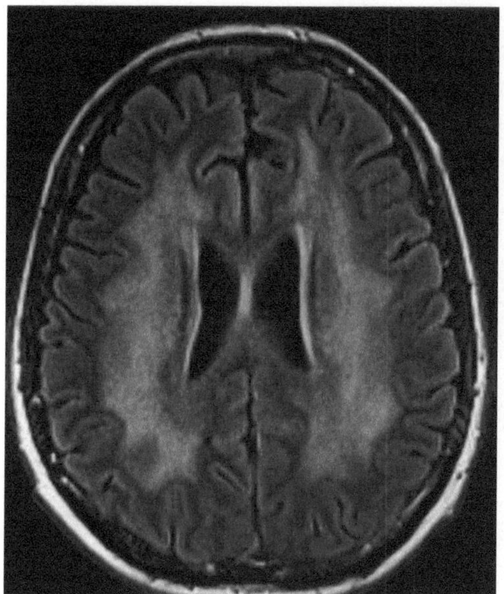

Fig. 27.4 This fluid-attenuated inversion recovery MRI sequences shows extensive areas of white matter abnormality consistent with the patient's prior chemotherapy. There is also evidence of overall brain atrophy.

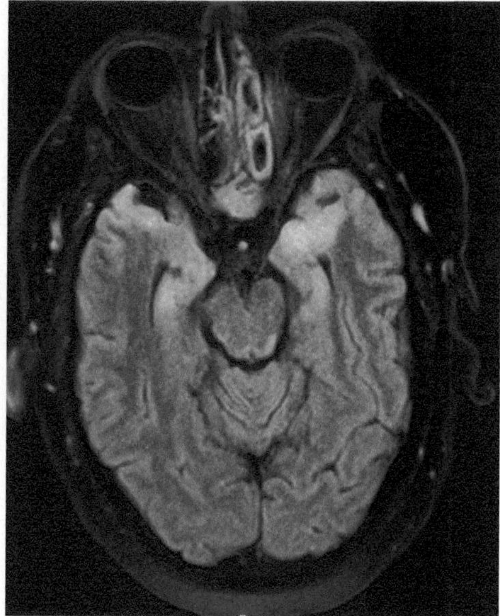

Fig. 27.5 A 62-year old man with melanoma treated with ipilimumab and nivolumab had rapid cognitive decline with cerebrospinal fluid showing cellularity and bands. The patient had some modest improvement in mentation after steroids, intravenous immunoglobulin, and rituximab.

2. There is emerging clinical experience with some patients who are receiving immune checkpoint inhibitors who may experience accelerated cognitive decline with immune-mediated encephalitis as the underlying pathophysiology and often a limbic encephalitis pattern on MRI (Fig. 27.5).

CASE 27.6 POSTTREATMENT CEREBROVASCULAR COMPLICATIONS—CAN THE DRUG BE GIVEN AGAIN?

Case. A 63-year-old woman was diagnosed with high-grade serous papillary cancer involving the peritoneum with tumor implants in bowel and diaphragm 4 years before her neurological presentation. She was treated with standard dose-dense taxol/carboplatin for over 1 year followed by liposomal doxorubicin and bevacizumab, the latter of which she received in 13 courses over 10 months. A few days after the 13th infusion, she developed prosopagnosia (i.e., inability to recognize familiar faces) and spatial disorientation. MRI showed confluent T2/fluid-attenuated inversion recovery (FLAIR) signal in the temporal, occipital, and posterior parietal cortex without enhancement. This was consistent with posterior reversible encephalopathy syndrome (PRES) (Fig. 27.6A). Bevacizumab was discontinued and there was improvement in the PRES pattern by 2 months later. However, three small acute infarcts in left cerebral hemisphere had developed, and innumerable scattered foci of micro-hemorrhages were noted on gradient echo (GRE) sequences (Fig. 27.6B). The patient reported progressive short-term memory issues.

Teaching Points. PRES or reversible posterior leukoencephalopathy syndrome (RPLS) is a clinicoradiologic syndrome occurring in several clinical settings including hypertensive urgencies, preeclampsia, and after administration of various chemotherapeutic agents, including antiangiogenic agents. Headache, seizures, confusion, and cortical blindness develop acutely with accompanying posterior parieto-occipital white matter changes of vasogenic edema. Changes are most pronounced in the posterior hemispheres. Most patients recover with elimination of the offending drug, blood pressure control, and, if necessary, treatment of seizures.

Bevacizumab is a humanized IgG monoclonal antibody targeting angiogenesis. It is currently approved for a number of systemic malignancies and for recurrent high-grade glial brain tumors. Common, mild adverse events include fatigue, hypertension and proteinuria.[3] More serious complications include thrombotic events, poor wound healing, and bowel perforation. Concurrent anticoagulation for arterial or venous infarction and bevacizumab has been studied with the conclusion that the risk-benefit profile is acceptable.[2]

Clinical Pearls

1. PRES should be considered in many clinical settings, the common denominator often being elevated blood pressure

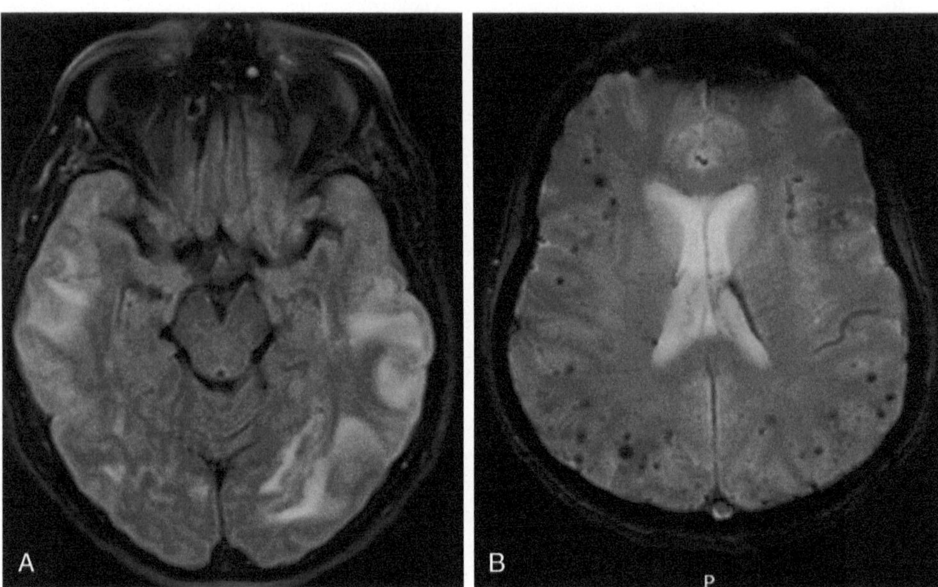

Fig. 27.6 (A) This fluid-attenuated inversion recovery sequence shows typical abnormalities of posterior reversible encephalopathy syndrome with hyperintensity involving primarily white matter, which were reversible after discontinuation of bevacizumab and treatment of hypertension.[8] The susceptibility weighted image (B) discloses numerous microhemorrhages (seen as dark spots on this image). Although they may not be directly related to the use of bevacizumab, the risk of hemorrhage from these areas precludes further antiangiogenic agent use.

and usually involves CT/MRI evidence of vasogenic edema predominantly in the posterior cerebral hemispheres.

2. Bevacizumab has been associated with both thrombotic and hemorrhagic events. Individualized decisions must be made about the risk/benefit of continuing this drug in the presence of arterial or venous thrombosis (see also this chapter, Case 27.7).

CASE 27.7 STROKE IN A CANCER PATIENT

Case. Twenty-three years after the diagnosis of an anaplastic astrocytoma treated with XRT and procarbazine, CCNU, and vincristine chemotherapy, a 52-year-old woman presented with recurrent tumor, now histologically a *IDH1/2*-negative, *MGMT*-promoter unmethylated glioblastoma. Repeat resection was followed by a year of temozolomide. Another recurrence was treated with repeat resection, followed by cycles of bevacizumab. After the 11th cycle of bevacizumab, she developed sudden left hemiparesis and right gaze preference. MRI showed a large area of diffusion restriction in the right hemisphere (Fig. 27.7).

Teaching Points. The presentations and etiologies of stroke in cancer patients differ from those in the non-cancer stroke populations (Table 27.3, Ref 2). Cancer patients with stroke more often have multi-vessel disease and may have altered levels of consciousness rather than a focal deficit as a presenting feature. Some drugs predispose to thrombophilic states (e.g., L-asparaginase and methotrexate). Stroke mimes such as seizure or stroke-like migraine after radiation therapy (SMART syndrome, see Chapter 26, Case 26.2 for further description) must be considered in the differential diagnosis. Infectious or nonbacterial thrombotic endocarditis, as well as rare tumor embolism, must be considered as well.

Thrombolytic agents for pulmonary embolism or ischemic stroke are contraindicated in patients with brain tumors. Risk of recurrent thromboembolic events after ischemic stroke in cancer patients is high. Up to one-third of stroke patients with cancer may have a recurrent thromboembolic event. Adenocarcinoma of the lung is the most common underlying cancer in patients with cancer-associated stroke. To judge the risk of anticoagulation, choice of agent, and duration of therapy, clinicians should consider clinical status, tumor type, and stroke mechanism.

Clinical Pearls

1. There are multiple mechanisms of hemorrhagic and ischemic stroke in cancer patients whose presentation may appear to be more of a mental status change than the onset of a focal deficit.
2. There are no firm guidelines for the use of direct oral anticoagulants in cancer patients with brain metastases or primary brain tumors.
3. Bevacizumab has been associated with both thrombotic and hemorrhagic cerebral events as well as venous thromboembolism (see this Chapter, Case 27.6).

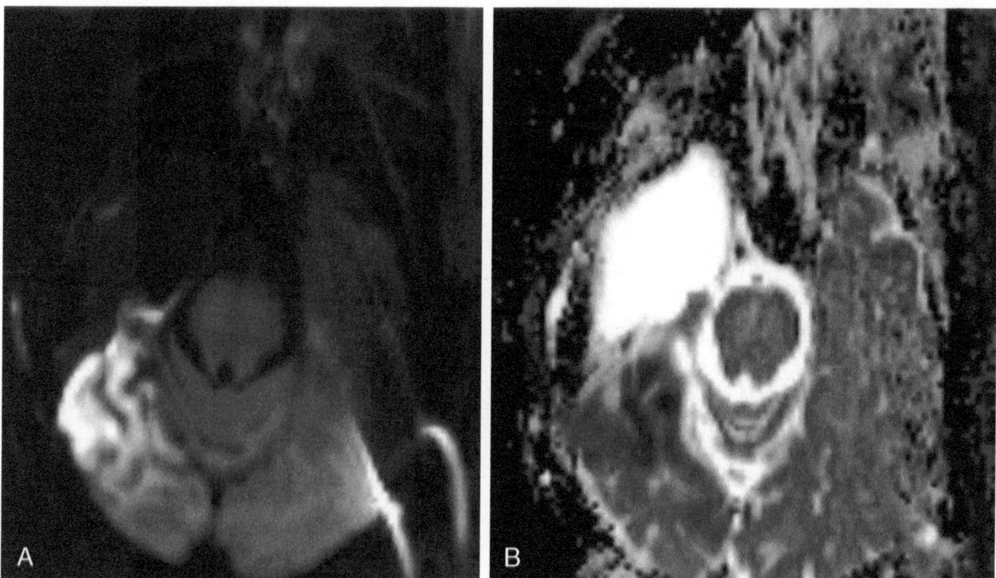

Fig. 27.7 (A) Diffusion-weighted image shows an area of hyperintensity consistent with recent stroke. (B) This was confirmed on apparent diffusion coefficient sequence where the dark area is clearly posterior to the original resection cavity.

CASES 27.8 AND 27.9 POSTTREATMENT MALIGNANCY

The final two cases illustrate the myriad of long-term sequelae of chemotherapy and radiation therapy, including secondary neoplasms, endocrinopathies, seizures, and cognitive changes. Many patients experience more than one long-term treatment adverse consequence and have influenced modification of treatment protocols.

CASE 27.8 TREATMENT-INDUCED BRAIN TUMORS

Case. A 61-year-old woman was treated for non-Hodgkin lymphoma at age 27 years with "prophylactic radiation" to the brain and MOPP chemotherapy. Twenty years later she was found to have multiple meningiomas, WHO grades I/II. In her late 40s, she also developed cognitive changes requiring retirement at age 50 years. Follicular thyroid cancer was diagnosed at age 48 years and melanoma at age 52 years. Bladder cancer, likely due to her prior alkylating agent therapy, required cystectomy at age 61 years. She began having seizures at age 60 years and at age 61 years had two episodes of SMART syndrome.

Teaching Points. This patient has radiation-induced meningiomas which often postdate treatment by many decades and are usually low grade. Her thyroid cancer is also likely due to prior radiation, but the bladder cancer is probably a consequence of her alkylating chemotherapy. SMART syndrome has been described in young adult survivors of medulloblastoma treatment and in older patients with supratentorial radiation as well. A combination of reversible focal neurological deficits can last hours to days, often with headache that is accompanied by MRI findings of gyral swelling in a nonvascular distribution[19] (Fig. 27.8).

CASE 27.9 TREATMENT-INDUCED SYSTEMIC MALIGNANCIES

Case. A 56-year-old woman complained of memory problems 42 years after treatment for leukemia/lymphoma presenting in the maxillary sinus. Around the time of the diagnosis she had a single right body seizure with dysphasia. CT, electroencephalography and lumbar puncture were negative, and she remained on phenobarbital with occasional right facial twitching. Her last reported seizure was 28 years ago during pregnancy with a low phenobarbital level. She has not had a dual energy x-ray absorptiometry (DEXA) scan in the last 2 years. Leukemia treatment included vincristine, prednisone, L-asparaginase and cyclophosphamide, and intrathecal methotrexate along with 2200 cGy craniofacial radiation to the maxillary and sphenoid sinuses.

Four years after the original diagnosis she had acute lymphoblastic leukemia (ALL) treated with vincristine, daunomycin, cytosine arabinoside, methotrexate, hydroxyurea, BCNU, and cyclophosphamide. Five years later, a mass in the right breast thought to be related to her original leukemia was treated with 2700 cGY. At that time, now age 24 years, she was treated with autologous bone marrow transplant (BMT) with conditioning with cytosine arabinoside, cyclophosphamide, and VP 16. She was diagnosed with ductal carcinoma in situ at age 48 years and treated with lumpectomy and radiation. She sees a cardiologist, dermatologist (wears 40–60 SPF sunscreen), and

Table 27.3 Stroke mechanisms in cancer patients

Ischemic stroke
Coagulopathy Nonbacterial thrombotic endocarditis Disseminated intravascular coagulation Hyperviscosity (polycythemia vera, multiple myeloma)
Paradoxical embolus (lung tumors, venous thromboembolism)
Venous sinus thrombosis (dehydration, tumor invasion)
Infection VZV vasculopathy Bacterial or fungal endocarditis Fungal vascular invasion *(Mucoraceae, Aspergillus)*
Direct neoplastic invasion Intravascular lymphoma Vascular compression (dural, leptomeningeal, parasellar) Tumor emboli (myxoma, lung tumors)
Radiation-induced vasculopathy Small vessel ischemic disease Moyamoya disease Angiitis Carotid stenosis after neck irradiation
Chemotherapy and targeted molecular agents L-Asparaginase Bevacizumab and other VEGF or VEGF receptor inhibitors Thalidomide Tamoxifen Ponatinib
Hemorrhagic stroke
Coagulopathy Thrombocytopenia or abnormal platelets Disseminated intravascular coagulation VEGF or VEGF receptor inhibitors Hemorrhage into cerebral mass (melanoma, germ cell tumors, thyroid, renal) Infectious aneurysm Head trauma (subdural, subarachnoid) Therapeutic anticoagulation

VEGF, Vascular endothelial growth factor; *VZV*, varicella-zoster virus.

ophthalmologist regularly. She feels chronically tired and, for the past 5 years, has complained of word-finding difficulty.

MRI scan was notable for diffuse white matter changes, a brainstem cavernous angioma, and volume loss. There is also severe cerebellar atrophy (Fig. 27.9).

Teaching Points. This case illustrates a host of sequelae of treatment in young adulthood for survivable malignancy complicated by unrelated seizures and the sequelae of their treatment. This patient had radiation-induced breast cancer and her MRI showed many of the sequelae of prior cancer treatment. Longitudinal follow-up requires multidisciplinary care and careful consideration of the need for continued antiepileptic drugs, which may contribute to osteopenia and bone fractures. Appropriate interventions for this patient include cognitive testing, measurement of bone density and vitamin D level, and consideration of tapering and discontinuation of phenobarbital. She may need more extensive neuropsychologic testing to differentiate mood problems from less correctable cognitive deficits.

Late mortality after allogeneic blood or marrow transplantation in childhood continues to shorten life expectancy in this population. Among 1388 patients living greater than 2 years after allogeneic BMT in childhood with median age at transplantation of 14.6 years, overall survival rate at 20 years was 79.3%. Leading causes of death are infection, chronic graft-versus-host disease, recurrence of primary disease, and subsequent malignant neoplasms. Overall, there was a 14.4-fold increased risk of death consistent with the general population, though the cumulative incidence of late mortality decreased over time and non-relapse-related mortality exceeded that of relapse-related mortality.[20]

Long-term follow-up and supportive care of cancer survivors necessitates a multidisciplinary coordinated program. Survivors of childhood brain cancer between 14–39 years of age and their caregivers commonly suffer from social isolation, impaired memory and attention, endocrine dysfunction, and fatigue, symptoms that also impact other family members. Adolescent and young adult survivors are less likely than their healthy peers to be employed or have children. They require age-specific psychosocial services.[21]

A large Scandinavian study looked at 4858 5-year or greater survivors of CNS tumor diagnosis in childhood.[22] A neurologic disorder was present in 27% of patients with an absolute excess risk (AER) of 20 hospitalizations per 1000 persons per year, risks which remained increased more than 20 years after diagnosis. The most frequent diagnoses were epilepsy and hydrocephalus. Survivors also had elevated risk for CNS infectious diseases, including meningitis, encephalitis, and intracranial abscesses as well as second malignancies.[23,24]

Although radiation is clearly the major culprit in long-term cognitive disabilities among cancer survivors, those who have chemotherapy alone are at risk for deficits in processing speed, executive function, and attention that impact real-world function.

ALL is the most common childhood malignancy, accounting for nearly 30% of childhood cancer diagnoses, and prognosis has improved over the last several decades, with current 10-year overall survival reaching 90%. Thus, ALL survivors represent a substantial proportion of survivors requiring continuity of neurological care.[25]

Conclusion

Notable from the cases in this chapter are the often-multifactorial problems with considerable overlap among clinical outcomes after treatment for different neoplasms. Optimal QOL and even length of overall survival depend

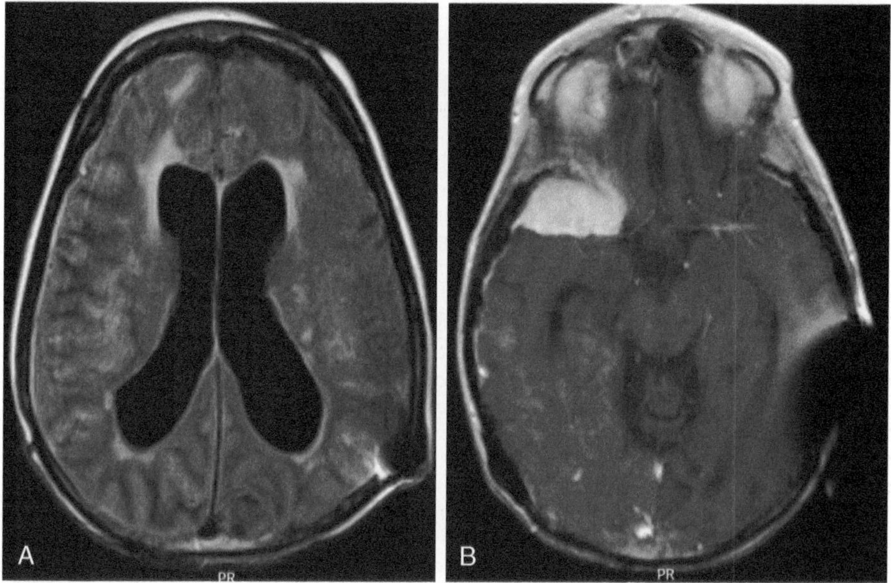

Fig. 27.8 (A) Fluid attenuated inversion recovery image is obtained during an episode of prolonged right hemisphere dysfunction (i.e., stroke-like migraine after radiation therapy syndrome) and shows rather diffusely swollen gyri. (B) The contrast-enhanced MRI sequence shows curvilinear enhancement in the affected right hemisphere, as well as a large radiation-induced meningioma.

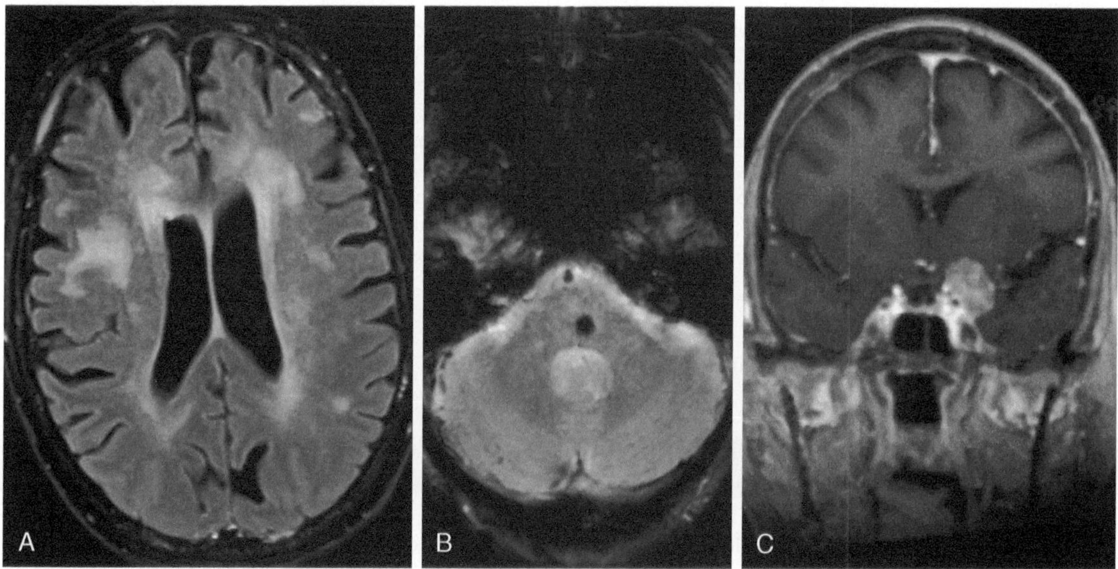

Fig. 27.9 These images from Case 27.9 show many of the sequelae of prior treatment. (A) Fluid-attenuated inversion recovery sequence shows diffuse white matter hyperintensities and brain atrophy. (B) Gradient echo sequence shows a brainstem cavernous angioma. (C) Demonstrates a sphenoid radiation-induced meningioma on coronal view and also illustrates diffuse dural enhancement, the MRI correlate of prior ventriculoperitoneal shunting.

Table 27.4 Clinicians' checklist for cancer survivorship evaluation

Consequences of antiepileptic drugs, corticosteroids, and/or chemotherapy
Musculoskeletal: osteoporosis, avascular necrosis **Endocrine:** impaired fertility, thyroid disease, weight gain, metabolic syndrome **Ocular:** cataracts, dry eye **Autoimmune conditions:** sarcoidosis-like syndrome, paraneoplastic encephalitides **Infections:** VZV, PML, PJP, hepatitis B or C reactivation, re-vaccination indications **Cognitive:** mood, executive dysfunction, short-term memory deficit ("chemo brain") **Secondary neoplasms:** AML, other myelodysplastic syndromes, melanoma, basal cell carcinoma, meningioma, glioma
Consequences of radiation therapy to central or peripheral nervous system
Musculoskeletal: osteoporosis, avascular necrosis, cervical disc disease, osteonecrosis of the jaw **Endocrine:** hypothalamic/pituitary dysfunction, melatonin deficiency, metabolic syndrome **Ocular:** radiation retinopathy, cataracts, dry eye **Hearing loss:** particularly after posterior fossa radiation **Cognitive:** leukoencephalopathy, communicating hydrocephalus **Vascular:** cavernous angiomas, microangiopathy with lacunar strokes, pseudoaneurysms, large vessel atherosclerosis after neck irradiation or mantle radiation **Secondary neoplasms**: meningioma, sarcoma, glioma, thyroid cancer, breast cancer (after radiation involving thorax)
Other syndromes
Other radiation-associated syndromes: Stroke-like migraines (SMART or ALERT syndrome), superficial siderosis (hearing loss ataxia, myelopathy)

ALERT, Acute late-onset encephalopathy after radiation therapy; *AML*, acute myelogenous leukemia; *PJP*, *Pneumocystis jirovecii* pneumonia; *PML*, progressive multifocal leukoencephalopathy; *SMART*, stroke-like migraine after radiation therapy; *VZV*, varicella-zoster virus.

on supportive management of multiple evolving complications in this growing population.

Clinicians should collaborate in survivorship management with colleagues from many disciplines and should consider developing checklists to ensure thorough follow-up, early detection of long-term treatment complications, and best evidence-based therapies to improve quality of survival[26] (Table 27.4).

Clinical pearls

1. Lifelong monitoring includes attention to vascular, endocrinologic, dermatologic, dental, cardiac, and pulmonary function.
2. Neurological monitoring should include inquiry about both CNS (cognitive, vascular) and PNS problems (peripheral neuropathy, pain).
3. Psychosocial problems can be addressed with appropriate neuropsychologic testing and education plans.
4. Secondary cancers include both primary brain tumors and systemic neoplasms that can be related both to prior radiation therapy and to antecedent chemotherapy.

References

1. Pruitt AA. Epidemiology, treatment and complications of central nervous system metastases. *Continuum*. 2017;23(6):1580–1600.
2. Pruitt AA. Medical management of patients with brain tumors. *Continuum*. 2015;21(2):314–331.
3. Schiff D, Lee EQ, Nayak L, Norden AD, Reardon DA, Wen PY. Medical management of brain tumors and the sequelae of treatment. *Neuro Oncol*. 2015;17(4):488–504.
4. Pruitt AA. Central nervous system infections complicating immunosuppression and transplantation. *Continuum*. 2018;24(5):1370–1396.
5. Miaskowski C, Mastick J, Paul SM, et al. Impact of chemotherapy-induced neurotoxicities on adult cancer survivors' symptom burden and quality of life. *J Cancer Surviv*. 2018;12(2):234–245.

6. Kolb NA, Smith AG, Singleton JR, et al. The association of CIPN symptoms and the risk of falling. *JAMA Neurol.* 2016;73(7):860–866.
7. Seretny M, Currie GL, Sena ES, et al. Incidence prevalence and predictors of chemotherapy-induced peripheral neuropathy: a systematic review and meta-analysis. *Pain.* 2014;155(12):2461–2470.
8. Kandula T, Farrar MA, Cohn RJ, et al. Chemotherapy-induced peripheral neuropathy in long-term survivors of childhood cancer: clinical neurophysiological, functional and patient-reported outcomes. *JAMA Neurol.* 2018;75(8):980–988.
9. Staff NP, Grisold A, Grisold W, Windebank AJ. Chemotherapy-induced peripheral neuropathy: a current review. *Ann Neurol.* 2017;81(6):772–781.
10. Smith EM, Pang H, Cirrincione C, et al. Effect of duloxetine on pain, function and quality of life among patients with chemotherapy-induced painful peripheral neuropathy: a randomized clinical trial. *J Am Med Assoc.* 2013;309(13):1359–1367.
11. Chan A, Hertz DL, Morales M, et al. Biological predictors of chemotherapy-induced peripheral neuropathy (CIPN): MASCC neurological complications working group overview. *Support Care Cancer.* 2019;27:3729–3737. https://doi.org/10.1007/s00520-019-04987-8.
12. Cortese I, Muranski P, Enose-Akahata Y, et al. Pembrolizumab treatment for progressive multifocal leukoencephalopathy. *N Engl J Med.* 2019;380(17):1597–1605.
13. Gilden D, Mahalingam R, Nagel MA. Varicella zoster virus vasculopathies: diverse clinical manifestations, laboratory features, pathogenesis, and treatment. Lancet Neurol 2009, Aug 8(8):731–740.
14. Hermelink K, Bühner M, Sckopke P, et al. Chemotherapy and posttraumatic stress in the causation of cognitive dysfunction in breast cancer patients. *J Natl Cancer Inst.* 2017;109(10).
15. Janelsins MC, Heckler CE, Peppone LJ, et al. Cognitive complains in survivors of breast cancer after chemotherapy compared with age-matched controls: an analysis from a nationwide, multicenter, prospective longitudinal study. *J Clin Oncol.* 2017;35:506–514. https://doi.org/10.1200/JCO.2016.68.5826.
16. Koppelmans V, Vernooij MW, Boogerd W, et al. Prevalence of cerebral small-vessel disease in long-term breast cancer survivors exposed to both adjuvant radiotherapy and chemotherapy. *J Clin Oncol.* 2015;33(6):588–593.
17. Chu G, Salzman J. Hyperammonemia after capecitabine associated with occult impairment of the urea cycle. *Cancer Med.* 2019;8(5):1996–2004.
18. Gibson EM, Nagaraja S, Ocampo A, et al. Methotrexate chemotherapy induces persistent tri-glial dysregulation that underlies chemotherapy-related cognitive impairment. *Cell.* 2019;176:43–55.
19. Pruitt A, Dalmau J, Detre J, Alavi A, Rosenfeld MR. Episodic neurologic dysfunction with migraine and reversible imaging findings after radiation. *Neurology.* 2006;67(4):676–678.
20. Holmqvist AS, Chen Y, Wu J, et al. Assessment of late mortality risk after allogeneic blood or marrow transplantation performed in childhood. *JAMA Oncol.* 2018;4(12):e182453.
21. Nicklin E, Velikova G, Hulme C, et al. Long-term issues and supportive care needs of adolescent and young adult childhood brain tumour survivors and their caregivers: a systematic review. *Psycho Oncol.* 2019;28:477–487.
22. Kenborg L, Winther JF, Linnet KM, et al. Neurologic disorders in 4858 survivors of central nervous system tumors in childhood—an Adult Life After Childhood Cancer in Scandinavia (ALiCCS) study. *Neuro Oncol.* 2019;21(1):125–136.
23. Schaapveld M, Aleman BM, van Eggemond AM, et al. Second cancer risk up to 40 years after treatment of Hodgkin lymphoma. *N Engl J Med.* 2015;373(26):2499–2511.
24. Momota H, Narita Y, Miyakita Y, Shibui S. Secondary hematological malignancies associated with temozolomide in patients with glioma. *Neuro Oncol.* 2013;15(10):1445–1450.
25. Jacola LM, Krull KR, Pui CH, et al. Longitudinal assessment of neurocognitive outcomes in survivors of childhood acute lymphoblastic leukemia treated on a contemporary chemotherapy protocol. *J Clin Oncol.* 2016;34:1239–1247.
26. Stone JB, DeAngelis LM. Cancer-treatment-induced neurotoxicity—focus on newer treatments. *Nat Rev Clin Oncol.* 2016;13(2):92–105.

Chapter | **28** |

Approach to chemotherapy-induced peripheral neuropathy

Taylor Brooks and Roy E. Strowd, III

CHAPTER OUTLINE

Introduction

Chemotherapy-induced peripheral neuropathy (CIPN) is one of the most common side effects of cytotoxic chemotherapy and presents as a distal, symmetric polyneuropathy (Table 28.1). Rates of CIPN depend on the agent being used but tend to occur in 60–70% of patients who receive neurotoxic agents.[1,2] According to one metaanalysis, the aggregate prevalence of CIPN is estimated to be 48%.[1] Incidence is highest among patients receiving platinum-based drugs and taxanes, and slightly lower for bortezomib and vinca alkaloids.[1,2]

Clinical presentation

CIPN is generally a small fiber, sensory predominant polyneuropathy that is dose-dependent. Patients develop neuropathic symptoms in a distal, symmetric distribution, which typically include numbness, tingling, cramping, and at times weakness or burning pain in the feet and hands. When large fiber proprioceptive afferents are involved, patients may also develop impaired balance and falls, which can further impair quality of life.[3–6] If CIPN is not recognized and chemotherapy doses not adjusted, delayed, or discontinued, permanent disability will occur. Most patients develop numbness first in the feet and hands. Neuropathic pain, motor weakness, or autonomic dysfunction are uncommon but may be seen with continued treatment as symptoms progress.[7]

Clinical manifestations vary with the type of neurotoxic agent. For example, taxane chemotherapies, commonly used in treating breast, gynecologic, head/neck, and thoracic malignancies, tend to cause a sensory neuropathy with prominent numbness and tingling. Burning neuropathic pain occurs in only about 30–40% of taxane-induced CIPN.[8] Neuropathy starts in the mid-to-late portion of the treatment and persists after patients complete their chemotherapy, often for weeks to months after the final dose. In contrast, oxaliplatin, which is commonly employed in regimens for gastrointestinal cancers, causes immediate cold hypersensitivity that occurs after each infusion as well as neuropathic pain, numbness, and tingling that worsens over time.[9]

Table 28.1 Chemotherapies associated with peripheral neuropathy[7]

	Cisplatin	Oxaliplatin	Oxaliplatin	Vincristine	Taxanes	Bortezomib
Neuropathy type	Chronic peripheral neuropathy	Acute neuropathy	Chronic peripheral neuropathy, cramps and fasciculations at high doses, rare autonomic neuropathy	Chronic peripheral neuropathy, muscle cramps, autonomic neuropathy	Chronic peripheral neuropathy, myalgia, and myopathy at high doses, rare autonomic neuropathy	Chronic peripheral neuropathy, painful small fiber damage, rare myopathy, causes autonomic neuropathy
Incidence	≥90%		70%	60–70%	70–90%	20–30%
Cumulative dose	>350 mg/m²	Infusional	>550 mg/m²	>2–6 mg/m²	>300 mg/m² (PTX) >100 mg/m² (TXT)	>16 mg/m²
Unique clinical features	Dose-dependent	Resolved between cycles	Coasting	Progressive worsening	Worse with higher cumulative and single doses	
Other common side effects	Ototoxicity	Myelotoxicity	Myelotoxicity		Myalgias, myelotoxicity	

PTX, Paclitaxel (Taxol); *TXT*, docetaxel (Taxotere)

CIPN frequently persists after completion of cytotoxic therapy in about half of patients where it becomes a significant source of survivorship morbidity. In one study, CIPN was present in 68.1% of individuals when measured in the first month after chemotherapy, 60% at 3 months, and 30% at 6 months or more.[1] Some patients even report neuropathic symptoms that persist for years after their last dose of chemotherapy.[10] In rare cases, patients with no symptoms or only mild neuropathy during treatment go on to develop CIPN or experience paradoxical intensification of symptoms following the cessation of chemotherapy, often referred to as "coasting."[11] Thus, predicting who is at risk for CIPN is a priority.

Risk factors

A number of clinical factors can increase the risk of developing CIPN. Age,[12,13] preexisting peripheral neuropathy,[14,15] higher cumulative chemotherapeutic doses,[7,12,14,16,17] smoking,[18] diabetes mellitus,[19] decreased creatinine clearance,[18] and cold allodynia/hyperalgesia[20] have all been shown to be associated with increased risk of CIPN. In addition, certain genetic polymorphisms may increase risk. Probably the most well-described genetic risk factor is *PMP22*, the gene that, when duplicated, causes Charcot–Marie–Tooth disease type 1A and, when deleted, causes hereditary neuropathy with liability to pressure palsies (HNLPP). These individuals suffer debilitating weakness after even a single dose of vincristine, prompting the Food and Drug Administration (FDA) to issue a black box warning of vincristine use in cancer patients with Charcot–Marie–Tooth disease.[21] In some studies, race and gender has been associated with higher risk of developing CIPN. African American women exhibited two to three times higher risk for developing CIPN relative to white women.[22,23] This increased risk has been associated with a unique, race-specific genetic haplotype in a DNA damage repair gene in women with taxane-induced CIPN.[24] African American race has also been associated with increased risk of developing CIPN in patients with colorectal cancer.[25] One study that investigated patients receiving platinum- and taxane-based chemotherapy for a variety of solid tumors in Hong Kong, Singapore, and the UK found that non–Chinese Asians had higher-risk of developing neuropathy than Chinese or Caucasians.[26] These associations need to be studied in larger samples while controlling for confounding variables before they will influence personalization of therapy.[27,28]

Numerous other genetic polymorphisms have been associated with the development of CIPN, many having a role in the pharmacokinetics, absorption, distribution, metabolism, or excretion of chemotherapeutics and other drugs. Genetic alterations in glutathione transferases, cytochrome P450 enzymes, and ATP binding cassette proteins could alter the cellular uptake of cytotoxic drugs and promote accumulation of these agents in sensory neurons, potentially leading to neurotoxicity and the development of CIPN.[29,30] Unfortunately, none of the above risk factors have been validated in large cohorts, limiting the clinical use of pharmacogenomics in pretreatment screening. Despite this, these candidate genes are consistent with postulated pathophysiologic mechanisms of CIPN and provide fertile ground in which clinical trials investigating diagnostic tools and therapies are cultivated.

Pathophysiologic mechanisms

The pathophysiologic mechanisms of CIPN are multifactorial: oxidative stress and apoptosis, aberrations in calcium homeostasis, axon degeneration, changes in neuronal excitability, and neuroinflammation all promote the development of CIPN with greater or lesser contributions depending on the chemotherapy being used.[30] Interestingly, despite similar mechanisms of action in their antiproliferative effect, the mechanisms of CIPN may differ among chemotherapeutic drugs within a class. For example, carboplatin toxicity predominantly affects the hematopoietic system, whereas cisplatin and oxaliplatin are much more neurotoxic. Similarly, among the vinca alkaloids, vincristine most commonly causes CIPN, whereas this is less common with vinblastine, vinflunine, and vinorelbine.[30,31]

Making the diagnosis

CIPN shares significant clinical overlap with other diseases of the peripheral nervous system. When there is motor involvement in CIPN, the differential diagnosis is broad (Table 28.2). However, correlating the timing of neuropathic symptoms with the onset of chemotherapy typically narrows etiologic considerations. CIPN is diagnosed clinically, often without the need for specialized testing (e.g., nerve conduction velocities). Unfortunately, there is no standardized approach to diagnosing CIPN. Clinician-reported grading is common with most providers using the National Cancer Institute (NCI) Common Terminology Criteria for Adverse Events (CTCAE) Neuropathy Sensory subscale. Grading is performed prior to each treatment, typically by the primary treating oncologist or nurse, and a neuropathy score is assigned using elements from the history and physical examination (Table 28.3). In general, grade 2 neuropathy indicates an impact on instrumental activities of daily living (IADLs), whereas grade 3 indicates impairment of routine ADLs. This scale is limited by inter-observer variability,[32] and it has been shown to be less sensitive to changes in the severity of CIPN.[33] Patient-reported outcome measures are frequently employed in clinical trials including the European Organization for Research and Treatment of Cancer (EORTC) QLQ-CIPN20 questionnaire. This instrument has good sensitivity to neuropathic symptoms and responsiveness to subtle changes in symptoms but correlates poorly with the degree of structural change or damage to the nerve itself.[34,35]

Neurology expertise is often sought in patients with an atypical presentation, when symptoms continue to worsen after discontinuation or completion of chemotherapy, or when other diagnoses (e.g., paraneoplastic or inflammatory neuropathy) are considered. Nerve conduction studies (NCS) can provide an objective assessment of clinical neuropathy but are often normal unless motor or large fiber sensory nerves are involved. NCS can be particularly helpful in differentiating CIPN from other peripheral neuropathies or paraneoplastic neuropathy when the diagnosis is in question.[36–39] Quantitative skin testing (QST) allows for the assessment of small fiber, sensory nerve function but is more commonly employed in the research setting and is rarely incorporated into clinical care algorithms. Skin biopsy for assessment of intraepidermal nerve fiber density (IENF) can be helpful in demonstrating underlying sensory nerve fiber loss but is rarely needed in the appropriate clinical setting.

Treatment

Clinical trials evaluating prevention or treatment of CIPN have generally failed to bring effective therapies into the clinic. Numerous substances with diverse mechanisms have been trialed: alpha-lipoic acid, acetyl-L-carnitine, and glutathione are all antioxidants that, despite promising results in pilot studies, failed to demonstrate efficacy in preventing CIPN in phase III trials.[40–42] Calcium and magnesium infusions were once routine in clinical practice but fell out of favor when large, randomized studies failed to show benefit.[43] Many clinicians consider the use

Table 28.2 Differential diagnosis of CIPN

Cause	Comments	Workup
HIV-associated neuropathy	Symmetric distal, demyelinating, polyradiculopathy, or mononeuropathy	HIV antibody, viral load
Paraneoplastic	Sensory. Often associated with encephalitis, cerebellar ataxia, opsoclonus-myoclonus syndrome, and Lambert-Eaton myasthenic syndrome, among others	Paraneoplastic panel (i.e., anti-Hu and -CV2 antibodies are relevant to neuropathy)
Diabetes mellitus	Can present as distal symmetric sensory/ sensorimotor polyneuropathy, autonomic neuropathy, mononeuropathy, or multiple mononeuropathies	Hemoglobin A1c, fasting plasma glucose
Hypothyroidism	Most typically carpal tunnel syndrome, rarely generalized, painful sensory polyneuropathy	TSH
Monoclonal gammopathy (e.g., Amyloidosis, MM, MGUS, WM, POEMS)	Typically painful dysesthesia of the hands and feet. Prominent autonomic involvement.	SPEP, UPEP, IF
Vitamin deficiency	Consider in patients with alcohol abuse, malabsorption, total parenteral nutrition, and bariatric surgery	B_1, B_6, B_{12}, homocysteine, vitamin E, copper level, methylmalonic acid levels
Toxic	Numerous agents, many of which confer reduced sensory nerve action potentials on NCS	Alcohol, lead, mercury, arsenic levels
Sjogren's syndrome	Length-dependent, pure small fiber and/or ganglionopathy	ANA, SS-A/Ro, SS-B/La
Vasculitis	Seen in a variety of conditions; RA, SLE, MCTD. Can be a mononeuropathy multiplex pattern or symmetric. Can be the result of drugs (e.g., leflunomide, tumor necrosis factor blockers)	
Hereditary neuropathy	HSAN, ALD/AMN, FAP, Tangier disease, all relatively rare, predominantly sensory	Genetic testing

ALD/AMN, adrenoleukodystrophy/adrenomyeloneuropathy; *ANA,* anti-nuclear antibody; *CIPN,* chemotherapy-induced peripheral neuropathy; *FAP,* familial amyloid polyneuropathy; *HSAN,* hereditary sensory and autonomic neuropathy; *IF,* immunofixation; *MCTD,* mixed connective tissue disease; *MGUS,* monoclonal gammopathy of uncertain significance; *MM,* multiple myeloma; *NCS,* nerve conduction studies; *POEMS,* polyneuropathy, organomegaly, endocrinopathy, monoclonal gammopathy, and skin changes syndrome; *RA,* rheumatoid arthritis; *SLE,* systemic lupus erythematosus; *SPEP,* serum protein electrophoresis; *TSH,* thyroid stimulating hormone; *UPEP,* urine protein electrophoresis; *WM,* Waldenstrom's macroglobulinemia

of neuropathic pain agents for symptomatic relief including gabapentin, pregabalin, tricyclic antidepressants, and others despite studies showing minimal benefit. Only venlafaxine[44] and duloxetine[45] have demonstrated efficacy for relief of painful paresthesias. Duloxetine is currently the only FDA-approved medication for the treatment of established CIPN.[46] As a result, CIPN is managed by treatment delay, dose reduction, or discontinuation of chemotherapy

Table 28.3 NCI common terminology criteria for adverse events (CTCAE)

	GRADE				
	1	2	3	4	5
Sensory neuropathy	Asymptomatic	Moderate symptoms; limiting instrumental ADL	Sensory alteration or severe symptoms; limiting self-care ADL	Life-threatening consequences; urgent intervention needed	Death
Motor neuropathy	Asymptomatic; clinical or diagnostic observation only	Moderate symptoms; limiting instrumental ADL	Sensory alteration or severe symptoms; limiting self-care ADL	Life-threatening consequences; urgent intervention needed	Death

ADL, Activities of daily living (i.e., bathing, dressing, grooming, toileting, transferring, walking, eating); instrumental *ADL* (i.e., shopping, cooking, medication management, using the telephone, housework, laundry, driving, managing finances); *NCI*, National Cancer Institute.

altogether, which limits the delivery of life-saving drugs and can result in poorer patient outcomes.[23]

Clinical cases

Although many antineoplastic agents have been associated with neurotoxicity, here we review four main groups of chemotherapeutic drugs that frequently cause CIPN: platinum-based antineoplastics (oxaliplatin), vinca alkaloids (vinblastine), taxanes (paclitaxel), and proteasome inhibitors (bortezomib). Each case provides a practical example for understanding the clinical presentation and management of CIPN and highlights clinical pearls that are common to all agents.

CASE 28.1 TAXANE-INDUCED PERIPHERAL NEUROPATHY

Case. A 65-year-old woman was diagnosed with invasive breast cancer after a screening mammogram revealed a focal asymmetry within the medial inferior right breast. Diagnostic mammogram revealed a BI-RADS IV, 8-mm solid mass in the upper inner right breast, suspicious for malignancy. Core biopsy showed invasive ductal carcinoma, grade 3, estrogen receptor 99%, progesterone receptor 60%, HER2/Neu+. She underwent a right lumpectomy with sentinel lymph node biopsy with negative margins and negative lymph node, pT1bN0M0. She received adjuvant chemotherapy with weekly paclitaxel and trastuzumab, which she initially tolerated well. After three cycles, she developed intermittent tingling in her fingers that spontaneously resolved after a few minutes. Throughout treatment, these symptoms progressed to involve the entire dorsal surface of the hands resolving prior to the next dose of treatment. After eight cycles of weekly paclitaxel, symptoms worsened from intermittent to constant, and she developed similar numbness and tingling in her toes and the soles of her feet. The patient also developed bilateral lower extremity edema, intermittent sensations of dyspnea, and a macular rash of the bilateral upper extremities. Because of these symptoms, her ninth cycle of chemotherapy was delayed and her subsequent cycle of paclitaxel was dose-reduced by 20%. Despite this, her sensory symptoms persisted, and after eleven cycles she began to experience intermittent, painful burning in her feet. She had no limitations in her ADLs or IADLs. Her physical examination was significant for normal gait, ambulation, and full strength of the upper and lower extremities. Sensory examination was normal except for subjective reduction in light touch and temperature in the distal legs bilaterally below the ankles and fingertips. The remainder of the examination was normal. Laboratory workup was normal, including normal blood glucose, hemoglobin A1c, folate, vitamin B_{12}, thyroid function studies, and rapid-plasma reagin. NCS revealed right lower leg sural nerve latency of 3.6 milliseconds, amplitude of 10 microvolts, and conduction velocity of 49 meters per second. She also underwent nerve ultrasound, which showed an enlarged right median nerve (cross-sectional area: 21.8 mm^2). Two months after her final dose of chemotherapy, the patient reported that her neuropathy had resolved.

Teaching Points. This case highlights two important principles of managing CIPN including: (1) additional contributors to peripheral nerve injury should be identified and managed in

CIPN patients, and (2) CIPN is a clinical diagnosis with objective measures of nerve function often used to rule out alternative etiologies.

Screen for treatable causes. The first principle is to evaluate and screen for treatable causes, contributors, and exacerbating conditions including diabetic neuropathy, vitamin B_{12} or folate deficiency, hypothyroidism, undiagnosed syphilis, or other readily treatable causes including alcohol consumption. Peripheral neuropathy as part of a paraneoplastic syndrome should be considered in selected patients with an atypical presentation, worsening of neuropathy after cessation of chemotherapy, and with selected cancers such as squamous and small-cell lung cancers, gynecologic cancers, and lymphoma which are the most common to be associated with this complication.[47] The patient in this case had none of these risk factors, had onset of symptoms after initiation of a neurotoxic agent, and worsening with increasing number of doses. Consideration of the route of administration and cumulative dose is important as well; for example, methotrexate rarely causes peripheral neuropathy except when administered via the intrathecal route,[48] and CIPN usually develops within the first 2 months of treatment, as in this patient.

Objectives measures of CIPN. The second important principle is the role of objective assessment measures. Objective measures of peripheral neuropathy provide valuable information about the extent of axonal loss in patients with CIPN. Although NCS is the gold standard for diagnosis of most toxic peripheral neuropathies, it is frequently normal in CIPN. Compound sensory action potentials (CSAP) and compound motor action potentials (CMAP), which are measured during NCS, provide information about large fiber nerve function. Reduction in action potential amplitude indicates axonal loss, whereas slowed conduction velocities and conduction block suggest demyelination and could indicate an immune-mediated cause (e.g., paraneoplastic). NCS is most sensitive to changes in larger fiber A-beta (6–12 μm, myelinated, altered touch detection to monofilaments) but not to changes in small A-delta fibers (1–5 μm, myelinated, altered sharpness detection) and nociceptors such as C-fibers (0.2–1.5 μm, unmyelinated, hot, cold, burning pain).[49]

Quantitative sensory testing. QST is a psychophysical assessment method that quantifies function of the somatosensory system. QST interrogates sensory nerve fibers of varying sizes by applying specific, calibrated stimuli and recording the subject's response. QST differs from the usual NCS and somatosensory-evoked potentials in that it requires a response from the subject to judge whether or not a stimulus is felt and/or whether or not the stimulus is perceived as painful.[50] QST has been used in over 1000 patients treated with neurotoxic chemotherapies and represents a complimentary assessment tool for evaluating the clinical impact of small fiber neuropathy but has principally been used in research studies.[51] Patient-reported outcomes include the EORTC QLQ-CIPN20, which has been shown to be more sensitive than NCI grading with good internal validity.[34,52] The total neuropathy score (TNS) combines symptom reporting with objective nerve assessment using NCS and has been used in clinical trials.[53,54] The TNS offers a wider range of values (0–40) compared with the CTCAE and may be more capable of discriminating between moderate and severe neuropathy in patients who experience no limitation in their ADLs. Skin biopsy is another technique that allows for objective quantification of IENF density. This minimally invasive technique has been validated across multiple different disorders of the peripheral nervous system and correlates well with clinical assessment.[55,56] Reduction in IENF density has been demonstrated in skin biopsies from patients with CIPN who received neurotoxic chemotherapies.[51] Taxane use has been associated with distal reduction in IENF density,[57,58] as in this patient (Fig. 28.1).

Studies are ongoing evaluating novel methods of predicting, screening, diagnosing, and tracking CIPN. We have previously explored the role of neuromuscular ultrasound to noninvasively assess gross nerve structure in CIPN (Fig. 28.2). The patient in this case was enrolled in a cross-sectional study comparing methods of objective assessment of CIPN and underwent NCS. Right median, right tibial, and right sural sensory conduction studies were normal. Her nerve ultrasound revealed an enlarged median nerve, which may have contributed to the early onset of symptoms in the hands. Anecdotally, this presentation is not uncommon in patients with taxane-induced CIPN. Whether treatment of carpal tunnel syndrome in these patients is beneficial is controversial.

Taxane-Induced Peripheral Neuropathy Summary. Taxanes, including paclitaxel, docetaxel, and cabazitaxel, have been used for nearly 30 years to treat a variety of cancers including breast, ovarian, non–small-cell lung cancer, and prostate cancer.[59] Frequency and intensity of CIPN is higher for paclitaxel than docetaxel and cabazitaxel.[60,61] Albumin-bound paclitaxel (Nab-paclitaxel) was developed to reduce toxicity, though the rate of CIPN is similar to the parent compound.[62] In patients treated with taxanes, neuropathy is typically sensory predominant. It classically is reported as a stocking-and-glove distribution, though many patients first describe numbness and tingling in the hands followed by symptoms in the feet bilaterally. Taxanes contribute to CIPN through several mechanisms. Microtubule disruption confers antineoplastic activity to taxanes but also impairs axonal transport of synaptic vesicles containing neurotransmitters.[63] Taxanes alter peripheral nerve excitability and calcium homeostasis, leading to hyperexcitability and hyperalgesia in rodent models of CIPN.[64,65] Paclitaxel is directly mitotoxic, promoting the formation of free radicals and reactive oxygen species that damage neuronal mitochondria. This promotes inflammatory cytokine production, disruption of the electron transport chain, demyelination, and apoptosis.[66–68] Finally, the role of the immune system in the pathogenesis of CIPN caused by taxanes is garnering interest, as paclitaxel has been shown to directly stimulate Toll-like receptors and promote the influx of inflammatory leukocytes, leading to demyelination and loss of nerves in the dorsal root ganglion.[69]

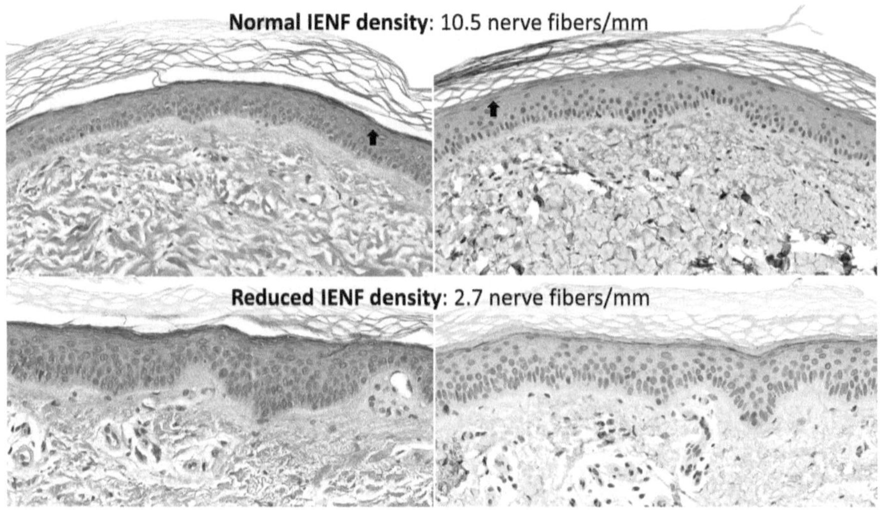

Fig. 28.1 Representative H&E *(left)* and PGP9.5 *(right)* images showing normal and reduced intraepidermal nerve (IENF) density. *H&E,* Hematoxylin and eosin.

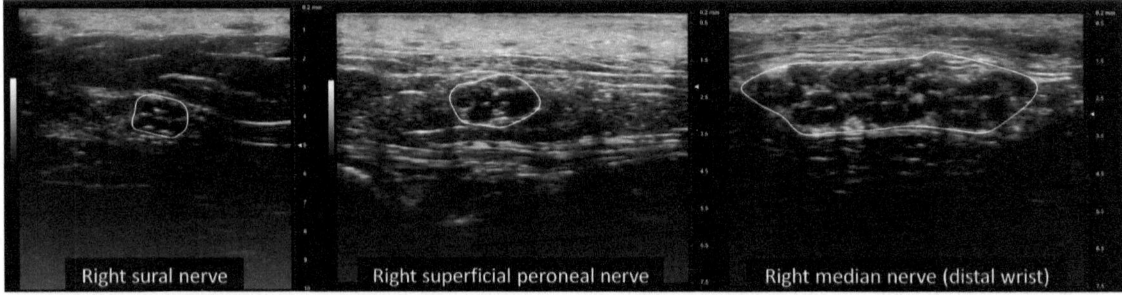

Fig. 28.2 Representative neuromuscular ultrasound images of the sural nerve *(left),* superficial peroneal nerve *(middle),* and median nerve at the distal wrist crease *(right).* The cross-sectional area (mm^2) of the sural nerve (3.34 mm^2) and superficial peroneal nerves (2.45 mm^2), whereas the median nerve (14.23 mm^2) is slightly enlarged. Yellow lines indicate a circumferential tracing inside the hyperechoic nerve sheath that is used to calculate the cross-sectional area.

CASE 28.2 OXALIPLATIN-INDUCED PERIPHERAL NEUROPATHY

Case. A 52-year-old man with a medical history of gout, chronic kidney disease, and HIV infection underwent screening colonoscopy, which revealed a circumferential firm mass at the splenic flexure completely obstructing the lumen of the colon. Biopsies revealed adenocarcinoma. Staging CT revealed locoregional, hypoattenuating lymph nodes up to 1.5 cm in diameter concerning for metastatic involvement. He underwent left hemicolectomy with lymph node dissection that showed poorly differentiated invasive colonic adenocarcinoma involving 4/36 lymph nodes sampled, pT3N2aM0. He was started on FOLFOX (folinic acid, fluorouracil, and oxaliplatin) therapy with weekly bolus and infusional 5-FU. Following the first infusion of FOLFOX, he developed new bilateral numbness and tingling of his fingertips that persisted for a few days and gradually resolved prior to his second infusion. He also experienced marked sensitivity of the hands to cold weather and perioral sensitivity to cold exposure. After five cycles, he developed grade III neutropenia (absolute neutrophil count 700) as well as worsening of his neuropathy; the latter progressed to constant numbness and tingling involving the toes in addition to the fingers. His sixth cycle was delayed by 1 week due to neutropenia, as were cycles nine and eleven. Prior to his final cycle of chemotherapy, his neuropathy worsened to the point of constant numbness and tingling of the fingers that was exacerbated by exposure to cold weather or cold substances. His neurologic examination was significant for 5/5 strength in the bilateral upper and lower extremities, no pronation or drift, 2+ deep tendon reflexes in all four extremities, and normal gait and ambulation. Coordination testing shows intact finger-to-nose, heel-to-shin, and rapid alternating movements. He had subjective decrease in sensation to light touch of the fingertips and toes, not extending past the fingers or balls of the feet and a negative Romberg test. The remainder of the physical examination was normal. Laboratory testing was significant for a baseline serum creatinine level of 1.5 mg/dL, estimated glomerular filtration rate of 60 mL/min, an HIV viral load of 20 copies/mL, and CD4 count of 680. His medications included levocarnitine supplement daily, oxycodone 5 mg as needed, and abacavir/dolutegravir/lamivudine multi-dose formulation daily. A trial of duloxetine was initiated.

Teaching Points. This case highlights several important aspects of oxaliplatin-induced CIPN including: (1) acute neuropathy is rare in CIPN but occurs with oxaliplatin, and (2) treatment with venlafaxine or duloxetine can improve patient symptoms. Oxaliplatin causes an acute as well as chronic peripheral neuropathy.

Acute oxaliplatin neuropathy. The acute neuropathy is an infusional hyperexcitability that results in cold allodynia and paresthesias of the hands and feet precipitated by cold exposure within 24 hours of the oxaliplatin infusion. This toxicity is exceedingly common, with 65–98% of patients experiencing cold-induced or cold-exaggerated neuropathic symptoms in the first 2 weeks of treatment with oxaliplatin.[70–72] Cold allodynia is unique to oxaliplatin-induced peripheral neuropathy, and this symptom can reliably distinguish this syndrome from other forms of peripheral neuropathy if there are other diagnostic considerations, as in this patient. His long-standing HIV infection increased the risk for developing HIV-associated peripheral neuropathy, a spectrum of diseases including a distal, symmetric polyneuropathy, demyelinating mono/polyneuropathy, and a sensory neuronopathy/ganglionopathy; cold allodynia is not a feature of any of the HIV-associated neuropathies. Other acute symptoms attributed to neurotoxicity include voice changes, visual alterations, pharyngo-laryngeal dysesthesia (i.e., lack of awareness of breathing), perioral or intraoral numbness, and muscle spasm, experienced by over 60% of patients.[73] These acute symptoms can prompt urgent consultations or considerations of stroke in patients and providers who are unfamiliar with them.

Chronic oxaliplatin neuropathy. Chronic oxaliplatin-induced CIPN is characterized by a pure sensory axonopathy that develops in a stocking-and-glove distribution.[74] Incidence varies, but chronic CIPN caused by oxaliplatin occurs in 26–46% of patients at 1 year.[75] Like other chemotherapeutic drugs, chronic peripheral neuropathy is dose-related,[76,77] and it can negatively impact quality of life.[78] Severe, chronic peripheral neuropathy caused by oxaliplatin resolves in approximately 13 weeks in over half of patients but may remain persistent in the remaining patients.[79] In this patient, he experienced both acute and chronic oxaliplatin-induced neuropathy that resolved approximately 8 weeks after he completed chemotherapy.

Numbness is the most common symptom experienced by patients with CIPN, and it is typically a chronic problem without much spontaneous improvement and often worsens after completion of chemotherapy. Paresthesias are less common, but when they do occur, they are less responsive to treatment. Pain is the least common manifestation of CIPN; however, it is often the most responsive to treatment. When symptoms arise, pharmacologic treatment of CIPN is indicated. Neuropathic pain and paresthesias are more common in oxaliplatin- than taxane-induced CIPN, which may explain the more favorable response to treatment for oxaliplatin-induced CIPN.

Treatment of CIPN—venlafaxine. Venlafaxine was shown to relieve the acute neuropathy from oxaliplatin when given 1 hour prior to the infusion.[44] In this study, oral venlafaxine was administered at 50 mg 1 hour prior to oxaliplatin infusion followed by 37.5 mg twice daily of the extended-release formulation through day eleven of chemotherapy. The proportion of patients experiencing full relief of acute neurotoxicity was 31.3% in the venlafaxine arm versus 5.3% in the placebo arm. At 3 months after the end of treatment, 38.5% of patients in the venlafaxine arm experienced grade 0 toxicity versus 5.6% in the placebo arm.[44] Unfortunately, this study was limited by small sample size (48 patients), and current guidelines do not support routine use of venlafaxine for treatment of established CIPN.

Treatment of CIPN—duloxetine. Duloxetine is an American Society of Clinical Oncology (ASCO)-recommended therapy for patients with established CIPN based on results of a phase III, randomized, double-blind, placebo-controlled crossover study where 231 patients were randomized to receive duloxetine at a target dose of 60 mg daily or placebo for 6 weeks. Patients receiving duloxetine experienced a significant decrease in pain scores within the first week of medication administration and experienced few side effects.[45]

Oxaliplatin-Induced Peripheral Neuropathy Summary. Oxaliplatin is used primarily in gastrointestinal malignancies, including advanced colorectal, esophageal, stomach, liver, and pancreatic cancers. Its antineoplastic activity is derived from its ability to form DNA-platinum adducts and inhibit DNA replication and RNA transcription. This leads to cell cycle arrest and induction of apoptosis.[80] Oxaliplatin also disrupts the electron transport chain of mitochondria leading to the production of radical oxygen species and apoptosis via the intrinsic pathway.[81] Oxaliplatin treatment leads to aberrant calcium homeostasis and unregulated intracellular proteolysis[82]; interestingly, disruption of voltage-gated sodium channel kinetics is thought to be responsible for the cold allodynia of acute oxaliplatin peripheral neuropathy.[83] Finally, enhanced inflammation and release of inflammatory cytokines by immune and nonimmune cells can cause both peripheral and central sensitization and promote the development of CIPN among patients receiving oxaliplatin.[29]

CASE 28.3 PERIPHERAL NEUROPATHY IN HEMATOLOGIC MALIGNANCIES (E.G., VINCA ALKALOIDS, BRENTUXIMAB)

Case. A 40-year-old man with no known medical history presented to urgent care for 2 months of cyclic fevers, malaise, and drenching night sweats. CT was obtained and revealed adenopathy involving the right inguinal and iliac chains as well as retroperitoneal lymphadenopathy. Excisional biopsy revealed classic Hodgkin lymphoma. PET scan showed tracer-avid disease in the retroperitoneum, bilateral iliac chains, and right pelvic sidewall, marked activity in the right thyroid, and diffuse uptake in the skeleton and marrow, consistent with stage IV disease. He underwent treatment with brentuximab-vedotin, dacarbazine, doxorubicin, and vinblastine. His first two cycles were complicated by severe fatigue, nausea, abdominal pain, and secondary to pulmonary embolism. On the day of his third cycle, he complained of occasional, intermittent numbness at the base of his hands with outward radiation. The numbness increased in frequency and duration after the third cycle, and he began having difficulty keeping firm grasp of things and with temperature discrimination. This prompted a 25% dose reduction of vinblastine and brentuximab. He continued to experience neuropathy despite this, as well as proximal muscle weakness. Follow-up PET scan after six cycles showed a complete response. Due to persistent neuropathic symptoms and proximal lower extremity weakness despite completion of therapy, he was referred to physical and occupational therapy. There, he was observed to have difficulty climbing stairs, rising from a seated position, and performing tasks requiring fine motor skills, like buttoning a shirt. He demonstrated good functional recovery after 10 sessions of physical and occupational therapy according to objective measures, but continued to have symptoms of numbness, tingling, and lower extremity weakness a full 2 months after his last chemotherapy dose.

Teaching Points. This case highlights the important aspects of CIPN from both vinblastine and brentuximab including (1) CIPN is sensory predominant but can affect motor fibers, and (2) limited preventive treatment options exist and current management focuses on symptom control.

Vinca alkaloids and brentuximab. The vinca alkaloids (e.g., vincristine, vinblastine, vinorelbine) and brentuximab are commonly used in treatment regimens for hematologic malignancies including leukemia and lymphoma. Peripheral neuropathy is most commonly associated with vincristine but can be seen to a lesser degree with the other vinca alkaloids. Brentuximab is a CD30-specific antibody-drug conjugate that has activity in relapsed or refractory Hodgkin lymphoma and anaplastic large cell lymphoma. Peripheral neuropathy is one of the most common treatment-related adverse events of these agents. Patients treated with vincristine may experience a coasting phenomenon, whereby neuropathic symptoms worsen upon discontinuation of the drug.[84] Motor neuropathies can also occur with these agents, characterized by muscle cramps and distal muscle weakness,[85] as well as an acute form of ascending paralysis clinically resembling acute inflammatory demyelinating polyneuropathy with loss of deep tendon reflexes, foot and wrist drop as well as profound weakness.[86] Autonomic neuropathy consists of heart rate variability, postural hypotension, and bladder and bowel disturbances.[87] Sensory neuropathy typically resolves within 2 months of cessation of treatment, but it can persist for years.

Both the acute and long-term manifestations of CIPN have prompted multiple clinical trials to prevent or treat this complication. There are two main goals when managing CIPN: the first is to prevent CIPN before it occurs; the second is to relieve symptoms once CIPN has set in. Regarding prevention, the ASCO practice guidelines stress that there are no established agents recommended for the prevention of CIPN in patients with cancer undergoing treatment with neurotoxic agents.[46] As such, when symptoms increase in severity and interfere with ADLs, dose reduction or discontinuation of the drug may be required, which limits the delivery of life-saving drugs and may result in poorer outcomes. Therefore, the most common approach is to maintain full doses of chemotherapeutic agents and treat symptoms once they occur.

Symptomatic management of CIPN. In addition to duloxetine and venlafaxine, multiple oral agents have been studied including tricyclic antidepressants amitriptyline and nortriptyline, but these investigations failed to demonstrate significant improvement in pain according to patient-reported outcome scores.[88,89] Similarly, gabapentin and lamotrigine to target doses of 2700 mg/day and 300 mg/day, respectively, were both unable to demonstrate benefit according to numeric rating scale and Eastern Cooperative Oncology Group neuropathy scale.[90,91] One group investigated a topical gel consisting of baclofen, amitriptyline, and ketamine applied to areas of pain twice daily for 4 weeks; they observed a trend toward decreased EORTC QLQ-CIPN20 scores that did not reach statistical significance, but found a significant improvement in the motor subscale.[92]

Complementary and alternative treatments for CIPN. Due to the failure of conventional approaches to the treatment of CIPN, approaches using complementary and alternative medicine have been investigated. Acupuncture is one such intervention that is increasingly used as an adjunctive treatment for CIPN. Reports often show benefit, but evidence is limited to a small number of randomized controlled trials, with the remainder of studies limited to heterogeneous, uncontrolled case reports or case series.[93] Neuromodulation seeks to "retrain" the brain to experience neuropathic pain as a nonpainful stimulus via electrical stimulation of peripheral nerves (e.g., transcutaneous electrical nerve stimulators, Scrambler therapy) or through modulation of the central processing of painful afferent impulses via real-time feedback using electroencephalography (EEG) (e.g., neurofeedback). To date, one randomized controlled trial examining neurofeedback for the treatment of CIPN reported improvement in Brief Pain Inventory worst-pain item scores with associated EEG correlates, an effect that persisted at 4 months following the intervention.[94,95] Results of Scrambler therapy for CIPN are mostly positive, but limited by heterogeneity and small sample sizes.[96,97] Finally, exercise[98] and cannabinoids[99] are two interventions with a growing body of clinical and preclinical evidence that supports their use in the treatment of CIPN. As cancer survivors are more likely to engage in complementary and alternative medicine therapies compared with individuals without a cancer diagnosis,[100] research in this area is needed.

Vinca Alkaloid-Induced and Brentuximab-Induced Peripheral Neuropathy Summary. Vinca alkaloids are drugs originally derived from the Madagascar periwinkle plant. These agents are the anti-microtubule agents most frequently associated with CIPN. The most common tumor types treated with these agents are Hodgkin and non-Hodgkin lymphoma, testicular cancer, and non–small-cell lung cancer.[101] This class of chemotherapeutic drug disrupts microtubules by binding to free tubulin dimers, the building blocks of microtubules. As such, they interfere with axonal transport in nerves and weaken the neuronal cytoskeleton, resulting in axonal degeneration, preferentially of sensory neurons.[102] Vincristine induces a dose-dependent peripheral sensory neuropathy that typically appears within 3 months of treatment. It presents with a stocking-and-glove distribution of numbness and tingling that can occur after the first dose. Overall, it manifests in 35–45% of patients receiving this drug, with higher risk conferred to patients receiving more than 2–6 mg/m^2.[84,85,103]

Newer anti-microtubule agents are being developed in an attempt to increase specificity, reduce toxicity, and improve outcomes of patients with cancer. Brentuximab-vedotin is one example. The CD30 antibody is conjugated to monomethyl auristatin E, an anti-microtubule synthetic polypeptide that is released intracellularly into malignant cells after endocytosis and lysosomal cleavage of the protease-cleavable linker. Grade I or II peripheral neuropathy occurs in up to 50% of patients receiving this drug, including 10% who develop motor neuropathy. Among those who develop CIPN, only around half experience resolution of symptoms.[104,105]

CASE 28.4 BORTEZOMIB-INDUCED PERIPHERAL NEUROPATHY

Case. A 60-year-old man with hypothyroidism was incidentally found to have an elevated serum protein level during a routine visit with his primary care doctor. Detailed workup with serum protein electrophoresis revealed a monoclonal (M)-spike of 3.16 g/dL with immunofixation showing IgG lambda. Bone marrow biopsy revealed hypercellular marrow with 15% clonal plasma cells, confirming multiple myeloma. He was treated with bortezomib, lenalidomide, and dexamethasone, achieving very good partial response. After undergoing autologous stem cell transplant, he was maintained on lenalidomide. Two years later, he suffered a relapse and was transitioned to subcutaneous bortezomib with oral lenalidomide and dexamethasone. After four cycles, he complained of mild to moderate numbness and tingling in his toes and feet. Treatment was continued and the patient developed new neuropathic pain, burning, and paresthesias in the legs to the ankles bilaterally and finger tips. Bortezomib was discontinued, and when repeat biopsy showed completed remission, a second stem cell transplant was pursued.

Teaching Points. This case highlights two key principles including (1) the common presentation of patients with bortezomib-induced peripheral neuropathy and (2) introduces the need to differentiate toxic CIPN from paraneoplastic or paraproteinemic neuropathy in patients with an underlying monoclonal gammopathy.

Bortezomib. Bortezomib is a proteasome inhibitor used in the treatment of multiple myeloma and mantle cell non-Hodgkin lymphoma. Its antineoplastic mechanism of action derives from its ability to inhibit the proteasome—the cellular degradation machinery—and promote the accumulation of unfolded proteins, triggering endoplasmic reticulum stress and eventually apoptosis. A painful, length-dependent, symmetric sensory neuropathy develops in around 34% of patients receiving this drug.[106] For unknown reasons, bortezomib preferentially damages unmyelinated C- and A-delta fibers with associated morphologic changes visible on biopsy.[107] Similar to other chemotherapeutic drugs, the mechanism of neurotoxicity is pleiotropic, involving alterations in intracellular calcium homeostasis,[108] ion channel opening, and inflammation.[109] Interestingly, low levels of vitamin D are associated with worse peripheral neuropathy in these patients, suggesting an immunomodulatory role of the vitamin.[110] The neurotoxicity is dose-dependent and the duration is variable; the painful peripheral neuropathy has resolved in some patients within weeks, and in other patients it has persisted for years.

Paraproteinemic neuropathy (PPN). PPN refers to a heterogeneous set of neuropathies associated with the presence of a clonal proliferation of immunoglobulin in the serum. Neuropathic typically presents as a length-dependent axonal sensorimotor polyneuropathy resulting in numbness, paresthesias, allodynia, cramping, or mild distal motor weakness. Symptoms may precede the clinical diagnosis of the antibody-producing syndrome which include monoclonal gammopathy of undetermined significance (MGUS) or multiple myeloma (MM). These conditions result in a proliferation of plasma cells and overabundance of monoclonal paraprotein (e.g., the M protein). Paraproteins are detected in approximately 10% of the general population. The prevalence of PPN increases with age, occurring in 5% of persons over 70 years such that serum protein immunofixation electrophoresis is recommended as an initial screening laboratory test along with blood glucose and vitamin B_{12} for patients presenting with new distal symmetric polyneuropathy.

Paraneoplastic Causes of Peripheral Neuropathy in Cancer Patients Summary. Paraneoplastic syndromes are a heterogeneous group of different disorders that are the systemic effects of cancers not necessarily attributable to the site of the primary tumor or metastases. The most common paraneoplastic syndromes involve the endocrine, hematologic, dermatologic, rheumatologic, and neurologic systems. Paraneoplastic neurologic syndromes (PNSs) are a rare occurrence, complicating around 0.01% of cancer diagnoses.[111] PNSs often present before the diagnosis of malignancy is established. Peripheral sensory neuropathy is a classic PNS presentation either characterized by a sensory-predominant polyneuropathy or mononeuritis multiplex that may be associated with painful dysesthesias. Distinguishing features that differentiate paraneoplastic sensory neuropathy from CIPN include rapid progression (weeks), asymmetric symptoms (often resembling radiculopathy or polyneuropathy), and association with ataxia, gait instability, and the development of pseudoathetoid movements. Notably, around 10% of patients with paraneoplastic sensory neuropathy exhibit an indolent course that is less severe.[112]

Paraneoplastic sensory neuropathy can be associated with any malignancy, but over 80% are found in patients with lung cancer, typically small-cell. The host antitumor immunity often results in the production of a humoral immune response that forms the bases for serologic corroboration of a suspected PNS. Of these antibodies, anti-Hu antibody (polyclonal, directed against a 35- to 40-kDa protein complex) is almost always found in serum of patients with small-cell lung cancer and a PNS; however, it is rare in other tumors.[113] Less common are antibodies to ampiphysin or CV2/CRMP5; patients in the latter group often demonstrate motor involvement and demyelination.[114]

New or worsening neuropathic symptoms in a patient with known cancer, particularly following the cessation of chemotherapy, requires evaluation to rule out a paraneoplastic process. Patients should have electromyography and NCS to assess inflammatory changes. If these suggest demyelination with or without a suspected inflammatory component, then lumbar puncture with cerebrospinal fluid (CSF) studies should be obtained. In a paraneoplastic neuropathy, CSF studies show pleocytosis, increased protein, and oligoclonal bands with intrathecal IgG; however, they can be normal as well. Negative studies suggest CIPN and support symptomatic management. Findings suggestive of a PNS should prompt treatment as such. Corticosteroids are often used to treat PNS. The efficacy of more aggressive therapies, such as intravenous immunoglobulin (IVIG), cyclophosphamide, rituximab, and plasma exchange, is limited to case reports.[115–117] Treatment of the underlying malignancy is the standard of care, with tumor regression correlating to resolution of neurologic symptoms.[118,119]

Conclusion

CIPN is a common, dose-limiting side effect of many chemotherapies which typically presents as a sensory-predominant distal, symmetric polyneuropathy. Symptoms frequently begin during the course of chemotherapy treatment but persist beyond the completion of therapy, resolving in about half of patients and resulting in long-term morbidity in the remaining patients. Clinicians should be aware of the typical presentations for patients receiving these agents and be able to screen for exacerbating conditions, differentiate paraneoplastic or paraproteinemic causes, and advise on potential treatment options, which are limited to symptom reducing interventions.

References

1. Seretny M, Currie GL, Sena ES, et al. Incidence, prevalence, and predictors of chemotherapy-induced peripheral neuropathy: a systematic review and meta-analysis. *Pain.* 2014;155(12):2461–2470.
2. Banach M, Juranek JK, Zygulska AL. Chemotherapy-induced neuropathies-a growing problem for patients and health care providers. *Brain Behav.* 2017;7(1):e00558.
3. Bao T, Basal C, Seluzicki C, Li SQ, Seidman AD, Mao JJ. Long-term chemotherapy-induced peripheral neuropathy among breast cancer survivors: prevalence, risk factors, and fall risk. *Breast Cancer Res Treat.* 2016;159(2):327–333.
4. Gewandter JS, Fan L, Magnuson A, et al. Falls and functional impairments in cancer survivors with chemotherapy-induced peripheral neuropathy (CIPN): a University of Rochester CCOP study. *Support Care Cancer.* 2013;21(7):2059–2066.
5. Kolb NA, Smith AG, Singleton JR, et al. The association of chemotherapy-induced peripheral neuropathy symptoms and the risk of falling. *JAMA Neurol.* 2016;73(7):860–866.
6. Mols F, Beijers T, Vreugdenhil G, van de Poll-Franse L. Chemotherapy-induced peripheral neuropathy and its association with quality of life: a systematic review. *Support Care Cancer.* 2014;22(8):2261–2269.
7. Park SB, Goldstein D, Krishnan AV, et al. Chemotherapy-induced peripheral neurotoxicity: a critical analysis. *CA Cancer J Clin.* 2013;63(6):419–437.
8. Loprinzi CL, Reeves BN, Dakhil SR, et al. Natural history of paclitaxel-associated acute pain syndrome: prospective cohort study NCCTG N08C1. *J Clinical Oncol.* 2011;29(11):1472–1478.
9. Alberti P. Platinum-drugs induced peripheral neurotoxicity: clinical course and preclinical evidence. *Expert Opin Drug Metab Toxicol.* 2019;15(6):487–497.
10. Kidwell KM, Yothers G, Ganz PA, et al. Long-term neurotoxicity effects of oxaliplatin added to fluorouracil and leucovorin as adjuvant therapy for colon cancer: results from National Surgical Adjuvant Breast and Bowel Project trials C-07 and LTS-01. *Cancer.* 2012;118(22):5614–5622.
11. Cavaletti G, Alberti P, Frigeni B, Piatti M, Susani E. Chemotherapy-induced neuropathy. *Curr Treat Options Neurol.* 2011;13(2):180–190.
12. Glendenning JL, Barbachano Y, Norman AR, Dearnaley DP, Horwich A, Huddart RA. Long-term neurologic and peripheral vascular toxicity after chemotherapy treatment of testicular cancer. *Cancer.* 2010;116(10):2322–2331.
13. Lavoie Smith EM, Li L, Chiang C, et al. Patterns and severity of vincristine-induced peripheral neuropathy in children with acute lymphoblastic leukemia. *J Peripher Nerv Syst.* 2015;20(1):37–46.
14. Alejandro LM, Behrendt CE, Chen K, Openshaw H, Shibata S. Predicting acute and persistent neuropathy associated with oxaliplatin. *Am J Clin Oncol.* 2013;36(4):331–337.
15. Dimopoulos MA, Mateos MV, Richardson PG, et al. Risk factors for, and reversibility of, peripheral neuropathy associated with bortezomib–melphalan–prednisone in newly

diagnosed patients with multiple myeloma: subanalysis of the phase 3 VISTA study. *Eur J Haematol.* 2011;86(1):23–31.
16. Beijers AJM, Mols F, Tjan-Heijnen VCG, Faber CG, van de Poll-Franse LV, Vreugdenhil G. Peripheral neuropathy in colorectal cancer survivors: the influence of oxaliplatin administration. Results from the population-based PROFILES registry. *Acta Oncol.* 2015;54(4):463–469.
17. Krarup-Hansen A, Helweg-Larsen S, Schmalbruch H, Rørth M, Krarup C. Neuronal involvement in cisplatin neuropathy: prospective clinical and neurophysiological studies. *Brain.* 2007;130(Pt 4):1076–1088.
18. Kawakami K, Tunoda T, Takiguchi T, et al. Factors exacerbating peripheral neuropathy induced by paclitaxel plus carboplatin in non-small cell lung cancer. *Oncol Res.* 2012;20(4):179–185.
19. Johnson C, Pankratz VS, Velazquez AI, et al. Candidate pathway-based genetic association study of platinum and platinum-taxane related toxicity in a cohort of primary lung cancer patients. *J Neurol Sci.* 2015;349(1–2):124–128.
20. Attal N, Bouhassira D, Gautron M, et al. Thermal hyperalgesia as a marker of oxaliplatin neurotoxicity: a prospective quantified sensory assessment study. *Pain.* 2009;144(3):245–252.
21. Graf WD, Chance PF, Lensch MW, Eng LJ, Lipe HP, Bird TD. Severe vincristine neuropathy in Charcot-Marie-Tooth disease type 1A. *Cancer.* 1996;77(7):1356–1362.
22. Schneider BP, Li L, Miller K, et al. Genetic associations with taxane-induced neuropathy by a genome-wide association study (GWAS) in E5103. *J Clin Oncol.* 2011;29(suppl 15): 1000–1000.
23. Speck RM, Sammel MD, Farrar JT, et al. Impact of chemotherapy-induced peripheral neuropathy on treatment delivery in nonmetastatic breast cancer. *J Oncol Pract.* 2013;9(5): e234–e240.
24. Sucheston LE, Zhao H, Yao S, et al. Genetic predictors of taxane-induced neurotoxicity in a SWOG phase III intergroup adjuvant breast cancer treatment trial (S0221). *Breast Cancer Res Treat.* 2011;130(3):993–1002.
25. Lewis MA, Zhao F, Jones D, et al. Neuropathic symptoms and their risk factors in medical oncology outpatients with colorectal vs. breast, lung, or prostate cancer: results from a prospective multicenter study. *J Pain Symptom Manage.* 2015;49(6):1016–1024.
26. Molassiotis A, Cheng HL, Leung KT, et al. Risk factors for chemotherapy-induced peripheral neuropathy in patients receiving taxane- and platinum-based chemotherapy. *Brain Behav.* 2019;9(6):e01312.
27. Hershman DL, Till C, Wright JD, et al. Comorbidities and risk of chemotherapy-induced peripheral neuropathy among participants 65 years or older in Southwest oncology group clinical trials. *J Clin Oncol.* 2016;34(25):3014–3022.
28. Miaskowski C, Mastick J, Paul SM, et al. Chemotherapy-induced neuropathy in cancer survivors. *J Pain Symptom Manage.* 2017;54(2):204–218.e202.
29. Zajaczkowska R, Kocot-Kepska M, Leppert W, Wrzosek A, Mika J, Wordliczek J. Mechanisms of chemotherapy-induced peripheral neuropathy. *Int J Mol Sci.* 2019;20(6):E1451.
30. Starobova H, Vetter I. Pathophysiology of chemotherapy-induced peripheral neuropathy. *Front Mol Neurosci.* 2017;10:174.
31. Grisold W, Cavaletti G, Windebank AJ. Peripheral neuropathies from chemotherapeutics and targeted agents: diagnosis, treatment, and prevention. *Neuro Oncol.* 2012;14(suppl 4):iv45–54.
32. Postma TJ, Heimans JJ, Muller MJ, Ossenkoppele GJ, Vermorken JB, Aaronson NK. Pitfalls in grading severity of chemotherapy-induced peripheral neuropathy. *Ann Oncol.* 1998;9(7):739–744.
33. Cavaletti G, Cornblath DR, Merkies IS, et al. The chemotherapy-induced peripheral neuropathy outcome measures standardization study: from consensus to the first validity and reliability findings. *Ann Oncol.* 2013;24(2):454–462.
34. Lavoie Smith EM, Barton DL, Qin R, Steen PD, Aaronson NK, Loprinzi CL. Assessing patient-reported peripheral neuropathy: the reliability and validity of the European Organization for Research and Treatment of Cancer QLQ-CIPN20 Questionnaire. *Qual Life Res.* 2013;22(10):2787–2799.
35. Postma TJ, Aaronson NK, Heimans JJ, et al. The development of an EORTC quality of life questionnaire to assess chemotherapy-induced peripheral neuropathy: the QLQ-CIPN20. *Eur J Cancer.* 2005;41(8):1135–1139.
36. Chaudhry V, Rowinsky EK, Sartorius SE, Donehower RC, Cornblath DR. Peripheral neuropathy from taxol and cisplatin combination chemotherapy: clinical and electrophysiological studies. *Ann Neurol.* 1994;35(3):304–311.
37. Lehky TJ, Leonard GD, Wilson RH, Grem JL, Floeter MK. Oxaliplatin-induced neurotoxicity: acute hyperexcitability and chronic neuropathy. *Muscle Nerve.* 2004;29(3):387–392.
38. LoMonaco M, Milone M, Batocchi AP, Padua L, Restuccia D, Tonali P. Cisplatin neuropathy: clinical course and neurophysiological findings. *J Neurol.* 1992;239(4):199–204.
39. Pietrangeli A, Leandri M, Terzoli E, Jandolo B, Garufi C. Persistence of high-dose oxaliplatin-induced neuropathy at long-term follow-up. *Eur Neurol.* 2006;56(1):13–16.
40. Guo Y, Jones D, Palmer JL, et al. Oral alpha-lipoic acid to prevent chemotherapy-induced peripheral neuropathy: a randomized, double-blind, placebo-controlled trial. *Support Care Cancer.* 2014;22(5):1223–1231.
41. Hershman DL, Unger JM, Crew KD, et al. Randomized double-blind placebo-controlled trial of acetyl-L-carnitine for the prevention of taxane-induced neuropathy in women undergoing adjuvant breast cancer therapy. *J Clin Oncol.* 2013;31(20):2627–2633.
42. Leal AD, Qin R, Atherton PJ, et al. North Central Cancer Treatment Group/Alliance trial N08CA-the use of glutathione for prevention of paclitaxel/carboplatin-induced peripheral neuropathy: a phase 3 randomized, double-blind, placebo-controlled study. *Cancer.* 2014;120(12):1890–1897.
43. Loprinzi CL, Qin R, Dakhil SR, et al. Phase III randomized, placebo-controlled, double-blind study of intravenous calcium and magnesium to prevent oxaliplatin-induced sensory neurotoxicity (N08CB/Alliance). *J Clin Oncol.* 2014;32(10):997–1005.
44. Durand JP, Deplanque G, Montheil V, et al. Efficacy of venlafaxine for the prevention and relief of oxaliplatin-induced acute neurotoxicity: results of EFFOX, a randomized, double-blind, placebo-controlled phase III trial. *Ann Oncol.* 2012;23(1):200–205.
45. Smith EM, Pang H, Cirrincione C, et al. Effect of duloxetine on pain, function, and quality of life among patients with chemotherapy-induced painful peripheral neuropathy: a randomized clinical trial. *JAMA.* 2013;309(13):1359–1367.
46. Hershman DL, Lacchetti C, Dworkin RH, et al. Prevention and management of chemotherapy-induced peripheral

neuropathy in survivors of adult cancers: American Society of Clinical Oncology clinical practice guideline. *J Clin Oncol.* 2014;32(18):1941–1967.
47. Rees JH. Paraneoplastic syndromes: when to suspect, how to confirm, and how to manage. *J Neurol Neurosurg Psychiatry.* 2004;75(suppl 2):ii43–ii50.
48. Brugnoletti F, Morris EB, Laningham FH, et al. Recurrent intrathecal methotrexate induced neurotoxicity in an adolescent with acute lymphoblastic leukemia: serial clinical and radiologic findings. *Pediatr Blood Cancer.* 2009;52(2):293–295.
49. Siegel A, Sapru H. *Essential Neuroscience.* 3rd ed. Lippincott Williams & Wilkins; 2015.
50. Backonja MM, Attal N, Baron R, et al. Value of quantitative sensory testing in neurological and pain disorders: NeuPSIG consensus. *Pain.* 2013;154(9):1807–1819.
51. Timmins HC, Li T, Kiernan MC, Horvath LG, Goldstein D, Park SB. Quantification of small fiber neuropathy in chemotherapy treated patients. *J Pain.* 2019;(19):5900–S1526.30765–5.
52. Wolf SL, Barton DL, Qin R, et al. The relationship between numbness, tingling, and shooting/burning pain in patients with chemotherapy-induced peripheral neuropathy (CIPN) as measured by the EORTC QLQ-CIPN20 instrument. *N06CA. Support Care Cancer.* 2012;20(3):625–632.
53. Cavaletti G, Bogliun G, Marzorati L, et al. Grading of chemotherapy-induced peripheral neurotoxicity using the total neuropathy scale. *Neurology.* 2003;61(9):1297–1300.
54. Cornblath DR, Chaudhry V, Carter K, et al. Total neuropathy score: validation and reliability study. *Neurology.* 1999;53(8):1660–1664.
55. Lauria G, Hsieh ST, Johansson O, et al. European Federation of Neurological Societies/Peripheral Nerve Society Guideline on the use of skin biopsy in the diagnosis of small fiber neuropathy. Report of a joint task force of the European Federation of Neurological Societies and the Peripheral Nerve Society. *Eur J Neurol.* 2010;17(7):903–912. e944–909.
56. Truini A, Biasiotta A, Di Stefano G, et al. Does the epidermal nerve fibre density measured by skin biopsy in patients with peripheral neuropathies correlate with neuropathic pain? *Pain.* 155(4):828–832.
57. Boyette-Davis JA, Cata JP, Driver LC, et al. Persistent chemoneuropathy in patients receiving the plant alkaloids paclitaxel and vincristine. *Cancer Chemother Pharmacol.* 2013;71(3):619–626.
58. Kroigard T, Schrøder HD, Qvortrup C, et al. Characterization and diagnostic evaluation of chronic polyneuropathies induced by oxaliplatin and docetaxel comparing skin biopsy to quantitative sensory testing and nerve conduction studies. *Eur J Neurol.* 2014;21(4):623–629.
59. Yared JA, Tkaczuk KH. Update on taxane development: new analogs and new formulations. *Drug Des Devel Ther.* 2012;6:371–384.
60. Cioroiu C, Weimer LH. Update on chemotherapy-induced peripheral neuropathy. *Curr Neurol Neurosci Rep.* 2017;17(6):47.
61. Di Lorenzo G, Bracarda S, Gasparro D, et al. Lack of cumulative toxicity associated with cabazitaxel use in prostate cancer. *Medicine.* 2016;95(2):e2299.
62. Peng L, Bu Z, Ye X, Zhou Y, Zhao Q. Incidence and risk of peripheral neuropathy with nab-paclitaxel in patients with cancer: a meta-analysis. *Eur J Cancer Care.* 2017;26(5).
63. Shemesh OA, Spira ME. Paclitaxel induces axonal microtubules polar reconfiguration and impaired organelle transport: implications for the pathogenesis of paclitaxel-induced polyneuropathy. *Acta Neuropathol.* 2010;119(2):235–248.
64. Siau C, Bennett GJ. Dysregulation of cellular calcium homeostasis in chemotherapy-evoked painful peripheral neuropathy. *Anesth Analg.* 2006;102(5):1485–1490.
65. Zhang H, Dougherty PM. Enhanced excitability of primary sensory neurons and altered gene expression of neuronal ion channels in dorsal root ganglion in paclitaxel-induced peripheral neuropathy. *Anesthesiology.* 2014;120(6):1463–1475.
66. Areti A, Yerra VG, Naidu V, Kumar A. Oxidative stress and nerve damage: role in chemotherapy induced peripheral neuropathy. *Redox Biol.* 2014;2:289–295.
67. Flatters SJ, Bennett GJ. Studies of peripheral sensory nerves in paclitaxel-induced painful peripheral neuropathy: evidence for mitochondrial dysfunction. *Pain.* 2006;122(3):245–257.
68. Griffiths LA, Flatters SJ. Pharmacological modulation of the mitochondrial electron transport chain in paclitaxel-induced painful peripheral neuropathy. *J Pain.* 2015;16(10):981–994.
69. Li Y, Zhang H, Zhang H, Kosturakis AK, Jawad AB, Dougherty PM. Toll-like receptor 4 signaling contributes to Paclitaxel-induced peripheral neuropathy. *J Pain.* 2014;15(7):712–725.
70. Argyriou AA, Cavaletti G, Briani C, et al. Clinical pattern and associations of oxaliplatin acute neurotoxicity: a prospective study in 170 patients with colorectal cancer. *Cancer.* 2013;119(2):438–444.
71. Gebremedhn EG, Shortland PJ, Mahns DA. The incidence of acute oxaliplatin-induced neuropathy and its impact on treatment in the first cycle: a systematic review. *BMC Cancer.* 2018;18(1):410.
72. Park SB, Goldstein D, Lin CS, Krishnan AV, Friedlander ML, Kiernan MC. Acute abnormalities of sensory nerve function associated with oxaliplatin-induced neurotoxicity. *J Clin Oncol.* 2009;27(8):1243–1249.
73. Leonard GD, Wright MA, Quinn MG, et al. Survey of oxaliplatin-associated neurotoxicity using an interview-based questionnaire in patients with metastatic colorectal cancer. *BMC Cancer.* 2005;5:116.
74. Park SB, Lin CS, Krishnan AV, Goldstein D, Friedlander ML, Kiernan MC. Long-term neuropathy after oxaliplatin treatment: challenging the dictum of reversibility. *Oncologist.* 2011;16(5):708–716.
75. Beijers AJ, Mols F, Vreugdenhil G. A systematic review on chronic oxaliplatin-induced peripheral neuropathy and the relation with oxaliplatin administration. *Support Care Cancer.* 2014;22(7):1999–2007.
76. Krishnan AV, Goldstein D, Friedlander M, Kiernan MC. Oxaliplatin-induced neurotoxicity and the development of neuropathy. *Muscle Nerve.* 2005;32(1):51–60.
77. Vatandoust S, Joshi R, Pittman KB, et al. A descriptive study of persistent oxaliplatin-induced peripheral neuropathy in patients with colorectal cancer. *Support Care Cancer.* 2014;22(2):513–518.
78. Tofthagen C, Donovan KA, Morgan MA, Shibata D, Yeh Y. Oxaliplatin-induced peripheral neuropathy's effects on health-related quality of life of colorectal cancer survivors. *Support Care Cancer.* 2013;21(12):3307–3313.
79. Grothey A. Oxaliplatin-safety profile: neurotoxicity. *Semin Oncol.* 2003;30(4 suppl 15):5–13.

80. Dasari S, Tchounwou PB. Cisplatin in cancer therapy: molecular mechanisms of action. *Eur J Pharmacol*. 2014;740:364–378.
81. Canta A, Pozzi E, Carozzi VA. Mitochondrial dysfunction in chemotherapy-induced peripheral neuropathy (CIPN). *Toxics*. 2015;3(2):198–223.
82. Wang JT, Medress ZA, Barres BA. Axon degeneration: molecular mechanisms of a self-destruction pathway. *J Cell Biol*. 2012;196(1):7–18.
83. Sittl R, Lampert A, Huth T, et al. Anticancer drug oxaliplatin induces acute cooling-aggravated neuropathy via sodium channel subtype Na(V)1.6-resurgent and persistent current. *Proc Natl Acad Sci U S A*. 2012;109(17):6704–6709.
84. Verstappen CC, Koeppen S, Heimans JJ, et al. Dose-related vincristine-induced peripheral neuropathy with unexpected off-therapy worsening. *Neurology*. 2005;64(6):1076–1077.
85. Haim N, Epelbaum R, Ben-Shahar M, Yarnitsky D, Simri W, Robinson E. Full dose vincristine (without 2-mg dose limit) in the treatment of lymphomas. *Cancer*. 1994;73(10):2515–2519.
86. Gonzalez Perez P, Serrano-Pozo A, Franco-Macias E, Montes-Latorre E, Gomez-Aranda F, Campos T. Vincristine-induced acute neurotoxicity versus Guillain-Barré syndrome: a diagnostic dilemma. *Eur J Neurol*. 2007;14(7):826–828.
87. Hancock BW, Naysmith A. Vincristine-induced autonomic neuropathy. *Br Med J*. 1975;3(5977):207.
88. Hammack JE, Michalak JC, Loprinzi CL, et al. Phase III evaluation of nortriptyline for alleviation of symptoms of cis-platinum-induced peripheral neuropathy. *Pain*. 2002;98(1–2):195–203.
89. Kautio AL, Haanpää M, Saarto T, Kalso E. Amitriptyline in the treatment of chemotherapy-induced neuropathic symptoms. *J Pain Symptom Manage*. 2008;35(1):31–39.
90. Rao RD, Flynn PJ, Sloan JA, et al. Efficacy of lamotrigine in the management of chemotherapy-induced peripheral neuropathy: a phase 3 randomized, double-blind, placebo-controlled trial, N01C3. *Cancer*. 2008;112(12):2802–2808.
91. Rao RD, Michalak JC, Sloan JA, et al. Efficacy of gabapentin in the management of chemotherapy-induced peripheral neuropathy: a phase 3 randomized, double-blind, placebo-controlled, crossover trial (N00C3). *Cancer*. 2007;110(9):2110–2118.
92. Barton DL, Wos EJ, Qin R, et al. A double-blind, placebo-controlled trial of a topical treatment for chemotherapy-induced peripheral neuropathy: NCCTG trial N06CA. *Support Care Cancer*. 2011;19(6):833–841.
93. Franconi G, Manni L, Schröder S, Marchetti P, Robinson N. A systematic review of experimental and clinical acupuncture in chemotherapy-induced peripheral neuropathy. *Evid Based Complement Alternat Med*. 2013;2013:516916.
94. Prinsloo S, Novy D, Driver L, et al. The long-term impact of neurofeedback on symptom burden and interference in patients with chronic chemotherapy-induced neuropathy: analysis of a randomized controlled trial. *J Pain Symptom Manage*. 2018;55(5):1276–1285.
95. Prinsloo S, Novy D, Driver L, et al. Randomized controlled trial of neurofeedback on chemotherapy-induced peripheral neuropathy: a pilot study. *Cancer*. 2017;123(11):1989–1997.
96. Loprinzi C, Le-Rademacher JG, Majithia N, et al. Scrambler therapy for chemotherapy neuropathy: a randomized phase II pilot trial. *Support Care Cancer*. 2019;28:1183–1197.
97. Majithia N, Smith TJ, Coyne PJ, et al. Scrambler therapy for the management of chronic pain. *Support Care Cancer*. 2016;24(6):2807–2814.
98. Dorsey SG, Kleckner IR, Barton D, et al. NCI Clinical Trials Planning Meeting for prevention and treatment of chemotherapy-induced peripheral neuropathy. *J Natl Cancer Inst*. 2019;111:531–537.
99. Wu BY, Liu CT, Su YL, Chen SY, Chen YH, Tsai MY. A review of complementary therapies with medicinal plants for chemotherapy-induced peripheral neuropathy. *Complement Ther Med*. 2019;42:226–232.
100. Mao JJ, Palmer CS, Healy KE, Desai K, Amsterdam J. Complementary and alternative medicine use among cancer survivors: a population-based study. *J Cancer Surviv*. 2011;5(1):8–17.
101. Liu YM, Chen HL, Lee HY, Liou JP. Tubulin inhibitors: a patent review. *Expert Opin Ther Pat*. 2014;24(1):69–88.
102. Kerckhove N, Collin A, Condé S, Chaleteix C, Pezet D, Balayssac D. Long-term effects, pathophysiological mechanisms, and risk factors of chemotherapy-induced peripheral neuropathies: a comprehensive literature review. *Front Pharmacol*. 2017;8:86.
103. Postma TJ, Benard BA, Huijgens PC, Ossenkoppele GJ, Heimans JJ. Long-term effects of vincristine on the peripheral nervous system. *J Neuro Oncol*. 1993;15(1):23–27.
104. Gopal AK, Ramchandren R, O'Connor OA, et al. Safety and efficacy of brentuximab vedotin for Hodgkin lymphoma recurring after allogeneic stem cell transplantation. *Blood*. 2012;120(3):560–568.
105. Younes A, Bartlett NL, Leonard JP, et al. Brentuximab vedotin (SGN-35) for relapsed CD30-positive lymphomas. *N Engl J Med*. 2010;363(19):1812–1821.
106. Saifee TA, Elliott KJ, Rabin N, et al. Bortezomib-induced inflammatory neuropathy. *J Peripher Nerv Syst*. 2010;15(4):366–368.
107. Carozzi VA, Renn CL, Bardini M, et al. Bortezomib-induced painful peripheral neuropathy: an electrophysiological, behavioral, morphological and mechanistic study in the mouse. *PloS One*. 2013;8(9):e72995.
108. Landowski TH, Megli CJ, Nullmeyer KD, Lynch RM, Dorr RT. Mitochondrial-mediated disregulation of Ca2+ is a critical determinant of Velcade (PS-341/bortezomib) cytotoxicity in myeloma cell lines. *Cancer Res*. 2005;65(9):3828–3836.
109. Stockstill K, Doyle TM, Yan X, et al. Dysregulation of sphingolipid metabolism contributes to bortezomib-induced neuropathic pain. *J Exp Med*. 2018;215(5):1301–1313.
110. Wang J, Udd KA, Vidisheva A, et al. Low serum vitamin D occurs commonly among multiple myeloma patients treated with bortezomib and/or thalidomide and is associated with severe neuropathy. *Support Care Cancer*. 2016;24(7):3105–3110.
111. Darnell RB, Posner JB. Paraneoplastic syndromes involving the nervous system. *N Engl J Med*. 2003;349(16):1543–1554.
112. Graus F, Bonaventura I, Uchuya M, et al. Indolent anti-Hu-associated paraneoplastic sensory neuropathy. *Neurology*. 1994;44(12):2258–2261.
113. Molinuevo JL, Graus F, Serrano C, Reñe R, Guerrero A, Illa I. Utility of anti-Hu antibodies in the diagnosis of paraneoplastic sensory neuropathy. *Ann Neurol*. 1998;44(6):976–980.
114. Antoine JC, Honnorat J, Camdessanché JP, et al. Paraneoplastic anti-CV2 antibodies react with peripheral nerve and are associated with a mixed axonal and demyelinating peripheral neuropathy. *Ann Neurol*. 2001;49(2):214–221.

115. Giometto B, Vitaliani R, Lindeck-Pozza E, Grisold W, Vedeler C. Treatment for paraneoplastic neuropathies. *Cochrane Database Syst Rev.* 2012;12:CD007625.
116. Shams'ili S, de Beukelaar J, Gratama JW, et al. An uncontrolled trial of rituximab for antibody associated paraneoplastic neurological syndromes. *J Neurol.* 2006;253(1):16–20.
117. Vernino S, O'Neill BP, Marks RS, O'Fallon JR, Kimmel DW. Immunomodulatory treatment trial for paraneoplastic neurological disorders. *Neuro Oncol.* 2004;6(1):55–62.
118. Graus F, Keime-Guibert F, Reñe R, et al. Anti-Hu-associated paraneoplastic encephalomyelitis: analysis of 200 patients. *Brain.* 2001;124(Pt 6):1138–1148.
119. Sillevis Smitt P, Grefkens J, de Leeuw B, et al. Survival and outcome in 73 anti-Hu positive patients with paraneoplastic encephalomyelitis/sensory neuronopathy. *J Neurol.* 2002;249(6):745–753.

Chapter 29

Neurologic complications of immune checkpoint inhibitors

Sarah E. Mancone and Roy E. Strowd, III

CHAPTER OUTLINE

Brief introduction to immunotherapy

Immune-based therapies have emerged as a promising modality in cancer treatment. These therapies use the body's immune system to fight cancer by harnessing the antitumor properties of the host immune system to eliminate the cancer. Several types of immunotherapy exist and can be broadly categorized into:

1. Cancer vaccines
2. Adoptive cell transfer therapies such as those using chimeric antigen receptor T-cells (see Chapter 30 on CAR T-cell therapies)
3. Immune checkpoint inhibitors (ICIs)

Cancer vaccines deliver a tumor-specific neoantigen or many tumor-associated antigens that are recognized by the host immune system and enhance the antitumor immune response. Adoptive cell transfer utilizes a host's T-cells, which are typically harvested by leukapheresis and enhanced *ex vivo* to make them more reactive to tumor-specific antigens. Chimeric antigen receptor (CAR) T-cells are a prototypical example where a patient's T-cells are collected and genetically modified to express a modified chimeric antigen receptor that traffics to the tumor, generates an antitumor cytolytic effect, or releases cytotoxins that induce cancer cell death when infused back into the patient.

This chapter focuses on the third category of immunotherapies, immune checkpoint inhibitors, which target the interaction between antigen presenting cells, T lymphocytes, and tumor cells to remove immunosuppressive signals. Here, we review their mechanism of action, efficacy, and indications, and then focus on the neurologic complications that occur in cancer patients undergoing ICI treatment.

Immune checkpoint inhibitors: mechanism, types, indications, and efficacy

Cancer growth and progression are characterized by immune suppression. ICIs work by releasing immunosuppressive signals that inhibit the antitumor immune response. In the normal state, immune checkpoints dampen the host immune response to protect normal tissues. Immune checkpoints keep T-cells inactive, prevent autoimmunity, and provide self-tolerance. Cancer cells take advantage of these checkpoints. By activating checkpoint molecules, cancers suppress T-cell activity and evade the antitumor immune response. ICIs are monoclonal antibodies that block checkpoint signals and reinvigorate the host immune responses to allow T-cells to infiltrate the tumor and improve outcomes.

Three categories of immune checkpoint inhibitors received initial approval from the Food and Drug Administration, including programmed cell death 1 (PD-1) inhibitors, programmed cell death ligand 1 (PD-L1) inhibitors, and cytotoxic T-lymphocyte-associated protein 4 (CTLA4) inhibitors (Table 29.1). Agents within each of these categories inhibit this substrate and prevent signaling at the immune checkpoint, allowing activated T-cells to infiltrate the tumor.

PD-1 inhibitors include pembrolizumab and nivolumab. Both are approved for the treatment of melanoma, non–small-cell lung cancer (NSCLC), classic Hodgkin lymphoma, squamous cell cancer of the head and neck, and urothelial carcinoma. Nivolumab is also approved for treating renal cell carcinoma (RCC) and colorectal carcinoma with high micro-satellite instability or mismatch-repair deficiency. Pembrolizumab is also approved for gastric cancer and solid tumors with high micro-satellite instability or mismatch-repair deficiency. PD-L1 inhibitors bind to the PD-1 ligand and include atezolizumab, avelumab, and durvalumab. Each of these therapies is approved for urothelial carcinoma. Additionally, atezolizumab is also approved for treating NSCLC, and avelumab for Merkel-cell carcinoma. Ipilimumab is a CTLA-4 inhibitor. As a monotherapy, it is approved for melanoma. In addition, it is used in combination with other checkpoint inhibitors for treating melanoma and various other cancer types.

ICIs are highly effective in treating patients with these cancers. Objective responses occur in 40–45% of patients with melanoma who are treated with pembrolizumab or nivolumab as first-line treatment. For patients with relapsed NSCLC who have failed chemotherapy, up to 20% will respond to ICIs. For RCC, 25% of patients had radiographic response to nivolumab.[1] This response is often enhanced by combination therapy. The median progression-free survival is up to 11.5 months with nivolumab plus ipilimumab, compared with 2.9 months with ipilimumab monotherapy and 6.9 months with nivolumab monotherapy.[2]

Non-neurologic immune-related adverse events

Despite their efficacy, ICIs can contribute to significant morbidity and even mortality from autoimmune-related complications. These immune-related adverse events (IRAEs) are common and can affect any organ system, including rarely the brain. Common manifestations include gastrointestinal, dermatologic, hepatic, endocrine, and pulmonary toxicities. Colitis occurs in approximately 25% of patients treated with ipilimumab and less than 5% of patients treated with PD-1 or PD-L1 inhibitors. Pneumonitis occurs in 2–5% of patients treated with ICIs. In these cases, both colitis and pneumonitis can be life-threatening. Hypophysitis occurs in up to 10% of patients treated with CTLA-4 inhibitors, and rarely in other types of ICIs. Early recognition is paramount, as this can result in adrenal/hypothalamic crisis and death. Hypothyroidism occurs in up to 20% of patients treated with checkpoint inhibitors, with hyperthyroidism being far less common. One percent of patients prescribed PD-1 or PD-L1 inhibitors and 10%

Table 29.1 Immune checkpoint inhibitor types and approved indications

Checkpoint inhibitor	Type	Approved indications
Pembrolizumab	PD-1 inhibitor	Melanoma, NSCLC, classic Hodgkin lymphoma, SCC of head and neck, urothelial carcinoma, gastric cancer, solid tumors with high micro-satellite instability or mismatch-repair deficiency
Nivolumab	PD-1 inhibitor	Melanoma, NSCLC, classic Hodgkin lymphoma, SCC of head and neck, urothelial carcinoma, RCC, colorectal carcinoma with high micro-satellite instability or mismatch-repair deficiency
Atezolizumab	PD-L1 inhibitor	Urothelial carcinoma, NSCLC
Avelumab	PD-L1 inhibitor	Urothelial carcinoma, Merkel-cell carcinoma
Durvalumab	PD-L1 inhibitor	Urothelial carcinoma
Ipilimumab	CTLA-4 inhibitor	Melanoma

CTLA-4, cytotoxic T-lymphocyte-associated protein 4; *NSCLC,* non–small-cell lung cancer; *PD-1,* programmed cell death 1; *PD-L1,* programmed cell death ligand 1; *RCC,* renal cell carcinoma; *SCC,* squamous cell cancer.

of patients prescribed CTLA-4 inhibitors will develop hepatitis. Skin manifestations are common and occur in up to 30% of patients treated with ICIs. Symptoms include pruritus, acneiform rash, and toxic epidermal necrolysis. Cardiac toxicity may also occur and commonly manifests as inflammatory myocarditis that is present in less than 1% of patients treated with ICIs.[3]

Neurologic adverse events are rare. Although headache occurs in 3–12% of patients, serious neurologic events occur in only 1% of patients treated with ICIs.[4] Despite their rarity, cases of neurologic adverse events with ICIs can be life-threatening, and thus a high index of suspicion is needed to identify these cases early and intervene appropriately. The following cases highlight the breadth and depth of neurologic adverse events and describe the evaluation and management decisions in these patients.

Clinical cases

CASE 29.1 NEUROLOGIC IRAEs ARE HIGHLY VARIABLE AND HAVE NO STANDARD CLINICAL PRESENTATION

Case. A man presents with rapid onset gait imbalance and bilateral lower extremity weakness 3 weeks following initiation of combination nivolumab and ipilimumab as first-line systemic therapy for metastatic melanoma.[5] Following cycle two, his gait dysfunction worsens, and he has numerous falls. ICIs are discontinued, but his weakness and numbness progresses from walking independently to being wheelchair bound over a few months. Physical examination is notable for loss of proprioception and vibration sense in bilateral toes and ankles, positive Romberg, symmetrically absent Achilles and diminished plantar reflexes, and intact motor strength (5/5) except for the right lower extremity (4/5). After failure of outpatient treatment with an oral prednisone taper, he is hospitalized. Workup includes MRI Brain with nonspecific T2-hyperintense white matter lesions and lumbar puncture with a mononuclear leukocytosis and two well-defined gamma restriction bands not present in the serum with normal IgG index, but no malignancy, significant B-cell or blast population on flow cytometry, negative paraneoplastic panel, and negative cytomegalovirus (CMV). Electromyography/nerve conduction velocity (EMG/NCV) show widespread subacute, severe sensory greater than motor neuropathy, with primarily demyelinating and secondary axonal features. These findings are consistent with a Common Terminology Criteria for Adverse Events (CTCAE) grade 4 sensorimotor demyelinating polyneuropathy. Treatment with intravenous corticosteroids as well as a 5-day course of intravenous immunoglobulin (IVIG) is pursued with minimal response. Despite ongoing treatment with oral prednisone and physical therapy, he remained wheelchair bound and died 5 months following initiation of ICI treatment from complications of a urinary tract infection.

Teaching Points. This case highlights several features of neurologic complications of ICIs including (1) the potential for life-threatening complications and (2) the concern for severe IRAEs in patients on combination treatment with two ICIs. There is no standard or typical presentation of a neurologic adverse event of immune checkpoint inhibitors. A spectrum of syndromes can occur ranging from mild neurologic symptoms such as headache to severe and life-threatening manifestations including encephalitis, myelitis, aseptic meningitis, meningoradiculitis, Guillain-Barré–like syndrome, myasthenic syndrome, and peripheral neuropathy, such as this case.[2,6] Mortality may be as high as 18%, but with prompt diagnosis and treatment, 70–80% of patients recover. Of note, higher incidence of IRAEs requiring drug discontinuation has been observed in patients on combination ICI therapy as well as more severe complications with long-term effects.[7] This has not been reliably demonstrated for patients with neurologic IRAEs but can be helpful to consider when evaluating a cancer patient with new neurologic symptoms undergoing ICI therapy. This is anticipated to be particularly relevant as more combination regimens are utilized.

Clinical Pearls

1. Serious neurologic IRAEs have been shown to occur in up to 1% of patients receiving ICIs.
2. In general, IRAEs have been shown to be more common and more severe in patients receiving combination therapy.

CASE 29.2 NEUROLOGICAL IRAEs FROM IMMUNE CHECKPOINT INHIBITORS ARE IDIOSYNCRATIC AND CAN BEGIN AT ANY TIME DURING TREATMENT

Case. A man with metastatic RCC presents with fever to 39.2°C and a transient speech disturbance.[6] He had completed four cycles of combination ipilimumab and nivolumab given every 3 weeks and then five cycles of nivolumab monotherapy given every 2 weeks, with symptom onset occurring 3 days after the fifth dose of nivolumab. The following day, he develops fluctuating confusion and becomes somnolent. Initial laboratory tests are only notable for increased serum creatinine, but MRI Brain shows mild diffuse dural enhancement. Cerebrospinal fluid (CSF) analysis from lumbar puncture demonstrates mononuclear pleocytosis, increased protein, and normal glucose. He is initially treated with intravenous acyclovir, ceftriaxone, and ampicillin for possible infectious meningoencephalitis, but shows no improvement and CSF cultures, cryptococcal antigen, and polymerase chain reaction

(PCR) for herpes simplex virus types 1 and 2, varicella zoster, CMV and Epstein-Barr viruses are all negative. CSF cytology is also negative for tumor cells. EEG shows diffuse non-specific slowing. As a result, an immune-related meningoencephalitis is suspected and treatment with high-dose prednisone is initiated. The patient shows significant clinical improvement and reaches full recovery.

Teaching Points. This case reveals the idiosyncratic onset of neurologic complications that is not dose-dependent and cannot be predicted by antecedent symptoms or red flag signs. The time to onset of neurologic IRAEs varies significantly and can occur at any point during treatment. The median time to onset of neurologic IRAE symptoms is 8 weeks following initiating ICI therapy. The median interval between the last dose of ICI and symptom onset is approximately 2 weeks.[6] In these studies, however, there was a wide range in time of onset observed. In this case, symptoms began at 19 weeks after initiation of ICI therapy and 3 days after the last ICI dose.

Clinical Pearls

1. Neurologic IRAEs from ICIs are idiosyncratic and can occur at any point during treatment.
2. Neurologic IRAEs are highly variable and have been shown to occur throughout the nervous system, with presentations including encephalitis, meningitis, myelitis, meningoradiculitis, myasthenic syndrome, Guillain-Barré–like syndrome, and peripheral neuropathy.

CASE 29.3 A HIGH INDEX OF SUSPICION IS NEEDED TO DIAGNOSE NEUROLOGIC IRAES

Case. A man presents to the clinic with 1 week of low back pain, bilateral hand numbness, and progressive lower extremity weakness approximately 9 months after initiating combination nivolumab and ipilimumab as first-line systemic therapy for metastatic melanoma.[5] He had completed four cycles of treatment prior to symptom onset. Physical examination is notable for bilateral lower extremity dysmetria, reduced sensation to light touch and pinprick with a sensory level to pinprick around the T8 dermatome on the back, and reduced to absent reflexes with full muscle strength, bulk, and range of motion throughout, creating a picture consistent with a thoracic myelopathy. As he is unable to safely ambulate without assistance, he is admitted to the hospital for further workup. An MRI of the brain is obtained and shows no acute pathology, and lumbar puncture is performed and demonstrates a mild mononuclear pleocytosis with no evidence of malignancy or infection. Somatosensory evoked potentials show prolonged P37 latency, consistent with myelopathy. Given a negative workup for infection and tumor progression, he is diagnosed with a CTCAE grade 4 transverse myelopathy secondary to nivolumab/ipilimumab therapy. His immunotherapy is discontinued, and he is treated with intravenous followed by oral corticosteroids. Symptoms improve significantly over the ensuing 4 weeks with only mild persistent lower extremity numbness.

Teaching Points. Neurologic IRAEs of ICIs are highly varied. Like in this case, when evaluating a patient who presents with a new neurologic syndrome and has been treated with these therapies, the general differential diagnosis must include: neurologic IRAE, central nervous system (CNS) infection, tumor progression, or a primary neurologic disease. As in many cases of drug toxicity, this is a diagnosis of exclusion, though if the concern is high, then that should not delay starting treatment, which is described in the following section. The initial workup will depend largely on the neurologic syndrome consistent with the presenting symptoms. The American Society of Clinical Oncology (ASCO) has published a clinical practice guideline regarding diagnosis and treatment of the most common and/or severe IRAEs, including neurologic toxicities.[8] The toxicities they address include myasthenia gravis, Guillain-Barré syndrome, peripheral neuropathy, autonomic neuropathy, aseptic meningitis, encephalitis, and transverse myelitis. These recommendations can be reviewed in Table 29.2.

In the case presented, the patient's symptoms being localized to the bilateral lower extremities and his sensory level on physical examination, amongst other findings, were most consistent with a spinal cord pathology, specifically transverse myelopathy. His differential diagnosis therefore needed to include neurologic IRAE, cancer progression with spinal or brain metastasis, and other primary neurologic syndromes that can cause this presentation in any host not necessarily receiving immunotherapy, depending on their risk factors. Based on both the clinical judgment of a neurologist and the ASCO guidelines, this therefore required CNS imaging, specifically an MRI of the brain and spinal cord, as well as a lumbar puncture, both of which were obtained. Results of CSF studies that are most consistent with neurologic IRAE will be nonspecific and likely feature inflammation with neutrophilic or lymphocytic predominance, as seen in this case.[4] Findings on neuroimaging are most likely to be nonspecific or unremarkable as well, but both imaging and lumbar puncture in this scenario serve the purpose to rule out other pathologies. Furthermore, as his symptoms raised some concern for peripheral involvement, EMG was obtained to further characterize the syndrome. Additional specific testing for conditions that could cause this presentation should be obtained and can depend on the patient's other symptoms and risk factors, such as if there was a concern for B_{12} deficiency, HIV, syphilis, thyroid disease, multiple sclerosis or neuromyelitis optica, or connective tissue diseases.[8]

Clinical Pearls

1. The differential diagnosis in a patient receiving ICIs and presenting with a new neurologic syndrome includes infection, tumor progression, primary neurologic syndrome, and neurologic IRAE. Infection and tumor progression in particular must be ruled out as part of the workup for a neurologic IRAE, often requiring neuroimaging and lumbar puncture.

Table 29.2 Management of neurologic IRAEs in patients treated with ICIs[8]

Grade	Management
Myasthenia gravis	
Clinical presentation: Fatigable or fluctuating muscle weakness, typically more proximal than distal. Frequently associated with ocular and/or bulbar involvement (i.e., ptosis, extraocular movement abnormalities resulting in diplopia, dysphagia, dysarthria, facial muscle weakness), and sometimes with neck and/or respiratory muscle weakness.	
Diagnostic workup: • Neurologic consultation • Serum AChR antibody and anti–striated muscle antibodies, if AChR antibodies are negative then consider serum muscle specific kinase and lipoprotein-related 4 antibodies • CPK, aldolase, CRP for possible concurrent myositis • Consider MRI of brain or spine to rule out CNS involvement of malignancy or alternative diagnoses • Electrodiagnostic studies, including neuromuscular junction testing with repetitive stimulation and/or jitter studies, as well as NCS to exclude neuropathy and needle EMG to assess for myositis • Pulmonary function assessment with NIF and VC • If respiratory insufficiency or elevated CPK or troponin T, perform cardiac examination with ECG and TTE for possible concomitant myocarditis	
Grade	Management
All grades warrant workup and intervention due to potential for respiratory compromise in progressive myasthenia gravis. There is no grade 1 myasthenia gravis.	
Grade 2: Some symptoms interfering with ADLs; exclusively ocular symptoms or mild generalized weakness	Withhold ICI, may resume if symptoms resolve Consult neurology Pyridostigmine starting at 30 mg PO three times a day and gradually increase to maximum of 120 mg PO four times a day as tolerated and based on symptoms Corticosteroids (PO prednisone 1–1.5 mg/kg daily), wean based on symptom improvement
Grade 3–4: Limiting self-care and requiring aides; weakness limiting walking; any dysphagia, facial weakness, or respiratory muscle weakness; rapidly progressive symptoms; moderate to severe generalized weakness to myasthenic crisis	Permanently discontinue ICI Admit patient, may need ICU-level monitoring Consult neurology Corticosteroids (IV methylprednisolone 1–2 mg/kg daily), wean based on symptom improvement Initiate IVIG 2 g/kg IV over 5 days (0.4 g/kg per day) or plasmapheresis for 5 days Frequent pulmonary function assessment Daily neurologic review
Additional considerations: • Avoid medications that worsen myasthenia (beta blockers, IV magnesium, fluoroquinolones, aminoglycosides, macrolides) • Wean pyridostigmine based on improvement • Myasthenia gravis due to ICIs may be monophasic, and additional corticosteroid-sparing agents may not be required	

Continued

Table 29.2 Management of neurologic IRAEs in patients treated with ICIs[8]—cont'd

<table>
<tr><th colspan="2">Guillain-Barré syndrome</th></tr>
<tr><td colspan="2">Clinical presentation: Progressive, usually symmetrical muscle weakness with reduced or absent deep tendon reflexes. Symptoms often initially sensory/neuropathic pain localized to lower back and thighs. May involve extremities (classically ascending weakness but not always), facial, respiratory, and bulbar and oculomotor nerves. May also see autonomic dysregulation.</td></tr>
<tr><th colspan="2">Diagnostic workup:</th></tr>
<tr><td colspan="2">• Neurologic consultation
• MRI of spine with or without contrast to rule out compressive lesion and evaluate for nerve root enhancement/thickening
• Lumbar puncture
  o Unlike classic Guillain-Barré syndrome, CSF typically has elevated protein and WBCs
  o Cytology should be sent
• Serum antiganglioside antibody tests for Guillain-Barré syndrome and its subtypes (e.g., anti-GQ1b for Miller Fisher variant associated with ataxia and ophthalmoplegia)
• Electrodiagnostic studies to evaluate polyneuropathy
• Pulmonary function testing (NIF and VC)
• Frequent neurochecks</td></tr>
<tr><td>Grade</td><td>Management</td></tr>
<tr><td colspan="2">All grades warrant workup and intervention due to potential for respiratory compromise in progressive Guillain-Barré syndrome. There is no grade 1 Guillain-Barré syndrome.</td></tr>
<tr><td>Grade 2: Moderate; some interference with ADLs; symptoms concerning to patient
Grade 3–4: Severe; limiting self-care and requiring aides; weakness limiting walking; any dysphagia, facial weakness, respiratory muscle weakness; rapidly progressive symptoms</td><td>Discontinue ICI
Admit patient, may need rapid transfer to ICU-level monitoring
Initiate IVIG (0.4 g/kg per day for 5 days for total dose of 2 g/kg) or plasmapheresis
Though corticosteroids are usually not recommended for idiopathic Guillain-Barré syndrome, in ICI-related forms, a trial is reasonable with IV methylprednisolone (2–4 mg/kg per day) followed by a slow taper
Pulse corticosteroid dosing (methylprednisolone IV 2–3 mg/kg per day) along with IVIG or plasmapheresis may be considered for grades 3–4
Frequent neurochecks and pulmonary function testing
Monitor for autonomic dysfunction
Nonopioid management of neuropathic pain
Treatment of constipation/ileus</td></tr>
<tr><td colspan="2">Additional considerations:
• Slow prednisone taper after corticosteroid pulse plus IVIG or plasmapheresis
• May require multiple IVIG courses
• Would practice caution with re-challenging for severe cases</td></tr>
<tr><th colspan="2">Peripheral neuropathy</th></tr>
<tr><td colspan="2">Clinical presentation: Symmetric or asymmetric sensory, motor, or sensorimotor deficit. Focal mononeuropathies including cranial neuropathies (e.g., facial neuropathies, Bell's palsy) may be present. Numbness and paresthesias may be painful or painless. Reduced or absent reflexes may be present as well as sensory ataxia.</td></tr>
<tr><td colspan="2">Diagnostic workup:
• Screen for reversible etiologies of neuropathy: diabetic screen, B_{12}, folic acid, TSH, and HIV; can also consider serum protein electrophoresis and other vasculitis and autoimmune testing
• Consider MRI of spine with or without contrast
• For grade 2, in addition to above recommend spinal MRI as well as brain MRI if cranial nerves involved, consider EMG/NCS and consider neurology consultation
• For grade 3–4, go to Guillain-Barré syndrome algorithm</td></tr>
</table>

Table 29.2 **Management of neurologic IRAEs in patients treated with ICIs[8]—cont'd**

Grade	Management
Grade 1: Mild; no interference with function; symptoms not concerning to patient Note: any cranial nerve problem should be managed as moderate	Low threshold to withhold ICI and monitor symptoms for 1 week If planning to continue ICI, monitor closely for symptom progression
Grade 2: Moderate; some interference with ADLs, symptoms concerning to patient (i.e., pain but no weakness or gait limitation)	Withhold ICI and resume when return to grade 1 Initial observation or initiate prednisone 0.5–1 mg/kg (if progressing from mild) Gabapentin, pregabalin, or duloxetine for pain
Grade 3–4: Severe; limiting self-care and aides required; weakness limiting walking or respiratory problems (i.e., foot drop, leg weakness, rapidly ascending sensory changes) Note: severe may actually be Guillain-Barré and should be managed as such	Permanently discontinue ICI Admit patient Consult neurology Initiate IV methylprednisolone 2–4 mg/kg and proceed as per Guillain-Barré syndrome management
Autonomic neuropathy	
Clinical presentation: May present with dysregulation of blood pressure, temperature control, digestion, bladder function, and sexual function. Can present with new severe constipation, nausea, urinary problems, sexual difficulties, sweating abnormalities, sluggish pupil reaction, and orthostatic hypotension.	
Diagnostic workup: • Consult neurology or other relevant specialist depending on organ system involved • Screen for other causes of autonomic dysfunction: diabetic screen, adrenal insufficiency, HIV, paraproteinemia, amyloidosis, botulism, and consider chronic diseases such as Parkinson's and other autoimmune syndromes • Orthostatic vital signs • Consider electrodiagnostic studies for evaluating concurrent polyneuropathy • Consider paraneoplastic autoimmune dysautonomia testing (e.g., anti-ganglionic acetylcholine receptor, antineuronal nuclear antibody type 1 [ANNA-1], and N-type voltage gated calcium channel antibodies)	
Grade	Management
Grade 1: Mild; no interference with function; symptoms not concerning to patient	Low threshold to withhold ICI and monitor symptoms for 1 week If planning to continue ICI, monitor closely for symptom progression
Grade 2: Moderate; some interference with ADLs; symptoms concerning to patient	Withhold ICI and resume when return to grade 1 Initial observation or initiate prednisone 0.5–1 mg/kg (if progressing from mild) Consult neurology
Grade 3–4: Severe; limiting self-care and requiring aides	Permanently discontinue ICI Admit patient Initiate methylprednisolone 1 g daily for 3 days followed by PO corticosteroid taper Consult neurology

Continued

Table 29.2 Management of neurologic IRAEs in patients treated with ICIs[8]—cont'd

<table>
<tr><th colspan="2">Aseptic meningitis</th></tr>
<tr><td colspan="2">Clinical presentation: May present with headache, photophobia, neck stiffness. Often afebrile but may be febrile. May have nausea and/or vomiting. Mental status should be normal (as distinguished from encephalitis, seen below).</td></tr>
<tr><td colspan="2">Diagnostic workup:
• MRI of brain with or without contrast and pituitary protocol
• AM cortisol, ACTH to rule out adrenal insufficiency
• Consider lumbar puncture: measure opening pressure, cell count, protein, glucose, gram stain, culture, PCR or HSV and other viral PCRs depending on suspicion, cytology
o May see elevated WBC count and normal glucose, normal culture and gram stain, may see reactive lymphocytes or histiocytes on cytology</td></tr>
<tr><td>Grading</td><td>Management</td></tr>
<tr><td>Grade 1: Mild; no interference with function; symptoms not concerning to patient
Note: any cranial nerve problem should be managed as moderate
Grade 2: Moderate; some interference with function; symptoms concerning to patient (i.e., pain but no weakness or gait limitation)
Grade 3–4: Severe; limiting self-care and requiring aides</td><td>Withhold ICI and discuss resumption with patient after taking into account the risks and benefits
Consider empiric antiviral (IV acyclovir) and antibacterial therapy until CSF results
Once bacterial and viral infection are negative, may closely monitor off corticosteroids or consider PO prednisone 0.5–1 mg/kg or IV methylprednisolone 1 mg/kg if moderate/severe symptoms</td></tr>
<tr><th colspan="2">Encephalitis</th></tr>
<tr><td colspan="2">Clinical presentation: Confusion, altered behavior, headaches, seizures, short-term memory loss, depressed level of consciousness, focal weakness, speech abnormality</td></tr>
<tr><td colspan="2">Diagnostic workup:
• MRI of brain with or without contrast, may reveal T2/FLAIR changes typically of that seen in autoimmune encephalopathies or limbic encephalitis or may be normal
• Lumbar puncture: check cell count, protein, glucose, gram stain, culture, PCR for HSV and other viral PCRs depending on suspicion, cytology, oligoclonal bands, autoimmune encephalopathy and paraneoplastic panels
• May see elevated WBC count with lymphocytic predominance and/or elevated protein
• EEG to evaluate for subclinical seizures
• Serum: metabolic, CBC, ESR, CRP, ANCA (if suspecting vasculitic process), thyroid panel including TPO and thyroglobulin
• Rule out concurrent anemia/thrombocytopenia, which can present with headaches and confusion
• Consult neurology</td></tr>
<tr><td>Grade</td><td>Management</td></tr>
<tr><td>Grade 1: Mild; no interference with function; symptoms not concerning to patient
Note: any cranial nerve problem should be managed as moderate
Grade 2: Moderate; some interference with function; symptoms concerning to patient (i.e., pain but no weakness or gait limitation)
Grade 3–4: Severe; limiting self-care and requiring aides</td><td>Withhold ICI and discuss resumption with patient after taking into account the risks and benefits
As above for aseptic meningitis, suggest concurrent IV acyclovir until PCR results obtained and negative
Trial of methylprednisolone 1–2 mg/kg
If severe, progressing, or oligoclonal bands present, consider pulse corticosteroids (methylprednisolone 1 g IV daily for 3–5 days) plus IVIG 2 g/kg over 5 days
If positive for autoimmune encephalopathy antibody and limited or no improvement, consider rituximab or plasmapheresis in consultation with neurology</td></tr>
</table>

Table 29.2 Management of neurologic IRAEs in patients treated with ICIs[8]—cont'd

<table>
<tr><th colspan="2">Transverse myelitis</th></tr>
<tr><td colspan="2">Clinical presentation: Acute or subacute weakness or sensory changes, bilateral, often with increased deep tendon reflexes</td></tr>
<tr><td colspan="2">Diagnostic workup:
• MRI of spine (with thin axial cuts through the region of suspected abnormality) and MRI of brain
• Lumbar puncture: check cell count, protein, glucose, oligoclonal bands, viral PCRs, cytology, onconeural antibodies
• Serum: B_{12}, HIV, ANA, Ro/La, TSH, aquaporin-4 IgG
• Consult neurology
• Evaluate for urinary retention, constipation</td></tr>
<tr><td>Grade</td><td>Management</td></tr>
<tr><td>Grade 1: Mild; no interference with function; symptoms not concerning to patient
Note: any cranial nerve problem should be managed as moderate
Grade 2: Moderate; some interference with function; symptoms concerning to patient (i.e., pain but no weakness or gait limitation)
Grade 3–4: Severe; limiting self-care and requiring aides</td><td>Permanently discontinue ICI
Initiate methylprednisolone IV 2 mg/kg
Strongly consider higher doses of 1 g per day for 3–5 days
Strongly consider IVIG</td></tr>
</table>

AChR, Acetylcholine receptor; *ACTH,* adrenocorticotropic hormone; *ADL,* activities of daily living; *AM,* morning; *ANA,* antinuclear antibody; *ANCA,* antineutrophil cytoplasmic antibodies; *CBC,* complete blood count; *CNS,* central nervous system; *CPK,* creatine phosphokinase; *CRP,* C-reactive protein; *CSF,* cerebrospinal fluid; *ECG,* electrocardiogram; *EEG,* electroencephalogram; *EMG,* electromyography; *ESR,* erythrocyte sedimentation rate; *FLAIR,* fluid attenuated inversion recovery; *HIV,* human immunodeficiency virus; *HSV,* herpes simplex virus; *ICI,* immune checkpoint inhibitor; *ICU,* intensive care unit; *IgG,* immunoglobulin G; *IV,* intravenous; *IVIG,* intravenous immunoglobulin; *IRAE,* immune-related adverse event; *MRI,* magnetic resonance imaging; *NCS,* nerve conduction study; *NIF,* negative inspiratory force; *PCR,* polymerase chain reaction; *PO,* oral; *RPR,* rapid plasma reagin; *TPO,* thyroid peroxidase; *TSH,* thyroid-stimulating hormone; *TTE,* transthoracic echocardiogram; *VC,* vital capacity; *WBC,* white blood cell.

CASE 29.4 TREATMENT OF NEUROLOGIC IRAES VARIES BY THE GRADE OF THE ADVERSE EVENT

Case. A man with metastatic melanoma presents with diplopia.[6] He is currently being treated with pembrolizumab following surgical resection of a right frontal metastasis and stereotactic radiosurgery for additional right frontal and left thalamic metastases, and has received two cycles of treatment. On physical examination, he is noted to have a left-sided ptosis and borderline left esophoria. Brain MRI is obtained and shows stable known parenchymal lesions without leptomeningeal or cranial nerve enhancement. As diurnal fluctuation is noted and concern is raised for immune-related etiology, he is treated with oral prednisone and pembrolizumab treatment is withheld. Though serum anti-acetylcholine receptor antibodies are negative, single-fiber EMG shows pathologic jitter compatible with a myasthenic syndrome. His diplopia gradually improves, and he is treated with a 1-month prednisone taper. Complete symptom resolution is noted 6 weeks following initial presentation, and pembrolizumab is later resumed with continuous low-dose prednisone, and no further neurologic deterioration is observed.

Teaching Points. Treatment of neurologic IRAEs can vary depending on the type and severity of complication, but if diagnosed and treated early, there can be significant response, as demonstrated in this case. In a 2017 systematic review of the literature, 73% of cases reported showed partial or complete neurologic recovery. Clinical improvement was only reported with drug discontinuation, however, with an additional 44% receiving steroids alone and 30% receiving steroids and IVIG or plasma exchanges.[4] In a review of 12 clinical trials, 74% of patients had clinical recovery, with a median time to resolution of symptoms of 32 days.[2] Specific treatment recommendations based on type and severity of IRAE per ASCO guidelines can be seen in Table 29.2. In the case described, his presentation would be consistent with a grade 2 ocular myasthenia gravis, therefore his treatment of withholding ICI and starting PO steroids with resumption of ICI later upon symptom resolution is largely consistent with ASCO recommendations.

The decision regarding if and when to resume immunotherapy, however, is one that requires discussion of the risks and benefits between the neurology and oncology providers as well as the patient. In one case series, two patients on ICIs who suffered neurologic IRAEs were able to be restarted on their immunotherapy after resolution of the adverse event without additional neurologic complications.[6] In the case above, ICI therapy was resumed—consistent with ASCO recommendations based on the localized nature of his symptoms—along with PO corticosteroids, and he did not experience further neurologic deficits. Case 29.3 demonstrates another example of the need to make a re-challenge decision on a case-by-case basis. The symptoms of this patient in Case 29.3 would be categorized as grade 3–4 transverse myelitis, and per ASCO recommendations (Table 29.2), the ICI should be permanently discontinued. However, for this patient, upon tumor progression 4 weeks after discharge from the hospital he was successfully re-challenged with nivolumab as monotherapy and experienced only mild recurrence of symptoms. These symptoms improved with a prednisone pulse with taper, and he went on to complete a total of 12 cycles of nivolumab treatment.[5] Therefore, the decision to resume ICIs after a neurologic IRAE should be made cautiously, with consideration of the risks and benefits as well as the patient's wishes.

Clinical Pearls

1. The treatment of neurologic IRAEs varies by the grade of adverse event, but for IRAEs of grade 2 or higher, will typically require oral or intravenous corticosteroids and delay in, or discontinuation of, immunotherapy.

Conclusion

In summary, immunotherapy is a very promising area of cancer therapy, showing efficacy in a variety of types of cancers, including many that have been unresponsive to traditional chemotherapy. In contrast to chemotherapy, which targets rapidly dividing cancer cells and can lead to side effects in organ systems with rapid cell turnover, immunotherapies activate the immune system, thus potentially leading to IRAEs, including in the nervous system. Though neurologic IRAEs are rare, their presentations are variable and can be severe. Therefore, neurologists and oncologists evaluating these patients must have a high index of suspicion in a patient receiving immune checkpoint inhibitors and presenting with a new neurologic syndrome, so that recognition and treatment can be promptly initiated.

References

1. Gibney GT, Weiner LM, Atkins MB. Predictive biomarkers for checkpoint inhibitor-based immunotherapy. *Lancet Oncol.* 2016;17(12):e542–e551.
2. Larkin J, Chiarion-Sileni V, Gonzalez R, et al. Combined nivolumab and ipilimumab or monotherapy in untreated melanoma. *N Engl J Med.* 2015;373:23–34.
3. Johnson DB, Chandra S, Sosman JA. Immune checkpoint inhibitor toxicity in 2018. *JAMA.* 2018;320(16):1702–1703.
4. Cuzzubbo S, Javeri F, Tissier M, et al. Neurological adverse events associated with immune checkpoint inhibitors: review of the literature. *Eur J Cancer.* 2017;73:1–8.
5. Fellner A, Makranz C, Lotem M, et al. Neurologic complications of immune checkpoint inhibitors. *J Neurooncol.* 2018;137(3):601–609.
6. Mancone S, Lycan TW, Ahmed T, et al. Severe neurologic complications of immune checkpoint inhibitors: a single-center review. *J Neurol.* 2018;265(7):1636–1642.
7. Postow MA, Sidlow R, Hellmann MD. Immune-related adverse events associated with immune checkpoint blockade. *N Engl J Med.* 2018;378:158–168.
8. Brahmer JR, Lacchetti C, Schneider BJ, et al. Management of immune-related adverse events in patients treated with immune checkpoint inhibitor therapy: American Society of Clinical Oncology Clinical Practice Guideline. *J Clin Oncol.* 2018;36(17):1714–1768.

Chapter 30

Neurologic complications associated with CAR T-cell therapy

Stephen J. Bagley

CHAPTER OUTLINE

Introduction

Immune-based therapies have revolutionized cancer treatment. These agents enhance the immune system's ability to seek out and attack tumor cells. One such treatment, CAR T-cells or chimeric antigen receptor T-cells, are a type of adoptive cell transfer therapy where a patient's own T-cells are collected, genetically modified to treat their cancer, and reinfused. CAR T-cell therapy starts with collecting autologous T lymphocytes from a patient via leukapheresis. These cells are genetically engineered to express a modified T-cell receptor known as a chimeric antigen receptor (CAR), which binds to a specific cancer antigen such as CD19. Once CAR T-cells express the chimeric receptor of interest in vitro, they are expanded, purified, and infused back into the patient after the patient has received lymphodepleting chemotherapy. Once infused, cancer antigens stimulate the CAR T-cells to release cytotoxins, inducing cancer cell death, and resulting in treatment responses.

Structure, function, and administration of CAR T-cells

CARs are genetically engineered fusion proteins that redirect the specificity and function of T-cells. The CAR protein is composed of an extracellular antigen-recognition domain, a transmembrane domain, and an intracellular signaling module derived from T-cell signaling proteins.[1] Each CAR contains the CD3ζ protein which plays a role in the activation of a T-cell.

- First-generation CARs contain CD3ζ
- Second-generation CARs possess a costimulatory endodomain (e.g., CD28 or 4-1BB) fused to CD3ζ[2]
- Third-generation CARs consist of two costimulatory domains linked to CD3ζ

After a CAR construct is transfected into autologous or allogeneic peripheral blood T-cells using plasmid transfection, mRNA, or viral vector transduction, the T-cells are infused into the patient to target whichever surface-exposed tumor antigen is specified by the CAR's extracellular targeting moiety, usually in the form of a single-chain variable fragment.[3] Upon CAR engagement of its associated antigen, primary T-cell activation occurs and leads to cytokine release, cytolytic degranulation, and T-cell proliferation.[4] Unlike vaccines and immunomodulatory agents that rely on in vivo priming of endogenous tumor-reactive cells and are therefore human leukocyte-antigen (HLA) restricted, CAR T-cells are capable of inducing durable antitumor responses in a universal, HLA-independent manner.[5]

Leukapheresis. Leukapheresis is the first step in developing CAR T-cells for use in an individual patient. First, blood is removed from the patient, leukocytes are separated, and the remainder of the blood is returned to the circulation.[6] After a sufficient number of leukocytes have been harvested, the leukapheresis product is enriched for T-cells. Next, the T-cells undergo an activation process during which they are incubated with the viral vector encoding the CAR, and after several days, the vector is washed out of the culture. Lentiviral vectors are used most frequently, but other methods of gene transfer are being explored.[7,8] When the cell expansion process is finished, the cell culture is concentrated to a volume that can be infused into the patient and is cryopreserved in infusible medium.[9] Finally, when the product is released for treatment, the frozen cells are transported to the treatment site and thawed prior to administration. In patients with hematologic malignancies, lymphodepleting chemotherapy is typically administered prior to the CAR T-cell reinfusion. Lymphodepletion can substantially increase the in vivo expansion of the infused CAR T-cells by multiple effects, including reducing the patient's lymphoid cell pool to make "space" for the CAR T-cells, increasing homeostatic cytokines, and ameliorating the tumor inhibitory microenvironment.[10–13]

Efficacy and toxicity of CAR T-cell therapy

Efficacy. The greatest advances for CAR T-cells have occurred in the treatment of hematologic malignancies, with the United States Food and Drug Administration (FDA) having approved two therapies as of the writing of this chapter. Tisagenlecleucel, a CD19-targeted CAR T-cell therapy formerly known as CTL019, was first approved for the treatment of patients up to 25 years of age with B-cell precursor acute lymphoblastic leukemia (ALL) that is refractory or in second or later relapse.[14] Tisagenlecleucel was subsequently approved for adult patients with relapsed or refractory large B-cell lymphoma after two or more lines of systemic therapy, including diffuse large B-cell lymphoma (DLBCL), high-grade B-cell lymphoma, and DLBCL arising from follicular lymphoma. The second CAR T-cell therapy approved by the FDA was axicabtagene ciloleucel, which is also targeted against CD19 and is approved for adult patients with relapsed or refractory large B-cell lymphoma patients who have failed at least two prior therapies, including DLBCL, primary mediastinal large B-cell lymphoma, high-grade B-cell lymphoma, and DLBCL arising from follicular lymphoma.[15] Remarkably, both of these CAR products have led to durable remissions in patients with B-cell malignancies refractory to standard salvage therapies, with an overall response rate of 50–90% across multiple trials.[16–21]

Cytokine release syndrome. CAR T-cell therapies for hematologic malignancies have unique toxicities that are distinct from those of cytotoxic chemotherapy, small-molecule targeted therapies, and even from other immunotherapies. The most commonly observed toxicity with CAR T-cells is cytokine-release syndrome (CRS), which manifests as high fever, hypotension, hypoxia, and/or multiorgan toxicity.[15] Rarely, cases of CRS progress to fulminant hemophagocytic lymphohistiocytosis (also known as macrophage-activation syndrome), which is characterized by severe immune activation, lymphohistiocytic tissue infiltration, and immune-mediated multisystem organ failure.[22,23] CRS is triggered by the activation of T-cells upon engagement of their CARs with cognate antigens expressed by tumor cells. When this occurs, both the activated T-cells, as well as bystander immune cells including monocytes and macrophages, release cytokines and chemokines that lead to a systemic inflammatory state that resembles sepsis physiology.[24] CRS usually manifests with constitutional symptoms, such as fever, malaise, anorexia, and myalgias, but can ultimately impact any organ in the body, including the heart, lungs, gut, liver, kidneys, bone marrow, or nervous system.[25] CRS should be managed in accordance with the grade of this toxicity, which can be determined using established guidelines.[15] Detailed discussion of the management of CRS is beyond the scope of this chapter, but interventions typically include supportive care such as intravenous fluid boluses, anti-interleukin (IL)-6 therapy with tocilizumab or siltuximab, and/or corticosteroids in cases refractory to anti-IL6 therapy.[24]

In addition to ALL and DLBCL, CAR T-cells have shown promise in early phase trials in other hematologic malignancies, including multiple myeloma.[26,27] In solid tumors, however, response rates have been much less favorable. Some of the most significant challenges for CAR T-cell immunotherapy in solid cancers include (1) identification of unique tumor target antigens, (2) improved CAR T-cell trafficking to tumor sites, (3) addressing tumor heterogeneity and antigen loss, and (4) manipulating the immunosuppressive tumor microenvironment to allow for effective CAR T-cell expansion and tumor cell killing.[28] While improved efficacy of CAR T-cells in solid tumors is eagerly awaited, patients enrolled on solid tumor CAR T-cell trials are at risk of many of the same complications as patients with hematologic malignancies. Thus, it is imperative that CRS and other compilations of CAR T-cells are recognized and managed appropriately by neurologists and other members of the care team. The remainder of this chapter will focus specifically on the neurotoxicity associated with CAR T-cell therapies.

Clinical case

CASE 30.1 NEUROLOGIC COMPLICATIONS OF CAR T-CELL THERAPY

Case. A 69-year-old male with a history of refractory DLBCL presented with progression of his tumor despite two recent cycles of salvage chemotherapy with R-ICE (rituximab, ifosfamide, carboplatin, and etoposide). He was recommended for CAR T-cell therapy with axicabtagene ciloleucel. T-cells were collected, and he was admitted to the hospital for CAR T-cell infusion. He received lymphodepleting chemotherapy with fludarabine and cyclophosphamide followed by infusion of CAR T-cells. He was initiated on seizure prophylaxis with levetiracetam 750 mg by mouth twice daily, which is standard. On day +1 following the infusion, he became febrile to 101.0°F. An infectious workup was initiated and was negative. On day +2, he developed an increasing oxygen requirement requiring a nonrebreather mask and was given a single dose of tocilizumab 8 mg/kg intravenously (IV) and dexamethasone 10 mg IV for presumed CRS. His hypoxia and fevers improved, but on day +5 following the infusion, he developed expressive aphasia, increased somnolence and confusion, and bowel/bladder incontinence. His somnolence and confusion progressed rapidly and he was transferred to the neurological intensive care unit. A non-contrast head CT was unremarkable and showed no evidence of intracranial hemorrhage or cerebral edema. MRI of the brain with and without contrast demonstrated diffuse, nonspecific T2-weighted and fluid-attenuated inversion recovery (FLAIR) signal abnormality in the periventricular and subcortical white matter. He was initiated on dexamethasone 10 mg IV every 6 hours. Despite this intervention, his mental status continued to decline, and he was intubated for airway protection. A lumbar puncture was performed. Cerebrospinal fluid (CSF) protein was elevated at 509 mg/dL, but other CSF studies were within normal limits. A 24-hour continuous electroencephalogram (EEG) was performed without any seizures or clinical events captured and demonstrated generalized slowing and sharp waves with triphasic morphology. He remained intubated for 2 days and was extubated on day +8 following CAR T-cell infusion when his mental status began to improve. He showed continued daily clinical improvement, and his corticosteroids were tapered rapidly. By day +20, his neurotoxicity had completely resolved, and by day +24, he was no longer on steroids.

Teaching Points. This case describes a typical presentation for a patient suffering from neurologic toxicity from CAR T-cell therapy. Neurotoxicity in the setting of CAR T-cell therapy has been referred to both as immune effector-cell associated neurotoxicity syndrome (ICANS)[29] and CAR-related encephalopathy syndrome (CRES).[15] Neurotoxicity is thought to develop either as a result of systemic cytokine release propagating into the central nervous system (CNS) or from direct migration of CAR-T-cells into the CNS. There is a bimodal distribution with neurotoxicity either developing early after CAR-T infusion usually in the setting of CRS or occurring several weeks after the infusion often without evidence of CRS. Nonspecific neurologic symptoms such as headache, malaise, nausea, and fatigue are not necessarily indicative of ICANS. However, red flag symptoms include encephalopathy, aphasia, dysgraphia, and tremor which should prompt urgent evaluation as they correlate with electrographic seizure activity, cerebral edema, and life-threatening elevated intracranial pressure (ICP). Like the patient in this case, all patients are treated empirically with prophylactic anticonvulsants for the first 30 days after CAR T-cell infusion. Patients who develop signs of neurotoxicity should be promptly evaluated for signs of seizure or cerebral edema. Administration of the anti-IL-6 therapy tocilizumab is used for treating CRS. Prompt initiation of corticosteroids is the treatment of choice for neurotoxicity.

Clinical presentation, grading, and general management of CAR T-cell neurotoxicity

Incidence and risk factors. Along with CRS, the other significant toxicity observed after CAR T-cell therapy is neurotoxicity. The published incidence rates range from 20–64%[30] and occurrence of ICANS may be a negative prognostic factor for overall survival.[31] Although neurotoxicity can occur alone in some patients, this toxicity generally tracks with CRS severity, and both are correlated with enhanced CAR T-cell expansion.[32] Patients at high risk of CAR T-cell–related neurotoxicity are generally the same patients who are at high risk of CRS. Thus, well-established factors associated with elevated risk of neurotoxicity include higher peak CAR T-cell expansion and high pretreatment disease burden.[33] Less well-established factors that may predispose to neurotoxicity include higher infused CAR T-cell dose,[34] high intensity lymphodepletion regimens,[35] preexisting neurologic comorbidities,[34] younger age,[34] and thrombocytopenia,[31] which may be a surrogate for preexisting endothelial activation.[36]

Pathophysiology. The pathophysiologic mechanism underlying CAR T-cell-related neurotoxicity is not fully understood, but passive diffusion of cytokines into the brain, as well as trafficking of T-cells into the CNS, have been postulated.[37,38] In humans, it has been shown that endothelial dysfunction and increased blood-brain barrier permeability are present in patients who develop neurotoxicity.[34] In nonhuman primates with CAR T-cell–related neurotoxicity, CAR and non–CAR T-cell infiltration into the CSF and brain, as well as increased levels of proinflammatory cytokines, have been observed.[39]

Laboratory tests and neuroimaging. Correlation between the development of CAR T-cell–related neurotoxicity and laboratory parameters is imperfect, and identification of predictive biomarkers for severe toxicity is needed. One study demonstrated that serum ferritin levels peak with the onset of neurologic symptoms, and higher ferritin levels were associated with higher neurotoxicity grade.[31] As with the patient in the presented case, protein levels in the CSF are often elevated in patients with CAR T-cell–related neurotoxicity, but other CSF studies are typically normal.[40] MRI and CT scan of the brain are usually negative for anatomic pathology. However, cases of reversible T2/FLAIR MRI hyperinstensity[40] and cerebral edema[38,41] have been reported.

Signs and symptoms of CAR T-cell–related neurotoxicity. The onset of neurotoxicity from CAR T-cell therapy either occurs:

1. Acutely within the first 5 days after CAR T-cell delivery, often accompanied by fever and other CRS symptoms
2. Delayed neurotoxicity occurring after fever and other CRS symptoms have subsided, more than a week after cell infusion[15]

The clinical presentation of CAR T-cell–related neurotoxicity is similar to that of other toxic encephalopathies. The earliest signs include tremor, dysgraphia, mild expressive aphasia, impaired attention, apraxia, and mild lethargy.[29] Headache sometimes occurs but is not specific for CAR T-cell–related neurotoxicity. Conversely, difficulty with speech, which often begins with mild expressive aphasia and can progress to global aphasia with both expressive and receptive difficulty, is highly specific for this condition.[33] Thus, while certain features of CAR T-cell–related neurotoxicity may overlap with other encephalopathies frequently observed in cancer patients (e.g., hepatic, toxic/metabolic, etc.), an awake patient who is mute and does not respond verbally or physically to an examiner is likely to have neurotoxicity from CAR T-cell therapy.[29] Other symptoms and signs of neurotoxicity from CAR T-cells include confusion, disorientation, agitation, and somnolence.[15] In severe cases, seizures and increased ICP can occur, and these are covered in more detail in subsequent sections of this chapter. Once the first signs of neurotoxicity are observed, progression to more severe symptoms can occur over the course of hours to days.

Grading of CAR T-cell–related neurotoxicity. Neurotoxicity from CAR T-cell therapy was initially graded using Common Terminology Criteria for Adverse Events (CTCAE) criteria.[42] However, as more trials have been conducted and clinical experience with neurotoxicity has increased, more specific grading systems have been published and are increasingly utilized.[15,29] First, a multi-institutional group of oncologists leading CAR T-cell trials across the United States published the CARTOX criteria for adults on grading of neurotoxicity (Table 30.1).[15] The CARTOX system grades neurotoxicity by assessing multiple neurologic domains that span the constellation of signs and symptoms associated with neurotoxicity. CARTOX incorporates a 10-point screening tool called the CARTOX-10, which includes the components of the Mini-Mental State Examination (MMSE) that are most specifically affected by the encephalopathy observed in patients with CAR T-cell–related neurotoxicity. The CARTOX grading system also includes other domains, such as level of consciousness, motor symptoms, seizures, and signs of elevated ICP. More recently, Lee et al. published the American Society for Blood and Marrow Transplantation (ASBMT) ICANS grading scheme (Table 30.1).[29] This grading scheme was intended to improve the objectivity, reproducibility, and practicality of assessing neurotoxicity in CAR T-cell–treated patients. The updated encephalopathy grading tool used in the ASBMT ICANS scheme, referred to as the Immune Effector Cell-Associated Encephalopathy (ICE) score, is nearly identical to the original CARTOX-10 scoring system; the main change is the addition of an element for assessing the receptive aphasia that is seen in these patients. In addition to this minor change in the scoring tool, the ASBMT ICANS seizure and ICP grading schema have been simplified (Table 30.1).

General management of CAR T-cell–related neurotoxicity. Similar to CRS, the management of CAR T-cell-related neurotoxicity is based on the toxicity grade. In general, supportive care alone is adequate for grade 1 neurotoxicity. This includes IV hydration, elevation of the head of bed to minimize aspiration risk, neurology consultation, avoidance of medications that cause central nervous system depression, daily 30-minute EEG until toxicity symptoms resolve, and fundoscopic examination to rule out papilledema. Low doses of lorazepam or haloperidol can be used with careful monitoring for agitated patients. Anti-IL-6 therapy (tocilizumab 8 mg/kg IV or siltuximab 11 mg/kg IV) is recommended for patients with grade ≥1 neurotoxicity who also have concurrent CRS. If neurotoxicity is not associated with CRS, corticosteroids are the preferred treatment for grade ≥2 neurotoxicity, and can be tapered rapidly after improvement of the neurotoxicity to grade 1. Dexamethasone 10 mg IV every 6 hours or methylprednisolone 1 mg/kg IV every 12 hours can be used. For grade 4 neurotoxicity, anti-IL-6 therapy should also be used regardless of whether concurrent CRS is present. Monitoring in the ICU is recommended for patients with grade 3 neurotoxicity and required for patients with grade 4 neurotoxicity. Detailed management of seizures and elevated ICP in patients with CAR T-cell–related neurotoxicity is outlined in the following sections.

Diagnosing and managing seizures from CAR T-cell neurotoxicity

In patients with neurotoxicity from CAR T-cell therapy, secondary cortical irritation may manifest with EEG findings of epileptiform discharges or nonconvulsive electrographic

Table 30.1 Published CAR T-cell neurotoxicity grading systems

	Neurotoxicity domain	Grade 1	Grade 2	Grade 3	Grade 4
CARTOX criteria[15]	Neurologic Assessment Score (CARTOX-10)[a]	7–9 (mild impairment)	3–6 (moderate impairment)	0–2 (severe impairment)	Patient in critical condition, and/or obtunded and cannot perform assessment of tasks
	Elevated ICP	N/A	N/A	Stage 1–2 papilledema or CSF opening pressure <20 mmHg	Stage 3–5 papilledema, or CSF opening pressure ≥20 mmHg, or cerebral edema
	Seizures or motor weakness	N/A	N/A	Partial seizure or nonconvulsive seizures on EEG with response to benzodiazepine	Generalized seizures or convulsive or nonconvulsive status epilepticus, or new motor weakness
ASBMT ICANS criteria[30]	ICE score[b]	7–9	3–6	0–2	0 (patient is unarousable and unable to perform ICE)
	Depressed level of consciousness	Awakens spontaneously	Awakens to voice	Awakens only to tactile stimulus	Patient is unarousable or requires vigorous or repetitive tactile stimuli to arouse. Stupor coma
	Seizure	N/A	N/A	Any clinical seizure, focal or generalized, that resolves rapidly or nonconvulsive seizures on EEG that resolve with intervention	Life-threatening prolonged seizure (>5 min); or repetitive clinical or electrical seizures without return to baseline in between
	Motor findings	N/A	N/A	N/A	Deep focal motor weakness such as hemiparesis or paraparesis
	Elevated ICP, cerebral edema	N/A	N/A	Focal/local edema on neuroimaging	Diffuse cerebral edema on neuroimaging; decerebrate or decorticate posturing; or cranial nerve VI palsy; or papilledema; or Cushing's triad

[a]In the CARTOX-10, 1 point is assigned for each of the following tasks that is performed correctly (normal cognitive function is defined by an overall score of 10): orientation to year, month, city, hospital, and President/Prime Minister of country of residence (total of 5 points); name three objects—for example, point to clock, pen, button (maximum of 3 points); write a standard sentence—for example, "our national bird is the bald eagle" (1 point); count backwards from 100 in tens (1 point).

[b]ICE adds a command-following assessment (e.g., "Show me two fingers" or "Close your eyes and stick out your tongue") in place of one of the CARTOX-10 orientation questions. The scoring system remains the same.

ASBMT, American Society for Blood and Marrow Transplantation; *CSF,* cerebrospinal fluid; *EEG,* electroencephalography; *ICANS,* immune effector-cell associated neurotoxicity syndrome; *ICE,* immune effector cell-associated encephalopathy; *ICP,* intracranial pressure; *N/A,* not applicable.

seizures.[15] Seizure prophylaxis with levetiracetam 750 mg orally or intravenously every 12 hours is recommended for 30 days starting on the day of the CAR T-cell infusion. EEG should be obtained for patients with any grade of suspected neurotoxicity. Common findings on EEG include diffuse generalized slowing with or without triphasic waves at 1–2 Hz, consistent with encephalopathy.[31] When seizures occur, it is typically after the development of severe (global) aphasia.[29]

The reported incidence of nonconvulsive status epilepticus in patients treated with CAR T-cell therapy is about 10%, with a small subgroup of those patients developing convulsive status epilepticus.[15] Nonconvulsive and convulsive status epilepticus should be managed with benzodiazepines and additional antiepileptics, preferably levetiracetam, as needed. The response to benzodiazepines is rapid in many patients, with resolution of EEG findings and improvement in mental status. However, if nonconvulsive status epilepticus persists after benzodiazepines and levetiracetam administration, the patient should be transferred to an ICU and treated with a loading dose of 60 mg IV phenobarbital, followed by maintenance antiepileptic therapy. For convulsive status epilepticus that persists after initial benzodiazepine and levetiracetam, a phenobarbital loading dose of 15 mg/kg IV should be administered, followed by maintenance antiepileptic therapy. In addition, continuous EEG monitoring should be performed if seizures are refractory to treatment. Lacosamide and phenytoin should be avoided in patients with CAR T-cell–related seizures due to higher risk of cardiovascular adverse effects (e.g., arrhythmias, hypotension), which is already heightened in patients with CRS.

Diagnosing and managing elevated ICP from CAR T-cell neurotoxicity

Assessment for papilledema by fundoscopy can be challenging in patients with altered mental status and difficulty cooperating with an examination. Neuroimaging and CSF opening pressure, if available, are typically better surrogates of increased ICP and possible cerebral edema. Lumbar puncture can be performed to obtain a CSF opening pressure, but can be limited by patient restlessness and/or coagulopathy. Alternatively, in patients with an Ommaya reservoir, the opening pressure can be measured in the supine position with the base of the manometer at heart level.

Clinicians should have a low threshold for obtaining neuroimaging in patients with suspected CAR T-cell–related neurotoxicity. In patients with grade 3 or 4 neurotoxicity or in patients with rapid changes in the grade of neurotoxicity, MRI of the brain (or CT if MRI is unable to be performed due to patient's clinical status) must be obtained to detect early signs of cerebral edema. Cerebral edema is most commonly encountered in patients who have other acute and clinically significant neurological changes, such as low CARTOX-10 score and/or seizures.[15]

Patients with stage 1 or 2 papilledema (according to the modified Frisén scale[43]) and CSF opening pressure of <20 mmHg without cerebral edema can be managed with acetazolamide only. Acetazolamide should be started with a 1000 mg IV dose, followed by 250–1000 mg IV every 12 hours with dosing adjusted based on renal function and acid-base balance (which should be monitored one to two times daily). For patients with stage 3 or higher papilloma, any signs of cerebral edema on imaging, or a CSF opening pressure of over 20 mmHg, high-dose corticosteroids should be administered using methylprednisolone IV 1 g/day. In addition, hyperventilation should be initiated to achieve target partial pressure of arterial carbon dioxide ($PaCO_2$) of 28–30 mmHg, although this should not be maintained for any longer than 24 hours. Hyperosmolar therapy with either mannitol (20 g/dL solution) or hypertonic saline (3% or 23.4%) should also be administered. Mannitol can be started at an initial dose of 0.5–1 g/kg, followed by maintenance dosing of 0.25–1 g/kg every 6 hours while monitoring the patient's metabolic profile and serum osmolality every 6 hours. Mannitol should be withheld if serum osmolality is ≥320 mOsm/kg, or the osmolality gap is ≥40. For hypertonic saline, initial dosing of 250 mL of 3% solution can be given, followed by maintenance at 50–75 mL/hour with electrolyte monitoring every 4 hours. Hypertonic infusion should be withheld if serum sodium levels reach ≥155 mEq/L. For patients with imminent herniation, initial 30 mL of 23.4% hypertonic saline should be administered and can be repeated after 15 minutes if needed. Neurosurgery should be consulted and IV anesthetics considered if the patient has burst-suppression pattern on EEG. Although elevated ICP from CAR T-cell therapy is generally reversible, fatal cases have been reported.[44,45]

Lastly, given that patients currently receiving CAR T-cell therapy outside of clinical trials have refractory hematologic malignancies, it is critical that a broad differential diagnosis is considered when neurologic symptoms are encountered following administration of CAR T-cells. Considerations beyond CAR T-cell–related toxicity include but are not limited to intracranial bleeding in the setting of thrombocytopenia, opportunistic infections, and CNS involvement of the patient's tumor.

Conclusion

In summary, CAR T-cells have emerged as a promising class of cell-based immunotherapy in refractory hematologic malignancies. Neurotoxicity represents a common and potentially life-threatening adverse effect of CAR T-cells, and its pathophysiology remains inadequately understood. Until more effective treatment and preventative strategies for CAR T-cell therapy-associated neurotoxicity are available, it is imperative that practicing oncologists and neurologists recognize this phenomenon promptly and understand the supportive care strategies that should be instituted.

Clinical pearls

1. Fatal neurotoxicity has been described in clinical studies of CAR T-cell therapies.
2. Neurotoxicity from CAR T-cells is highly correlated with manifestation of CRS, and neurologic symptoms are preceded by fever in most patients.
3. Common signs and symptoms of CAR T-cell-associated neurotoxicity including lethargy, somnolence, impaired attention, headache, tremor, dysgraphia, aphasia, focal weakness, seizures, and elevated ICP. Of these signs and symptoms, only expressive aphasia is highly specific for neurotoxicity from CAR T-cells, often manifesting as an awake patient who is mute and does not respond verbally or physically to an examiner.
4. Neuroimaging is frequently unrevealing in patients with neurotoxicity from CAR T-cells, but may reveal nonspecific T2/FLAIR signal abnormality and/or cerebral edema in severe cases. Serum levels of inflammatory markers may correlate with severity.
5. CAR T-cell-associated neurotoxicity is graded based on assessing multiple neurologic domains that span the constellation of signs and symptoms associated with this phenomenon; CARTOX and the ASBMT ICANS Consensus Grading systems are the most commonly utilized.
6. Management of neurotoxicity from CAR T-cell therapy is primarily supportive in nature and is based on the toxicity grade. Anti-IL-6 therapy is recommended for patients with grade ≥1 neurotoxicity with concurrent CRS; if not associated with CRS, corticosteroids are the preferred treatment for grade ≥2 neurotoxicity, and can be tapered after improvement of ICANS to grade 1.
7. Both seizure-like activity and nonepileptic myoclonus are common in patients with neurotoxicity from CAR T-cells, and EEG typically demonstrates diffuse background slowing. For patients who progress to nonconvulsive or convulsive status epilepticus, benzodiazepines and levetiracetam are preferred; phenobarbital is added if seizures persist.
8. CAR T-cell–associated neurotoxicity with raised ICP should be managed promptly with corticosteroids and acetazolamide; patients who develop grade 4 neurotoxicity with cerebral edema should also receive hyperventilation and hyperosmolar therapy.
9. Patients who receive CAR T-cell therapy are often heavily pretreated for their malignancies and may have significant medical comorbidities. Therefore, it is critical that a broad differential diagnosis beyond CAR T-cell–related neurotoxicity is considered when neurologic symptoms are encountered in these patients. Diagnostic considerations include but are not limited to intracranial bleeding in the setting of thrombocytopenia, opportunistic infections, and CNS involvement of the patient's tumor.

References

1. Sadelain M, Brentjens R, Rivière I. The basic principles of chimeric antigen receptor design. *Cancer Discov*. 2013;3(4):388–398.
2. June CH, O'Connor RS, Kawalekar OU, Ghassemi S, Milone MC. CAR T cell immunotherapy for human cancer. *Science*. 2018;359(6382):1361–1365.
3. Eshhar Z, Waks T, Bendavid A, Schindler DG. Functional expression of chimeric receptor genes in human T cells. *J Immunol Methods*. 2001;248(1–2):67–76.
4. Hombach A, Wieczarkowiecz A, Marquardt T, et al. Tumor-specific T cell activation by recombinant immunoreceptors: CD3 zeta signaling and CD28 costimulation are simultaneously required for efficient IL-2 secretion and can be integrated into one combined CD28/CD3 zeta signaling receptor molecule. *J Immunol*. 2001;167(11):6123–6131.
5. Chen D, Yang J. Development of novel antigen receptors for CAR T-cell therapy directed toward solid malignancies. *Transl Res*. 2017;187:11–21.
6. Smith JW. Apheresis techniques and cellular immunomodulation. *Ther Apher*. 1997;1(3):203–206.
7. Huls MH, Figliola MJ, Dawson MJ, et al. Clinical application of Sleeping Beauty and artificial antigen presenting cells to genetically modify T cells from peripheral and umbilical cord blood. *J Vis Exp*. 2013;(72):e50070.
8. Singh H, Figliola MJ, Dawson MJ, et al. Manufacture of clinical-grade CD19-specific T cells stably expressing chimeric antigen receptor using Sleeping Beauty system and artificial antigen presenting cells. *PloS One*. 2013;8(5):e64138.
9. Levine BL, Miskin J, Wonnacott K, Keir C. Global manufacturing of CAR T cell therapy. *Mol Ther Methods Clin Dev*. 2017;4:92–101.
10. Muranski P, Boni A, Wrzesinski C, et al. Increased intensity lymphodepletion and adoptive immunotherapy—how far can we go? *Nat Clin Pract Oncol*. 2006;3(12):668–681.
11. Anthony SM, Rivas SC, Colpitts SL, Howard ME, Stonier SW, Schluns KS. Inflammatory signals regulate IL-15 in response to lymphodepletion. *J Immunol*. 2016;196(11):4544–4552.
12. Gattinoni L, Finkelstein SE, Klebanoff CA, et al. Removal of homeostatic cytokine sinks by lymphodepletion enhances the

efficacy of adoptively transferred tumor-specific CD8+ T cells. *J Exp Med*. 2005;202(7):907–912.
13. Heczey A, Louis CU, Savoldo B, et al. CAR T cells administered in combination with lymphodepletion and PD-1 inhibition to patients with neuroblastoma. *Mol Ther*. 2017;25(9):2214–2224.
14. Buechner J, Grupp SA, Maude SL, et al. Global registration trial of efficacy and safety of CTL019 in pediatric and young adult patients with relapsed/refractory (R/R) acute lymphoblastic leukemia (ALL): update to the interim analysis. *Haematologica*. 2017;102(suppl 2):1–882.
15. Neelapu SS, Tummala S, Kebriaei P, et al. Chimeric antigen receptor T-cell therapy—assessment and management of toxicities. *Nat Rev Clin Oncol*. 2018;15(1):47–62.
16. Kochenderfer JN, Wilson WH, Janik JE, et al. Eradication of B-lineage cells and regression of lymphoma in a patient treated with autologous T cells genetically engineered to recognize CD19. *Blood*. 2010;116(20):4099–4102.
17. Porter DL, Levine BL, Kalos M, Bagg A, June CH. Chimeric antigen receptor-modified T cells in chronic lymphoid leukemia. *N Engl J Med*. 2011;365(8):725–733.
18. Grupp SA, Kalos M, Barrett D, et al. Chimeric antigen receptor-modified T cells for acute lymphoid leukemia. *N Engl J Med*. 2013;368(16):1509–1518.
19. Maude SL, Frey N, Shaw PA, et al. Chimeric antigen receptor T cells for sustained remissions in leukemia. *N Engl J Med*. 2014;371(16):1507–1517.
20. Kochenderfer JN, Dudley ME, Kassim SH, et al. Chemotherapy-refractory diffuse large B-cell lymphoma and indolent B-cell malignancies can be effectively treated with autologous T cells expressing an anti-CD19 chimeric antigen receptor. *J Clin Oncol*. 2015;33(6):540–549.
21. Turtle CJ, Hay KA, Hanafi LA, et al. Durable molecular remissions in chronic lymphocytic leukemia treated with CD19-specific chimeric antigen receptor-modified T cells after failure of Ibrutinib. *J Clin Oncol*. 2017;35(26):3010–3020.
22. Maude SL, Barrett D, Teachey DT, Grupp SA. Managing cytokine release syndrome associated with novel T cell-engaging therapies. *Cancer J*. 2014;20(2):119–122.
23. Ishii K, Shalabi H, Yates B, et al. Tocilizumab-refractory cytokine release syndrome (CRS) triggered by chimeric antigen receptor (CAR)-transduced T cells may have distinct cytokine profiles compared to typical CRS. *Blood*. 2016;128(22). 3358–3358.
24. Lee DW, Gardner R, Porter DL, et al. Current concepts in the diagnosis and management of cytokine release syndrome. *Blood*. 2014;124(2):188–195.
25. Brudno JN, Kochenderfer JN. Toxicities of chimeric antigen receptor T cells: recognition and management. *Blood*. 2016;127(26):3321–3330.
26. Garfall AL, Maus MV, Hwang WT, et al. Chimeric antigen receptor T cells against CD19 for multiple myeloma. *N Engl J Med*. 2015;373(11):1040–1047.
27. Raje N, Berdeja J, Lin Y, et al. Anti-BCMA CAR T-cell therapy bb2121 in relapsed or refractory multiple myeloma. *N Engl J Med*. 2019;380(18):1726–1737.
28. Schmidts A, Maus MV. Making CAR T cells a solid option for solid tumors. *Front Immunol*. 2018;9:2593.
29. Lee DW, Santomasso BD, Locke FL, et al. ASTCT consensus grading for cytokine release syndrome and neurologic toxicity associated with immune effector cells. *Biol Blood Marrow Transplant*. 2019;25(4):625–638.
30. Wang Z, Han W. Biomarkers of cytokine release syndrome and neurotoxicity related to CAR-T cell therapy. *Biomark Res*. 2018;6(1):4.
31. Karschnia P, Jordan JT, Forst DA, et al. Clinical presentation, management, and biomarkers of neurotoxicity after adoptive immunotherapy with CAR T-cells. *Blood*. 2019;133:2212–2221.
32. Mackall CL, Miklos DB. CNS endothelial cell activation emerges as a driver of CAR T cell-associated neurotoxicity. *Cancer Discov*. 2017;7(12):1371–1373.
33. Santomasso BD, Park JH, Salloum D, et al. Clinical and biologic correlates of neurotoxicity associated with CAR T cell therapy in patients with B-cell acute lymphoblastic leukemia (B-ALL). *Cancer Discov*. 2018;8:958–971.
34. Gust J, Hay KA, Hanafi LA, et al. Endothelial activation and blood-brain barrier disruption in neurotoxicity after adoptive immunotherapy with CD19 CAR-T cells. *Cancer Discov*. 2017;7(12):1404–1419.
35. Hay KA, Hanafi LA, Li D, et al. Kinetics and biomarkers of severe cytokine release syndrome after CD19 chimeric antigen receptor–modified T-cell therapy. *Blood*. 2017;130(21):2295–2306.
36. Park JH, Santomasso B, Riviere I, et al. Baseline and early post-treatment clinical and laboratory factors associated with severe neurotoxicity following 19-28z CAR T cells in adult patients with relapsed B-ALL. *J Clin Oncol*. 2017;35(suppl 15). 7024–7024.
37. Lee DW, Kochenderfer JN, Stetler-Stevenson M, et al. T cells expressing CD19 chimeric antigen receptors for acute lymphoblastic leukaemia in children and young adults: a phase 1 dose-escalation trial. *Lancet*. 2015;385(9967):517–528.
38. Hu Y, Sun J, Wu Z, et al. Predominant cerebral cytokine release syndrome in CD19-directed chimeric antigen receptor-modified T cell therapy. *J Hematol Oncol*. 2016;9(1):70.
39. Taraseviciute A, Tkachev V, Ponce R, et al. Chimeric antigen receptor T cell–mediated neurotoxicity in nonhuman primates. *Cancer Discov*. 2018;8:750–763.
40. Santomasso B, Park JH, Riviere I, et al. Biomarkers associated with neurotoxicity in adult patients with relapsed or refractory B-ALL (R/R B-ALL) treated with CD19 CAR T cells. *J Clin Oncol*. 2017;35(suppl 15). 3019–3019.
41. Harris J. Kite reports cerebral edema death in ZUMA-1 CAR T-Cell Trial. *OncLive*. 2017.
42. National Cancer Institute. *Common Terminology Criteria for Adverse Events (CTCAE) Version 4.0*. US Department of Health & Human Services; 2010.
43. Frisen L. Swelling of the optic nerve head: a staging scheme. *J Neurol Neurosurg Psychiatry*. 1982;45(1):13–18.
44. Teachey DT, Lacey SF, Shaw PA, et al. Identification of predictive biomarkers for cytokine release syndrome after chimeric antigen receptor T-cell therapy for acute lymphoblastic leukemia. *Cancer Discov*. 2016;6:664–679.
45. Schuster SJ, Svoboda J, Dwivedy Nasta S, et al. Sustained remissions following chimeric antigen receptor modified T cells directed against CD19 (CTL019) in patients with relapsed or refractory CD19+ lymphomas. *Blood*. 2015;126(23). 183–183.

Appendix 1

Summary of clinical pearls

1. Chapter 1: Fundamentals of neuropathology: introduction to neuropathology and molecular diagnostics

a. Classification of glioblastoma
   i. Microvascular proliferation and pseudopalisading necrosis are pathologic hallmarks of glioblastoma (GBM) and, when present, establish the diagnosis of GBM.
   ii. *IDH1/2* gene mutation is rare in GBM; *EGFR* amplification and MGMT promoter methylation are observed in approximately 40% of GBMs.
b. Classification of low-grade oligodendroglioma
   i. When molecular profiling of a brain tumor reveals the presence of 1p/19q co-deletion and *IDH1/2* mutation, a diagnosis of oligodendroglioma is made.
   ii. Histologically, oligodendrogliomas are characterized by the presence of round nuclei and perinuclear halo that has a "fried egg" appearance.
   iii. Grading of oligodendrogliomas is restricted to grade II and III tumors; there is no grade I or IV oligodendroglioma; oligodendrogliomas with necrosis and microvascular proliferation are grade III.
c. Classification of low-grade astrocytoma
   i. Grade I gliomas are generally well circumscribed, whereas grades II–IV are diffusely infiltrating.
   ii. Low-grade diffusely infiltrating gliomas that lack co-deletion of chromosomes 1p and 19q are molecularly defined as astrocytomas.
   iii. While *IDH1/2* gene mutation is common in low-grade diffuse astrocytomas, this is not a molecularly defining event and *IDH* wild-type low-grade diffuse astrocytomas also occur.
   iv. Low-grade gliomas (LGGs) can progress to higher-grade neoplasms and, when they recur as GBM, are considered "secondary" GBMs.
d. Classification of anaplastic astrocytoma
   i. The presence of mitoses (a marker of cell division) in a diffuse glioma warrants upgrading to an anaplastic glioma (grade III).
   ii. The presence of chromosome 10q loss combined with polysomy of chromosome 7 favors a molecular diagnosis of a higher-grade glioma.
e. Classification of meningioma
   i. Meningiomas are the most common primary brain tumor and appear as dural-based lesions often with an area of adjacent thickened dura, termed a dural "tail."
   ii. Up to 95% of meningiomas are benign WHO grade I lesions, but rarely grade II and grade III tumors can present and require additional treatment.

2. Chapter 2: Surgical considerations for brain and spine tumors

a. Surgical management of posterior fossa lesions and increased intracranial pressure
   i. Clinicians must be aware of symptoms of increased intracranial pressure (ICP) including early morning headache, unexplained nausea, vision changes, bilateral cranial nerve VI palsies, and papilledema.
   ii. Obstructive hydrocephalus from a posterior fossa mass requires urgent or emergent surgical evaluation for resection or ventricular decompression.
   iii. Children with posterior fossa pilocytic astrocytomas generally have excellent outcomes, particularly when gross total resection (GTR) is achieved.
b. Surgical management of resectable brain lesions
   i. Gross or near GTR with >90% of tumor resected is consistently associated with improved outcomes in uncontrolled studies of glioma.

ii. In general, surgery plays three roles in the management of glioma patients including: (1) tissue diagnosis, (2) cytoreduction of tumor, and (3) symptom relief from cerebral edema.

c. Surgical management of unresectable brain lesions

i. Tumors in deep locations, adjacent to eloquent structures, or crossing the midline may not be amenable to open resection.

ii. In selected cases, laser interstitial thermal therapy (LITT) is a surgical option for tissue ablation and can be performed at the time of tissue biopsy.

d. Surgical management of spinal cord lesions

i. GTR is consistently associated with improved outcomes for patients with ependymoma and should be pursued aggressively.

ii. Extramedullary tumors such as metastases, meningiomas, and schwannomas carry a different surgical risk from intramedullary lesions such as astrocytomas or ependymomas.

e. Surgical management of brain metastasis

i. When evaluating a patient with a known cancer diagnosis and multiple brain lesions, surgery may be beneficial when there is a single, large (>3 cm) lesion with symptomatic cerebral edema.

f. Surgical management of meningioma

i. For meningiomas that cannot be observed, surgical resection should be considered, particularly when there is brain infiltration, mass effect, or clinical symptoms.

ii. Extent of surgical resection for WHO grade 1 meningiomas is guided by the Simpson grade scale where greater extent of resection predicts lower rates of tumor recurrence.

g. Surgical management of epidural spinal cord compression

i. Management of patients with osseous metastasis to the spinal cord should include assessment of new neurological symptoms, degree of spinal cord compression on axial T2-weighted MRI images at the point of greatest compression, and treatment responsiveness of the tumor type.

ii. Spinal cord decompression improves neurological outcomes for patients with new deficits including paralysis, bowel or bladder dysfunction, or sensory loss that have been present for no more than 48 hours from onset.

3. Chapter 3: Introduction to radiation therapy

a. Radiation therapy for high-grade glioma (HGG)

i. The standard of care for HGG is maximal safe resection followed by combined modality therapy consisting of adjuvant radiation therapy and temozolomide. The typical radiation regimen is 60 Gy in 30 fractions (2 Gy per fraction) delivered over 6 weeks.

ii. Among the elderly or those with poor performance status, hypofractionated radiation therapy (for example, 40.05 Gy in 15 fractions delivered over 3 weeks) with temozolomide, radiation therapy alone, or temozolomide alone may be appropriate in certain patients. This decision is often guided by *MGMT* methylation status.

iii. External beam radiotherapy for HGG may be planned and delivered with 3D-conformal radiotherapy, intensity-modulated radiotherapy, or volumetric-modulated arc radiotherapy.

iv. Imaging follow-up should occur 1 month after completion of radiation therapy to establish a new baseline prior to continuation of additional adjuvant chemotherapy. The possibility of pseudoprogression instead of early disease progression should be considered, particularly in patients treated with concurrent temozolomide.

b. Stereotactic radiosurgery (SRS) for brain metastasis

i. Among patients with a limited number of brain metastases and good prognosis, SRS is preferred over whole brain radiation therapy (WBRT). SRS achieves high rates of local control and is associated with improved cognitive function and quality of life compared to WBRT.

ii. Because of the risk of developing new brain metastases after SRS, patients should have routine surveillance imaging every 2–3 months following treatment and with longer intervals with longer time of central nervous system disease stability.

iii. Radiation necrosis is a late toxicity of SRS that develops months to years after treatment and is most commonly asymptomatic but can have associated symptoms ranging from focal neurologic deficits to generalized cognitive symptoms depending upon the location. Steroids, bevacizumab, or surgical resection are used to treat symptomatic radiation necrosis.

iv. The risk of radiation necrosis is associated with brain metastasis size and radiation dose. Fractionated radiation therapy should be considered for high-risk lesions. Alternatively, SRS can be delivered with a reduced dose or in few fractions (between two and five) to reduce risk of toxicity.

c. Whole Brain Radiation Therapy (WBRT) for Brain Metastasis

i. WBRT is generally recommended for patients with diffuse brain metastases and reduces the risk of new brain metastases compared to management by SRS.

ii. WBRT improves survival for only limited sets of patients. Patients who are elderly, debilitated, or with

a very poor prognosis may not benefit from WBRT in terms of survival or quality of life. Best supportive care is a reasonable alternative for these groups of patients.
   iii. WBRT is most commonly delivered as 30 Gy in 10 fractions over 2 weeks.
   iv. WBRT harbors significant risk of toxicity, the most severe of which is irreversible cognitive decline that may occur months to years after treatment.
   v. Delivery of WBRT with intensity-modulated radiotherapy and/or volumetric-modulated arc radiotherapy allows dose adjustment to specific intracranial structures, including dose reduction to the hippocampus. This approach is termed hippocampal avoidance whole brain radiation therapy (HA-WBRT) and may reduce cognitive decline following treatment.

d. Radiation therapy for spinal cord tumors
   i. Radiation therapy for intramedullary spinal cord tumors is standard after surgery or at the time of progressive disease.
   ii. Patients are most commonly treated with a dose between 45 to 54 Gy in 1.8 Gy daily fractions over the course of 5–6 weeks.
   iii. Chronic progressive myelopathy is the most serious complication of spinal cord irradiation. It results in permanent and often progressive neurologic deficits, ranging from minor sensory and motor deficits to complete paraplegia in severe cases. There are no proven effective treatments.
   iv. Proton therapy for intramedullary spinal cord tumors may be considered in some clinical scenarios, particularly for children who are at highest risk of long-term treatment-associated toxicity.

4. Chapter 4: Evidence-based approaches to chemotherapy for gliomas

a. General principles of chemotherapy for gliomas
   i. In general, chemotherapy has been use as a neoadjuvant, adjuvant, or concurrent treatment defined as: *neoadjuvant* chemotherapy is administered prior to the main or definitive treatment which is usually surgery (i.e., before surgery); *adjuvant* chemotherapy is administered after the main or definitive treatment; *concurrent* chemotherapy may be administered simultaneously with radiation therapy.
   ii. Temozolomide (TMZ) is used commonly in many central nervous system (CNS) regimens due to its many favorable characteristics including good oral bioavailability, limited binding protein, and good CNS penetration with measurable levels being achieved in the cerebrospinal fluid (CSF) and in brain parenchyma following oral administration.
   iii. The most frequent side effects of TMZ are nausea/vomiting and fatigue. However, approximately 20% of patients discontinue TMZ due to myelosuppression, in particular for thrombocytopenia ($<100,000/mm^3$).
   iv. Procarbazine (PC), lomustine (CCNU), and vincristine (PCV) is a combined therapy used frequently to treat patients with oligodendrogliomas including both low-grade and anaplastic.

b. Chemotherapy for co-deleted anaplastic oligodendrogliomas
   i. *IDH* mutant, 1p19q co-deleted oligodendrogliomas are among the most chemosensitivity gliomas with several clinical trials having demonstrated prolonged median survival of more than 10 years by adding PCV chemotherapy to radiotherapy (RT).
   ii. Clinicians should be aware of the risk of a tyramine reaction in patients taking procarbazine (included in the PCV chemotherapy regimen). This catecholamine-like reaction can occur in patients who ingest or consume tyramine-containing foods or pharmacologic agents while taking procarbazine.

c. Chemotherapy for non–co-deleted anaplastic gliomas
   i. The standard of care for 1p/19q non–co-deleted anaplastic gliomas includes maximal safe resection, RT, and TMZ-based chemotherapy.
   ii. To date, data show that a trend toward a benefit of concomitant chemoradiation is observed in *IDH* mutated tumors, but not in *IDH* wild-type tumors.

d. Chemotherapy for low-grade gliomas
   i. LGGs are a heterogeneous group of tumors that include pure oligodendrogliomas, *IDH* mutant astrocytomas, and *IDH* wild-type astrocytomas.
   ii. Selected LGGs are chemosensitive to alkylating therapy with recent clinical trials showing favorable outcomes in patients with 1p19q co-deleted oligodendrogliomas and frequently for *IDH* mutant astrocytomas, compared to *IDH* wild-type LGGs, which have largely not been responsive to chemotherapy.

e. Chemotherapy for glioblastoma
   i. Standard of care for patients with GBM includes concurrent chemotherapy followed by six cycles of adjuvant temozolomide chemotherapy and tumor treating field therapy.
   ii. Methylation of the *MGMT* gene promoter is both prognostic of improved survival as well as predictive of a more favorable response to chemotherapy.

f. Chemotherapy for recurrent gliomas
   i. Treatment options for patients with recurrent gliomas are limited and generally include temozolomide, nitrosoureas, and bevacizumab.

5. Chapter 5: Evaluation of a dural-based lesion

a. Clinical pearls for evaluating dural-based lesions
   i. Most are T1 iso-hypointense on MRI. If they are T1 hyperintense, consider etiologies that contain methemoglobin (subacute hemorrhage), high protein, fat, melanin, or calcium.
   ii. Some dural-based lesions are T2 hyperintense due to high water content. Others are T2 hypointense due to their high cellularity (particularly if the tumor cells have a high nuclear-to-cytoplasmic ratio, such as lymphoma). Some meningiomas can be fibrous and these have lower T2 signal.
   iii. Diffusion restriction in dural-based lesions is variable. Diffusion restriction is an evaluation of how freely water molecules can move in a given medium. If restricted diffusion is present, then consider highly cellular tumors, such as lymphoma, cellular meningiomas, or metastases.
   iv. Enhancement is a product of disruption of the blood-brain barrier. Extraaxial lesions do not have a blood-brain barrier and most avidly enhance. Meningiomas, the most common dural-based neoplasm, typically diffusely and homogeneously enhance. They often have adjacent dural enhancement/thickening that is referred to as a "dural tail." Most other dural-based neoplasms also avidly enhance, so the presence of enhancement does not exclude more aggressive neoplasms. If the enhancement pattern is heterogenous, a low-grade meningioma is less likely.
   v. Evaluate the relationship of the dural-based lesion with the brain. To establish the lesion is truly extraaxial, look for CSF between the margins of the tumor and the adjacent brain parenchyma (also called a CSF cleft). If there is an indistinct interface between the dural-based mass and the brain or if there is a large amount of edema in the brain, there is a higher likelihood that the mass will be a higher meningioma grade or a more aggressive neoplasm.

6. Chapter 6: Evaluation of a supratentorial parenchymal lesion

a. Imaging features of supratentorial GBM
   i. The imaging differential for a single ring-enhancing supratentorial lesion includes HGG, solitary brain metastasis, cerebral abscess, tumefactive demyelination, and subacute stroke.
   ii. For such a lesion, surgical consultation and evaluation is required to establish a tissue diagnosis and guide treatment decisions.

b. Imaging features of supratentorial low-grade glioma
   i. The differential diagnosis of a non-enhancing supratentorial lesion on MRI includes LGG and subacute ischemia, cerebritis, an arteriovenous malformation, or herpes encephalitis

c. Imaging features of CNS lymphoma
   i. The imaging differential diagnosis for an enhancing lesion consistent with CNS lymphoma includes CNS lymphoma, GBM, infections (i.e., abscess, toxoplasmosis), progressive multifocal leukoencephalopathy (PML), demyelinating disorders, or metastases.
   ii. Compared to malignant glioma, treatment response is considerable higher for patients with CNS lymphoma even without cytoreduction. Thus, stereotactic biopsy is favored.

d. Imaging features of brain metastasis
   i. The imaging differential for multifocal brain metastasis includes multifocal GBM, abscess, demyelinating disease, or CNS lymphoma (in immunocompromised patients).
   ii. Multidisciplinary evaluation including radiology, neurosurgery, radiation oncology, medical oncology, and neuro-oncology help determine an optimal treatment plan.

7. Chapter 7: Evaluation of an infratentorial lesion

a. General tips for imaging of the posterior fossa
   i. MRI offers higher soft-tissue resolution with more qualitative data on posterior fossa lesions, though it is not available at all centers, requires a degree of technical expertise, is slower, may necessitate sedation for younger and unstable patients, and is more expensive than CT.
   ii. CT is fast, less expensive, and more widely available than MRI, and offers insights into calcifications and boney involvement of lesions though with limited resolution and narrow lesion characteristics. Additionally, CT can be used to rapidly assess potentially life-threatening complications of posterior fossa masses, including hydrocephalus, acute hemorrhage, or pending herniation.
   iii. In pediatric patients with space-occupying posterior fossa lesions, a primary brain tumor is by far the most likely diagnosis, with metastatic lesions in this population being exceedingly rare.
   iv. In older adults, a space-occupying lesion in the posterior fossa is more likely to be a metastatic tumor

or acute hemorrhage, and should prompt a comprehensive history and physical examination and consideration of additional body imaging to evaluate for a primary tumor or risk factors for stroke.

   v. Location and characteristics of pediatric tumors can guide the clinician regarding a most likely diagnosis, which may include LGG, HGG, medulloblastoma, ependymoma, atypical teratoid/rhabdoid tumor, or others.

b. Differential diagnosis of a midline fourth ventricular lesion
   i. The imaging differential of a midline posterior fossa lesion in a child should include medulloblastoma (e.g., "M" for midline) and ependymoma. Pilocytic astrocytomas tend to occur in the lateral cerebellum.

c. Differential diagnosis of a lateral cerebellar lesion
   i. Lateral cerebellar cystic lesion with a mural nodule should raise suspicion for a pilocytic astrocytoma in children and for a cerebellar hemangioblastoma in adults.

d. Differential diagnosis of a non-enhancing pontine lesion
   i. The imaging differential diagnosis for an intrinsic pontine brainstem glioma should include causes of rhombencephalitis (e.g., infectious, inflammatory, paraneoplastic) including *Listeria* infection, enterovirus, other viral encephalitis (e.g., herpes simplex virus, Epstein-Barr virus [EBV], human herpesvirus 6), Behcet disease, Erdheim-Chester disease, or other etiologies.
   ii. Pontine gliomas are typically expansile with enlargement of the central pons, often with the basilar artery displaced anteriorly or with the tumor appearing to engulf the artery.

e. Differential diagnosis of an enhancing cerebellar lesion
   i. The cerebellum is the second most common parenchymal location for brain metastasis.
   ii. Management of cerebellar metastasis should include definitive tumor treatment as well as a consideration for reducing brainstem compression, maintaining CSF flow, and providing a tissue diagnosis when there is no contributory systemic malignancy present.

f. Differential diagnosis of a non-enhancing cerebellar lesion
   i. Acute cerebellitis is a heterogeneous clinical syndrome characterized by cerebellar ataxia or dysfunction that is attributable to a recent or concurrent infection, a recent vaccination, or an ingestion of medication.
   ii. MRI imaging of typical acute bilateral cerebellitis includes metabolic diseases, demyelinative disorders, and meningitis.
   iii. In cases of hemicerebellitis when imaging findings are asymmetric, the imaging differential includes dysplastic cerebellar gangliocytoma (Lhermitte-Duclos), vasculitis, and inflammatory processes related to cytarabine or other toxicities.

8. Chapter 8: Imaging of spinal lesions

a. Imaging findings of spinal cord astrocytoma
   i. Intramedullary spinal cord tumors account for ~10% of primary spinal cord tumors and are most often ependymomas, which are slightly favored over astrocytomas.
   ii. Most intramedullary WHO grade 1 pilocytic astrocytomas enhance on neuroimaging and may be confused with higher-grade lesions without a tissue diagnosis.

b. Imaging findings of spinal cord ependymoma
   i. Enhancing spinal cord tumors can mimic inflammatory and infectious lesions in the spinal cord including transverse myelitis, multiple sclerosis, neuromyelitis optic spectrum disorder, infectious myelitis, and other related conditions.

c. Imaging findings of spinal cord hemangioblastoma
   i. Spinal hemangioblastomas are the prototypical tumor associated with von Hippel Lindau (vHL) disease.
   ii. Hemangioblastomas associated with vHL have earlier onset of disease, and are often solitary but can be multiple, including the cerebellum.

d. Imaging findings of peripheral nerve sheath tumors
   i. Schwannomas and neurofibromas account for up to one-third of intradural spinal cord tumors and appear as homogeneously enhancing extramedullary masses.

9. Chapter 9: Evaluation of peripheral nerve lesions

a. Imaging findings of a solitary neurofibroma
   i. The vast majority of neurofibromas are sporadic and not associated with neurofibromatosis type 1 (NF1).
   ii. Characteristic MRI features include heterogeneous enhancement on T1-weighted post-contrast and hyperintensity on T2-weighted and short tau inversion recovery (STIR) sequences. A target and/or split-fat sign may be seen.
   iii. The main differential diagnosis for a neurofibroma is schwannoma, and these two entities may be difficult to distinguish based on MRI alone.

b. Imaging findings of plexiform neurofibromas in NF1
   i. Plexiform neurofibromas (pNFs) affect up to 60% of patients with NF1.
   ii. Although histologically benign and typically slow growing, pNFs can cause significant morbidity due to local mass effect and infiltration of vital anatomic structures. A small proportion of pNFs can transform into malignant peripheral nerve sheath tumors.
   iii. A regional MRI with contrast-enhanced and STIR sequences of the affected region should be obtained. Whole-body MRI may be useful to assess a patient's baseline tumor burden.
c. Imaging findings of malignant peripheral nerve sheath tumors (MPNSTs)
   i. Rapid development or changes of symptoms (e.g., tumor growth, pain, or neurologic dysfunction) in a patient with NF1 should prompt evaluation for MPNST.
   ii. Initial workup should include a contrast-enhanced regional MRI of the affected body region. Diffusion-weighted imaging with apparent diffusion coefficient (ADC) mapping may aid in the detection of malignant foci. If the history or MRI is suggestive of malignancy, an ^{18}F-fluorodeoxyglucose (FDG) positron emission tomography (PET)/CT should be obtained to identify metabolically active areas suitable for biopsy and histologic confirmation of malignancy.
   iii. Patients should be referred to a surgeon for an image-guided biopsy and managed by an experienced multidisciplinary team including a surgeon, radiation oncologist, and medical oncologist.
   iv. Prognosis is poor even with treatment, particularly for patients with advanced or metastatic disease.
d. Diffuse lumbosacral nerve root thickening
   i. The etiology of nerve root thickening and enhancement on spine MRI includes inflammatory/autoimmune, hereditary, infectious, and neoplastic causes.
   ii. The degree of thickening, presence of significant nodularity, and degree of enhancement, and clinical and family history can help narrow down the differential diagnosis.
   iii. Additional studies should be patient-specific and may include brain MRI, systemic body imaging, electromyography/nerve conduction studies, and CSF analysis.
e. Non-vestibular schwannomas in NF2
   i. Most schwannomas are solitary and occur sporadically. The presence of multiple schwannomas should prompt evaluation for an underlying genetic syndrome such as NF2 or schwannomatosis (SWN).
   ii. A contrast-enhanced MRI of the entire brain and with thin cuts through the internal auditory canals to evaluate for vestibular schwannomas should be obtained. Similarly, a spine MRI with and without contrast is required to assess for the presence of spinal schwannomas, ependymomas, and meningiomas.
   iii. Non-vestibular schwannomas may be difficult to distinguish from neurofibromas on MRI but the patient's history and examination can help establish the diagnosis.
f. Schwannomas in schwannomatosis
   i. Schwannomas in SWN patients most commonly involve the spinal and peripheral nerves.
   ii. Evaluation of a patient presenting with possible NF2 or SWN should include a brain MRI with thin cuts through the internal auditory canal to exclude the presence of bilateral vestibular schwannomas as well as a spine MRI.
   iii. Benign schwannomas can display FDG avidity on PET/CT and mimic malignancy.
   iv. Genetic testing for mutations in the *NF2*, *SMARCB1*, and *LZTR1* genes is recommended given the significant phenotypic overlap between NF2 and SWN.
   v. Management should focus on pharmacologic and non-pharmacologic treatment of pain, and if medically refractory, surgical resection of symptomatic or compressive tumors.

10. Chapter 10: Approach to the meningioma patient

a. Approach to patients without a tissue diagnosis
   i. The decision for observation or surgery of a meningioma should be made on an individual basis after discussions with the patient, taking into account the patient's clinical presentation, imaging characteristics, tumor growth patterns, and other medical history and comorbidities.
   ii. In symptomatic patients or patients with rapidly enlarging tumors without tissue diagnosis, surgery is the main treatment modality for both symptomatic relief and pathologic diagnosis.
b. Approach to WHO grade I meningioma
   i. GTR is the goal of any meningioma surgery.
   ii. Extent of resection after meningioma surgery is determined by the Simpson grading scale with Simpson grades I–III indicating total/near total resection of tumor and Simpson grades IV–V indicating partial/minimal resection of tumor.
   iii. For WHO grade I meningiomas, tumors can be monitored with serial imaging after GTR if the patient remains asymptomatic.
c. Approach to WHO grade II meningioma
   i. Evidence supports safe GTR of WHO grade II meningiomas as the first-line treatment for surgically resectable lesions.

ii. Retrospective data supports a trend toward adjuvant radiation following resection of WHO grade II meningiomas in favorable locations; however, the strength of radiation as an effective adjuvant therapy in these patients is still unclear.
iii. At 5 years, 60–90% of patients will be free of meningioma recurrence after GTR and 30–70% of patients will be recurrence free after subtotal resection.
iv. If GTR is not feasible for a WHO grade II meningioma, subtotal resection with adjuvant RT should be considered.

d. Approach to WHO grade III meningioma
   i. WHO grade III meningiomas are aggressive malignant neoplasms.
   ii. Safe maximal resection should be pursued for WHO grade III meningiomas followed by RT.
   iii. Even with maximal aggressive therapy, rates of recurrence are as high as 60–90%.

e. Approach to Recurrent Meningioma
   i. If recurrent meningioma is detected that poses a significant risk to neighboring brain structures or patient quality of life, the patient and clinician can choose between repeated surgery or radiation therapy.
   ii. Systemic therapies have not been shown to improve outcomes in newly diagnosed meningiomas but are often considered in multiply recurrent, treatment-refractory, or metastatic meningiomas.
   iii. In recent years, several clinical trials of systemic therapies have become available for patients with grade II and III meningiomas refractory to surgery and radiation.

11. Chapter 11: Approach to the low-grade glioma patient

a. Classification of low-grade gliomas
   i. Most diffuse LGGs can be separated into three molecularly, prognostically, and clinically distinct groups: 1p/19q co-deleted, *IDH* mutant, and *IDH* wild-type gliomas.

b. Timing of treatment for low-grade gliomas
   i. Observation of low-risk asymptomatic patients, including patients with controlled seizures, is reasonable and typically includes MRI every 3 months, which is gradually lengthened in patients whose gliomas show stability.
   ii. High-risk features in LGG patients include age >40 years, subtotal resection and, in some cases, tumor-related symptoms, poor performance status, preoperative tumor size (worse if ≥5 cm), astrocytic histology, and high proliferative index (poor if MIB-1 is >3%).

c. Approaches to treatment protocols for low-grade gliomas
   i. For low-grade 1p/19q co-deleted oligodendrogliomas, evidence-based treatment is radiation plus PCV.
   ii. For low-grade *IDH*-mutant non–co-deleted astrocytomas, the optimal treatment regimen is not as clear but some clinicians will add temozolomide to radiation therapy either concurrently and/or adjuvantly.
   iii. Despite their low-grade, *IDH*-wild type gliomas follow an aggressive clinical course and patients tend to have worse outcomes with poorer response to chemotherapy.

12. Chapter 12: Approach to the high-grade glioma patient

a. Approach to anaplastic oligodendroglioma
   i. Oligodendrogliomas are defined by co-deletion of chromosomes 1p/19q and respond well to radiation and PCV chemotherapy.
   ii. Maximum safe resection may prolong survival but is never curative and may not be feasible in deeply infiltrative lesions that cross the midline or are adjacent to eloquent structures.
   iii. New or worsening seizures are an indicator of tumor progression in HGGs and should be evaluated with contrast-enhanced MRI and, if necessary, biopsy or resection.
   iv. Besides antiepileptic drugs (AEDs), antineoplastic therapy may help improve seizure control.

b. Approach to anaplastic astrocytoma
   i. High-grade astrocytomas are treated with RT with concurrent and adjuvant temozolomide chemotherapy.
   ii. IDH mutant astrocytomas have a more favorable prognosis and response to treatment than those with wild-type IDH.

c. Approach to glioblastoma
   i. High-grade diffuse gliomas include GBMs, anaplastic astrocytomas, and oligodendrogliomas.
   ii. Diagnosis of a HGG begins with histologic assessment and integrates molecular alterations to identify HGG subgroups that have distinct prognoses and therapy responses.
   iii. MGMT promoter methylation predicts favorable response to temozolomide in *IDH* wild-type astrocytomas.

d. Approach to neurological complications of high-grade glioma
   i. Multidisciplinary symptom-oriented care may provide improved quality-of-care in complex cases.

ii. Corticosteroids are used to manage symptoms caused by tumor-induced edema.
iii. Corticosteroids can be effectively administered in one or two doses a day and evening doses should be avoided to minimize steroid-related insomnia.
iv. Bevacizumab can be utilized as a steroid-sparing agent in select cases.

e. Approach to non-neurological complications of HGG
i. Thirty percent of patients with IDH wild-type gliomas develop venous thromboembolisms (VTEs).
ii. Anticoagulation is safe in most glioma patients with VTE.
iii. Lymphopenia is a common complication of chemoradiation and is associated with shorter survival and increased risk for infection.
iv. *Pneumocystis jirovecii* pneumonia prophylaxis is recommended in lymphopenic patients.

f. Approach to imaging surveillance and recurrence in HGG
i. Guidelines recommend surveillance imaging of a HGG every 2–4 months for the first 3 years and these recommendations are often individualized based on prognostic factors and risk of early recurrence.
ii. Virtually all HGGs will recur, at which time repeat surgery, radiation, salvage chemotherapy, or clinical trials are considered.
iii. There is currently no known second-line systemic therapy that prolongs overall survival for GBM.
iv. Palliative care is optimally integrated into the management of HGGs early and contemporaneously with aggressive tumor-directed therapy, particularly once these tumors recur.

13. Chapter 13: Approach to the patient with CNS lymphoma

a. Approach to the diagnosis of CNS lymphoma
i. Immunosuppression and older age are the major risk factors for the development of primary central nervous system lymphoma (PCNSL).
ii. The typical clinical presentation of PCNSL involves progressive and relatively rapid focal neurological symptoms associated with the neuroanatomic localization of the tumor.
iii. Treatment with corticosteroids should be deferred until pathologic confirmation.

b. Differentiating primary and secondary CNS lymphoma
i. Ninety to ninety-five percent of cases of PCNSL are classified histologically as diffuse large B-cell lymphoma (DLBCL).
ii. MRI with contrast is the most sensitive imaging modality for the detection of PCNSL.
iii. Diagnosis and staging require a HIV serology, full body CT or PET-CT; detailed ophthalmologic examination, lumbar puncture, and, in older males, a testicular ultrasound.

c. Treatment of primary CNS lymphoma
i. High-dose methotrexate is the single most important treatment agent for PCNSL. Current therapy consists of a methotrexate-based combination chemotherapy with rituximab for B-cell lymphomas. Intrathecal therapy may be considered in patients with evidence of leptomeningeal involvement.
ii. In patients who achieve a complete response to induction therapy, high-dose chemotherapy with autologous stem cell rescue should be offered as consolidation to fit patients.
iii. In patients who achieve a complete response to induction therapy and are not candidates for autologous stem cell rescue, consolidation chemotherapy is considered or in some cases clinicians may consider WBRT.

d. Approach to PCNSL in immunocompromised patients
i. Patients with AIDS-related PCNSL require highly active antiretroviral therapy and chemotherapy.
ii. An elevated CSF EBV polymerase chain reaction in the setting of a typical brain lesion on MRI or FDG-avid CNS lesion on PET is highly specific for primary CNS lymphoma and may justify treatment initiation.

e. Posttransplant lymphoproliferative disease (PTLD)
i. Patients with PTLD and PCNSL require reduction in immunosuppression and chemotherapy.

f. Approach to recurrent primary CNS lymphoma
i. More than half of PCNSL patients who respond to treatment suffer from relapse. PCNSL relapse is treated with chemotherapy, immunotherapy, or WBRT.

g. Bing-Neel syndrome
i. Bing-Neel syndrome is a rare and slowly progressing complication of Waldenström macroglobulinemia whereby malignant lymphoplasmacytic cells invade the CNS.
ii. Treatment of Bing-Neel syndrome aims at treating neurological symptoms of the disease.

h. Primary T-cell lymphoma
i. T-cell primary CNS lymphoma (TPCNSL) is a rare form of PCNSL. The clinical picture and treatment modalities for TPCNSL are similar to DLBCL with similar agents used in treatment.

i. Diagnosis and management of neurological complications of PCNSL treatment
i. Treatment related neurotoxicity including neurocognitive dysfunction after WBRT, delayed-onset leukoencephalopathy after methotrexate, or progressive multifocal leukoencephalopathy are major complications of PCNSL treatment and require frequent follow-up after treatment.

14. Chapter 14: Approach to a patient with brain metastasis

a. Fundamentals of brain metastasis
   i. Brain metastases are the most common CNS malignancy with approximately 160,000 new cases per year.
   ii. Patients who experience a seizure due to brain metastases should be managed with brain metastases and advised to not drive an automobile for at least 6 months after last seizure.
b. Craniotomy for brain metastasis
   i. Craniotomy is indicated for patients with large, symptomatic lesions or those without a known diagnosis of cancer.
   ii. Cavity-directed SRS is indicated to reduce the risk of recurrence after craniotomy for brain metastases.
c. Radiosurgery for brain metastasis
   i. SRS for intact brain metastases is preferred for treatment of a limited number of brain metastases, as it preserves quality of life and neuro-cognition.
   ii. Patients who are managed with SRS are more likely to develop new brain metastases than those with WBRT, but these can be managed with a second session of SRS.
d. WBRT for brain metastasis
   i. WBRT is useful for patients with too many brain metastases to effectively treat with SRS.
   ii. WBRT contributes to decline in quality of life and neurocognitive decline, and is avoided when possible due to side effects.
e. Neurological complications of brain metastasis treatment
   i. Follow-up for brain metastases with MRI is critical in order to detect new brain metastases prior to developing symptoms and to detect radiation necrosis after SRS.
   ii. Neurocognitive dysfunction is common after WBRT with up to 90% of patients developing a decline in neurocognitive testing after WBRT.
   iii. In patients who do undergo WBRT, clinicians may consider strategies to avoid long-term neurocognitive dysfunction including hippocampal avoidance and prophylactic pharmacologic therapy (e.g., memantine, donepezil), though the benefits of these interventions have not been confirmed in large, randomized phase III studies.

15. Chapter 15: Approach to the patient with leptomeningeal metastasis

a. The role of spinal tap in the diagnosis and management of leptomeningeal disease (LMD)
   i. CSF cytology is the gold standard for diagnosing LMD.
   ii. Common solid tumors that metastasize to the leptomeninges include melanoma, breast cancer, small-cell lung cancer, and non–small-cell lung cancer.
   iii. CSF cytology has a high false negative rate; in patients with a high index of suspicion for LMD, a second or third dural puncture may be needed if CSF cytology is negative after the first spinal tap.
   iv. In patients with suspected LMD, CSF studies should include cell count, glucose, protein, and cytology.
   v. In patients with known or suspected hematologic malignancies, CSF flow cytometry should be performed as it is two to three times more sensitive than cytology for the detection of leukemic or lymphomatous meningitis.
b. The role of neuroimaging in the diagnosis and management of LMD
   i. The most frequent MRI findings of LMD are focal or diffuse enhancement of leptomeninges along the sulci, cranial nerves, and spinal nerve roots, linear or nodular enhancement of the cord, and thickening of lumbosacral roots.
   ii. Neuroimaging also helps define the extent of disease and the presence of bulky/nodular disease that may require radiation or selected high-dose systemic therapies.
c. Approach to the treatment for LMD
   i. Cancer-directed treatment is individualized based on various factors including the type of malignancy (e.g., solid versus hematologic malignancy), performance status, type and state of systemic cancer, burden of LMD, and clinical symptoms.
   ii. Symptomatic treatments include management of elevated ICP seizure treatment, supportive care for cranial neuropathies, and pain control.
   iii. WBRT is used for treating diffuse LMD in patients with symptoms of high ICP to improve CSF flow.
   iv. Focal conformal radiation therapy or SRS are used for treating bulky lesions that impair CSF flow (noncommunicating hydrocephalus) or symptomatic nodules that result in impaired neurological function.
   v. In LMD patients with active systemic therapy, clinicians should explore systemic chemotherapy or targeted therapies with favorable blood-brain barrier penetrating properties.
   vi. In LMD patients without bulky, nodular disease, intrathecal chemotherapy is a treatment consideration, particularly for patients without active systemic disease.
   vii. Intrathecal chemotherapy is administered either by lumbar puncture or intraventricular administration via a surgically implanted Ommaya reservoir.
   viii. Intrathecal chemotherapy is generally well tolerated, though up to 20% of patients will develop aseptic meningitis and present with abrupt onset of headache, stiff neck, nausea, vomiting, lethargy, and fever several hours after the injection.

16. Chapter 16: Approach to patients with the neoplasms associated with neurofibromatosis type 1, neurofibromatosis type 2, and schwannomatosis

a. Approach to NF1 associated plexiform neurofibroma
   i. Clinically, changes in the severity or nature of pain or rapid growth warrants evaluation for possible malignant conversion with imaging and biopsy.
   ii. Currently, in a person with NF1 with a growing plexiform neurofibroma that is increasingly symptomatic and has findings that could be consistent with malignant degeneration based on a distinct nodular appearance on anatomic MRI, low ADC on functional MRI, and elevated standardized uptake value maximum on FDG-PET, biopsy of the most atypical region on imaging should be pursued if feasible.
   iii. It is important to distinguish plexiform neurofibroma from cutaneous and subcutaneous neurofibromas that can involve the skin; cutaneous neurofibromas do not require regular surveillance.
   iv. Increasingly good medical options are available for both adults and children with plexiform neurofibroma.

b. Approach to NF1 associated optic pathway glioma
   i. Optic pathway gliomas (OPGs) are seen in 15–20% of NF1 patients.
   ii. Vision should be followed with yearly eye examination in all NF1 children and, if deficits are observed, MRI and regular ophthalmology examination should be performed to follow patients found to have an OPG.
   iii. Symptoms and signs that warrant treatment include vision loss, proptosis, or endocrinopathy.

c. Approach to brainstem or cerebellar glioma in NF1
   i. Three imaging characteristics favor that a brain lesion in an NF1 patient is LGG and not a benign focal area of signal abnormality (FASI) including: contrast enhancement, mass effect on surrounding tissue, or T1-weighted hypointensity relative to gray matter.
   ii. Lesions concerning for tumor should be followed by an oncologist familiar with NF1.
   iii. For NF1-associated LGG, surgical resection is the mainstay of therapy. Tumors that have been completely or nearly resected often require no further therapy. Subtotally resected or recurrent tumors are treated with chemotherapy or targeted systemic therapies.

d. Management of vestibular schwannomas in NF2
   i. Bilateral vestibular schwannomas (VS) are pathognomonic for NF2. VSs present with hearing loss, tinnitus, and balance difficulty. Vertigo is rare.
   ii. NF2 patients should be monitored with neuroimaging of suspicious lesions and audiometry initially at 6-month intervals to determine tumor growth rate and hearing.
   iii. Removal of every tumor in NF2 is usually not feasible or necessary. Treatment focuses on preserving hearing, maintaining function, and maximizing quality of life.
   iv. Bevacizumab has been studied at multiple dose schedules, each showing a hearing improvement rate of around 40–50% and radiographic response rate of 30–50% in NF2 patients.

e. Diagnosis of schwannomatosis
   i. SWN is characterized by germline pathogenic variants in *SMARCB1* or *LZTR1* genes and likely additional unidentified genes.
   ii. Tumor formation in SWN is caused by mutational inactivation of two genes including the *NF2* gene as well as either *SMARCB1* or *LZTR1*.

f. Management of pain in schwannomatosis
   i. Chronic pain is the most common symptom reported by over 65% of patients with SWN.
   ii. Managing chronic pain is challenging in SWN as no class of pain medication has been associated with consistent benefit.
   iii. Referral to pain specialists may be helpful for comprehensive pain management. Treatment of concomitant anxiety and depression is strongly recommended.

17. Chapter 17: Approach to the patient with tuberous sclerosis

a. Diagnosis of tuberous sclerosis
   i. Cutaneous findings are present in approximately 90% of tuberous sclerosis complex (TSC) patients.
   ii. The first cutaneous sign is often hypopigmented macules called Ash leaf spots that are first apparent in infancy.
   iii. Between 10% and 25% of patients who fulfill the clinical criteria for TSC will have no identified mutation on genetic testing.
   iv. Several important TSC findings manifest later in life including pulmonary lymphangioleiomyomatosis, which occurs more commonly in adult women.

b. TSC-associated epilepsy
   i. Seizures occur in approximately 85% of TSC patients, often beginning as infantile spasms and progressing to include multiple seizures types.
   ii. Vigabatrin is the only AED with TSC-specific data supporting its efficacy in TSC.
   iii. In the EXIST-3 study, treatment with the oral mTOR inhibitor everolimus resulted in improvement in seizures in 50% of patients at 2 years.

c. Brain MRI findings in TSC
   i. Cortical tubers occur in 90% of TSC patients, have no malignant potential, but can contribute to epilepsy.
   ii. Subependymal nodules are hyperintense lesions adjacent to the ventricular surface that do not enhance with gadolinium contrast.
   iii. Subependymal giant cell astrocytomas (SEGAs) are a WHO grade 1 glioma that occur within the ventricular system often around the foramen of Munro and enhance with gadolinium contrast.
d. Renal angiomyolipomas in TSC
   i. Angiomyolipomas (AMLs) are benign kidney tumors that are present in up to 80% of patients with TSC.
   ii. AMLs rarely develop into renal cell carcinoma but can be complicated by renal hemorrhage, which is rare.
   iii. When treatment of an AML is indicated, mTOR inhibitors (e.g., everolimus) are first-line therapy, with an overall response rate of 58%.

18. Chapter 18: Approach to von Hippel Lindau, Cowden disease, and other inherited conditions

a. von Hippel Lindau
   i. vHL is tumor-predisposition syndrome characterized by neoplasms of the nervous system, kidneys, and other organs.
   ii. Cerebellar, spinal, and retinal hemangioblastomas are the most common nervous system manifestations.
   iii. Cerebellar hemangioblastomas are benign, slow-growing, highly vascular, cystic WHO grade I neoplasms.
b. Cowden syndrome
   i. Cowden syndrome is a rare autosomal dominant disorder that results from germline mutation in the *phosphatase and tensin homolog* (*PTEN*) gene.
   ii. Neurologic manifestations in Cowden syndrome frequently include benign CNS tumors such as meningiomas, macrocephaly, heterotopias, vascular abnormalities, and developmental delay.
   iii. The most common CNS neoplasm is the dysplastic gangliocytoma of the cerebellum which, when present, is known as *Lhermitte-Duclos disease* (LDD). In adults, LDD is pathognomonic for Cowden syndrome.
c. Li-Fraumeni syndrome
   i. Li-Fraumeni is a rare autosomal dominant disease that results from inactivating mutation in the *TP53* gene which predisposes patients to a wide array of neoplasms.
   ii. CNS neoplasms occur in approximately 10% of patients with Li-Fraumeni syndrome and include supratentorial tumors, neuroectodermal tumors, choroid plexus carcinomas, and medulloblastoma.
d. Lynch syndrome
   i. Lynch syndrome (e.g., hereditary nonpolyposis colorectal cancer syndrome) is a multi-tumor syndrome caused by germline mutation in DNA mismatch repair genes.
   ii. Lynch syndrome is characterized by a significantly increased risk of colorectal and endometrial cancer along with a fourfold higher risk of GBM.

19. Chapter 19: Neurologic complications of cancer

a. Neurological side effects of brain tumors
   i. Dexamethasone is the preferred corticosteroid for treating cerebral edema. Treatment decisions should be based on the degree of neurologic symptoms and not on imaging findings.
   ii. Patients should be managed on the lowest dose of dexamethasone that controls their symptoms. Given the long-term side effects, efforts should continually be made to taper or discontinue corticosteroids when symptomatically possible.
   iii. Brain tumor patients presenting with a seizure should be treated with an antiepileptic medication. Enzyme-inducing AEDs should be avoided due to interactions with chemotherapy and corticosteroids.
   iv. There is no evidence to support the use of prophylactic anticonvulsants in brain tumor patients.
   v. Brain tumor patients are at increased risk for hemorrhagic and ischemic stroke. Patients with acute onset of neurologic symptoms should be urgently evaluated for stroke.
   vi. Endocrinologic complications are common in brain tumor patients and can present with variable symptoms. Hypopituitarism and syndrome of inappropriate antidiuretic hormone should be considered in the differential of fatigue and encephalopathy.
b. Non-neurological side effects in brain tumor patients
   i. Venous thromboembolism is common in brain tumor patients. Patients with new lower extremity swelling, shortness of breath, or hypoxia should be urgently evaluated for deep venous thrombosis or pulmonary embolism with lower extremity ultrasound or CT angiogram of the chest.
   ii. Prophylactic anticoagulation is only indicated for brain tumor patients in the perioperative setting.
   iii. Therapeutic anticoagulation with low-molecular-weight heparin is preferred for prevention of recurrent venous thromboembolism in cancer patients.

- iv. The etiology of fatigue and cognitive dysfunction in brain tumor patients is multifactorial. Assessment includes evaluation of antitumor treatments, supportive care medications, metabolic and endocrine abnormalities, mood disturbance, and sleep dysregulation.
- v. All patients should be screened for depression throughout their disease course and treated when appropriate.

20. Chapter 20: Paraneoplastic neurologic disorder syndromes

- a. Broadly, paraneoplastic neurologic disorder (PND) syndromes can be classified by whether the target is an intracellular antigen (e.g., anti-Hu, anti-Yo, anti-CV2, anti-Ri, anti-Ma, and others) or a neuronal cell surface antigen (e.g., anti-NMDA receptor, anti-VGCC, and others).
- b. PND may manifest in typical ways such as encephalitis, myelitis, cerebellar degeneration, neuropathy, myoclonus/opsoclonus, Lambert-Eaton myasthenic syndrome, and dermatomyositis.
- c. Typical findings in PND involving the CNS include CSF pleocytosis, elevated CSF protein, increased CSF immunoglobulin synthesis and presence of oligoclonal bands.
- d. The first approach to PND should be source control with tumor treatment as appropriate for the given malignancy.
- e. First-line immunotherapies include corticosteroids, intravenous immunoglobulins, and plasma exchange. Second-line immunosuppressant medications include rituximab, cyclophosphamide, azathioprine, and mycophenolate.

21. Chapter 21: Perineural spread of cancer

- a. General principles of perineural invasion
  - i. Perineural invasion (PNI) refers to a rare type of contiguous spread of neoplastic cells from their primary site along the potential space between or beneath the layers of perineurium.
  - ii. PNI can be broadly divided into microscopic PNI and clinical PNI.
  - iii. Classically, PNI presents in a patient with a history of head and neck cancer who develops cranial neuropathy, with cranial nerve V and VII being the most commonly affected.
- b. Brachial plexus invasion of malignancy
  - i. Contrast-enhanced MRI is the gold standard for establishing an imaging diagnosis of PNI but false-negative rates are high and may fail to demonstrate active disease in at least 45% of patients.
  - ii. A combination of CT and MRI with selected use of FDG-PET may increase the detection rate and improve the understanding of disease extent.
  - iii. The differential diagnosis of a new-onset brachial plexopathy in a cancer patient includes perineural spread and radiation-induced brachial plexopathy.
  - iv. For these patients, the presence of pain should favor perineural spread or locoregional cancer recurrence, while the absence of pain should favor radiation-induced brachial plexopathy.
- c. Perineural cranial neuropathy
  - i. Early diagnosis of PNI is critical for prompt initiation of treatment as neurological deficits are poorly rescued once significant dysfunction has developed.
  - ii. Surgical resection with the goal of clear margins must be balanced against the risk of postoperative morbidity from neurological insult.
  - iii. Five-year survival in patients treated with surgical resection and adjuvant RT is 55% for patients with microscopic PNI and 50% for symptomatic patients.

22. Chapter 22: Cancer-associated plexopathy

- a. Neoplastic brachial plexopathy
  - i. The presentation of a neoplastic brachial plexopathy is frequently in the form of worsening pain in the neck, shoulder, or arm over the span of weeks to months.
  - ii. In such cases, Horner syndrome may be present, especially with the involvement of the lower trunk.
  - iii. The lower plexus is most often involved in cancer-related brachial plexopathies and electrodiagnostic studies can be helpful to confirm localization.
  - iv. MRI images of the cervical spine and plexus are required to assess for bulky locoregional disease that may be amenable to treatment with surgery or radiation therapy.
- b. Radiation-induced brachial plexopathy (RIBP)
  - i. RIBP can occur years following the initial course of radiation therapy.
  - ii. The progression of symptoms may occur in an indolent fashion over months and even years and is typically in the form of sensory symptoms, pain, and worsening weakness and atrophy.
  - iii. Although classically thought to involve the upper plexus, RIBP can also involve the lower plexus or entire plexus, as is the case in this scenario.

iv. Imaging of the brachial plexus may reveal RT-related changes in other adjacent anatomic structures such as the lung, bones, and connective tissue.

c. Lumbosacral plexopathy
   i. A prior history of a pelvic floor tumor and new lower extremity symptoms should raise the concern for a lumbosacral plexopathy related to local disease recurrence or metastasis.
   ii. Electrodiagnostic studies are not required to confirm localization if the imaging findings can account for the localization suggested by the clinical examination.

23. Chapter 23: Cancer complications in patients with hematologic malignancies

a. Lymphomatous meningitis
   i. Lymphomatous infiltration of the leptomeninges is the most common neurologic complication of non-Hodgkin lymphoma (NHL).
   ii. The clinical presentation of leptomeningeal metastases is characterized by multifocal neurological signs and symptoms affecting the brain, cranial nerves, spinal cord, and exiting nerve roots. It may also cause obstructive hydrocephalus.
   iii. MRI demonstrating leptomeningeal enhancement and CSF analysis including cytology and flow cytometry are typically needed for diagnosis of leptomeningeal involvement.
   iv. Treatment strategies for leptomeningeal disease typically include a combination of intrathecal and systemic chemotherapy.

b. CNS recurrence of systemic lymphoma
   i. Parenchymal metastases are less common than leptomeningeal disease in secondary CNS lymphoma, with the exception of DLBCL.
   ii. Treatment of secondary CNS lymphoma with parenchymal disease is similar to that of primary CNS lymphoma, including systemic high-dose methotrexate, rituximab, and temozolomide as primary treatment options. Emerging treatment agents include lenalidomide, ibrutinib, and immune therapies.

c. Epidural spinal cord compression
   i. Red flag symptoms of spinal cord compression in a patient with known cancer such as back pain, lower extremity weakness, incontinence, and gait instability should prompt urgent neurologic evaluation and spinal MR imaging.
   ii. Initial treatment includes intravenous dexamethasone 10 mg IV followed by 4 mg every 6 hours to reduce vasogenic edema with close monitoring of patient's symptoms and neurological examination.
   iii. Hematologic malignancies are radiosensitive and urgent treatment should be provided to reduce the risk of permanent neurological injury.

d. Neurolymphomatosis
   i. Neurolymphomatosis is a rare manifestation of lymphoma, and may manifest as a painful radiculopathy, cranial neuropathy, painless polyneuropathy, or mononeuropathy.
   ii. MR imaging is useful for diagnosis; however, nerve biopsy is the gold standard of diagnosis and will show lymphomatous cell infiltration in the perineurium and endoneurium.
   iii. Treatment of neurolymphomatosis involves high-dose IV methotrexate with ibrutinib and lenalidomide as possible options for refractory cases.

e. CNS prophylaxis for high-risk systemic lymphoma
   i. The prevalence of CNS involvement in acute lymphoblastic leukemia is sufficiently high that all patients should routinely receive CNS prophylaxis.
   ii. CNS prophylaxis in DLBCL is reserved for high-risk patients.
   iii. The best prophylactic strategy is yet to be determined, but regimens typically include intrathecal chemotherapy in combination with systemic chemotherapy. Ommaya reservoir placement for intrathecal therapy may be desirable in some patients due to the need of frequent injections and superior distribution of the drug after intraventricular administration.

f. Paraneoplastic disorders in hematologic malignancies
   i. Paraneoplastic syndromes are rarely associated with Hodgkin and non-Hodgkin lymphoma and most cases have negative onconeural antibodies.
   ii. Patients with low-grade lymphomas may have accompanying devastating paraneoplastic neurological disorders. Some of these patients respond to immunotherapy.
   iii. PCA-Tr, mGluR1, and mGluR5 are well-recognized biomarkers of paraneoplastic neurological syndromes associated with Hodgkin lymphoma.
   iv. Granulomatous angiitis is a unique paraneoplastic syndrome associated with Hodgkin lymphoma.

24. Chapter 24: Approach to the patient with radiation necrosis

a. Pseudoprogression in glioma
   i. Pseudoprogression is an earlier and reversible form of radiation necrosis that typically occurs within 3 months of chemoradiotherapy for glioma and resolves spontaneously.

ii. Although there is no imaging modality proven to provide accurate diagnosis of radiation necrosis, MR perfusion, MR spectroscopy, or PET may be considered to help supplement the diagnostic workup.

b. Radiation necrosis in glioma
   i. Delayed radiation necrosis can occur months or years after fractionated RT and can continue to wax and wane even after surgical resection.
   ii. Surgical resection or prolonged follow-up of clinical course remains the best way to establish the diagnosis of radiation necrosis at the current time.
   iii. In cases of suspected radiation necrosis, early involvement of a multidisciplinary team that includes neurosurgeons, radiation oncologists, and neuro-oncologists is recommended.
   iv. Asymptomatic cases should be initially observed with close monitoring.
   v. For symptomatic cases, corticosteroids are the initial mainstay of treatment.
   vi. Additional treatment options for mild cases include Vitamin E and pentoxifylline; for more severe cases, surgery, interstitial laser ablation, bevacizumab, or hyperbaric oxygen may be considered.

25. Chapter 25: Neurological complications of radiation

a. Neurocognitive dysfunction from radiation (beamo-brain)
   i. The neuropsychologic evaluation should include an assessment of fatigue and depression as both occur at high rates within the brain tumor patient population and can impact cognitive functioning.
   ii. Neuropsychologic evaluation should be performed by a board-certified neuropsychologist who is experienced in working with brain tumor patients.
   iii. Neurologists and neuro-oncologists should use the neuropsychology report to guide treatment interventions that can include pharmacologic and nonpharmacologic interventions.
   iv. Cognitive impairment can indicate disease recurrence or progression so imaging should be obtained if a patient has a significant and sudden decline in cognitive performance.
   v. However, cognitive impairment often increases over time after treatment for brain tumors in the absence of disease progression as a result of treatment-related damage to neural circuitry.
   vi. Shortened neuropsychologic examinations may be appropriate for brain tumor patients who are older or have poorer performance status as they may not have the stamina to complete a full evaluation.
   vii. Patients with severe cognitive impairment may not be capable of living independently. Consideration should be given in these cases to home safety evaluations or assisted living should be discussed with the patient's family.
   viii. Preventive strategies are an area of very active research and include radioprotective agents, use of radiosurgery, and hippocampal-avoidance.

26. Chapter 26: Uncommon radiation-induced neurological syndromes

a. Radiation myelitis
   i. Radiation myelitis is the most common of the rare complications of spinal cord irradiation and can present as a transient early or irreversible late reaction.
   ii. Other rare complications include paralysis secondary to ischemia, hemorrhage, and lower motor neuron syndrome.

b. Stroke-like migraine attacks after radiation therapy (SMART) syndrome
   i. SMART syndrome is a delayed complication of brain irradiation characterized by recurrent episodes of complicated migraines.
   ii. This is a rare entity with approximately 40 reported cases.
   iii. Time to onset in these cases ranges from 1–35 years with a median of 14 years post-irradiation.
   iv. Common symptoms include headache, seizure, hemianopsia, hemiparesis, and aphasia.
   v. Symptoms are often recurrent over a period of hours to weeks but generally considered reversible, although incomplete neurologic recovery has been reported.

c. Hypothalamic dysfunction
   i. Dysfunction of the hypothalamus most often involves the hypothalamic-pituitary axis but can also be limited to the hypothalamus alone.
   ii. The hypothalamus is located in the ventral brain above the pituitary gland and may fall within the radiation field during cranial irradiation for numerous indications including prophylactic irradiation (≤30 Gy), total-body irradiation (10–14 Gy), and treatment of primary brain, nasopharyngeal, sinonasal, skull base, and metastatic lesions (≤60 Gy).
   iii. The hypothalamus releases hormones that act on the pituitary gland, forming the hypothalamic-pituitary axis to regulate multiple endocrine systems and is also involved in nonendocrine functions of temperature, appetite, and autonomic nervous system regulation.

iv. Disruptions of either the hypothalamic or pituitary component of the axis can lead to endocrine dysfunction, both of which require care coordination with endocrinology, with a focus on managing hormonal derangements.

d. Post-radiation vasculopathy and stroke
   i. Post-radiation vasculopathy is a late-onset complication potentially manifesting as ischemic or hemorrhagic cerebrovascular accidents (CVA), vascular occlusive disease, vascular malformations, or intracranial hemorrhage.
   ii. Incidence is higher among those who received radiation as children compared to adults.
   iii. The pathophysiology of radiation-induced vascular injury is complex and attributed to multiple changes including progressive endothelial loss, disruption of the blood-brain barrier, inflammation, vasogenic edema, and thrombosis, followed by long-term effects on vascular remodeling including atheroma formation, endothelial proliferation, adventitial fibrosis, basement membrane thickening, and eventual vessel dilation.

e. Radiation-induced meningioma
   i. Meningiomas are tumors arising from the meninges surrounding the brain and spinal cord and are the most common primary CNS tumors, accounting for approximately one-third of cases.
   ii. While the vast majority of meningiomas arise spontaneously, prior exposure to ionizing radiation is an established acquired risk factor for development of meningioma, and meningiomas are in fact the most common secondary CNS tumors following cranial RT.

f. Radiation-induced glioblastoma
   i. Radiation-induced gliomas (RIG) are a rare but known entity following cranial irradiation, second to radiation-induced meningiomas.
   ii. Criteria for RIG are similar to those for other secondary neoplasms per modified Cahan criteria, including occurrence within the irradiated field, sufficient latency between radiation and new neoplasm development, distinct tumor histology compared to the primary lesion, and absence of genetic predisposition to tumor development.

27. Chapter 27: Approach to the patient with a delayed posttreatment CNS neurotoxicity

a. Posttreatment PML
   i. The risk for infection continues well beyond the active treatment period.
   ii. CSF can be negative for John Cunningham (JC) virus when tested by commercially available methods.
   iii. CSF formulas in immunocompromised patients can fail to reflect inflammation in the presence of cytopenias or impaired immune response.
   iv. PML can have variable appearances with or without contrast enhancement.
   v. Immunocompromised patients should have screening CT/MRI before lumbar puncture.
   vi. There is no established therapy for PML, but pembrolizumab is being investigated.

b. Posttreatment meningoencephalitis
   i. Up to 15% of leukemia and lymphoma patients will have symptomatic dermatomal varicella zoster virus infection. Post-herpetic neuralgia is more than three times as frequent in cancer patients as in those without cancer who develop shingles.
   ii. Systemic neurologic syndromes from zoster include the well-known dermatomal or disseminated skin lesions, focal segmental weakness, acute encephalitis or myelitis, vasculopathy with large and small vessel arteritis—40% of whom have no history of rash and up to one-third who have no CSF pleocytosis.
   iii. Ocular manifestations of varicella zoster virus include Ramsay-Hunt syndrome, pontine myelitis infarction of one or more cranial nerves, acute monocular visual loss with temporal arteritis-like presentation, and acute outer retinal necrosis.
   iv. The new varicella zoster virus subunit vaccine (Shingrix) is appropriate for immunocompromised patients.

c. Chemo brain
   i. Radiation in childhood leads to many long-term sequelae including endocrinopathies, vasculopathy, neurocognitive dysfunction, and risk of second malignancy among others. The patient (in Case 27.3) did not have cavernous angiomata or communicating hydrocephalus and had no evidence of a secondary neoplasm, both differential considerations in this situation.
   ii. Superficial siderosis is a syndrome usually appearing many years after cranial surgery or traumatic brain injury, particularly in the posterior fossa. The pathophysiology is deposition of hemosiderin around the brainstem and cerebellar folia; the MRI signature is a rim of hypointensity around the basal cisterns and in the cerebellum.
   iii. Differential diagnosis of late-onset cognitive change after cancer treatment, as in this patient, should include interrogation of endocrine status for further discussion of evaluating patients with treatment-induced neurocognitive dysfunction.
   iv. Chronic cytopenias raise the risk of a myelodysplastic syndrome and such patients require lifelong surveillance.

v. Chemo brain is not explained exclusively by affective disorder or post-traumatic stress disorder.
vi. Early detection of cerebral micro-hemorrhages requires attention to specific susceptibility-weighted imaging MRI sequences and may represent an opportunity to adjust therapeutic strategies before cognitive impairment becomes clinically detectable.
vii. Specific attention to rigorous hypertension and other vascular risk factor treatment is indicated.

d. Delayed posttreatment leukoencephalopathy
i. Delayed leukoencephalopathy has been seen in transplant recipients receiving cyclosporine or tacrolimus.
ii. There is emerging clinical experience with some patients who are receiving immune checkpoint inhibitors who may experience accelerated cognitive decline with immune-mediated encephalitis as the underlying pathophysiology and often a limbic encephalitis pattern on MRI.

e. Posttreatment stroke
i. Posterior reversible encephalopathy syndrome should be considered in many clinical settings, the common denominator often being elevated blood pressure and usually involves CT/MRI evidence of vasogenic edema predominantly in the posterior cerebral hemispheres.
ii. Bevacizumab has been associated with both thrombotic and hemorrhagic events. Individualized decisions must be made about the risk/benefit of continuing this drug in the presence of arterial or venous thrombosis.
iii. There are multiple mechanisms of hemorrhagic and ischemic stroke in cancer patients whose presentation may appear to be more of a mental status change than the onset of a focal deficit.
iv. There are no firm guidelines for the use of direct oral anticoagulants in cancer patients with brain metastases or primary brain tumors.
v. Bevacizumab has been associated with both thrombotic and hemorrhagic cerebral events as well as venous thromboembolism.

f. Treatment-induced malignancies
i. Lifelong monitoring includes attention to vascular, endocrinologic, dermatologic, dental, cardiac, and pulmonary function.
ii. Neurological monitoring should include inquiry about both central (cognitive, vascular) and peripheral (peripheral neuropathy, pain) nervous system problems.
iii. Psychosocial problems can be addressed with appropriate neuropsychologic testing and education plans.
iv. Secondary cancers include both primary brain tumors and systemic neoplasms that can be related both to prior radiation therapy and to antecedent chemotherapy.

28. Chapter 28: Approach to chemotherapy-induced peripheral neuropathy

a. Taxane-induced chemotherapy-induced peripheral neuropathy (CIPN)
i. Taxanes, including paclitaxel, docetaxel, and cabazitaxel, have been used for nearly 30 years to treat a variety of cancers including breast, ovarian, non–small-cell lung cancer, and prostate cancer.
ii. Skin biopsy is another technique that allows for objective quantification of intraepidermal nerve fiber density in small fiber sensory neuropathies like CIPN.

b. Oxaliplatin-induced CIPN
i. Acute oxaliplatin neuropathy is an infusional hyperexcitability that results in cold allodynia and paresthesias of the hands and feet precipitated by cold exposure within 24 hours of the oxaliplatin infusion.
ii. Chronic oxaliplatin-induced CIPN is characterized by a pure sensory, axonopathy that develops in a stocking-and-glove distribution.
iii. Venlafaxine was shown to relieve the acute neuropathy from oxaliplatin when given 1 hour prior to the infusion.
iv. Duloxetine is an American Society of Clinical Oncology (ASCO) recommended therapy for patients with established CIPN based on results of a phase III, randomized, double-blind, placebo-controlled crossover study where 231 patients were randomized to receive duloxetine at a target dose of 60 mg daily or placebo for six weeks.

c. CIPN in hematologic malignancies
i. Peripheral neuropathy is most commonly associated with vincristine but can be seen to a lesser degree with the other vinca alkaloids.
ii. Brentuximab is a CD30-specific antibody-drug conjugate that has activity in relapsed or refractory Hodgkin lymphoma and anaplastic large cell lymphoma. Peripheral neuropathy is one of the most common treatment-related adverse events of this agent.
iii. There are two main goals when managing CIPN: the first is to prevent CIPN before it occurs; the second is to relieve symptoms once CIPN has set in.

d. Bortezomib-induced peripheral neuropathy
i. Bortezomib is a proteasome inhibitor used in the treatment of multiple myeloma and mantle cell non-Hodgkin lymphoma.
ii. The neurotoxicity is dose-dependent and the duration is variable; the painful peripheral neuropathy has resolved in some patients within weeks, and in other patients it has persisted for years.

iii. Paraproteinemic neuropathy refers to a heterogeneous set of neuropathies associated with the presence of a clonal proliferation of immunoglobulin in the serum.
iv. Neuropathic pain typically presents as a length-dependent axonal sensorimotor polyneuropathy resulting in numbness, paresthesias, allodynia, cramping, or mild distal motor weakness.

29. Chapter 29: Neurologic complications of immune checkpoint inhibitors

a. Serious neurologic immune-related adverse events (IRAEs) have been shown to occur in up to 1% of patients receiving immune checkpoint inhibitors (ICIs).
b. In general, IRAEs have been shown to be more common and more severe in patients receiving combination therapy.
c. Neurologic IRAEs from ICIs are idiosyncratic and can occur at any point during treatment.
d. Neurologic IRAEs are highly variable and have been shown to occur throughout the nervous system, with presentations including encephalitis, meningitis, myelitis, meningoradiculitis, myasthenic syndrome, Guillain–Barre-like syndrome, and peripheral neuropathy.
e. The differential diagnosis in a patient receiving ICIs and presenting with a new neurologic syndrome includes infection, tumor progression, primary neurologic syndrome and neurologic IRAE. Infection and tumor progression in particular must be ruled out as part of the workup for a neurologic IRAE, often requiring neuroimaging and lumbar puncture.
f. The treatment of neurologic IRAEs varies by the grade of adverse event, but for IRAEs of grade 2 or higher, will typically require oral or intravenous corticosteroids and delay in, or discontinuation of, immunotherapy.

30. Chapter 30: Neurologic complications associated with CAR T-cell therapy

a. Fatal neurotoxicity has been described in clinical studies of chimeric antigen receptor (CAR) T-cell therapies.
b. Neurotoxicity from CAR T-cells is highly correlated with manifestation of cytokine release syndrome (CRS), and neurologic symptoms are preceded by fever in most patients.
c. Common signs and symptoms of CAR T-cell–associated neurotoxicity include lethargy, somnolence, impaired attention, headache, tremor, dysgraphia, aphasia, focal weakness, seizures, and elevated ICP. Of these signs and symptoms, only expressive aphasia is highly specific for neurotoxicity from CAR T-cells, often manifesting as an awake patient who is mute and does not respond verbally or physically to an examiner.
d. Neuroimaging is frequently unrevealing in patients with neurotoxicity from CAR T-cells, but may reveal nonspecific T2/fluid attenuated inversion recovery (FLAIR) signal abnormality and/or cerebral edema in severe cases. Serum levels of inflammatory markers may correlate with severity.
e. CAR T-cell–associated neurotoxicity is graded based on assessing multiple neurologic domains that span the constellation of signs and symptoms associated with this phenomenon; CARTOX and the American Society for Blood and Marrow Transplantation (ASBMT) immune effector-cell associated neurotoxicity syndrome (ICANS) Consensus Grading systems are the most commonly utilized.
f. Management of neurotoxicity from CAR T-cell therapy is primarily supportive in nature and is based on the toxicity grade. Anti-IL-6 therapy is recommended for patients with grade ≥1 neurotoxicity with concurrent CRS; if not associated with CRS, corticosteroids are the preferred treatment for grade ≥2 neurotoxicity, and can be tapered after improvement of ICANS to grade 1.
g. Both seizure-like activity and non-epileptic myoclonus are common in patients with neurotoxicity from CAR T-cells, and EEG typically demonstrates diffuse background slowing. For patients who progress to nonconvulsive or convulsive status epilepticus, benzodiazepines and levetiracetam are preferred; phenobarbital is added if seizures persist.
h. CAR T-cell–associated neurotoxicity with raised ICP should be managed promptly with corticosteroids and acetazolamide; patients who develop grade 4 neurotoxicity with cerebral edema should also receive hyperventilation and hyperosmolar therapy.
i. Patients who receive CAR T cell therapy are often heavily pre-treated for their malignancies and may have significant medical comorbidities. Therefore, it is critical that a broad differential diagnosis is considered beyond CAR T-cell–related neurotoxicity is considered when neurologic symptoms are encountered in these patients. Diagnostic considerations include but are not limited to intracranial bleeding in the setting of thrombocytopenia, opportunistic infections, and CNS involvement of the patient's tumor.

Appendix 2

Reference list of clinical cases covered in this book

1. Brain metastasis

a. General approach
   i. Chapter 14, Case 1: Approach to large, symptomatic brain metastasis—surgery
   ii. Chapter 14, Case 2: Approach to innumerable multifocal brain metastasis—whole brain radiation
   iii. Chapter 14, Case 3: Approach to multifocal brain metastasis—stereotactic radiosurgery
   iv. Chapter 23, Case 2: Intracranial metastases from systemic lymphoma (hematologic malignancy)
   v. Chapter 23, Case 3: Epidural metastases
b. Surgical management
   i. Chapter 2, Case 5: New symptomatic multifocal brain lesions in a known cancer patient
   ii. Chapter 2, Case 7: Bony metastatic lesion with spinal cord compression
c. Imaging
   i. Chapter 5, Case 6: Dural-based metastasis
   ii. Chapter 6, Case 4: Multifocal enhancing parenchymal lesion
   iii. Chapter 7, Case 4: Enhancing cerebellar lesion in an adult
   iv. Chapter 8, Case 6: Extradural spinal vertebral metastasis
d. Radiation therapy
   i. Chapter 3, Case 2: Stereotactic radiosurgery for a patient with a solitary brain metastasis
   ii. Chapter 3, Case 3: Whole brain radiation therapy for diffuse brain metastases
e. Special populations
   i. Cerebellar—Chapter 7, Case 4: Enhancing cerebellar lesion in an adult
   ii. Radiation necrosis—Chapter 24, Case 3: Radiation necrosis after radiosurgery
   iii. Spinal cord—Chapter 8, Case 6: Extradural spinal vertebral metastasis

2. Ependymoma

a. General approach
   i. Chapter 8, Case 2: Spinal cord ependymoma

3. Ganglion cell tumors (ganglioglioma, gangliocytoma)

a. Chapter 18, Case 2: Cowden syndrome

4. Glioma: Glioblastoma

a. General approach
   i. Chapter 12, Case 2: Approach to anaplastic astrocytoma: patchy contrast enhancement in a high-grade brain lesion
   ii. Chapter 12, Case 3a: Approach to glioblastoma: acute-onset neurologic deficit from a high-grade brain lesion
b. Histopathologic classification
   i. Chapter 1, Case 1: Characteristic histopathologic and molecular features of glioblastoma
c. Imaging
   i. Chapter 6, Case 1: Rim-enhancing parenchymal lesion
   ii. Chapter 24, Case 1: Pseudoprogression in glioma
   iii. Chapter 24, Case 2: Delayed radiation necrosis in glioma
d. Surgical management
   i. Chapter 2, Case 2: New symptomatic supratentorial high-grade lesion
   ii. Chapter 2, Case 3: Recurrent unresectable supratentorial high-grade glioma

e. Radiation therapy
   i. Chapter 3, Case 1: Radiation therapy for high-grade glioma
f. Chemotherapy
   i. Chapter 4, Case 4: Newly diagnosed glioblastoma
g. Recurrence
   i. Chapter 4, Case 6: Recurrent high-grade glioma
   ii. Chapter 12, Case 3d: Recurrent disease and end-of-life care in high-grade glioma
h. Treatment complications
   i. Chapter 12, Case 3b: Seizures, edema, and post-treatment neurological complications in high-grade glioma
   ii. Chapter 12, Case 3c: Venous thrombosis, *Pneumocystis*, steroid myopathy, and non-neurological complications of glioma
   iii. Chapter 19, Case 1: Neurological complications (e.g., cerebral edema, epilepsy, stroke, hydrocephalus, syndrome of inappropriate antidiuretic hormone [SIADH])
   iv. Chapter 19, Case 2: Non-neurological treatment complications (e.g., venous thromboembolism, hypercoagulability, neurocognitive dysfunction, fatigue, sleep dysfunction)
i. Special populations
   i. Elderly— Chapter 4, Case 5: Glioblastoma in the elderly
   ii. End-of-life care—Chapter 12, Case 3d: Recurrent disease and end-of-life care in high-grade glioma
   iii. Lynch syndrome—Chapter 18, Case 4: Lynch syndrome
   iv. Radiation-inducedglioblastoma—Chapter26,Case6: Radiation-induced glioma/glioblastoma

5. Glioma: Anaplastic gliomas

a. General approach
   i. Chapter 12, Case 1: Progression from low-grade to anaplastic oligodendroglioma
b. Histopathologic classification
   i. Chapter 1, Case 4: Histopathologic and molecular findings for WHO grade 3 anaplastic astrocytoma
c. Imaging
   i. Chapter 6, Case 1: Rim-enhancing parenchymal lesion
   ii. Chapter 24, Case 1: Pseudoprogression in glioma
   iii. Chapter 24, Case 2: Delayed radiation necrosis in glioma
d. Radiation therapy
   i. Chapter 3, Case 1: Radiation therapy for high-grade glioma
e. Chemotherapy
   i. Chapter 4, Case 1: Anaplastic 1p19q co-deleted oligodendrogliomas
   ii. Chapter 4, Case 2: Anaplastic non–co-deleted astrocytomas
f. Recurrence
   i. Chapter 4, Case 6: Recurrent high-grade glioma
g. Treatment complications
   i. Chapter 12, Case 3b: Seizures, edema, and post-treatment neurological complications in high-grade glioma
   ii. Chapter 12, Case 3c: Venous thrombosis, *Pneumocystis*, steroid myopathy, and non-neurological complications of glioma
   iii. Chapter 19, Case 1: Direct effects of brain tumors (e.g., cerebral edema, epilepsy, stroke, hydrocephalus, SIADH)
   iv. Chapter 19, Case 2: Non-neurological treatment complications (e.g., venous thromboembolism, hypercoagulability, neurocognitive dysfunction, fatigue, sleep dysfunction)

6. Glioma: Low-grade gliomas

a. General approach
   i. Chapter 11, Teaching point #1: How to determine an integrated histologic and molecular diagnosis of low-grade glioma
   ii. Chapter 11, Teaching point #2: How to differentiate high-risk and low-risk low-grade glioma
   iii. Chapter 11, Teaching point #3: How to determine whether to observe or initiate treatment at diagnosis of low-grade glioma
   iv. Chapter 11, Teaching point #4: How to determine a patient-specific treatment plan for low-grade glioma
   v. Chapter 11, Teaching Point #5: How to select a patient-specific chemotherapy regimen for low-grade glioma
b. Histopathologic classification
   i. Chapter 1, Case 3: Use of genomic profiling to establish a diagnosis of WHO grade 2 astrocytoma
   ii. Chapter 1, Case 2: Use of molecular testing to define the diagnosis of WHO grade 2 oligodendroglioma
c. Imaging
   i. Chapter 6, Case 2: Non-enhancing parenchymal lesion
d. Chemotherapy
   i. Chapter 4, Case 3: Low-grade gliomas
e. Special populations
   i. *H3K27M* mutant glioma—Chapter 12, Final section after cases: Approach to *H3K27M* mutant diffuse midline gliomas
   ii. *IDH* mutant—Chapter 11, Clinical pearl 1: Approach to *IDH*-mutant low-grade gliomas

iii. *IDH* wild type—Chapter 11, Clinical pearl 2: Approach to *IDH* wild-type low-grade gliomas
iv. Neurologic complications—Chapter 11, Clinical pearl 4: Approach to the diagnosis and management of neurological complications for low-grade gliomas
v. Seizure management—Chapter 11, Clinical pearl 3: Approach to seizure management in low-grade gliomas

7. Hemangioblastoma

a. General approach
   i. Chapter 8, Case 3: Spinal cord hemangioblastoma in a patient with von Hippel Lindau disease
   ii. Chapter 18, Case 1: von Hippel Lindau disease

8. Hemangiopericytoma or solitary fibrous tumor

a. General approach
   i. Chapter 5, Case 5: Dural-based lesion diagnosed as hemangiopericytoma

9. Leptomeningeal metastasis

a. Chapter 15, Case 1: Diagnosis of leptomeningeal disease (LMD) in a patient with metastatic lung cancer
b. Chapter 15, Case 2: Diagnosis of LMD in a patient with a hematologic malignancy
c. Chapter 15, Case 3: Radiographic diagnosis of LMD in a breast cancer patient with cranial neuropathy
d. Chapter 15, Case 4: Management of LMD in a breast cancer patient with symptomatic bulky disease
e. Chapter 15, Case 5: Management of LMD in a small-cell cancer patient without bulky LMD
f. Chapter 23, Case 1: Leptomeningeal recurrence

10. Lhermitte-Duclos disease

a. Chapter 18, Case 2: Cowden syndrome

11. Lymphoma

a. Secondary central nervous system (CNS) lymphoma
   i. Chapter 23, Case 5: Central nervous system prophylaxis
   ii. Chapter 23, Case 1: Leptomeningeal recurrence of systemic lymphoma
   iii. Chapter 23, Case 2: Intracranial metastases from systemic lymphoma
b. Primary CNS lymphoma
   i. Chapter 6, Case 3: Homogeneously enhancing parenchymal lesion
   ii. Chapter 13, Case 1 (only case): Approach to CNS lymphoma
c. Leptomeningeal lymphoma
   i. Chapter 15, Case 2: Diagnosis of LMD in a patient with a hematologic malignancy
   ii. Chapter 23, Case 1: Leptomeningeal recurrence of systemic lymphoma
d. Dural-based lymphoma
   i. Chapter 5, Case 7: Dural-based lymphoma
e. Special population
   i. Chapter 23, Case 4: Neurolymphomatosis

12. Medulloblastoma

a. Chapter 7, Case 1: Midline fourth ventricular lesion
b. Chapter 18, Case 3: Li-Fraumeni syndrome

13. Meningioma

a. General approach
   i. Chapter 10, Case 1: Approach to the patient without a tissue diagnosis
   ii. Chapter 10, Case 2: Approach to the patient with WHO grade I meningioma
   iii. Chapter 10, Case 3: Approach to the patient with WHO grade II meningioma
   iv. Chapter 10, Case 4: Approach to the patient with WHO grade II meningioma with residual postoperative disease
   v. Chapter 10, Case 5: Approach to the patient with WHO grade III meningioma
   vi. Chapter 10, Case 6: Approach to recurrent meningioma
b. Histopathologic classification
   i. Chapter 1, Case 5: Pathologic assessment of dural-based meningioma
c. Imaging
   i. Chapter 5, Case 1: Small incidentally discovered dural-based meningioma
   ii. Chapter 5, Case 2: Large atypical dural-based meningioma

   iii. Chapter 5, Case 3: Skull-based lesion concerning for meningioma vs inflammatory lesion
   iv. Chapter 8, Case 4: Intradural extramedullary spinal meningioma
d. Surgical management
   i. Chapter 2, Case 6: Large dural-based lesion with symptoms
e. Recurrence
   i. Chapter 10, Case 6: Approach to recurrent meningioma
f. Special populations
   i. Cerebellopontine angle—Chapter 5, Case 4b: Cerebellopontine angle (CPA) meningioma
   ii. Radiation-induced meningioma—Chapter 26, Case 5: Radiation-induced meningioma
   iii. Radiation-induced meningioma—Chapter 27, Case 8: Treatment-induced meningioma
   iv. Spinal cord—Chapter 8, Case 4: Intradural extramedullary spinal meningioma
   v. Spinal cord—Chapter 8, Case 4: Imaging of intradural extramedullary spinal meningioma

14. Neuronal tumors (e.g., ganglioglioma, gangliocytoma)

a. Or see Ganglion Cell Tumors above
b. Chapter 18, Case 2: Cowden syndrome

15. Paraneoplastic syndromes

a. Chapter 20, Case 1: Encephalitis and limbic encephalitis
b. Chapter 20, Case 2: Encephalomyelitis
c. Chapter 20, Case 3: Paraneoplastic subacute cerebellar degeneration
d. Chapter 20, Case 4: Opsoclonus-myoclonus
e. Chapter 20, Case 5: Paraneoplastic sensory neuronopathy
f. Chapter 20, Case 6: Lambert-Eaton myasthenic syndrome
g. Chapter 20, Case 7: Paraneoplastic dermatomyositis
h. Chapter 23, Case 6: Paraneoplastic neurological syndrome in patients with hematologic malignancy

16. Peripheral nerve sheath tumors (excluding vestibular schwannoma)

a. Histopathologic classification
   i. Chapter 1, Case 6: Histopathology of a benign peripheral nerve sheath tumor: schwannoma vs neurofibroma
b. General approach
   i. Chapter 8, Case 5: Intradural extramedullary spinal cord schwannoma
   ii. Chapter 9, Case 1: Sporadic solitary peripheral nerve sheath tumor diagnosed as neurofibroma
   iii. Chapter 9, Case 2: Benign plexiform neurofibroma in neurofibromatosis type 1 (NF1)
   iv. Chapter 9, Case 3: Malignant peripheral nerve sheath tumor
   v. Chapter 9, Case 4: Diffuse lumbosacral nerve root thickening
   vi. Chapter 9, Case 5: Peripheral nerve schwannomas in patients with NF2
   vii. Chapter 9, Case 6: Peripheral nerve schwannomas in schwannomatosis
c. Special populations
   i. NF1—Chapter 9, Case 2: Benign plexiform neurofibroma in neurofibromatosis type 1
   ii. NF1—Chapter 9, Case 3: Malignant peripheral nerve sheath tumor
   iii. NF2—Chapter 9, Case 5: Peripheral nerve schwannomas in patients with NF2
   iv. Plexiform neurofibroma—Chapter 16, Case 1: Approach to an adult with NF1-associated plexiform neurofibroma
   v. Schwannomatosis—Chapter 9, Case 6: (Imaging of) peripheral nerve schwannomas in schwannomatosis
   vi. Schwannomatosis—Chapter 16, Case 5: Diagnosis of schwannomatosis
   vii. Schwannomatosis—Chapter 16, Case 6: Management of pain in adults with schwannomatosis

17. Pilocytic astrocytomas and other low-grade astrocytomas

a. Imaging
   i. Chapter 7, Case 2: Lateral cerebellar cystic lesion
   ii. Chapter 8, Case 1: Spinal cord astrocytoma
b. Special populations
   i. Lhermitte-Duclos disease—Chapter 18, Case 2: Cowden syndrome
   ii. Optic pathway glioma—Chapter 16, Case 2: Diagnosis and management of NF1-associated optic pathway glioma
   iii. Pilocytic astrocytoma in NF1—Chapter 16, Case 3: Management of brain lesions in children with NF1
   iv. Subependymal giant cell astrocytoma—Chapter 17, Case 4: Diagnosis and management of subependymal giant cell astrocytoma (SEGA)

18. Pituitary tumors

a. Chapter 19, Case 1: Approach to endocrinopathy

19. Plexiform neurofibroma

a. Chapter 16, Case 1: Approach to an adult with NF1-associated plexiform neurofibroma

20. Posterior fossa tumors

a. Surgical management
   i. Chapter 2, Case 1: Elevated intracranial pressure from a posterior fossa mass
b. Diffuse intrinsic pontine glioma or midline glioma
   i. Chapter 7, Case 3: Non-enhancing pontine lesion
   ii. Chapter 12, Final section after cases: Approach to *H3K27M* mutant diffuse midline gliomas
c. Ependymoma
   i. Chapter 8, Case 2: Spinal cord ependymoma
d. Medulloblastoma
   i. Chapter 7, Case 1: Midline fourth ventricular lesion
   ii. Chapter 18, Case 3: Li-Fraumeni syndrome
e. Meningioma
   i. Chapter 5, Case 4b: Cerebellopontine angle (CPA) meningioma
f. Metastasis
   i. Chapter 7, Case 4: Enhancing cerebellar lesion in an adult
g. Non-neoplastic posterior fossa or cerebellar lesions
   i. Chapter 7, Case 5: Non-enhancing cerebellar lesion
h. Pilocytic astrocytoma
   i. Chapter 7, Case 2: Lateral cerebellar cystic lesion
i. Vestibular schwannoma
   i. Chapter 5, Case 4a: Cerebellopontine angle (CPA) vestibular schwannoma
   ii. Chapter 5, Case 4b: Cerebellopontine angle (CPA) meningioma

21. Spinal cord tumors

a. Imaging
   i. Chapter 8, Case 1: Spinal cord astrocytoma
   ii. Chapter 8, Case 2: Spinal cord ependymoma
   iii. Chapter 8, Case 3: Spinal cord lesions in a patient with von Hippel Lindau disease
   iv. Chapter 8, Case 4: Intradural extramedullary spinal meningioma
   v. Chapter 8, Case 5: Intradural extramedullary spinal cord schwannoma
   vi. Chapter 8, Case 6: Extradural spinal vertebral metastasis
b. Surgical management
   i. Chapter 2, Case 7: Bony metastatic lesion with spinal cord compression
   ii. Chapter 2, Case 4: Recurrent symptomatic intramedullary spinal cord tumor
c. Radiation therapy
   i. Chapter 3, Case 4: Radiation therapy for a primary intramedullary spinal cord tumor

22. Subependymal giant cell astrocytoma (SEGA)

a. Chapter 17, Case 4: Diagnosis and management of subependymal giant cell astrocytoma (SEGA)

23. Treatment complications

a. Brachial plexopathy
   i. Chapter 21, Case 1: Brachial plexus involvement in breast cancer patient: perineural spread vs radiation-induced plexopathy
   ii. Chapter 22, Case 1: Neoplastic brachial plexopathy
   iii. Chapter 22, Case 2: Radiation-induced brachial plexopathy
b. Chemotherapy induced peripheral neuropathy
   i. Chapter 28, Case 1: Taxane-induced peripheral neuropathy
   ii. Chapter 28, Case 2: Oxaliplatin-induced peripheral neuropathy
   iii. Chapter 28, Case 3: Peripheral neuropathy in hematologic malignancies (e.g., vinca alkaloids, brentuximab)
   iv. Chapter 28, Case 4: Bortezomib-induced peripheral neuropathy
c. Cranial neuropathy
   i. Chapter 21, Case 2: Trigeminal neuralgia pain in a patient with head and neck cancer
d. Endocrinopathy
   i. Chapter 26, Case 3: Hypothalamic dysfunction
e. Fatigue
   i. Chapter 19, Case 2ii: Fatigue, cognitive dysfunction, and sleep disturbances in brain tumor patients
f. Hypercoagulability

i. Chapter 19, Case 2i: Venous thromboembolism and hypercoagulability

g. Immunotherapies
   i. Chapter 29, Case 1–4: Neurological immune-related adverse events from immune checkpoint inhibitors
   ii. Chapter 30, Case 1 (only 1 case): Immune effector-cell–associated neurotoxicity syndrome from CAR T-cell therapy
h. Leukoencephalopathy
   i. Chapter 27, Case 5: Delayed posttreatment leukoencephalopathy
i. Lumbosacral plexopathy
   i. Chapter 22, Case 3: Lumbosacral plexopathy
j. Meningoencephalitis
   i. Chapter 27, Case 2: Posttreatment VZV meningoencephalitis
k. Neurological complications
   i. Chapter 19, Case 1: Neurological complications (e.g., cerebral edema, epilepsy, stroke, hydrocephalus, SIADH)
l. Neurocognitive dysfunction
   i. Chapter 19, Case 2: Neurocognitive dysfunction
   ii. Chapter 25, Case 1: Neurocognitive dysfunction in a patient with associated mood symptoms
   iii. Chapter 25, Case 2: Management of neurocognitive dysfunction in a patient with sleep dysfunction
   iv. Chapter 27, Case 3: Treatment-induced neurocognitive dysfunction and cavernomas
   v. Chapter 27, Case 4: Chemo brain
m. Progressive multifocal leukoencephalopathy (PML)
   i. Chapter 27, Case 1: Posttreatment PML in hematologic malignancy patient
n. Stroke
   i. Chapter 26, Case 4: Post-radiation vasculopathy and stroke
   ii. Chapter 27, Case 6: Posttreatment cerebrovascular complications
   iii. Chapter 27, Case 7: Posttreatment stroke
o. Radiation complications
   i. Chapter 26, Case 1: Radiation myelitis
   ii. Chapter 26, Case 2: SMART syndrome: stroke-like migraine attacks after radiation therapy
p. Sleep dysfunction
   i. Chapter 19, Case 2ii: Fatigue, cognitive dysfunction, and sleep disturbances in brain tumor patients

24. Vestibular schwannoma

a. Sporadic
   i. Chapter 5, Case 4a: Cerebellopontine angle (CPA) vestibular schwannoma
   ii. Chapter 5, Case 4b: Cerebellopontine angle (CPA) meningioma
b. Associated with NF2
   i. Chapter 16, Case 4: Approach to management of NF2-associated bilateral vestibular schwannomas

Index

Page numbers followed by "*f*" indicate figures, "*t*" indicate tables, and "*b*" indicate boxes.

O

P